GENOMIC DISORDERS

GENOMIC DISORDERS

The Genomic Basis of Disease

Edited by

JAMES R. LUPSKI, MD, PhD
PAWEŁ STANKIEWICZ, MD, PhD

Department of Molecular and Human Genetics
Baylor College of Medicine, Houston, TX

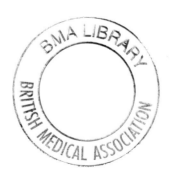

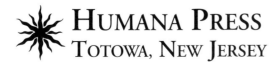

HUMANA PRESS
Totowa, New Jersey

© 2006 Humana Press Inc.
999 Riverview Drive, Suite 208
Totowa, New Jersey 07512

www.humanapress.com

Production Editor: Melissa Caravella

Cover design by Patricia F. Cleary

Cover Illustration: From Fig. 2 in Chapter 7, "Genetic Basis of Olfactory Deficits," by Idan Menashe, Ester Feldmesser, and Doron Lancet; Fig. 2 in Chapter 9, "Primate Chromosome Evolution," by Stefan Müller; Figs. 1 and 4 in Chapter 20, "Inversion Chromosomes," by Orsetta Zuffardi, Roberto Ciccone, Sabrina Giglio, and Tiziano Pramparo; Fig. 1 in Chapter 23, "Mechanisms Unlerlying Neoplasia-Associated Genomic Rearrangements," by Thoas Fioretos.

For additional copies, pricing for bulk purchases, and/or information about other Humana titles, contact Humana at the above address or at any of the following numbers: Tel.: 973-256-1699; Fax: 973-256-8341, E-mail: orders@humanapr.com; or visit our Website: www.humanapress.com

Printed in Singapore. 10 9 8 7 6 5 4 3 2 1
eISBN 1-59745-039-1

Library of Congress Cataloging-in-Publication Data

Genomic disorders : the genomic basis of disease / edited by James R. Lupski, Paweł Stankiewicz.
      p. ; cm.
   Includes bibliographical references and index.
   ISBN 1-58829-559-1 (alk. paper)
   1. Genetic disorders--Molecular aspects.
   [DNLM: 1. Genetic Diseases, Inborn. 2. Chromosome Aberrations. 3. Genome Components. 4. Genome. 5. Genomics--methods. QZ 50 G3354 2006] I. Lupski, James R., 1957- II. Stankiewicz, Paweł.
   RB155.5.G465 2006
   616'.042--dc22
                                              2005020461

Dedication

To our many mentors who have nurtured our intellectual curiosity and to our dedicated families for their love and support.

—J. R. L. and P. S.

In Memorium

In memory of Carlos A. Garcia (1935–2005) and his passion for medicine, science, and the patients and families for whom he cared.

Preface

Uncovering Recurrent Submicroscopic Rearrangements As a Cause of Disease

For five decades since Fred Sanger's *(1)* seminal discovery that proteins have a specific structure, since Linus Pauling's *(2)* discovery that hemoglobin from patients with sickle cell anemia is molecularly distinct, and since Watson and Crick's *(3)* elucidation of the chemical basis of heredity, the molecular basis of disease has been addressed in the context of how mutations affect the structure, function, or regulation of a gene or its protein product. Molecular medicine has functioned in the context of a genocentric world. During the last decade it became apparent, however, that many disease traits are best explained not by how the information content of a single gene is changed, but rather on the basis of genomic alterations. Furthermore, it has become abundantly clear that architectural features of the human genome can result in susceptibility to DNA rearrangements that cause disease traits. Such conditions have been referred to as genomic disorders *(4,5)*.

It remains to be determined to what extent genomic changes are responsible for disease traits, common traits (including behavioral traits), or perhaps sometimes represent benign polymorphic variation. The widespread structural variation of the human genome, alternatively referred to as large-copy number polymorphisms, large-scale copy number variations, or copy number variants has begun only recently to be appreciated *(6–9)*. High-resolution analysis of the human genome has enabled detection of genome changes heretofore not observed because of technology limitations. Whereas agarose gel electrophoresis enables detection of changes of the genome up to 25–30 kb in size, and cytogenetic banding techniques can resolve deletion rearrangements only greater than 2–5 Mb in size, alterations of the genome between more than 30 kb and less than 5 Mb defied detection until pulsed-field gel electrophoresis and fluorescence *in situ* hybridization became available to resolve changes in the human genome of such magnitude *(10–12)*. Those methods were limited to detection of specific genomic regions of interest and could not evaluate genomic rearrangements in a global way.

The availability of a "finished" human genome sequence *(13)* and genomic microarrays *(14)* have enabled approaches to resolve changes in the genome heretofore impossible to assess on a global genome scale (i.e., simultaneously examining the entire genome rather than discreet segments). Array comparative genome hybridization (aCGH) is one powerful approach to high-resolution analysis of the human genome. The CGH determines differences by comparisons to a reference "normal genome," whereas the array enables detection of such changes at essentially any resolution that is desired, limited only by imagination and cost. Furthermore, the application of bioinformatic analyses to the finished human genome sequence and comparative genomic analysis enable information technology approaches to identify key architectural features throughout the entire genome that are associated with known recurrent rearrangements causing genomic disorders.

An increasing number of human diseases are recognized to result from recurrent DNA rearrangements involving unstable genomic regions. A combination of high-resolution genome analysis with informatics capabilities to examine individuals with well-characterized phenotypic traits is a powerful approach to address the question: To what extent are constitutional DNA rearrangements in the human genome responsible for human traits? Such approaches may also yield insights into recurrent somatic rearrangements *(15)*.

Genomic Disorders: The Genomic Basis of Disease attempts to survey the subject area of genomic disorders in the beginning of the postgenomic era. After a short historical presentation (Part I) describing the trials and tribulations involved in uncovering the recurrent submicroscopic duplication associated with Charcot-Marie-Tooth disease type 1A, the book is organized into parts on genome structure (II), genome evolution (III), genomic rearrangements and disease traits (IV), functional aspects of genome structure (V), and modeling and assays for genomic disorders (VI). Finally, Part VII includes appendices that delineate disease traits and genomic features (listed in tabular form) for well-characterized genomic disorders as well as clinical phenotypes for which chromosome microarray analysis may be used to detect the responsible rearrangement mutation. We believe that the topics chosen for individual chapters illustrate the genomic basis of disease.

James R. Lupski, MD, PhD
Paweł Stankiewicz, MD, PhD

REFERENCES

1. Sanger F. The terminal peptides of insulin. Biochem J 1949;45:563–574.
2. Pauling L, Itamo HA, Singer SJ, Wells IC. Sickle cell anemia, a molecular disease. Science 1949;110:64–66.
3. Watson DA, Crick FHC. Molecular structure of nucleic acids. A structure for deoxyribose nucleic acids. Nature 1953;171:737–738.
4. Lupski JR. Genomic disorders: structural features of the genome can lead to DNA rearrangements and human disease traits. Trends Genet 1998;14:417–422.
5. Stankiewicz P, Lupski JR. Genome architecture, rearrangements and genomic disorders. Trends Genet 2002;18:74–82.
6. Shaw-Smith C, Redon R, Rickman L, et al. Microarray based comparative genomic hybridisation (array-CGH) detects submicroscopic chromosomal deletions and duplications in patients with learning disability/mental retardation and dysmorphic features. J Med Genet 2004;41:241–248.
7. Iafrate AJ, Feuk L, Rivera MN, et al. Detection of large-scale variation in the human genome. Nat Genet 2004;36:949–951.
8. Sebat J, Lakshmi B, Troge J, et al. Large-scale copy number polymorphism in the human genome. Science 2004;305:525–528.
9. Tuzun E, Sharp AJ, Bailey JA, et al. Fine-scale structural variation of the human genome. Nat Genet 2005;37:727–732.
10. Schwartz DC, Cantor CR. Separation of yeast chromosome-sized DNAs by pulsed field gradient gel electrophoresis. Cell 1984;37:67–75.
11. Pinkel D, Straume T, Gray JW. Cytogenetic analysis using quantitative, high-sensitivity, fluorescence hybridization. Proc Natl Acad Sci USA 1986;83:2934–2938.
12. Lupski JR. 2002 Curt Stern Award Address. Genomic disorders: recombination-based disease resulting from genomic architecture. Am J Hum Genet 2003;72:246–252.
13. International Human Genome Sequencing Consortium. Finishing the euchromatic sequence of the human genome. Nature 2004;431:931–945.
14. Carter NP, Vetrie D. Applications of genomic microarrays to explore human chromosome structure and function. Hum Mol Genet 2004;13:R297–R302.
15. Barbouti, A., Stankiewicz, P., Birren, B., et al. The breakpoint region of the most common isochromosome, i(17q), in human neoplasia is characterized by a complex genome architecture with large palindromic low-copy repeats. Am J Hum Genet 2004;74:1–10.

Contents

CONTRIBUTORS

NICOLETTA ARCHIDIACONO, PhD • *Department of Genetics and Microbiology, University of Bari, Bari, Italy*

ALBINO BACOLLA, PhD • *Center for Genome Research, Texas A & M University System Health Science Center, Texas Medical Center, Houston, TX*

BLAKE C. BALLIF, PhD • *Signature Genomic Laboratories, LLC, Spokane, WA*

ARTHUR L. BEAUDET, MD • *Department of Molecular and Human Genetics, Baylor College of Medicine, Houston, TX*

WEIMIN BI, PhD • *Department of Molecular and Human Genetics, Baylor College of Medicine, Houston, TX*

NIGEL P. CARTER, DPhil • *The Sanger Institute, Wellcome Trust Genome Campus, Cambridge, UK*

SAU W. CHEUNG, PhD • *Department of Molecular and Human Genetics, Baylor College of Medicine, Houston, TX*

ROBERTO CICCONE, PhD • *Biologia Generale e Genetica Medica, Universita di Pavia, Pavia, Italy*

PRESCOTT DEININGER, PhD • *Department of Epidemiology, Tulane Cancer Center, Tulane University Health Sciences Center, New Orleans, LA*

EVAN E. EICHLER, PhD • *Department of Genome Sciences, University of Washington, Seattle, WA*

ESTER FELDMESSER, MSc • *Department of Molecular Genetics and the Crown Human Genome Center Weizmann Institute of Science, Rehovot, Israel*

HEIKE FIEGLER, PhD • *The Sanger Institute, Wellcome Trust Genome Campus, Cambridge, UK*

THOAS FIORETOS, MD, PhD • *Department of Clinical Genetics, Lund University Hospital, Lund, Sweden*

SABRINA GIGLIO, MD, PhD • *Ospedale San Raffaele, Milano, Italy*

SUSAN GRIBBLE, PhD • *The Sanger Institute, Wellcome Trust Genome Campus, Cambridge, UK*

AMY E. HULME, BS, MS • *Department of Human Genetics, The University of Michigan Medical School, Ann Arbor, MI*

MATTHEW E. HURLES, PhD • *The Sanger Institute, Wellcome Trust Genome Campus, Cambridge, UK*

KEN INOUE, MD, PhD • *Department of Mental Retardation and Birth Defect Research, National Institute of Neuroscience, National Center of Neurology and Psychiatry, Kodaira, Tokyo, Japan*

JERZY JURKA, PhD • *Genetic Information Research Institute, Mountain View, CA*

DEANNA A. KULPA, BS, MS • *Department of Human Genetics, The University of Michigan Medical School, Ann Arbor, MI*

NAOHIRO KUROTAKI, MD, PhD • *Department of Molecular and Human Genetics, Baylor College of Medicine, Houston, TX*

DORON LANCET, PhD • *Department of Molecular Genetics and the Crown Human Genome Center, Weizmann Institute of Science, Rehovot, Israel*

PENTAO LIU, PhD • *The Sanger Institute, Wellcome Trust Genome Campus, Cambridge, UK*

JAMES R. LUPSKI, MD, PhD • *Department of Molecular and Human Genetics, Department of Pediatrics, Baylor College of Medicine, Houston, TX*

NAOMICHI MATSUMOTO, MD, PhD • *Department of Human Genetics, Yokohama City University Graduate School of Medicine, Fukuura, Yokohama, Japan*

HEATHER E. MCDERMID, PhD • *Department of Biological Sciences, University of Alberta, Edmonton, Alberta, Canada*

IDAN MENASHE, MSc • *Department of Molecular Genetics and the Crown Human Genome Center, Weizmann Institute of Science, Rehovot, Israel*

JOHN V. MORAN, PhD • *Department of Human Genetics and Internal Medicine, The University of Michigan Medical School, Ann Arbor, MI*

BERNICE E. MORROW, PhD • *Department of Molecular Genetics, Albert Einstein College of Medicine, Bronx, NY*

STEFAN MÜLLER, PhD • *Department of Biology II, Ludwig, Maximilians University, Munich, Germany*

LUCY R. OSBORNE, PhD • *Departments of Medicine and Molecular & Medical Genetics, University of Toronto, Toronto, Canada*

ADAM PAVLICEK, PhD • *Genetic Information Research Institute, Mountain View, CA*

JOSÉ LUIS GARCIA PEREZ, PhD • *Department of Human Genetics, The University of Michigan Medical School, Ann Arbor, MI*

TIZIANO PRAMPARO, PhD • *Biologia Generale e Genetica Medica, Universita di Pavia, Pavia, Italy*

RICHARD REDON, PhD • *The Sanger Institute, Wellcome Trust Genome Campus, Cambridge, UK*

MARIANO ROCCHI, PhD • *Department of Genetics and Microbiology, University of Bari, Bari, Italy*

M. KATHARINE RUDD, PhD • *Institute for Genome Sciences & Policy, Duke University, Durham, NC*

STEPHEN W. SCHERER, PhD • *Program in Genetics & Genomic Biology, Sick Kids Hospital, Toronto, Canada; Department of Molecular & Medical Genetics, University of Toronto, Toronto, Canada*

LISA G. SHAFFER, PhD • *Signature Genomic Laboratories, LLC, Spokane, WA; Sacred Heart Medical Center, Spokane, WA; Health Research and Education Center, Washington State University, Spokane, WA*

ANDREW J. SHARP, PhD • *Department of Genome Sciences, University of Washington, Seattle, WA*

PAWEŁ STANKIEWICZ, MD, PhD • *Department of Molecular and Human Genetics, Baylor College of Medicine, Houston, TX*

KAREN STEPHENS, PhD • *Departments of Medicine and Laboratory Medicine, University of Washington, Seattle, WA*

VINCENT TIMMERMAN, PhD • *Molecular Genetics Department, Flanders Interuniversity Institute for Biotechnology, University of Antwerp, Antwerpen, Belgium*

CHRIS TYLER-SMITH, PhD • *The Sanger Institute, Wellcome Trust Genome Campus, Cambridge, UK*

ROBERT D. WELLS, PhD • *Center for Genome Research, Texas A & M University System Health Science Center, Texas Medical Center, Houston, Texas*

RACHEL WEVRICK, PhD • *Department of Medical Genetics, University of Alberta, Edmonton, Alberta, Canada*

HUNTINGTON F. WILLARD, PhD • *Institute for Genome Sciences & Policy, Duke University, Durham, NC*

PAULINE H. YEN, PhD • *Institute of Biomedical Sciences, Academia Sinica, Taipei, Taiwan*

ORSETTA ZUFFARDI, PhD • *Biologia Generale e Genetica Medica, Universita di Pavia, Pavia, Italy*

I Introduction

1

The CMT1A Duplication

A Historical Perspective Viewed From Two Sides of an Ocean

James R. Lupski, MD, PhD
and Vincent Timmerman, PhD

CONTENTS

FROM THE UNITED STATES

I came to Houston, Texas in 1986 with one goal being to identify "the gene" for Charcot-Marie-Tooth (CMT) disease. I was peripherally aware of the paper by Botstein and colleagues *(1)* proposing the genetic mapping of human "disease genes" using linked restriction fragment length polymorphisms (RFLPs) to position the gene within the human genome and indeed became very excited as a graduate student when Gusella's paper *(2)* appeared in *Nature* linking the Huntington disease locus to markers on chromosome 4. It was a natural extension to think this "positional cloning" approach might be applied to a host of other human traits. There was a personal, one might say egocentric, reason to choose CMT because I have the disease *(3)* and, in fact, the first blood samples collected for DNA linkage studies were from my own family wherein CMT segregated as an apparent autosomal recessive trait.

The year 1986 was also somewhat historic for the opportunity to attend the Cold Spring Harbor Symposium on Quantitative Biology, which that year was on "The Molecular Biology of *Homo sapiens*" *(4)*. It was there that Kary Mullis first announced publicly the polymerase chain reaction (PCR) technique, and also some of the first "scientific public" debates surrounding the initiation of the Human Genome Project took place. I distinctly remember Kary Mullis arguing during these discussions that if there was going to be a huge amount of DNA sequence determined (like the three billion basepair human genome) then the "G" symbol for the base guanine should be changed to "W" to distinguish it from "C," which was difficult to do because of the typewriters and printers available at the time. He argued that Crick already had one of the symbols ("C" for cytocine) named after him and Watson should have one. I vaguely remember Jim Watson smiling on the sidelines of the audience. I was married that week in Huntington, New York.

From: *Genomic Disorders: The Genomic Basis of Disease*
Edited by: J. R. Lupski and P. Stankiewicz © Humana Press, Totowa, NJ

The move to Houston was also because of the decision to continue my clinical training and begin internship and residency in pediatrics at Texas Children's Hospital. This occupied my time immensely and, thus, I was fortunate to be able to join Pragna Patel, a junior faculty member in the Institute for Molecular Genetics, to bank CMT family samples and initiate our genetic linkage studies.

Family collections began in earnest towards the end of my residency (1988–1989). Pragna had known of a physician, Carlos Garcia (New Orleans), who followed a number of families with CMT in Louisiana and we also contacted Jim Killian (Houston), at the time co-chairman of Neurology at Baylor College of Medicine, who published a huge French Acadian pedigree segregating CMT a decade earlier (5). He had also made the intriguing observation that apparent homozygosity for the dominant CMT gene, a child of two affected parents, resulted in a significantly more severe phenotype (5). Thus, like many other human traits, CMT is probably better characterized as a semi-dominant disorder.

Carlos Garcia directed the *Muscular Dystrophy Association* clinics in New Orleans, Baton Rouge, and Lafayette, LA. Once a month, Carlos' wife Mona would always remark "It's that time of the month again," I would fly to New Orleans and stay overnight Monday at the Garcia's. Carlos and I would awaken and drive a couple of hours to Baton Rouge and see patients from morning until just after lunch, drive to Lafayette (where Carlos followed several hundred CMT patients) and see patients until dinner time. We would have a wonderful Cajun dinner, stay overnight in Lafayette, and the next day start seeing patients early in the morning until late afternoon, then he would drive me back to the New Orleans airport with a suitcase of blood samples in hand. Carlos would clinically examine and oversee nerve conduction velocity (NCV) testing (NCVs are an objective laboratory test for type 1 CMT [CMT1]) while I would draw pedigrees and obtain blood for DNA samples and to make permanent transformed lymphoblastoid cell lines on my return to Houston.

One particular blood collection sticks out in my mind. It took place in a hospital clinic adjacent to the emergency room of a local hospital in Lafayette. We first collected blood from a teenage man distinguished by an unusual haircut and tattoos dressed in an outfit becoming of a punk rocker. When we next began collecting blood from his younger sister, she passed out and started to have myoclonic jerks. Her older brother started to shout "she is throwing a fit." He then proceeded to stand, look at both Dr. Garcia and I, and stated, "I am going to go get a REAL doctor" and proceeded to the emergency room next door. Needless to say both he and she were just fine and Dr. Garcia and I recovered from our ego bruising.

These monthly trips continued for a few years, but for the collection of very large families we would sometimes arrange a family reunion. It was remarkable how there would be one family member, often an unaffected individual, who could mobilize the entire family because of their belief in the research efforts. Importantly, we had to perform the electrical studies (NCVs) and collect blood samples from all family members. This included unaffected individuals, who were sometimes hesitant, or required further explanation of the need for their samples. I often thought of the irony of the situation. At these reunion parties, Dr. Garcia would oversee the administration of the electrical shocks accompanying nerve conduction studies, I would draw blood from each family member, and they would feed us wonderful Cajun barbeque. We similarly collected the large family reported by Dr. Killian using the family reunion approach. In this case, Jim Killian rented the town hall of a small town in the French Acadian countryside of Louisiana. I remember Dr. Killian asking other family members about one particular family member, expressing some concern during the inquiry. Apparently, during the examinations and home visits that led to the 1979 paper of Killian and Kloepfer *(5)*, this family member drew a gun on Dr. Killian thinking that he was either "the law," or a tax collector.

Meanwhile in Houston, Pragna had collected several polymorphic DNA markers from the laboratory of Dr. Ray White in Utah and we analyzed systematically the family material that was available. We began with the smaller chromosomes and essentially had ruled out several, including initially chromosome 17, using sparse markers when Jeff Vance (Durham, NC) *(6)* reported linkage of CMT1A to chromosome 17 using the same marker that revealed linkage to *NF1* on chromosome 17. We and others confirmed this chromosome 17 linkage *(7)*.

Much effort was now focused on identifying, and/or making more informative, DNA markers for the pericentromeric region of chromosome 17. Yusuke Nakamura (Tokyo, Japan) had provided some chromosome 17 cosmid clones, which were used to identify chromosome 17 polymorphic markers. Also, Pragna developed a novel method to obtain region specific chromosome 17 markers using differential *Alu*-PCR *(8)*. At the time *Alu*-PCR had been recently developed in our Institute for Molecular Genetics by David Nelson in Tom Caskey's lab *(9)*. To identify region specific markers, *Alu*-PCR was performed on somatic cell hybrids that retain either intact human chromosome 17 or a deleted chromosome from a patient with Smith-Magenis syndrome (SMS) [del(17)(p11.2p11.2)] *(10)*. Amplification products were compared and if a band was present in the amplification from the hybrid retaining intact chromosome 17, but not from the amplification of the hybrid with the deletion chromosome, then this was surmised to physically come from the specific deleted region. Of course, one also identifies *Alu* polymorphisms this way. We found that the procedure could be remarkably simplified by first reducing the genome complexities using restriction endonuclease digestion before the *Alu*-PCR. This, in turn, lead to the development of "restricted-*Alu* PCR" *(11)*. By 1989 we had accumulated extensive mapping data to show that the CMT1A locus was on the short arm of chromosome 17 and most tightly linked to markers that were physically located within the common SMS deletion interval in 17p11.2.

Here I must digress to say that much of our daily business was centered around marker genotyping using RFLPs. It was clear that some markers worked better than others, for some the segregating alleles were easier to score than for others, and in general each DNA marker had its own "personality." There were clearly certain DNA markers that appeared to show an artifact of different hybridization intensities for cross-hybridizing bands on genomic Southern blots. However, individuals from the same families were not always run adjacent to each other on the genomic Southerns. By no means did we initially recognize that the presumed artifact of "dosage differences between cross-hybridizing bands" segregated in a Mendelian fashion. Scoring of alleles was done independent of knowledge of affection status. Linkage analyses were performed in collaboration with Aravinda Chakravarti (Baltimore, MD), and I worked mostly with his student Susan Slaugenhaupt, who would input the data from the scoring sheets for the analyses.

Although RFLP mapping was proceeding, much effort was also expended on screening the proximal 17p linked probes for the presence of simple sequence repeats (SSR; e.g., $[GT]_n$) because these were just identified in the human genome *(12,13)*, determined to be highly polymorphic, and could be rapidly analyzed by PCR. Odila Saucedo-Cardenas cloned and sequenced several different SSRs from CMT1A-linked markers and developed flanking primer sets with Roberto Montes de Oca-Luna that could be used in the PCR to type CMT1A families. Odila and Roberto were, at the time, both Research Technicians in the laboratory. Roberto

T G C A

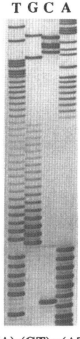

(TA)₅(GT)₁₇(AT)₈

Fig. 1. Nucleotide sequence of the simple sequence repeat RM11-GT. Autoradiogram of a DNA sequencing gel showing the repeat, which lies at the basis of the polymorphic DNA marker RM11-GT. Initial evidence for the Charcot-Marie-Tooth type 1A (CMT1A) duplication was revealed by this marker that showed three alleles (i.e., triallelic) in fully informative CMT patients.

made an interesting observation for one of the SSR markers, termed RM11-GT with SSR $(TA)_5(GT)_{17}(AT)_8$ (*see* Fig. 1) *(14)*. When primers were used to type the CMT1A families for this marker, one often found three alleles rather than the usual two expected with one inherited from each parent. Three alleles were observed in many individuals with CMT1A, but not in all—the marker was not always fully informative. Three alleles were not observed in unaffected family members with the exception of three individuals who were asymptomatic; however, these latter three seemingly unaffected individuals had not had nerve conduction studies. Subsequent NCV studies revealed decreased motor NCVs consistent with CMT1 and confirmed our suspicion that these individuals had subclinical, not yet penetrant disease.

Roberto examined some of the Southern blots that utilized an RFLP marker from the same locus and noted that often when there were three alleles revealed by RM11-GT *(14)*, a dosage difference could be observed between the two alleles if the affected individual was heterozygous for that RFLP. These initial observations suggested that there may be three copies of the genomic region that was being assayed, potentially reflecting genomic duplication at the CMT1A locus. The entire laboratory now focused on the "duplication hypothesis" and, to keep our hypothesis quiet, it was referred to as the "D" word within the laboratory because we all focused on gathering data to support or refute the duplication hypothesis using multiple independent molecular approaches. When now correcting for diagnosis (i.e., making sure that all apparent unaffected individuals did not have subclinical disease by performing NCVs and systematically examining CMT1A families), the putative duplication appeared to cosegregate with the CMT1A phenotype as determined by objective NCV measurements *(15)*.

To reconcile dosage differences of heterozygous RFLP alleles with the three RM11-GT alleles observed in CMT1A duplication patients, Pragna performed an important experiment. For one of the RFLP markers revealing dosage differences, and from which the PCR-typeable RM11-GT marker was derived, the *Msp*I alleles were separated on preparative agarose gels and used as templates for PCR amplifications of RM11-GT. As anticipated, from the RFLP allele showing increased dosage she could amplify 2 RM11-GT alleles, whereas only one was found from the PCR of the other RFLP allele that displayed normal dosage *(15)*. Similar types of experiments, to examine the molecular basis for the dosage differences of alleles, were performed by first physically separating the two chromosome homologs in rodent somatic cell hybrids *(15)*.

The allele dosage differences revealed by RFLP analyses could also be observed, although it was much more difficult to see and less informative, for two other CMT1A-linked markers that by genetic mapping studies were adjacent to the initial marker revealing duplication. This suggested the putative duplication might be large and we, thus, attempted to obtain further, physical evidence for its existence. Pentao Liu applied pulsed-field gel electrophoresis (PFGE) as a means to try to resolve a potentially large genomic change. Indeed, he was able to identify a 500-kb apparent junction fragment in CMT1A patients that was not observed in controls. Furthermore, he showed that this junction fragment cosegregated with CMT1A *(15)*. Interestingly, this junction fragment was increased in dosage in a patient, whom we presumed was homozygous for the CMT mutation given the severe clinical picture, where both parents had CMT1A. In collaboration with Barbara Trask (Seattle, WA), we attempted to resolve the duplication by fluorescence *in situ* hybridization of metaphase spreads from lymphoblastoid cell lines constructed from CMT1A patients and controls. The metaphase analysis failed, but on interphase spreads she could identify duplication on one of the two chromosome 17 homologs *(15)*. Moreover, she identified an apparent duplication on both homologous chromosomes in the patient presumed to be homozygous on clinical grounds. Because these were interphase cells, it was important to distinguish duplication from replication and this was done by comparison to a nearby control probe. To our knowledge, this was the first time that a common autosomal dominant human disease trait was diagnosed using a microscopic technique. Although it was 55 years later, I think we were probably as excited as Calvin Bridges was when he initially applied the then new technique of polytene chromosomes to the study of fruit fly traits and found that the *Bar* gene was a duplication *(16)*.

We had accumulated very strong physical evidence thus far; 3 GT alleles, dosage differences of heterozygous RFLP alleles, a PFGE junction fragment, and interphase fluorescence *in situ* hybridization revealing a duplicated signal, for the CMT1A duplication. However, what remained was reconciliation with the genetic data. The marker VAW409, from which RM11-GT was derived and which physically revealed the duplication by virtue of dosage differences of heterozygous RFLP alleles in CMT1A patients, also appeared to reveal recombinants in the genetic analysis. We thought it would be hard to publish our CMT1A duplication findings without reconciling the physical and genetic data. Through conversations I was having with Markus Grompe (Portland, OR), a then clinical genetics fellow with me at Baylor, it became clear that the duplication could have consequences for the interpretation of marker genotypes and thus linkage analyses. The failure to account for the duplication in linkage analyses produces false recombinants (Fig. 2A). Linkage programs score

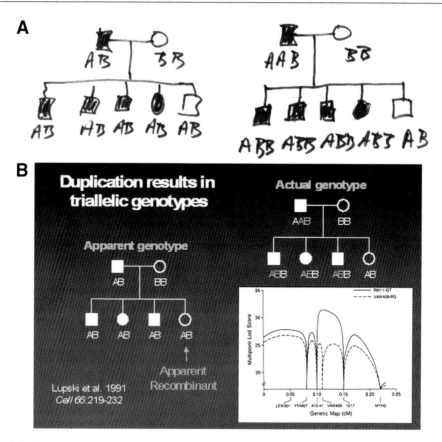

Fig. 2. Triallelic marker genotypes and false recombinants. (A) Actual note paper wherein biallelic marker genotype scoring was compared to triallelic marker genotype scoring to reveal the molecular genetic basis of false recombinants. (B) The effects of molecular duplication on the interpretation of marker genotypes and linkage mapping. Standard pedigree symbols are used; females depicted as circles and males by squares. Filled-in symbols denote affected individuals. On the left is a simple pedigree with marker genotypes scored as a usual biallelic system with one of the two alleles inherited from each parent. One unaffected daughter is an apparent recombinant (false recombinant) because she has the same apparent genotype as her three affected siblings. To the right is shown the actual genotypes scored as a triallelic system accounting for the molecular duplication. The lower right shows how the different scoring biallelic (dashed line) vs triallelic (bold line), affects the multipoint LOD-score. Note the differences in peak LOD scores and the fact that the failure to account for three alleles (or dosage differences in heterozygous restriction fragment length polymorphisms) results in an erroneous map position.

genetic transmission data using a biallelic system—one inherits one allele from each of two parents. However, the duplication produces three alleles. The failure to account for dosage differences at a two allele (biallelic) RFLP in linkage analysis, when it exists, leads to the misinterpretation of the parental origin of alleles (Fig. 2B). Importantly, when we rescored the marker genotypes as a triallelic system, both the genetic data and the physical duplication data converged on the same locus *(15)*.

We now thought that the problem was solved, but convincing one's colleagues and peer reviewers is another challenge. Pragna and I initially showed all the data to our Chairman Tom Caskey. He said that he was not completely convinced, but we better be absolutely sure if we were going to publish this from his department. Art Beaudet, a senior colleague, seemed to be convinced and made some helpful comments on both of the manuscripts. I say two manuscripts because the amount of accumulated data was extensive; there was one entire paper that covered the genetic analyses and the second manuscript described the physical evidence for duplication.

We sent both manuscripts to *Science* and they were both rejected. Interestingly, I subsequently learned from Christine Van Broeckhoven (Antwerp, Belgium), whose laboratory independently identified the CMT1A duplication in Europe, that she had submitted their paper to *Science* the same month that we submitted our papers. There were referees' and editors' comments to both of us from a couple of journals that we "had not identified the gene." This pretty clearly showed that the reviewers completely misunderstood the novelty of our findings, as did the editor handling the manuscript, thus, the burden was on us to make it clearer. At the time, I certainly do not think that I understood the implications of the CMT1A duplication for other human diseases that result from genome rearrangements; a class of conditions subsequently referred to as genomic disorders that represent recombination-based disease resulting form DNA rearrangements owing to genome architecture *(17,18)*. Nor did I anticipate that the requirement for three alleles to manifest a trait, triallelic inheritance, might apply to the genetic transmission of other conditions *(19)*. A revision and resubmission of both manuscripts to *Cell* was met with more favorable reviews. They each insisted on condensation to one large paper, because of the interdependence of the genetic and physical data, and suggested the deletion of some material. Although heated discussions concerning authorships and positions on the paper ensued, Pragna, Aravinda, and I agreed with the reviewers' ideas that because of interdependence of the data, it would be best presented as a single paper. Whether Pragna or I would be first or last author was mainly settled by which person would now condense these two papers into one and address each of the reviewer's thoughtful comments.

We first presented the data for the CMT1A duplication at a small CMT meeting in Tucson, AZ hosted by the Muscular Dystrophy Association (MDA). Christine Van Broeckhoven spoke first about a duplication they identified in CMT patients from Europe *(20)*. I felt immediate relief and excitement—our hypothesis and supporting data were already reproduced in another part of the world. I spoke after her and described the multiple methods we used to obtain evidence in support of the duplication and how this genomic rearrangement affected the interpretation of marker genotypes. During the lunch break that followed our talks, multiple audience members called their respective laboratories and, indeed, review of their Southern blots revealed RFLP dosage differences for the appropriate markers. The existence of the CMT1A duplication had now almost instantaneously been confirmed around the world.

FROM EUROPE

I started my PhD in October 1988 at the University of Antwerp, Belgium in the laboratory of Christine Van Broeckhoven, currently the scientific director of the Molecular Genetics Department affiliated to the Flanders Interuniversity Institute for Biotechnology. I became interested in her molecular genetic research of neurological disorders, after reading a paper in *Nature* on Alzheimer's disease *(21)*. I selected this paper as a topic for a course in the frame of my master studies in biotechnology (applied in agriculture) at the University of Leuven, Belgium. When I joined the Antwerp team, Peter Raeymaekers was the only other PHD student, performing molecular genetics on a multi-generation Belgian CMT family with autosomal dominant transmission. In fact, Peter initially started his PHD on genetics of Alzheimer disease, but because the families were still being sampled, he initially spent a lot of effort in developing protocols for isolating human DNA, and in cloning probes that recognized RFLPs. When Peter De Jonghe and Jan Gheuens, clinical neurologists at the Neurology Department of the University Hospital Antwerp, presented to him the large pedigree of a CMT family, he decided to switch to research into genetics of CMT. It became apparent that the pedigree of this CMT family was huge, with more than 350 family members in five generations. In total we sampled 51 affected and 60 healthy relatives for linkage studies. Because we were convinced that CMT was a very rare disorder at that time, we used alphabetical letters in the acronyms of the CMT families we ascertained in Belgium. Still, we had not changed our opinion of the disease frequency when we reached the letter Z, and considered starting again with A-A, in retrospect it is fortunate that we decided to switch to numbers. At this moment we have nearly 2000 CMT families under investigation, either sampled in Belgium or obtained through international collaboration, particularly within the European CMT consortium founded in 1991. However, looking back it seems like the alphabetical letters had some magic value: the CMT-A family turned out to belong to the CMT1A subtype *(22)*, family CMT-B belongs to the CMT1B subtype *(23)*, and CMT-M has a pure motor phenotype *(24)*.

Fortunately, Belgium is a small country (you can hardly drive 2 hours by car without ending up in a neighboring country), in which people tend to continue living in the village where they were born. Every week Peter De Jonghe and his wife Gisèle Smeyers, at that time the research nurse on the project, made many trips visiting family members of family CMT-A at their homes to collect blood samples. Gisèle made the first contact with the patients and relatives to explain the aims of the study and to ask whether she could visit again, but now with the neurologist Peter De Jonghe, who was leading the project. What she did not tell was that the neurologist was in fact her husband, because she wanted the family members to feel free to criticize doctors because of lack of attention for the problems of a CMT patient. However, there soon came a moment when she had to disclose the husband–wife relationship. When visiting a CMT patient whose husband was a forester, she was offered a rabbit to take home. The next visit, the man offered her again a rabbit but said "and here is one for the doctor too." Not to look greedy, she disclosed that the doctor was her husband Peter De Jonghe, but still received the two rabbits.

In the Belgian CMT-A family, Peter Raeymaekers used RFLPs to exclude the first CMT locus on chromosome 1-designated CMT1B in 1982 *(25)*, and initiated a genome search using some of his in-house developed RFLPs. However, shortly before Peter Raeymaekers' PhD thesis defense June 1989, Jeffery Vance (Durham, NC) reported linkage with two chromosome 17p markers (*D17S58* and *D17S71*) in CMT1A families *(6)*. We confirmed the linkage with the two 17p DNA markers in the Belgian CMT-A family, and obtained a log of the odd (LOD) score of 10.67 (significant linkage is obtained when the LOD > 3) *(22)*. We proceeded with the genetic analysis of eight additional chromosome 17 markers, and showed that the CMT1A mutation was mapped in the 17p11.2-p12 region between the marker *D17S71* and the gene coding for myosin heavy polypeptide 2 (*MYH2*) *(26)*.

At that time only partial genetic maps were available for linkage studies *(27,28)*. To fine-map the CMT1A locus, we genotyped additional RFLPs and detected informative recombinants in family CMT-A. However, the genotypes obtained for two DNA markers (pVAW409R1 and pVAW409R3), representing the same locus *D17S122*, were hard to interpret on RFLP analysis. For one marker we obtained a significant LOD score of 16.20, but it recombined with the second marker at *D17S122*. These results were hard to believe, and our first reaction was that we had misinterpreted the genotypes. The autoradiograms of the Southern blots were messy, with high backgrounds owing to the presence of repetitive sequences that made it

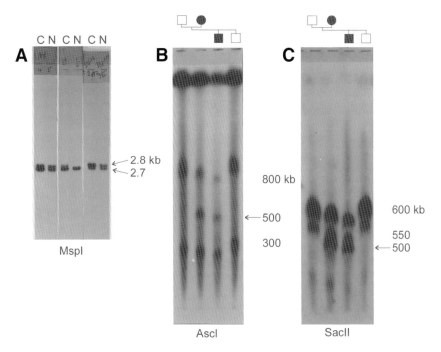

Fig. 3. Hybridization signals obtained with probe pVAW409R3a (*D17S122*). (A) Southern blot of genomic DNA digested with *Msp*I of Charcot-Marie-Tooth neuropathy type 1A (CMT1A) duplication patients (C) and healthy relatives (N) of three different CMT families. Dosage differences between the alleles are seen in each patient, either in the upper allele (2.8 kb) or lower allele (2.7 kb). (B,C) Southern patterns of genomic DNA digested with rare cutter restriction enzymes *Asc*I and *Sac*II. DNA fragments were separated by pulsed-field gel electrophoresis. The 500-kb junction fragment (arrow) is only present in the CMT1A duplication patients belonging to a small branch of the Belgian family CMT-A.

difficult to "read" the *Msp*I alleles. To avoid these "dirty blots," we decided to "clean up" the pVAW409R1 and pVAW409R3 clones, by recloning the non-repetitive restriction fragments into derivative probes designated pVAW409R1b and pVAW409R3a. The hybridization results were squeaky clean; however, much to my amazement, in each genotype one allele had the double density of the other. There was also no consistency because in one patient it was the upper band and in another patient the lower band revealing the increased dosage intensity. After checking and rechecking, I realized that the data could only be explained if one of the alleles was duplicated. I reinterpreted the genotypes, and yes, the recombinants had disappeared.

I can still feel the excitement that went through my body that summer in 1990. Although I was convinced that the data were true, I refrained from telling Peter Raeymaekers and my supervisor Christine. Could it still be that I mixed up samples? I redid the entire experiment, but no, the same results appeared (Fig. 3A). Now it was time to share my findings! Suddenly, the project became the hottest one in the group, we worked hard and step-by-step discovered that the duplication had to be >1 Mb in size based on other duplicated markers in the region (pVAW412R3 [*D17S125*] and pEW401 [*D17S61*]) and PFGE data. We wrote the paper and submitted it to *Nature*. While under editorial review, we continued the work and found the real genetic proof that it was the duplication that caused the disease, namely in one family we observed the duplication appearing *de novo* together with the disease. In this family (CMT-G), the grandparents were unaffected, and among their six children there was only one patient, who transmitted CMT to his son.

Peter Raeymaekers, Peter De Jonghe and I attended the seventh International Congress on Neuromuscular Diseases in Münich, September 1990. During this meeting our excitement about the finding of the CMT1A duplication gradually turned into sheer paranoia. Jeffery Vance was giving the plenary lecture on CMT; did he not know about the duplication, or did he and would not tell? Who was chatting to whom during the poster session and what about? Could it be that the CMT1A duplication would be revealed in the "surprise box," the last presentation of the meeting? To us shareholders of the CMT1A duplication an extraordinary event took place at this meeting. During the poster session, authors had to present their poster in three slides in a session chaired by Peter James Dyck (Rochester, NY) one of the forefathers of the entire field of peripheral neuropathies. At some point, there was a heated discussion regarding controversial data presented by Victor Ionascescu (Iowa City, IA). To change the subject and calm the audience, P. J. Dyck suddenly asked, "in all these fancy molecular genetic studies, has someone of you ever seen something special like a duplication?" Peter Raeymaekers turned pale and almost fainted. However, nobody noticed the remark, and later it became apparent that P. J. Dyck had absolutely no knowledge of the CMT1A duplication at that time.

Nature did not send our paper for review. Christine, my supervisor, had many hours of discussion with the associate editor Kevin Davies handling the paper; she added new data to the paper (e.g., the *de novo* duplication data, the size of the duplication estimated at around 1 Mb, additional CMT1A duplication families), but nothing helped. The final verdict was "since we were so close to the gene we might consider coming back when we found it." This illustrated the disbelief in the scientific community that an autosomal dominant disease could result from a gene dosage defect, a genetic mechanism that now is commonly accepted! Also, in 1990 we did not have available the technology we have today, and cloning a gene from a larger than 1 Mb region was still a major challenge. Later, Kevin Davies became editor of *Nature Genetics*, and invited Christine to tell the story of the CMTA duplication at the first International Conference of *Nature Genetics* on "Human Genetics: Mapping the Future," Washington, April 1993.

We sent the paper to *Science* and *Lancet* and neither were prepared to send it for review and comments ranged from "not interesting for the larger public" to "the duplication does not provide insight in the identity of the genetic defect causing CMT1A." By now it was spring 1991, we were desperate and terribly disappointed, while running into another problem.

Christine was organizing and chairing the eighth workshop on "The Genetics of Hereditary Motor and Sensory Neuropathies" sponsored by the European NeuroMuscular Center (ENMC), in May 1991, in The Netherlands. The paper was not yet resubmitted, and thus we were confronted with a major dilemma: should we be quiet while the workshop aimed at defining criteria for sampling CMT families using strict diagnostic criteria of CMT1 for mapping and cloning of the CMT1A defect, although we knew about the duplication? We decided not, what could we lose at this point. Also, if it became later known to the participants that we as organizers had this information at the time of the workshop, all European CMT researchers would feel deceived. We decided to share the exciting, although still unpublished data, having it presented by Peter Raeymaekers.

While Peter was gradually building the story towards the discovery of the CMT1A duplication, one could notice the increasing excitement among the participants who became silent, stopped taking notes and started whispering "they found it." After the applause, Alan Emery, former research director of the ENMC stood up, congratulated the Antwerp researchers with their important and fascinating finding that they were sharing prepublication. He asked all participants to keep all the presented data confidential, to remember they heard about this unpublished data at the ENMC workshop, and refrain from publishing their data on the duplication obtained without crediting the Antwerp group. To us, he suggested to publish our manuscript in *Neuromuscular Disorders*, a new journal of his good friend Victor Dubowitz *(20)*. This explains why our most cited paper was published in the second issue of a journal that had not yet had an impact factor in 1991. Later on in June 1991, my supervisor Christine Van Broeckhoven attended the MDA-organized workshop on CMT in Tucson, AZ, chaired by Kurt Fischbeck (Bethesda, MD). Here, again there was the dilemma, but now all European researchers that were present at the workshop had brought data from their families confirming that the duplication was the major CMT1A mutation. The evening before the workshop Christine informed Kurt Fischbeck. Also, present in the bar was Garth Nicholson (Sidney, Australia) who bought a bottle of champagne, and made a phone call to his co-workers who, while he was asleep, collected all the data on the Australian families. The next day, Christine presented the Antwerp data and referenced the data of the European groups. Next there was a presentation by Jim Lupski (Houston, TX) who had similar data that was in press in *Cell (15)*. A more extreme difference in journal impact factors, is hard to imagine. Though, we had not published this major finding in a major journal, we did receive substantial recognition thanks to the many European and American colleagues who always cited, and still do, our paper in *Neuromuscular Disorders (20)*. Also, since the MDA workshop in 1991, the Antwerp and Houston labs had a special bond based on mutual respect and friendship, and have been collaborating on the genetics of different inherited peripheral neuropathies ever since.

After the discovery of the CMT1A duplication many labs requested our "clean" RFLP probes for research and DNA-diagnosis of CMT neuropathies. I remember the many tubes we had to prepare to distribute the clones around the world. In the same year we reported our findings to the patients in Belgium. Since then, we organize yearly meetings for the Belgian CMT organization. In some families, such as CMT-G, the disease appeared simultaneously with a *de novo* duplication originating from an unequal crossover event between two homologous chromosomes *(20)*. These findings indicated that the CMT1A duplication in 17p11.2 was the disease-causing mutation. At that time it was thought that isolated cases of hereditary motor and sensory neuropathies represented autosomal recessive traits. We and others demonstrated that the CMT1A duplication was responsible for most cases of autosomal dominant CMT1, but that *de novo* mutations occurred in 9 out of 10 sporadic patients. This finding became important for genetic counseling of isolated CMT patients *(29)*.

Because the duplicated markers in CMT1A spanned a minimal distance of approx 10 cM on the genetic map of chromosome 17p11.2-p12, we constructed a physical map of the CMT1A region using rare cutter restriction enzymes in combination with PFGE. This was a very laborious undertaking that resulted in determining the size of the CMT1A duplication to about 1.5 Mb. The discrepancy between the genetic and physical map distances suggested that the 17p11.2 region was extremely prone to recombination events, and that the high recombination rate could be a contributing factor to the genetic instability of this chromosomal region. We also determined by PFGE mapping the position of the duplication breakpoints. The discovery of extra restriction fragments or "duplication junction fragments" with the markers in 1.5-Mb region, provided a more accurate DNA-diagnostic tool for the screening of CMT1A patients (Fig. 3B,C). In addition to the unequal crossover resulting into the CMT1A duplication, we also observed in some of our CMT1 families recombination between DNA markers located on the chromosome transmitting the CMT1A duplication, making our research a puzzling event *(30)*.

After the proposed genetic mechanism causing the CMT1A duplication was determined to be owing to unequal crossover during meiosis, we studied the parental origin of the duplication in genetically sporadic CMT1A patients. We demonstrated that in all cases the mutation was the product of an unequal nonsister chromatid exchange during spermatogenesis. The fact that only paternal *de novo* duplications were observed in the sporadic CMT1A patients, suggested that male-specific factors may be operating during spermatogenesis that either aid in the formation of the duplication and/or stabilize the duplicated chromosome *(31)*. Later, *de novo* duplications were also described on the maternal chromosome.

The next step was to identify the gene interrupted by the duplication, or to find a dosage-sensitive gene (three copies instead of two copies), or one in which a position effect on one or more genes is involved. One year after the discovery of the CMT1A duplication, Ueli Suter (Zürich, Switzerland) reported two independent mutations in the transmembrane domain of the mouse peripheral myelin protein 22 (*PMP22*) gene. These missense mutations occurred spontaneously in the *trembler* (Tr) and *trembler-j* (Tr[j]) mouse mutants *(32,33)*. These mice were considered a model for CMT neuropathy owing to weakness and atrophy of distal limb muscles and hypomyelination of peripheral nerves. Interestingly, *PMP22* was expressed in the myelin of peripheral nerves and shown to be identical in DNA sequence to the growth arrest specific gene *Gas3*. The *Gas3* gene was mapped to mouse chromosome 11 in a region syntenic to human chromosome 17p11.2. Using our pulsed-field mapping data, we demonstrated that the human *PMP22* gene was located in the middle of the duplicated CMT1A region and that this gene was not interrupted by the duplication. Eva Nelis, who joined our small CMT research group as a PhD student, demonstrated that the *PMP22* gene showed a dosage-effect because density differences were observed in the hybridization signals on Southern blots. This finding indicated that *PMP22* was a good candidate gene for CMT1A. I remember my first trip to the United States, where we presented our physical CMT1A mapping data at a Chromosome 17 workshop in Park City. There it was decided between the participating teams to submit the *PMP22* gene data as site-by-site manuscripts.

Finally, the work was published in the first issue of *Nature Genetics (34–37)*. The proof that *PMP22* was the disease-causing gene for CMT1A was made after the identification of point mutations in some rare patients *(38–40)*.

After my PhD defense in 1993, Phillip Chance (Seattle, WA) demonstrated that the condition known as hereditary neuropathy with liability to pressure palsies (HNPP) was associated with an interstitial deletion of the same 1.5-Mb region that is duplicated in CMT1A patients *(41)*. The mechanism for unequal crossover was explained by the misalignment at flanking repeat sequences (CMT1A-REPs) leading to a tandem duplication in CMT1A and the reciprocal deletion in HNPP *(42,43)*, and subsequently confirmed by many labs. As a result of another paper by Lupski's team *(44)*, Jim invited me in 1995 as a visiting scientist at the Baylor College of Medicine in Houston, to screen markers located within the CMT1A-REP. Our joint effort allowed analyzing a large group of unrelated CMT1A duplication and HNPP deletion patients from different European countries for the presence of a recombination hotspot in the CMT1A-REP sequences. We confirmed the hotspot for unequal crossover between the misaligned flanking CMT1A-REP elements, and detected novel junction fragments in more than 70% of the unrelated patients. This recombination hotspot was also present in *de novo* CMT1A duplication and HNPP deletion patients. Our data also indicated that the hotspot of unequal crossover occurred in several populations independent of ethnic background. We concluded that the detection of junction fragments from the CMT1A-REP element on Southern blots could be used as a novel and reliable DNA-diagnostic tool in most patients *(45)*. Nowadays, the Southern blot method (Fig. 3A) has been replaced by PCR methods making use of highly informative short tandem repeat markers in the CMT1A region or specific primers located within the CMT1A-REP region.

At the second CMT workshop, sponsored by the ENMC in The Netherlands, researchers from several European countries agreed to contribute to a large study with the aim to estimate the frequency of the CMT1A duplication and HNPP deletion, and to make the first inventory of mutations in the myelin genes causing CMT. I remember the many phone calls (e-mail was not yet available in all 28 centers involved in the study) Eva Nelis made to find out that the CMT1A duplication was present in more than 70% of 800 unrelated CMT1 patients, and the deletion in 84% of more than 150 unrelated HNPP patients. In CMT1 patients negative for the duplication, mutations were identified in *PMP22*, myelin protein zero (*MPZ*), and connexin 32 (*GJB1/Cx32*) *(46)*. These data resulted in the *Inherited Peripheral Neuropathy Mutation Database* developed and maintained by Eva Nelis (http://www.molgen.ua.ac.be/CMTMutations/).

Without the excellent contacts between our lab and the many CMT patients and their families involved in this research, we could have never detected the CMT1A duplication and the many disease-causing genes currently involved in distinct types of inherited peripheral neuropathies. Professor Alan Emery said at the first European CMT workshop: "This is another step towards discovery of the causes of all these disorders, which will open doors to possible treatments in the future." The CMT1A duplication mechanism is now referred to in many textbooks on Human Molecular Genetics.

ACKNOWLEDGMENTS

I appreciate the help of both Christine Van Broeckhoven and Peter De Jonghe for their input on this historical perspective.

REFERENCES

1. Botstein D, White RL, Skolnick M, Davis RW. Construction of a genetic linkage map in man using restriction fragment length polymorphisms. Am J Hum Genet 1980;32:314–331.
2. Gusella JF, Wexler NS, Conneally PM, et al. A polymorphic DNA marker genetically linked to Huntington's disease. Nature 1983;306:234–238.
3. Breo DL. Researchers Lupski and Chance study a baffling genetic disease–their own. J Am Med Assoc 1993;270:2374–2375.
4. Molecular biology of *Homo sapiens*. Cold Spring Harb Symp Quant Biol 1986;51:1–702.
5. Killian JM, Kloepfer HW. Homozygous expression of a dominant gene for Charcot-Marie-Tooth neuropathy. Ann Neurol 1979;5:515–522.
6. Vance JM, Nicholson GA, Yamaoka LH, et al. Linkage of Charcot-Marie-Tooth neuropathy type 1a to chromosome 17. Exp Neurol 1989;104:186–189.
7. Patel PI, Franco B, Garcia C, et al. Genetic mapping of autosomal dominant Charcot-Marie-Tooth disease in a large French-Acadian kindred: identification of new linked markers on chromosome 17. Am J Hum Genet 1990;46:801–809.
8. Patel PI, Garcia C, Montes de Oca-Luna R, et al. Isolation of a marker linked to the Charcot-Marie-Tooth disease type IA gene by differential Alu-PCR of human chromosome 17-retaining hybrids. Am J Hum Genet 1990;47:926–934.
9. Nelson DL, Ballabio A, Victoria MF, et al. Alu-primed polymerase chain reaction for regional assignment of 110 yeast artificial chromosome clones from the human X chromosome: identification of clones associated with a disease locus. Proc Natl Acad Sci USA 1991;88:6157–6161.
10. Greenberg F, Guzzetta V, Montes de Oca-Luna R, et al. Molecular analysis of the Smith-Magenis syndrome: a possible contiguous-gene syndrome associated with del(17)(p11.2). Am J Hum Genet 1991;49:1207–1218.

11. Guzzetta V, Montes de Oca-Luna R, Lupski JR, Patel PI. Isolation of region-specific and polymorphic markers from chromosome 17 by restricted Alu polymerase chain reaction. Genomics 1991;9:31–36.

12. Litt M, Luty JA. A hypervariable microsatellite revealed by in vitro amplification of a dinucleotide repeat within the cardiac muscle actin gene. Am J Hum Genet 1989;44:397–401.

13. Weber J, May P. Abundant class of human DNA polymorphisms which can be typed using the polymerase chain reaction. Am J Hum Genet 1989;44:388–396.

14. Montes de Oca-Luna R. Localization of the Charcot-Marie-Tooth Type 1A Disease Locus: A DNA Duplication Associated With Disease, PHD thesis. Monterrey, Mexico: Universidad Antóma de Neuvo León. 1991.

15. Lupski JR, de Oca-Luna RM, Slaugenhaupt S, et al. DNA duplication associated with Charcot-Marie-Tooth disease type 1A. Cell 1991;66:219–232.

16. Bridges C. The *Bar* "gene" duplication. Science 1936;83:210–211.

17. Lupski JR. Genomic disorders: structural features of the genome can lead to DNA rearrangements and human disease traits. Trends Genet 1998;14:417–422.

18. Lupski JR. 2002 Curt Stern Award Address. Genomic disorders recombination-based disease resulting from genomic architecture. Am J Hum Genet 2003;72:246–252.

19. Katsanis N, Ansley SJ, Badano JL, et al. Triallelic inheritance in Bardet-Biedl syndrome, a Mendelian recessive disorder. Science 2001;293:2256–2259.

20. Raeymaekers P, Timmerman V, Nelis E, et al. Duplication in chromosome 17p11.2 in Charcot-Marie-Tooth neuropathy type 1a (CMT 1a). The HMSN Collaborative Research Group. Neuromuscul Disord 1991;1:93–97.

21. Van Broeckhoven C, Genthe AM, Vandenberghe A, et al. Failure of familial Alzheimer's disease to segregate with the A4-amyloid gene in several European families. Nature 1987;329:153–155.

22. Raeymaekers P, Timmerman V, De Jonghe P, et al. Localization of the mutation in an extended family with Charcot-Marie-Tooth neuropathy (HMSN I). Am J Hum Genet 1989;45:953–958.

23. Nelis E, Timmerman V, De Jonghe P, Muylle L, Martin JJ, Van Broeckhoven C. Linkage and mutation analysis in an extended family with Charcot-Marie-Tooth disease type 1B. J Med Genet 1994;31:811–815.

24. Timmerman V, De Jonghe P, Simokovic S, et al. Distal hereditary motor neuropathy type II (distal HMN II): mapping of a locus to chromosome 12q24. Hum Mol Genet 1996;5:1065–1069.

25. Stebbins NB, Conneally PM. Linkage of dominantley inherited Charcot-Marie-Tooth neuropathy to the Duffy locus in an Indiana family. Am J Hum Genet 1982;34:A195.

26. Timmerman V, Raeymaekers P, De Jonghe P, et al. Assignment of the Charcot-Marie-Tooth neuropathy type 1 (CMT1A) gene to 17p11.2-p12. Am J Hum Genet 1990;47:680–685.

27. Nakamura Y, Lathrop M, O'Connell P, et al. A mapped set of DNA markers for human chromosome 17. Genomics 1988;2:302–309.

28. Wright EC, Goldgar DE, Fain PR, Barker DF, Skolnick MH. A genetic map of human chromosome 17p. Genomics 1990;7:103–109.

29. Hoogendijk JE, Hensels GW, Gabreels-Festen AA, et al. *De-novo* mutation in hereditary motor and sensory neuropathy type I. Lancet 1992;339:1081–1082.

30. Raeymaekers P, Timmerman V, Nelis E, et al. Estimation of the size of the chromosome 17p11.2 duplication in Charcot-Marie-Tooth neuropathy type 1a (CMT1a). HMSN Collaborative Research Group. J Med Genet 1992;29:5–11.

31. Palau F, Lofgren A, De Jonghe P, et al. Origin of the de novo duplication in Charcot-Marie-Tooth disease type 1A: unequal nonsister chromatid exchange during spermatogenesis. Hum Mol Genet 1993;2:2031–2035.

32. Suter U, Welcher AA, Ozcelik T, et al. *Trembler* mouse carries a point mutation in a myelin gene. Nature 1992;356:241–244.

33. Suter U, Moskow JJ, Welcher AA, et al. A leucine-to-proline mutation in the putative first transmembrane domain of the 22-kDa peripheral myelin protein in the *trembler-J* mouse. Proc Natl Acad Sci USA 1992;89:4382–4386.

34. Patel PI, Roa BB, Welcher AA, et al. The gene for the peripheral myelin protein *PMP-22* is a candidate for Charcot-Marie-Tooth disease type 1A. Nat Genet 1992;1:159–165.

35. Valentijn LJ, Bolhuis PA, Zorn I, et al. The peripheral myelin gene *PMP-22/GAS-3* is duplicated in Charcot-Marie-Tooth disease type 1A. Nat Genet 1992;1:166–170.

36. Timmerman V, Nelis E, Van Hul W, et al. The peripheral myelin protein gene *PMP-22* is contained within the Charcot-Marie-Tooth disease type 1A duplication. Nat Genet 1992;1:171–175.

37. Matsunami N, Smith B, Ballard L, et al. *Peripheral myelin protein-22* gene maps in the duplication in chromosome 17p11.2 associated with Charcot-Marie-Tooth 1A. Nat Genet 1992;1:176–179.

38. Valentijn LJ, Baas F, Wolterman RA, et al. Identical point mutations of *PMP-22* in *Trembler-J* mouse and Charcot-Marie-Tooth disease type 1A. Nat Genet 1992;2:288–291.

39. Roa BB, Garcia CA, Suter U, et al. Charcot-Marie-Tooth disease type 1A. Association with a spontaneous point mutation in the *PMP22* gene. N Engl J Med 1993;329:96–101.

40. Nelis E, Timmerman V, De Jonghe P, Van Broeckhoven C. Identification of a 5′ splice site mutation in the *PMP-22* gene in autosomal dominant Charcot-Marie-Tooth disease type 1. Hum Mol Genet 1994;3:515–516.

41. Chance PF, Alderson MK, Leppig KA, et al. DNA deletion associated with hereditary neuropathy with liability to pressure palsies. Cell 1993;72:143–151.

42. Pentao L, Wise CA, Chinault AC, Patel PI, Lupski JR. Charcot-Marie-Tooth type 1A duplication appears to arise from recombination at repeat sequences flanking the 1.5 Mb monomer unit. Nat Genet 1992;2:292–300.

43. Chance PF, Abbas N, Lensch MW, et al. Two autosomal dominant neuropathies result from reciprocal DNA duplication/deletion of a region on chromosome 17. Hum Mol Genet 1994;3:223–228.

44. Reiter LT, Murakami T, Koeuth T, et al. A recombination hotspot responsible for two inherited peripheral neuropathies is located near a mariner transposon-like element. Nat Genet 1996;12:288–297.

45. Timmerman V, Rautenstrauss B, Reiter LT, et al. Detection of the CMT1A/HNPP recombination hotspot in unrelated patients of European descent. J Med Genet 1997;34:43–49.

46. Nelis E, Van Broeckhoven C, De Jonghe P, et al. Estimation of the mutation frequencies in Charcot-Marie-Tooth disease type 1 and hereditary neuropathy with liability to pressure palsies: a European collaborative study. Eur J Hum Genet 1996;4:25–33.

II | GENOMIC STRUCTURE

2   *Alu* Elements

Prescott Deininger, PhD

CONTENTS

INTRODUCTION

Alu elements represent one of the most successful mobile elements found in any genome. They have reached a copy number in excess of one million copies, making up more than 10% of the human genome. The level of amplification required to reach this high copy number has created an enormous number of insertion mutations resulting in human disease and genome evolution. They also add extensive diversity to the genome by introducing alternative splicing and editing to a wide range of RNA transcripts. In addition, after insertion *Alu* elements contribute to a high level of genetic instability through recombination. This instability contributes to a significant number of germ-line mutations and may be an even bigger factor in cancer and/or aging.

ALU ELEMENTS

Alu elements have reached a copy number in excess of 1×10^6, representing more than 10% of the human genome *(1)*. They are widely distributed across the entire genome, with only a relatively few regions that have few of them. *Alu* elements tend to be enriched in the GC-rich, gene-rich regions, with many *Alu* elements located in the introns of genes.

The current rate of *Alu* amplification has been estimated to be in the range of one new insertion per 20–200 human births *(2,3)*. The *Alu* insertion process has the potential to damage the genome both through insertional mutagenesis, and through facilitation of unequal, homologous recombination events *(2)*. Insertional mutagenesis by *Alu* causes approx

From: *Genomic Disorders: The Genomic Basis of Disease*
Edited by: J. R. Lupski and P. Stankiewicz © Humana Press, Totowa, NJ

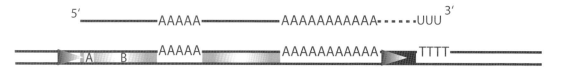

Fig. 1. Structure of an *Alu* element. A typical *Alu* element is schematized with the arrowheads representing the short, direct repeats formed at the point of insertion. The left half of *Alu* contains the A and B boxes of the RNA polymerase III promoter. The two halves of the *Alu* dimer are separated by an A-rich region and the 3' end of the *Alu* contains a variable, A-rich region. The line above represents a typical *Alu* transcript, which terminates in the downstream flanking sequence at a terminator that generally contains four or more T residues in a row. The dotted portion of the line represents sequences downstream of the *Alu* element that will be variable between transcripts from different genomic loci.

0.1% of human genetic disease, whereas recombination processes contribute to a much higher level. Little is known about the influence of *Alu* insertions in somatic or transformed cells. They have the potential to contribute to genetic instability in tumorigenesis, aging, and other somatic disorders.

MECHANISM OF INSERTION

Understanding the mechanism of *Alu* insertion is critical to understanding how they influence genetic instability. A typical *Alu* element, shown schematically in Fig. 1, contains an internal, RNA polymerase III promoter that allows transcription through the element and into the flanking sequence. *Alu* elements have a dimer structure, with both halves having an ancestral derivation from the 7SL RNA gene and have no capacity to code for proteins. At the 3' end of each *Alu* element is an A-rich sequence of variable length and the elements are generally flanked by short, direct repeats of 5–20 bp in length that are formed from duplications of the target site during insertion. It has been shown that the 3' A-rich region is routinely lengthened by the insertion process *(4,5)*, and rapidly shrinks after insertion *(6)*.

It is thought that the RNA polymerase III-transcribed *Alu* RNA must associate in some way with at least the ORF2 product of L1, which codes for endonuclease and reverse transcriptase activities. Thus, *Alu* is considered a nonautonomous mobile element, which is dependent on the autonomous L1 elements. The endonuclease then cleaves the genomic DNA at a loose consensus sequence, and the genomic site primes reverse transcription of the *Alu* RNA, using the 3' oligo-A region of the *Alu* RNA as a template. It has been hypothesized that *Alu* elements with longer A-tails are more active in the retrotransposition process *(6)*. The typical integration is then finished off by the formation of a second-strand nick and integration of the end of the cDNA (Fig. 2A). However, significant portions of the events appear to complete the integration process by recombining with another upstream *Alu* element *(7)* (Fig. 2B). This would cause sequences between the point of insertion and the upstream *Alu* element to be deleted. It also seems likely that many *Alu* elements may not complete the insertion process. Thus, the initiation of the insertion may create genomic nicks that contribute to mutation and recombination processes in the cell, but show no evidence of *Alu* insertion.

Although *Alu* amplification is clearly dependent on L1 elements for their retroposition, there are definite differences in their amplification process. The most notable difference is that, using a tagged *Alu* reporter system, *Alu* insertion was found to not require exogenous L1 ORF1 expression *(5)*.

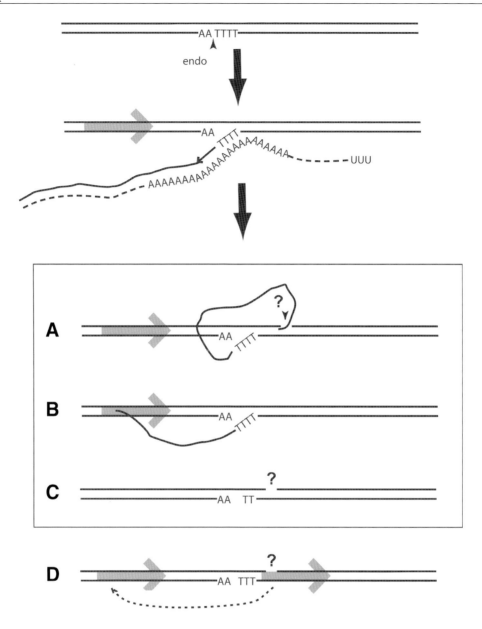

Fig. 2. Integration of *Alu* elements into genomic sites. The basic mechanism of *Alu* insertion is thought to involve a target-primed reverse transcription (TPRT) in which the endonuclease provided by L1 elements creates a nick in the genomic DNA at a consensus sequence resembling TTTT'AA. The nicked strand with the T residues can then prime reverse transcription from the 3' A-rich region of the *Alu* RNA. The second-strand integration process is poorly understood. The typical integration is schematized in (A) with a second nick occurring from an unknown source, probably allowing integration of the 3' end of the cDNA using some sort of microhomology-driven priming. (B) An alternative mechanism that occurs occasionally where the 5' end finds a homology with another *Alu* element upstream. (C) It is possible that the integration process may abort prematurely, possibly with the intervention of DNA repair processes, leading to DNA damage. (D) *Alu* elements may undergo unequal recombination with other *Alu* elements nearby. We hypothesize that nicking by L1 endonuclease at consensus sites adjacent to *Alu* elements may facilitate this recombination process.

EVOLUTION OF *ALU*

Alu elements began to amplify early in primate evolution *(8)*. A precursor to *Alu* elements may have predated the primate/rodent divergence. Rodents have B1 elements that are also derived from the 7SL RNA gene. However, the B1 elements have a monomer structure, whereas the *Alu* elements have a dimer structure that formed early in primate evolution. *Alu* elements are found even in the prosimian primates. *Alu* elements began to accumulate in primates about 65 million years ago. Because there is no specific mechanism for removal of *Alu* elements, their copy number has continued to increase throughout primate evolution.

As the copy number increased, the sequence of *Alu* elements has evolved as well. Figure 3 shows a schematic of *Alu* insertions during primate evolution. There were very high levels of *Alu* retroposition early in primate evolution. The current rate in human is nearly 100-fold lower than at the peak of *Alu* insertion. At different stages of primate evolution, the *Alu* elements that amplified had distinct sequence differences that allowed them to be classified into subfamilies *(8)*. Recent studies suggest that there has been a modest increase of *Alu* insertions in the human lineage relative to the other great apes *(9)*.

The most likely explanation for the formation of different *Alu* subfamilies at different evolutionary times is that there are extremely few "active" *Alu* elements at any one time. This allows the sequence of active elements to drift with time. Various hypotheses have been proposed for the features that limit *Alu* element activity. These include the flanking sequences of *Alu* elements influencing transcription rates *(10,11)* and subfamily-specific changes interacting with the retrotransposition machinery *(12)*. Currently, we favor the length of the A-tail as the most important factor *(6)*. The A-tail grows on insertion but shrinks rapidly in evolutionary terms, potentially silencing individual *Alu*s. In addition, older *Alu* elements accumulate mutations that lessen their expression, as well as potentially their interaction with the retroposition proteins. Thus, only progeny from the most recent insertions are likely to maintain activity.

Because the most recent inserts are also the most likely to be active elements, many of the most active elements will be polymorphic in the human population. Thus, different individuals in a population may be more or less prone to *Alu* amplification and it is the entire population that serves as a reservoir for potentially active elements.

Chromosomal Distribution

Although *Alu* elements are spread throughout the human genome, they show some regions of higher density. In particular, *Alu* elements appear to be preferentially located in GC-rich genomic "isochores," while L1 elements are located in AT-rich isochores. However, most recent data suggest that *Alu* elements insert relatively randomly with respect to GC content *(1)*, and are selectively lost from the AT-rich regions *(13,14)*, creating the bias seen. Thus, *Alu* elements are likely to have a fairly random insertional mutagenesis potential, but are more likely to contribute to postinsertional recombination events (*see* below) in the GC- and gene-rich regions of the chromosomes.

INSERTIONAL MUTAGENESIS

Alu elements create an approx 300-bp insertion mutation at any new genomic insertion site. If *Alu* insertion occurs in a coding exon, or near a splice junction, they are likely to disrupt the appropriate expression of a gene *(2)*. Table 1 shows a collection of most of the known cases

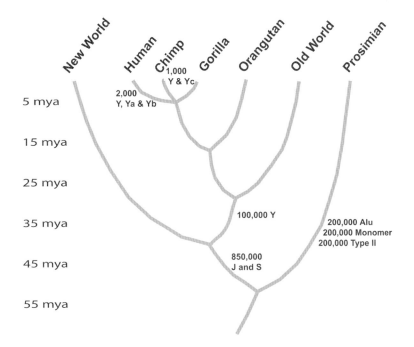

Fig. 3. Insertion history of *Alu* elements in the primate lineage. The times and approximate copy numbers of some of the major subfamilies of *Alu* elements are listed on a primate tree to illustrate the approximate times of formation of *Alu* elements, primarily for the human lineage, but also including several SINEs identified in prosimians.

of human diseases, caused fairly equally by these two types of insertions. Although these represent a number of different diseases, reflecting the broad distribution of *Alu* elements throughout the human genome, there are multiple independent cases in four different loci. This is probably largely a case of ascertainment bias because those genes have been very heavily studied. However, there is also a strong preference seen for diseases associated with the X chromosome (10/23 cases). There is much less of a bias for the X chromosome than has been seen for L1 element insertions, and probably also largely represents an ascertainment bias in favor of sex-linked diseases.

In a few rare cases, *Alu* elements have inserted into an exon coding for the carboxy-terminus of a protein and has not destroyed the function of the protein *(15,16)*. In these cases, the *Alu* element has incorporated a portion of its sequence into the coding region of the protein, likely because that portion of the protein was not critical for function, but novel proteins can evolve this way.

Insertions in the middle of introns or between genes appear to be well-tolerated and to have minimal effects on genes. Many genes have introns that include dozens of *Alu* elements that make up more than half of their DNA. However, as discussed next, many of these initially harmless *Alu* insertions can become deleterious by contributing to recombination events, or through further mutation altering their properties.

As illustrated in Fig. 2C, it is possible that *Alu* elements sometimes begin the insertion process, but that cellular repair processes remove the initial primed element. This would result in a nicked DNA that could serve as a free end in a recombination event (Fig. 2D), as well as

Table 1
Alu Insertions Causing Human Disease

Locus	CHR	Disease	Refs.
3X HEMB (IX)	X	Hemophilia B	*3,61,62*
2X HEMA (VIII)	X	Hemophilia A	*63,64*
2X CLCN5	X	Dent disease	*65,66*
BTK	X	X-linked γ-globulinaemia	*67*
IL2RG	X	XSCID	*67*
GK	X	Glycerol kinase deficiency	*68*
BCHE	3	Cholinesterase deficiency	*69*
CASR	3	Hypocalciuric hypercalcemia and hyperparathyroidism	*70*
MLVI2	5	Leukemia	*71*
APC	5	Hereditary desmoid disease	*72*
EYA1	8	Branchio-oto-renal syndrome	*73*
2X FGFR2	10	Apert syndrome	*74*
FASL	10	Autoimmune lymphoproliferative syndrome	*75*
C1NH	11	Complement deficiency	*76*
AIP	11	AI porphyria	*77*
BRCA2	13	Breast cancer	*78*
NF1	17	Neurofibromatosis	*79*

CHR refers to the chromosome for the insertion.
2X and 3X refer to genes that have had two or three insertions, respectively.

lead to mistakes in DNA repair and other DNA damage. Such events would be the result of an attempted *Alu* insertion, but would leave no evidence of the role of the *Alu* element. Thus, at this point we believe that we underestimate the role of mobile elements in recombining and damaging the human genome.

POSTINSERTION DAMAGE

Recombination

Alu elements may continue to contribute to genetic instability even if they do not initially damage a gene. A common form of secondary damage is owing to unequal homologous recombination, but several other types of mutations can alter the properties of *Alu* elements to create damage.

Alu elements may contribute to recombination events in several ways. The best understood is through either a deletion using the single-strand annealing reaction (Fig. 2D) or a reciprocal, unequal homologous recombination (Fig. 4A), which can cause either duplications or deletions of the segments between the *Alu* elements that recombine. The recombination event does not have to be reciprocal. For instance, if cells use the single-strand annealing pathway of recombination, nearby homologous *Alu* elements may recombine causing only deletions. These types of homologous recombination events have been estimated to cause at least 0.3% of human genetic disease *(2)*. However, as the majority of larger genomic rearrangements have not been characterized to this level, it seems likely that this represents an underestimate.

There are several studies suggesting that *Alu* elements located near one another in an inverted orientation may be even more destabilizing than those in a direct orientation *(17–19)*. How-

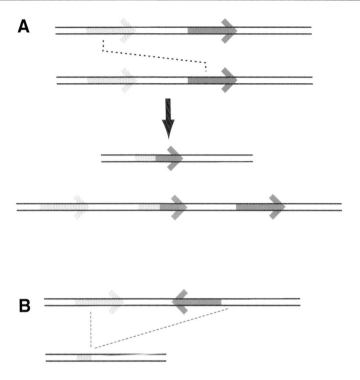

Fig. 4. Unequal *Alu–Alu* recombination. (A) When *Alu* elements are located in the same orientation near one another in the genome, it is possible for an unequal homologous recombination event to occur that can give rise to either a duplication or deletion of the sequences between the *Alu*s. A hybrid *Alu* element is usually formed at the point of recombination. (B) When *Alu* elements are in the inverted orientation, they also seem to trigger recombination in their vicinity, but the recombination junctions do not seem to be driven by recombination so that the resulting products can be variable.

ever, the instability caused by the inverted *Alu* elements (Fig. 4B) does not create a predictable junction that allows individual recombination events to be definitively defined as being caused by *Alu* elements. Recombination can occur at various locations around both *Alu* elements. Thus, it is difficult to distinguish between *Alu*-induced recombination events of this type, and *Alu*-unrelated nonhomologous end-joining events. However, it has been suggested that secondary structures may contribute to the majority of recombination junctions *(20)*, and *Alu* elements represent one of the most abundant elements that could consistently contribute to such secondary structures.

We have previously reported a broad range of genes that have undergone homologous recombination events leading to genetic defects *(2)*. These represent a broad variety of genes, as *Alu* elements are spread throughout essentially all genes. However, there are a few genes with unusually high levels of *Alu–Alu* recombination events. This includes a large number of events in the LDLR and C1 inhibitor loci. However, there are also seven different recombination events leading to breast cancer in the *BRCA1* gene *(21–25)*, three mutations in the *MSH2* gene that may represent as much as 10% of the defects in that gene *(26,27)*, and a duplication and a deletion in *MSH6 (28)*. The majority of cases of acute myelogenous leukemia that do not involve a visible translocation have been shown to involve *Alu–Alu*-mediated duplication events in the *MLL* gene *(29)*. Although inter-chromosomal translocations generally do not

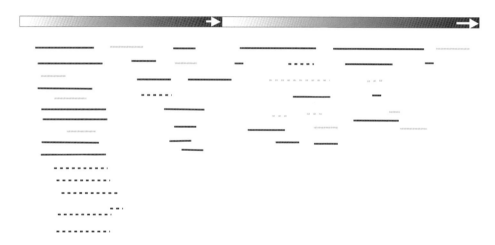

Fig. 5. Map of the *Alu–Alu* recombination junctions found in an assortment of recombination events. The darker dashed lines represent those occurring in the *LDLR* gene. The lighter dashed lines represent those occurring in the globin genes. The solid gray lines represent those that occurred in the *MLL* gene leading to acute myelogenous leukemia and the solid dark lines represent recombination events in an assortment of other genes. The length of the lines represents the uncertainty in the exact point of the recombination events relative to the schematic map of the *Alu* dimer shown. The arrows in the dimer portions represent the A-rich regions.

involve *Alu–Alu*-mediated translocations, there is now some evidence that many of these cases have additional, smaller rearrangements in the *MLL* gene that may be *Alu*-mediated *(30)*. Recently, it has been suggested that up to 30% of mutations in the Fanconi anemia gene (*FANCA*) may be caused by *Alu–Alu* recombination events and that these types of events are not typically detected using the polymerase chain reaction strategies commonly in use *(31)*. Thus, there is likely a strong ascertainment bias against detecting *Alu*-mediated genomic rearrangements.

Most of the *Alu–Alu* recombination events are between nearby elements, generally spanning distances of less than 50 kb and often only a few kb in length. There are also a number of cases of chromosomal translocations that suggest some involvement of *Alu* elements *(20,32)*, but very few that involve *Alu–Alu* homologous recombination.

It has been proposed that *Alu* elements may contain specific sequences that trigger recombination *(33)*. An analogy has been made to "chi-like" sites that may cause targeting of the recombination events within the upstream portion of the *Alu* element. The original data that triggered that hypothesis were mostly from recombination events in the *LDLR* gene that appear to cluster (Fig. 5). However, when a broader range of *Alu–Alu* recombination events are mapped, they occur dispersed throughout the *Alu* element, with only a modest predisposition to the left end. This includes both germline recombination events, as well as somatic events like those that contribute to AML *(29)*. The apparent predisposition for the upstream end of *Alu* may be caused by numerous factors. One is that none of the positions that define the *Alu* subfamilies occur toward the upstream end of *Alu* and therefore *Alu* elements from different subfamilies may show fewer mismatches with one another at that end. Also, that region includes the RNA pol III promoter for the element and may have a more open structure, particularly with specific *Alu* elements that may be in the appropriate chromatin environment to favor expression *(11)*.

Finally, whatever sequence features favored the insertion of the *Alu* at that location in the first place may lead to higher recombination rates near the end of the element.

Alternative Mutagenic Changes

In addition to a major contribution to genetic instability through insertion and recombination, *Alu* elements may also contribute to other forms of DNA damage. There are a growing number of reports that *Alu* elements may influence splicing of genes. *Alu* elements have inserted in a number of loci without causing any apparent defect, but point mutations in the *Alu* elements have led to activation of cryptic splice sites causing genetic defects *(34,35)*. In addition, there is growing evidence that even *Alu* elements that are tolerated in genes may be contributing to a significant level of alternative and aberrant splicing *(36–38)*. This leads to the inclusion of parts of *Alu* elements in a proportion of transcripts coming from the gene. In most cases these would be expected to result in defective RNAs and would, therefore, decrease the overall expression from those genes.

Although the A-tails of new *Alu* insertions appear to generally be homogeneous, they have been shown to commonly lead to the creation of more complex microsatellites over time *(39)*. Although such changes would lead to frequent genetic polymorphism, the vast majority would be expected to be relatively harmless. One important example of a disease-causing change occurred in the middle A-rich region of an *Alu* in the frataxin gene *(40)*. In one particular human, this region mutated into a GAA microsatellite. This GAA microsatellite created the permutation allele that grew through triplet repeat instability to a size where it somehow blocked transcription of the frataxin gene *(41–43)*, leading to Friedreich ataxia in those carrying this microsatellite.

Other changes within these A-rich regions commonly generate the potential polyadenylation signal, AATAAA *(44)*. This could lead to truncation of transcripts and disruption of gene expression.

EVOLUTIONARY CHANGES CAUSED BY *ALU*

In order to create the more than 1 million *Alu* elements fixed today in the human genome, there have had to be massive numbers of other insertions events that were not fixed. Thus, *Alu* elements have been a major contributor to genomic instability and evolution throughout primate history. One such event was an insertion-mediated deletion that inactivated the CMP-*N*-acetylneuraminic acid hydroxylase gene only in humans *(45)*. This led to altered protein glycosylation, which may have been a significant change helping to result in the speciation of humans from chimpanzees.

Alu–Alu recombination events have also played an important role in chromosomal evolution and potentially speciation. It appears that an *Alu–Alu*-mediated recombination in the gulonolactone oxidase gene occurred after the divergence of prosimians from the other primates *(46)*. This enzyme is a critical late step in the synthesis of vitamin C and resulted in the inability of primates to synthesize this vitamin, leading to the possibility of scurvy.

In a broader sense, *Alu* elements appear to have been involved in a number of recombination events that have helped lead to segmental duplications on human chromosomes *(47,48)*. These segmental duplications have in turn been associated with a number of different syndromes through instability of the segmental duplications *(49)*. Thus, *Alu* elements appear to have contributed to an overall rearrangement of the genome and chromosomes that has given rise to extra copies of genes, which may be beneficial for evolution, which on the other hand, can have negative impacts on the long-term genomic stability and function.

Gene Regulation and Stability

In addition to the evolutionary changes that *Alu* may cause that are related to its role in genetic instability, *Alu* elements have also been suggested to cause changes in gene structure and regulation. Transcriptional regulatory elements have been mapped to *Alu* elements near the promoters of genes (reviewed in ref. *50*), as well as *Alu* elements having been shown in several reporter systems to be able to contribute transcription factor binding sites to stimulate gene expression *(51,52)*, as well as insulator sequences to isolate genes from other nearby elements *(53)*. Thus, *Alu* elements have probably influenced expression of many genes through insertion near their promoters.

It also has been suggested that expression of *Alu* elements may contribute to a selective regulation of the initiation of translation *(54)*. Because expression of *Alu* elements is stimulated by viral infection *(55)*, transformation *(56,57)*, chemotherapeutic DNA-damaging agents *(58)*, and a number of cellular stresses *(59)*, leading to speculation that this may help regulate the translation process in those situations.

Alu elements may make up a large portion of the intronic sequence in RNAs, as well as being presented in 3' non-coding regions. It has recently been noted that there are high levels of adenine-to-inosine RNA editing in human cells, and that more than 90% of it occurs within *Alu* elements *(60)*. This is likely because of the ability of *Alu* elements in various orientations in the RNA to form duplex structures that make excellent substrates for the editing enzyme (ADAR). Whether there is a role for this editing of *Alu* elements, or whether they just compete with other RNA substrates, is currently not known. Through RNA editing, differential splicing, and other mechanisms, *Alu* elements may influence the processing and stability numerous cellular transcripts.

FUTURE DIRECTIONS

Although our understanding of both the mechanisms of *Alu* element amplification and their role in human disease have increased greatly, there are a number of important issues still to be resolved. In terms of human disease, one of the current problems is that many of the polymerase chain reaction-based strategies used to identify human disease mutations are biased against the detection of large sequence insertions or deletions. Thus, we are probably not detecting a significant proportion of the *Alu* element-induced damage in human disease.

As we learn more about the mechanism of *Alu* amplification, it will be important to focus on which cell types are involved in the amplification; germ line, somatic, and tumor cells. Also important are questions of how *Alu* elements interact with cellular gene products that may modulate, or respond to, their amplification. This will help determine whether different individuals are more or less susceptible to damage by these elements. Similarly, with evidence that expression of *Alu* elements being stimulated by numerous environmental factors, the possibility that different individuals are more or less prone to damage by *Alu* elements in response to genomic exposures will be an important issue. Finally, *Alu* elements apparently utilize the L1 machinery for their amplification more efficiently than does L1 itself. It will be important to delineate both the commonalities and differences in the actual mechanism of amplification of these elements, as well as their respective impacts once inserted in the genome, in order to fully assess the roles these elements play in human genetic instability. Ultimately, we must determine whether there is anything we can do to minimize the genetic instability caused by these elements.

SUMMARY

Alu elements have caused insertional mutation events throughout primate evolution and continue to cause a significant level of sporadic human genetic disease. Furthermore, the high copy number of *Alu* elements in the human genome contributes to secondary events, such as recombination events, that also contribute extensively to human disease. There are also a number of other ways in which *Alu* elements contribute to human genetic diversity (i.e., causing alternative splicing and changes in gene regulation).

REFERENCES

1. Lander ES, Linton LM, Birren B, et al. Initial sequencing and analysis of the human genome. International Human Genome Sequencing Consortium. Nature 2001;409:860–921.
2. Deininger PL, Batzer MA. Alu repeats and human disease. Mol Genet Metab 1999;67:183–193.
3. Li X, Scaringe WA, Hill KA, Roberts S, et al. Frequency of recent retrotransposition events in the human factor IX gene. Hum Mutat 2001;17:511–519.
4. Hagan CR, Sheffield RF, Rudin CM. Human Alu element retrotransposition induced by genotoxic stress. Nat Genet 2003;35:219–220.
5. Dewannieux M, Esnault C, Heidmann T. LINE-mediated retrotransposition of marked Alu sequences. Nat Genet 2003;35:41 48.
6. Roy-Engel AM, Salem AH, Oyeniran OO, et al. Active Alu element "A-tails"; size does matter. Genome Res 2002;12:1333–1344.
7. Xing J, Salem AH, Hedges DJ, et al. Comprehensive analysis of two Alu Yd subfamilies. J Mol Evol 2003;57:S76–S89.
8. Deininger P, Batzer MA. Evolution of retroposons. In: *Evolutionary Biology* (Heckht MK, et al., eds. New York, NY: Plenum Publishing, 1993; pp. 157–196.
9. Salem AH, Ray DA, Xing J, et al. Alu elements and hominid phylogenetics. Proc Natl Acad Sci USA 2003;100: 12,787–12,791.
10. Chesnokov I, Schmid CW. Flanking sequences of an Alu source stimulate transcription in vitro by interacting with sequence-specific transcription factors. J Mol Evol 1996;42:30–36.
11. Roy AM, West NC, Rao A, et al. Upstream flanking sequences and transcription of SINEs. J Mol Biol 2000;302:17–25.
12. Sinnett D, Richer C, Deragon JM, Labuda D. Alu RNA transcripts in human embryonal carcinoma cells. Model of post-transcriptional selection of master sequences. J Mol Biol 1992;226:689–706.
13. Brookfield JF. Selection on Alu sequences? Curr Biol 2001;11:R900–R901.
14. Deininger PL, Batzer MA. Mammalian retroelements. Genome Res 2002;12:1455–1465.
15. Makalowski W, Mitchell GA, Labuda D. Alu sequences in the coding regions of mRNA: a source of protein variability. Trends Genet 1994;10:188–193.
16. Britten RJ. Mobile elements inserted in the distant past have taken on important functions. Gene 1997;205: 177–182.
17. Gebow D, Miselis N, Liber HL. Homologous and nonhomologous recombination resulting in deletion: effects of p53 status, microhomology, and repetitive DNA length and orientation. Mol Cell Biol 2000;20:4028–4035.
18. Stenger JE, Lobachev KS, Gordenin D, Darden TA, Jurka J, Resnick MA. Biased distribution of inverted and direct alus in the human genome: implications for insertion, exclusion, and genome stability. Genome Res 2001;11:12–27.
19. Lobachev KS, Stenger JE, Kozyreva OG, Jurka J, Gordenin DA, Resnick MA. Inverted Alu repeats unstable in yeast are excluded from the human genome. Embo J 2000;19:3822–3830.
20. Chuzhanova N, Abeysinghe SS, Krawczak M, Cooper DN. Translocation and gross deletion breakpoints in human inherited disease and cancer II: Potential involvement of repetitive sequence elements in secondary structure formation between DNA ends. Hum Mutat 2003;22:245–251.

21. Puget N, Sinilnikova OM, Stoppa-Lyonnet D, et al. An Alu-mediated 6-kb duplication in the BRCA1 gene: a new founder mutation? Am J Hum Genet 1999;64:300–302.

22. Puget N, Torchard D, Serova-Sinilnikova OM, et al. A 1-kb Alu-mediated germ-line deletion removing BRCA1 exon 17. Cancer Research 1997;57:828–831.

23. Rohlfs EM, Chung CH, Yang Q, et al. In-frame deletions of BRCA1 may define critical functional domains. Hum Genet 2000;107:385–390.

24. Rohlfs EM, Puget N, Graham ML, et al. An Alu-mediated 7.1 kb deletion of BRCA1 exons 8 and 9 in breast and ovarian cancer families that results in alternative splicing of exon 10. Genes Chromosomes Cancer 2000;28:300–307.

25. Montagna M, Santacatterina M, Torri A, et al. Identification of a 3 kb Alu-mediated BRCA1 gene rearrangement in two breast/ovarian cancer families. Oncogene 1999;18:4160–4165.

26. Wang Y, Friedl W, Lamberti C, et al. Hereditary nonpolyposis colorectal cancer: frequent occurrence of large genomic deletions in MSH2 and MLH1 genes. Int J Cancer 2003;103:636–641.

27. Thiffault I, Hamel N, Pal T, et al. Germline truncating mutations in both MSH2 and BRCA2 in a single kindred. Br J Cancer 2004;90:483–491.

28. Plaschke J, Ruschoff J, Schackert HK. Genomic rearrangements of hMSH6 contribute to the genetic predisposition in suspected hereditary non-polyposis colorectal cancer syndrome. J Med Genet 2003;40:597–600.

29. Strout MP, Marcucci G, Bloomfield CD, Caligiuri MA. The partial tandem duplication of ALL1 (MLL) is consistently generated by Alu-mediated homologous recombination in acute myeloid leukemia. Proc Natl Acad Sci USA 1998;95:2390–2395.

30. Kolomietz E, Meyn MS, Pandita A, Squire JA. The role of Alu repeat clusters as mediators of recurrent chromosomal aberrations in tumors. Genes Chromosomes Cancer 2002;35:97–112.

31. Callen E, Tischkowitz MD, Creus A, et al. Quantitative PCR analysis reveals a high incidence of large intragenic deletions in the FANCA gene in Spanish Fanconi anemia patients. Cytogenet Genome Res 2004;104:341–345.

32. Wei, Y., Sun, M., Nilsson, G., et al. Characteristic sequence motifs located at the genomic breakpoints of the translocation t(X;18) in synovial sarcomas. Oncogene 2003;22:2215–2222.

33. Rudiger NS, Gregersen N, Kielland-Brandt MC. One short well conserved region of Alu-sequences is involved in human gene rearrangements and has homology with prokaryotic chi. Nucleic Acids Res 1995;23:256–260.

34. Knebelmann, B., Forestier, L., Drouot, L., et al. Splice-mediated insertion of an Alu sequence in the COL4A3 mRNA causing autosomal recessive Alport syndrome. Hum Mol Genet 1995;4:675–679.

35. Mitchell, G. A., Labuda, D., Fontaine, G., et al. Splice-mediated insertion of an Alu sequence inactivates ornithine delta-aminotransferase: a role for Alu elements in human mutation. Proc Natl Acad Sci USA 1991;88:815–819.

36. Sorek R, Shamir R, Ast G. How prevalent is functional alternative splicing in the human genome? Trends Genet 2004;20:68–71.

37. Lev-Maor G, Sorek R, Shomron N, Ast G. The birth of an alternatively spliced exon: 3' splice-site selection in Alu exons. Science 2003;300:1288–1291.

38. Kreahling J, Graveley BR. The origins and implications of Aluternative splicing. Trends Genet 2004;20:1–4.

39. Arcot S, Wang Z, Weber J, Deininger P, Batzer M. Alu repeats: a source for the genesis of primate microsatellites. Genomics 1995;29:136–144.

40. Montermini L, Andermann E, Labuda M, et al. The Friedreich ataxia GAA triplet repeat: premutation and normal alleles. Hum Mol Genet 1997;6:1261–1266.

41. Ohshima K, Montermini L, Wells RD, Pandolfo M. Inhibitory effects of expanded GAA.TTC triplet repeats from intron I of the Friedreich ataxia gene on transcription and replication in vivo. J Biol Chem 1998;273:14,588–14,595.

42. Bidichandani SI, Ashizawa T, Patel PI. The GAA triplet-repeat expansion in Friedreich ataxia interferes with transcription and may be associated with an unusual DNA structure. Am J Hum Genet 1998;62:111–121.

43. Patel PI, Isaya G. Friedreich ataxia: from GAA triplet-repeat expansion to frataxin deficiency. Am J Hum Genet 2001;69:15–24.

44. Roy-Engel AM, El-Sawy M, Farooq L, et al. Human retroelements may introduce intragenic polyadenylation sites. Cytogenet Genome Res 2004, in press.

45. Hayakawa T, Satta Y, Gagneux P, Varki A, Takahata N. Alu-mediated inactivation of the human CMP-N-acetylneuraminic acid hydroxylase gene. Proc Natl Acad Sci USA 2001;98:11,399–11,404.

46. Challem JJ, Taylor EW. Retroviruses, ascorbate, and mutations, in the evolution of Homo sapiens. Free Radic Biol Med 1998;25:130–132.

47. Bailey JA, Liu G, Eichler EE. An Alu transposition model for the origin and expansion of human segmental duplications. Am J Hum Genet 2003;73:823–834.

48. Babcock M, Pavlicek A, Spiteri E, et al. Shuffling of genes within low-copy repeats on 22q11 (LCR22) by Alu-mediated recombination events during evolution. Genome Res 2003;13:2519–2532.

49. Bailey JA, Yavor AM, Massa HF, Trask BJ, Eichler EE. Segmental duplications: organization and impact within the current human genome project assembly. Genome Res 2001;11:1005–1017.

50. Britten RJ. DNA sequence insertion and evolutionary variation in gene regulation. Proc Natl Acad Sci USA 1996;93:9374–9377.

51. Norris J, Fan D, Aleman C, et al. Identification of a new subclass of Alu DNA repeats which can function as estrogen receptor-dependent transcriptional enhancers. J Biol Chem 1995;270:22,777–22,782.

52. Vansant G, Reynolds WF. The consensus sequence of a major Alu subfamily contains a functional retinoic acid response element. Proc Natl Acad Sci USA 1995;92:8229–8233.

53. Thorey IS, Cecena G, Reynolds W, Oshima RG. Alu sequence involvement in transcriptional insulation of the keratin 18 gene in transgenic mice. Mol Cell Biol 1993;13:6742–6751.

54. Rubin CM, Kimura RH, Schmid CW. Selective stimulation of translational expression by Alu RNA. Nucleic Acids Res 2002;30:3253–3261.

55. Panning B, Smiley JR. Activation of expression of multiple subfamilies of human Alu elements by adenovirus type 5 and herpes simplex virus type 1. J Mol Biol 1995;248:513–524.

56. Carey MF, Singh K, Botchan M, Cozzarelli NR. Induction of specific transcription by RNA polymerase III in transformed Cells. Mol Cell Biol 1989;6:3068–3076.

57. Chu WM, Wang Z, Roeder RG, Schmid CW. RNA polymerase III transcription repressed by Rb through its interactions with TFIIIB and TFIIIC2. J Biol Chem 1997;272:14,755–14,761.

58. Rudin CM, Thompson CB. Transcriptional activation of short interspersed elements by DNA-damaging agents. Genes Chromosomes Cancer 2001;30:64–71.

59. Li TH, Schmid CW. Differential stress induction of individual Alu loci: implications for transcription and retrotransposition. Gene 2001;276:135–141.

60. Levanon EY, Eisenberg E, Yelin R, et al. Systematic identification of abundant A-to-I editing sites in the human transcriptome. Nat Biotechnol 2004;22:1001–1005.

61. Vidaud D, Vidaud M, Bahnak BR, et al. Haemophilia B due to a de novo insertion of a human-specific Alu subfamily member within the coding region of the factor IX gene. Eur J Hum Genet 1993;1:30–36.

62. Wulff K, Gazda H, Schroder W, Robicka-Milewska R, Herrmann FH. Identification of a novel large F9 gene mutation-an insertion of an Alu repeated DNA element in exon e of the factor 9 gene. Hum Mutat 2000;15:299.

63. Sukarova E, Dimovski AJ, Tchacarova P, Petkov GH, Efremov GD. An Alu insert as the cause of a severe form of hemophilia A Acta Haematol 2001;106:126–129.

64. Ganguly A, Dunbar T, Chen P, Godmilow L, Ganguly T. Exon skipping caused by an intronic insertion of a young Alu Yb9 element leads to severe hemophilia A Hum Genet 2003;113:348–352.

65. Claverie-Martin F, Gonzalez-Acosta H, Flores C, Anton-Gamero M, Garcia-Nieto V. De novo insertion of an Alu sequence in the coding region of the CLCN5 gene results in Dent's disease. Hum Genet 2003;113:480–485.

66. Thakker RV. Molecular pathology of renal chloride channels in Dent's disease and Bartter's syndrome. Exp Nephrol 2000;8:351–360.

67. Lester T, McMahon C, VanRegemorter N, Jones A, Genet S. X-linked immunodeficiency caused by insertion of Alu repeat sequences. J Med Gen Suppl 1997;34:S81.

68. Zhang Y, Dipple KM, Vilain E, et al. AluY insertion (IVS4-52ins316alu) in the glycerol kinase gene from an individual with benign glycerol kinase deficiency. Hum Mutat 2000;15:316–323.

69. Muratani K, Hada T, Yamamoto Y, et al. Inactivation of the cholinesterase gene by Alu insertion: Possible mechanism for human gene transposition. Proc Natl Acad Sci USA 1991;88:11,315–11,319.

70. Janicic N, Pausova Z, Cole DE, Hendy GN. Insertion of an Alu sequence in the Ca(2+)-sensing receptor gene in familial hypocalciuric hypercalcemia and neonatal severe hyperparathyroidism. Am J Hum Genet 1995;56:880–886.

71. Economou-Pachnis A, Tsichlis PN. Insertion of an Alu SINE in the human homologue of the Mlvi-2 locus. Nucleic Acids Res 1985;13:8379–8387.

72. Halling KC, Lazzaro CR, Honchel R, et al. Hereditary desmoid disease in a family with a germline Alu I repeat mutation of the APC gene. Hum Hered 1999;49:97–102.

73. Abdelhak S, Kalatzis V, Heilig R, et al. Clustering of mutations responsible for branchio-oto-renal (BOR) syndrome in the eyes absent homologous region (eyaHR) of EYA1. Hum Mol Genet 1997;6:2247–2255.

74. Oldridge M, Zackai EH, McDonald-McGinn DM,et al. De novo Alu-element insertions in FGFR2 identify a distinct pathological basis for apert syndrome. Am J Hum Genet 1999;64:446–461.

75. Tighe PJ, Stevens SE, Dempsey S, Le Deist F, Rieux-Laucat F, Edgar JD. Inactivation of the Fas gene by Alu insertion: retrotransposition in an intron causing splicing variation and autoimmune lymphoproliferative syndrome. Genes Immun 2002;3:S66–S70.

76. Stoppa-Lyonnet D, Duponchel C, Meo T,et al. Recombinational biases in the rearranged C1-inhibitor genes of hereditary angioedema patients. Am J Hum Genet 1991;49:1055–1062.

77. Mustajoki S, Ahola H, Mustajoki P, Kauppinen R. Insertion of Alu element responsible for acute intermittent porphyria. Hum Mutat 1999;13:431–438.

78. Miki Y, Katagiri T, Kasumi F, Yoshimoto T, Nakamura Y. Mutation analysis in the BRCA2 gene in primary breast cancers. Nat Genet 1996;13:245–247.

79. Wallace MR, Andersen LB, Saulino AM, Gregory PE, Glover TW, Collins FS. A de novo Alu insertion results in neurofibromatosis type 1. Nature 1991;353:864–866.

3

The Impact of LINE-1 Retrotransposition on the Human Genome

Amy E. Hulme, BS, MS, Deanna A. Kulpa, BS, MS, José Luis Garcia Perez, PhD, and John V. Moran, PhD

CONTENTS

BACKGROUND

Long interspersed element-1 (LINE-1 or L1) is an abundant retrotransposon that comprises approx 17% of human DNA. L1 retrotransposition events can lead to genome diversification and individual genetic variation by serving as insertional mutagens and by providing recombination substrates either during or long after their insertion. L1 retrotransposition also generates genomic variation by mobilizing DNA derived from its flanks, non-autonomous retrotransposons (e.g., *Alu* elements), and cellular mRNAs to new genomic locations. Together, these sequences comprise approx 15% of human genomic DNA. Thus, L1-mediated retrotransposition events are responsible for at least one-third of our genome. In this chapter, we discuss how innovative assays developed in recent years have increased our understanding of L1 biology and the impact of L1 on the human genome.

From: *Genomic Disorders: The Genomic Basis of Disease*
Edited by: J. R. Lupski and P. Stankiewicz © Humana Press, Totowa, NJ

Table 1
Mobile Elements in the Human Genome

Mobile element	Example	Percentage of genome	Functional
DNA transposons			
Transposons	Trigger/Pogo	Approx 3%	No
Retrotransposons			
Autonomous			
LTR	HERV-K	Approx 8%	No
Non-LTR	LINE-1	Approx 21%	Yes
Non-Autonomous	*Alu*	Approx 13%	Yes

Mobile elements found in the human genome can be subdivided into DNA transposons and retrotransposons. Retrotransposons can be classified based on whether they encode their own proteins (autonomous) or must rely on exogenous proteins (non-autonomous) for mobility. Autonomous retrotransposons are subclassified by whether they contain long terminal repeats (LTRs) or not (non-LTRs). Only non-LTR retrotransposons and non-autonomous retrotransposons are known to be currently active in the human genome. The percentage of the human genome that each mobile element class comprises and an example of that class is given. HERV, human endogenous retrovirus; LINE-1, long interspersed element-1.

INTRODUCTION

Approximately 1.5% of the human genome encodes proteins *(1,2)*. Much of the remaining DNA often is disparaged as "junk" owing to its assumed lack of function. Transposable elements account for nearly half of "junk DNA," and they are classified based on their mobility intermediate (Table 1). DNA transposons move (i.e., transpose) using a DNA intermediate, represent approx 3% of genomic DNA, but are now immobile *(3)*. Retrotransposons move (i.e., retrotranspose) using an RNA intermediate and account for approx 30% of human DNA *(4)*. They are subclassified based on whether they encode proteins required for their retrotransposition (autonomous retrotransposons) or rely on proteins to be supplied *in trans* (non-autonomous retrotransposons).

Autonomous retrotransposons are subdivided further based on their structure. Long terminal repeat (LTR)-containing retrotransposons, typified by human endogenous retroviruses (HERVs), resemble retroviruses, but generally lack or contain a nonfunctional envelope gene. Although they comprise approx 8% of genomic DNA, the vast majority of HERVs are immobile (Table 1). However, some HERVs are polymorphic with respect to presence and a few elements may have protein coding potential *(5,6)*. Thus, a few HERVs may remain retrotransposition-competent.

Non-LTR retrotransposons, exemplified by LINEs, lack LTRs and usually end in a poly (A) tail. They represent the largest class of transposable element derived repeats in the genome, accounting for approx 21% of human DNA *(1)*. LINE-1s (L1s), the most abundant retrotransposon, are present at more than 500,000 copies in the haploid genome, and some L1s remain retrotransposition-competent. In contrast, LINE-2 and LINE-3 elements are structurally distinct from L1s, are less abundant in human DNA, and are no longer retrotransposition-competent *(1)*.

The proteins encoded by retrotransposition-competent L1s also can function *in trans* to mobilize either non-autonomous retrotransposons (e.g., *Alu* and perhaps short interspersed element R-VNTR-*Alu* [SVA] elements) or cellular mRNAs, resulting in processed pseudogene formation *(7–9)*. Together, *Alu* elements, SVA elements, and processed pseudogenes comprise approx 15% of human genomic DNA *(1)*. Thus, either directly or through the promiscuous mobilization of cellular RNAs, the L1-encoded proteins are responsible for at least one billion of the three billion bases in human genomic DNA. Therefore, a detailed understanding of L1 biology will unveil important aspects of human genome evolution.

The purpose of this chapter is to review the impact of L1 retrotransposition on the human genome. When appropriate, we also will examine parallels that exist between L1s and other related non-LTR retrotransposons. Several outstanding reviews address the evolutionary dynamics of L1 retrotransposition in mammalian genomes *(10–12)* and other chapters in this book discuss the interrelatedness between L1s and other human transposable elements. We refer the reader to these references for additional information about L1 biology.

THE STRUCTURE OF A RETROTRANSPOSITION COMPETENT L1

Candidate retrotransposition-competent human L1s originally were identified as progenitors of mutagenic insertions into the *Factor VIII* and *Dystrophin* genes, respectively *(13–15)*. These L1s are approx 6.0 kb in length and contain a 5' untranslated region (UTR) that harbors an internal promoter *(16)*, two non-overlapping open reading frames (ORF1 and ORF2) *(13,17)*, and a 3' UTR that ends in a poly (A) tail (Fig. 1A). ORF1 encodes an RNA-binding protein (p40 or ORF1p) *(18,19)*, whereas ORF2 has the potential to encode a 150-kDa protein (ORF2p) with demonstrated endonuclease (L1 EN) and reverse transcriptase activities (L1 RT) *(20–22)*. ORF2p also contains a conserved cysteine-rich domain (C) of unknown function *(23)*. In addition, L1s usually are flanked by target site duplications that vary in length from 7 to approx 30 bp, which are generated on retrotransposition *(24)*.

METHODS TO STUDY L1 RETROTRANSPOSITION

A Cultured Cell Retrotransposition Assay

In 1996, an assay was developed to monitor L1 retrotransposition in cultured human cells *(25)*. In this assay, the 3' UTR of a candidate L1 was tagged with an indicator cassette designed to detect retrotransposition events (Fig. 1B). The initial retrotransposition indicator cassette (*mneoI*) consisted of a selectable marker (*NEO*) containing its own promoter and poly-adenylation signal. The *mneoI* cassette was introduced into the L1 so that the L1 and reporter gene were in opposite transcriptional orientations. The *mneoI* gene also was interrupted by an intron in the same transcriptional orientation as the L1 *(26)*. This arrangement ensured that G418-resistant foci would arise only when a transcript initiated from the promoter driving L1 expression underwent retrotransposition.

Using this assay, it was demonstrated that various L1s could retrotranspose at a high efficiency when expressed from an extrachromosomal expression vector in HeLa cells *(25,27)*. Subsequent characterization of the resultant retrotransposition events revealed L1 structural hallmarks, indicating that retrotransposition was faithfully reconstituted in HeLa cells *(25,28,29)*. Alternative retrotransposition indicator cassettes *(30)* and high throughput versions of the cultured cell retrotransposition assay *(27,31)* have been developed in recent years and these assays have been used to uncover several aspects of L1 biology:

1. Characterize functional domains in the L1-encoded proteins *(22,25,32)*.
2. Identify retrotransposition-competent L1s in the human and mouse genomes *(33–36)*.

A
Consensus structure of a retrotransposition competent L1

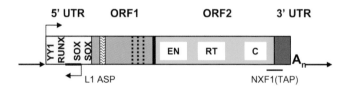

B
Cultured Cell Assay

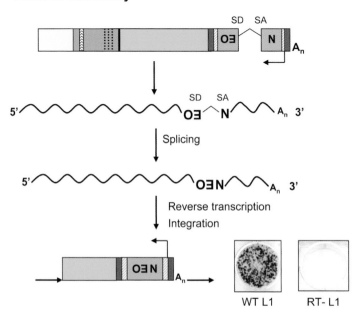

Fig. 1. (A) The structure of a retrotransposition competent L1 (not to scale). A retrotransposition competent L1 contains a 5' UTR (yellow), two open reading frames—ORF1 (blue) and ORF2 (green), a 3' UTR (red), and a poly (A) tail. The direction of transcription from both the L1 promoter and the antisense promoter in the 5' UTR (L1 ASP) are denoted with arrows. Transcription factor binding sites (YY1, RUNX3, and SOX) are indicated. ORF1 contains a leucine zipper domain near its amino terminus (wavy lined box) and several conserved basic amino acid motifs near its carboxyl terminus (dotted lines). A 63-bp intergenic region (black line) separates ORF1 and ORF2. ORF2 contains an endonuclease domain (EN), a reverse transcriptase domain (RT), and a cysteine-rich domain (C). A putative NXF1(TAP) binding site is located in the region spanning the end ORF2 and the beginning of the 3' UTR (underlined and labeled). L1 usually is flanked by variable length target site duplications in the genome (bold black arrows). (B) The cultured cell retrotransposition assay. A retrotransposition-competent L1 is tagged with a retrotransposition indicator cassette (*mneo*I; orange, labeled backwards neo) that has its own promoter and poly (A) signal (orange slashed). The cassette contains an intron in the same transcriptional orientation as the L1 (denoted by SD for splice donor and SA for splice acceptor). When this construct is transfected into HeLa cells, G418 resistant colonies will only be present if there is transcription from the L1 promoter, splicing, reverse transcription, and integration of the L1 transcript. Cells then are fixed and stained to view colonies. Representative results of this assay are shown in which HeLa cells were transfected with a wild type L1 construct (WT L1) or an L1 construct containing a mutation in the reverse transcriptase domain (RT- L1).

3. Demonstrate that the L1-encoded proteins exhibit a *cis*-preference for their encoding RNA *(7,9)*.
4. Show that the L1-encoded proteins can act *in trans* to mobilize nonautonomous retrotransposons and cellular mRNAs *(7–9)*.
5. Demonstrate that L1s can retrotranspose into genes and can mobilize sequences derived from their 5' and 3' flanks to new genomic locations *(1,29,37,38)*.
6. Uncover an endonuclease-independent (but RT-dependent) L1 retrotransposition pathway *(30)*.
7. Discover that L1 retrotransposition is associated with various forms of genetic instability in transformed cultured cells *(28–30)*.

Other Approaches to Study L1 Retrotransposition

In addition to characterizing disease-producing L1 insertions and employing the cultured cell retrotransposition assay, there are three principal ways to study L1 biology *(11)*. The first approach is to use biochemical and molecular biological techniques to characterize the L1-encoded proteins and L1 RNA. These experiments have been conducted primarily on active human and mouse L1s and have been instrumental in characterizing enzymatic activities encoded by the L1 proteins (*see* Functional Analyses).

The second approach is to utilize phylogenetic and evolutionary analyses to examine L1s present in whole genome sequences. These methodologies have allowed the classification of human L1 subfamilies *(39)* and have been instrumental in identifying candidate retrotransposition-competent L1s in the human, mouse, and rat genomes *(1,40,41)*. More recently, comparative genomics and molecular biological approaches have been useful in examining intra- and interorganism differences in L1 content that exist between available genome sequences *(42–47)*.

The third approach is to study L1 expression and/or retrotransposition in animal models. The use of animal models remains in its infancy, but their application has shown that full-length sense strand L1 RNA is expressed in both male and female germ cells and that human L1s can retrotranspose in the male germline prior to the onset of meiosis II *(48–51)*. A combination of the previously described approaches has led to a greater understanding of the mechanism of L1 retrotransposition and its effects on the genome.

FUNCTIONAL ANALYSES

The 5' UTR

Human L1s have a 910-bp 5' UTR that contains an internal RNA polymerase II promoter *(16)*. To remain autonomously mobile, the L1 promoter must be able to direct transcription such that an entire L1 transcription unit can be faithfully retrotransposed to a new genomic location. Transcription has been proposed to be a limiting step in retrotransposition and most promoter activity is attributed to the first 600 bases of the 5' UTR.

A YY1-binding site, located at +12 to +21 on the non-coding strand, is required for proper initiation of transcription at or near the first nucleotide of L1 (Fig. 1A) *(38,52,53)*. L1s lacking a functional YY1 binding site can initiate transcription and retrotranspose in cultured cells, but the resultant progeny likely will not regenerate the complete 5' UTR. Thus, it is predicted that over successive rounds of retrotransposition, L1s lacking a functional YY1-binding site will become progressively shorter and ultimately retrotransposition-defective.

The L1 5' UTR also contains two SOX binding sites at +472 to +477 and +572 to +577, as well as a RUNX3 binding site at +83 to +101 (Fig. 1A) *(54,55)*. These sequences can bind SOX and RUNX3 proteins in vitro, respectively. Moreover, mutations in the RUNX3 and SOX sites results in a decrease in L1 retrotransposition in cultured cells, whereas overexpression of RUNX3 protein in HeLa cells results in an increase in L1 transcription and a nearly twofold increase in retrotransposition (*[55]*; Athanikar and Moran, unpublished data). However, the mechanism by which the RUNX3 and SOX proteins affect L1 transcription and retrotransposition merits further study.

Finally, the 5' UTR contains a potent antisense promoter (L1 ASP) that can influence the expression of cellular genes (Fig. 1A) *(56,57)*. Transcripts of cellular genes originating from the L1 ASP have been identified in both cDNA libraries and expressed sequence tag databases. Most of these transcripts were spliced correctly, but the majority only contained part of the coding region of a gene. Thus, some L1 ASP-derived transcripts have the potential to encode alternative, perhaps functional, forms of a native cellular protein. It also is intriguing to speculate that some L1 ASP-derived transcripts may act to regulate the expression of their resident gene.

ORF1p

Human ORF1 encodes a 338 amino acid RNA binding protein (p40 or ORF1p) that co-localizes with L1 RNA in cytoplasmic ribonucleoprotein particles (RNPs), which are proposed retrotransposition intermediates *(18,19)*. Elegant biochemical studies conducted on mouse L1 ORF1p indicate that it possesses RNA binding and nucleic acid chaperone activities and can form a homotrimer in vitro *(58–61)*. The amino terminus of ORF1p is predicted to fold into a coiled-coil domain that is important for ORF1p–ORF1p interactions *(19,62)*. Human ORF1p contains a leucine zipper motif that is required for retrotransposition, perhaps by stabilizing L1 RNPs, by interacting with host factors important for retrotransposition, or by functioning at downstream steps in the retrotransposition process (*[19]*; Hulme and Moran, unpublished data). Interestingly, the amino terminus of ORF1p is evolving rapidly yet mouse, rabbit, and rat L1s lack the leucine zipper domain. This rapid evolution may reflect adaptive changes that have occurred in response to host repression mechanisms over the course of L1 evolution *(63)*.

The carboxyl terminus of ORF1p contains a number of conserved motifs that are rich in basic amino acids. Mutations in these amino acids severely reduce L1 retrotransposition in cultured cells and may affect RNA binding and nucleic acid chaperone activity of mouse ORF1p in vitro *(25,58,62)*. However, the carboxyl terminal domain of ORF1p lacks overt sequence similarity to any known RNA-binding proteins. Thus, more biochemical studies are required to elucidate the structural and functional role of ORF1p in L1 retrotransposition.

ORF2p

ORF2 has the potential to encode a 150-kDa protein that has been difficult to detect in vivo *(13,20)*. Sequence comparisons and crystallization studies indicated that the 5' terminus of L1 ORF2, as well as analogous sequences from related non-LTR retrotransposons, share homology with apurinic/apyrimidinic (AP) endonucleases *(22,64,65)*. Subsequent biochemical analyses revealed that the amino terminus of L1 ORF2p has endonuclease activity in vitro. L1 EN purified from *Escherichia coli* neither shows a preference for cleaving abasic substrates in vitro nor possesses 3'–5' exonuclease or RNase H activities that are common to other AP endonucleases *(66)*. Instead, it makes a site-specific single-stranded endonucleolytic nick at the degenerate consensus sequence (5'TTTT/A; where the "/" indicates the scissile phosphate), exposing a 3' hydroxyl residue and 5' monophosphate *(66,67)*. Mutations in the putative L1 EN active site abolish endonucleolytic cleavage activity in vitro and reduce L1 retrotransposition in HeLa cells by two to three orders of magnitude *(22,25)*.

The central region of ORF2p shares homology to the reverse transcriptase domains encoded by other non-LTR retrotransposons *(68,69)*. Biochemical studies demonstrated that ORF2p has RT activity that can extend homopolymer/oligonucleotide primer template complexes in vitro and requires divalent cations (Mg^{+2} is favored over Mn^{+2}) *(21,70)*. Mutations in the putative L1 RT active site abolish RT activity in vitro and reduce L1 retrotransposition in HeLa cells by approximately three orders of magnitude *(21,25)*.

The carboxyl terminus of ORF2p contains a conserved cysteine-rich motif ($CX_3CX_7HX_4C$) of unknown function *(23)*. Site-directed point mutations in conserved cysteine and histidine residues within the C-domain reduce human L1 retrotransposition in HeLa cells by two orders of magnitude, but do not affect L1 RT activity as measured in a yeast expression assay *(25,71)*. Thus, the C-domain provides a function required for retrotransposition that apparently is distinct from L1 EN or L1 RT.

The 3' UTR

The 3' UTR of mammalian L1s has a relatively weak poly (A) signal as well as a conserved guanosine-rich polypurine tract that, based on studies of rat L1s, is predicted to form an intrastrand tetraplex *(25,37,72)*. Sequence spanning the 3' end of ORF2 and the beginning of the 3' UTR contains at least two *cis*-acting repeats (5'-CACA [N5] GGGA-3') that can bind the nuclear export factor NXF1(TAP) and this sequence functions as a nuclear RNA export signal in vitro (Fig. 1A) *(73)*. Paradoxically, despite the presence of these conserved and/or functional sequences, the L1 3' UTR is dispensable for retrotransposition in HeLa cells *(25)*. Thus, the function of the L1 3' UTR in L1 retrotransposition remains enigmatic.

THE L1 RETROTRANSPOSITION CYCLE

Human L1 retrotransposition begins with transcription from an internal promoter located within its 5' UTR (Fig. 2). After transcription, the bicistronic L1 RNA is transported to the cytoplasm, where ORF1 and ORF2 undergo translation. Recent studies suggest that ORF2p is translated by an unconventional mechanism and that it is made at much lower levels than ORF1p (Alisch, Garcia Perez, and Moran, unpublished data). Indeed, it is possible that as few as one molecule of ORF2p is synthesized from a single L1 RNA *(74)*.

Genetic, biochemical, and phylogenetic studies indicate that ORF1p and ORF2p exhibit a strong *cis*-preference *(7,9)*, and preferentially associate with the RNA that encoded them to form an RNP, which is a proposed retrotransposition intermediate *(19,75)*. The L1 RNP enters the nucleus either by active import or passively, perhaps during mitotic nuclear envelope breakdown. The only non-LTR retrotransposon studied in this respect is the Tad element from *Neurospora crassa*, which gains access to the nucleus by active transport *(76)*.

Once in the nucleus, L1 retrotransposition likely occurs by target-site primed reverse transcription (TPRT), a mechanism first demonstrated for the R2 retrotransposon from *Bombyx mori* (R2Bm) *(77)*. During TPRT, L1 EN is thought to cleave genomic DNA, liberating a 3' hydroxyl, which then serves as a primer for reverse transcription of L1 RNA by the L1 RT, generating the first strand of L1 cDNA *(22,67,78)*. Recent in vitro biochemical data suggest that besides functioning in RNP assembly, the nucleic acid chaperone activity of ORF1p also may facilitate early steps of TPRT *(60)*. Second-strand synthesis and integration of the nascent L1 cDNA into

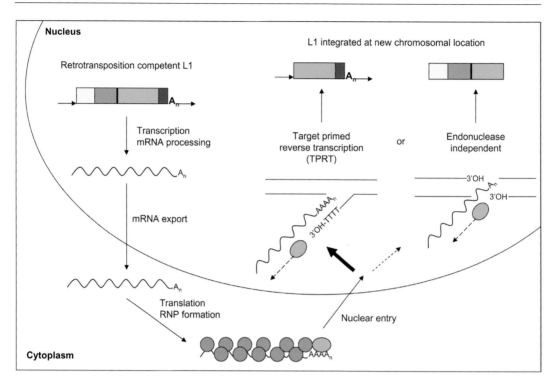

Fig. 2. Model of L1 retrotransposition cycle. A retrotransposition competent L1 is transcribed and the L1 RNA is transported to the cytoplasm. Here, ORF1p (blue circle) and ORF2p (green oval) are translated and bind back to the L1 RNA from which they were transcribed to form a ribonucleoprotein particle (RNP). This L1 RNP then translocates to the nucleus where target-site primed reverse transcription (TPRT) occurs to integrate the L1 at a new location in the genome. The newly integrated L1 exhibits characteristic structures including 5' truncation, a poly (A) tail, and variable length target site duplications (black arrows). A variation on TPRT is endonuclease independent retrotransposition, in which L1 integrates at pre-existing nicks in DNA. Endonuclease independent retrotransposition events sometimes lack a poly (A) tail, lack target sited duplications, and may be 3' truncated. TPRT is the prevalent route of integration into the genome (indicated by bold arrow), whereas endonuclease independent retrotransposition probably occurs at a much lower frequency in vivo (indicated by the dashed arrow).

genomic DNA completes retrotransposition and results in L1 structural hallmarks (i.e., frequent 5' truncations, a 3' A-tail, and variable-length target site duplications) *(24)*. However, the initiation of second strand synthesis and the completion of L1 integration remains a mystery.

TPRT: VARIATIONS ON A THEME

Approximately 99% of L1s present in the human genome working draft (HGWD) contain random 5' truncations and approx 20% of those L1s contain internal rearrangements (i.e., they have inversion/deletion structures; Fig. 3). It has been proposed that 5' truncation is owing to reduced processivity of the L1 RT *(79)*. However, it is counterintuitive that L1 would evolve a poorly processive RT when it requires this enzyme for its survival. Furthermore, studies on the related R2Bm RT show that it is a highly processive enzyme in vitro *(80)*. Thus, incomplete L1 cDNA synthesis may arise from host repair processes that act to suppress retrotransposition by disassociating the L1 RT from its nascent cDNA *(74)*.

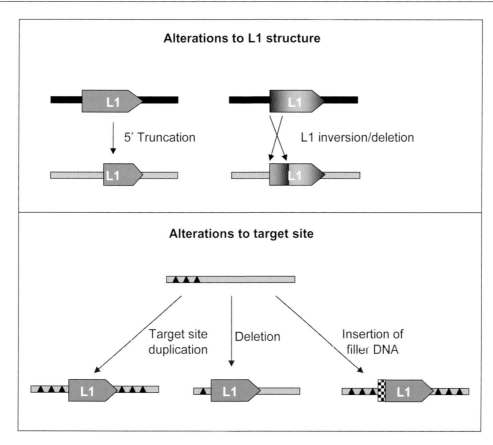

Fig. 3. L1-mediated changes on insertion. Insertion into a new site in the genome (gray bar) can result in 5' truncation of the L1 or inversion/deletion structures (breakpoints denoted by arrows) when compared with its progenitor L1 (black bar). L1 insertion can also result in changes to the target site (gray bar with three black triangles), such as target site duplications, deletions of target site nucleotides, and the insertion of small "filler" DNAs (checked box).

The "twin-priming" model can explain the formation of inversion/deletion L1s *(81)*. Twin priming evokes the use of the 3' OH on the top strand of target site DNA (after its cleavage) as a second primer for reverse transcription on the L1 RNA. Resolution of the convergent cDNAs followed by microhomology-mediated recombination then leads to the formation of the inversion/deletion. The twin-priming model is supported by both analyses of genome insertions from databases and cell culture experiments *(28,29)*.

In general, TPRT leads to minor alterations of target site DNA, including the generation of short target site duplications or small deletions, yet in some instances there is neither a gain or loss of target site nucleotides (Fig. 3). How TPRT can lead to these various outcomes requires further study, but it has been proposed that the variable placement of top strand cleavage can account for all the observed scenarios *(28)*. In fact, though there is a clear L1 EN consensus "bottom strand" cleavage site, there is little or no target site preference for top strand cleavage *(28,82)*. Thus, L1 EN either is an unusual enzyme that only displays cleavage specificity for a single DNA strand, or an undiscovered activity (encoded by either L1 or the host) is required for second (i.e., top) strand cleavage.

Various forms of genetic instability are associated with another approx 10% of L1 retrotransposition events in transformed cultured cells (Fig. 3). These alterations include the addition of "filler DNA" at the 5' genomic DNA/L1 junction, the generation of target site deletions or intrachromosomal duplications, the formation of chimeric L1s, and the possible generation of chromosomal inversions and interchromosomal translocations *(28,29)*. Although the relatively high incidence of these unusual rearrangements may reflect the transformed status of the cells used in these experiments, comparative genomic studies have identified rare deletion events associated with both L1 and *Alu* insertions in humans *(46,83,84)*. Moreover, deletions are associated with two of eight mutagenic L1 insertions in the mouse *(85,86)*. Thus, it is probable that genetic instability occasionally accompanies L1 retrotransposition in vivo and it is intriguing to speculate that these events may have impacted genome evolution *(87)*.

There also are variations in the standard TPRT model of retrotransposition. For example, it is hypothesized that pre-existing lesions in genomic DNA may be used as primers in place of the L1 endonuclease-generated sites, referred to as endonuclease-independent retrotransposition (Fig. 2) *(30,88)*. This phenomenon is most obvious in Chinese Hamster Ovary cells defective for nonhomologous end joining and can be considered a type of RNA-mediated DNA repair (i.e., a chromosomal "Band-Aid") that is a remnant from the "RNA world."

L1 AS A MUTAGEN

The fact that L1 retrotransposition is ongoing in the human genome was realized in 1988, when it was discovered that two unrelated patients afflicted with Hemophilia A acquired independent L1 retrotransposition events into exon 14 of the *Factor VIII* gene *(89)*. Extensive characterization of one of these mutations showed that it was not present in either parent and arose by a *de novo* retrotransposition event either in the maternal germline or soon after fertilization. Since that time, deleterious L1 insertions in the germ lines of both human and mouse have resulted in a variety of genetic disorders *(12)*. In humans, the majority of L1 insertions characterized have led to X-linked recessive diseases (Table 2). Although subject to ascertainment biases, it is estimated that deleterious L1 insertions are responsible for approx 1 in 1000 disease-producing mutations in man *(90)*, and that approx 1/10 to 1/100 male germ cells may harbor *de novo* retrotransposition events *(91,92)*.

Somatic L1 retrotransposition events also have the potential to cause disease (Table 2). In one instance, an L1 insertion into the adenomatous polyposis coli (*APC*) tumor suppressor gene was implicated in colon cancer because the mutagenic insertion was present only in the tumor and not the surrounding constitutional tissue *(93)*. Moreover, hypomethylation of the L1 promoter, an increase in the level of L1 transcription and elevated levels of ORF1p have been detected in a variety of tumor types, suggesting that retrotransposition may play a role in tumorigenesis and/or tumor progression *(94–98)*.

L1 insertions can alter gene expression by disrupting exons, by inducing mis-splicing or premature polyadenylation of primary transcripts, and by altering the transcriptional profile of a gene because of the potent anti-sense promoter located within the L1 5' UTR (*see* Fig. 4) *(12,56,57,99)*. In addition, it is proposed that L1 insertions in the same transcriptional orientation as genes may act as RNA polymerase II transcriptional pause sites that can attenuate gene expression by serving as "molecular rheostats" *(100)*. However, although intriguing, the "molecular rheostat" hypothesis awaits rigorous experimental proof.

Table 2
Disease-Producing L1 Insertions in the Human Genome

Disease	Disrupted gene	Insertion size	Ta subset	L1-mediated transduction
Hemopilia A	*Factor VIII*	3.8 kb	Yes	No
		2.2 kb	No	No
Duschene muscular dystrophy	*Dystrophin*	608 bp	Yes	No
		878 bp	Yes	Yes
		2.0 kb	Yes	No
		524 bp	Yes	No
B-Thalessemia	*B-globin*	6.0 kb	Yes	No
X-linked retinitis pigmentosa	*RP2*	6.0 kb	Yes	No
Chronic granulamatous	CYBB	1.7 kb	Yes	Yes
		940 bp	Yes	No
Fukuyama-type congenital muscular dystrophy	*FCMD*	1.2 kb	Yes	No
Hemophilia B	*Factor IX*	463 bp	Yes	No
Choroideremia	*CHM*	538 bp	Yes	Yes
Colon cancer	*APC*	538 bp	Yes	Yes

Human diseases resulting from L1 insertion into genes are noted. The size of the insertion and the subfamily that gave rise to the insertion are given *(12,121,129,130)*. Ta, transcribed active L1 *(98)*.

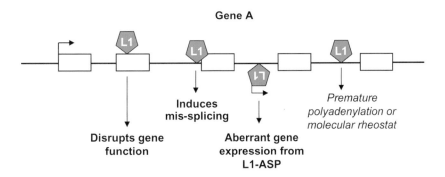

Fig. 4. L1 is an insertional mutagen. L1s can insert into many regions in ene A with exon (white boxes) and intron (bold lines) structure. When L1 inserts into exons it disrupts Gene A protein. Insertion into introns can lead to missplicing of Gene A mRNA. The L1 antisense promoter can facilitate transcription of partial Gene A transcripts when L1 inserts into an intron. The A-richness of L1 can lead to premature polyadenylation of Gene A mRNA when L1 inserts into an intron and may cause an arrest of transcriptional elongation as proposed by the molecular rheostat hypothesis. Text in bold represents processes that have been characterized in the human genome, and text in italics refers to proposed effects of L1 on gene expression.

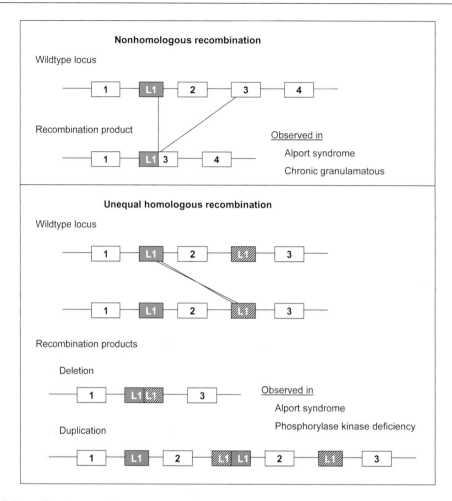

Fig. 5. L1-mediated recombination. Recombination can cause human disease when it occurs at L1 sequences located in introns. Nonhomologous recombination occurs between L1 sequence and sequence within the gene, where the L1 is located, resulting in a deletion of the intervening DNA. This process occurred to cause cases of Alport syndrome and chronic granulamatous disease *(101,131)*. Unequal homologous recombination occurs when there are at least two L1s within a gene. Recombination between different L1s results in deletion and/or duplication gene products. This type of recombination resulted in deletions in sporadic cases of Alport syndrome and phosphorylase kinase deficiency *(131,132)*.

Because L1 and *Alu* elements are widely distributed across the genome, they also can serve as substrates for unequal homologous or nonhomologous DNA recombination either during or long after their insertion (Fig. 5) *(11)*. Unequal recombination events between *Alu* elements have resulted in a variety of genetic diseases (*see* Chapter 1). Although less common, recombination events between homeologous L1 sequences have resulted in sporadic cases of Alport syndrome and chronic granulomatous disease *(101,102)*. Similarly, molecular biological and DNA sequence analyses indicate that both L1 and *Alu* elements can act as substrates for gene conversion and/or recombinational repair *(103,104)*. Thus, it is tempting to speculate that similar events can lead to the genome instability that frequently is observed in many tumors.

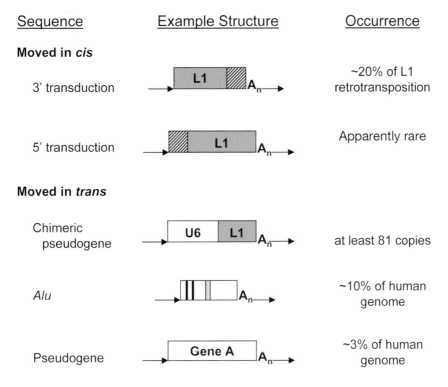

Fig. 6. L1-mediated movement of other sequences. L1s can move other sequences in *cis* and *in trans*. 3' transduction occurs when transcription reads through the L1 poly (A) signal in favor of a stronger downstream poly (A) signal, resulting in insertion of 3' flanking DNA (bold slashed rectangle) with L1 at a new genomic location. Similarly, 5' transduction occurs when transcription is initiated upstream of L1, resulting insertion of 5' flanking material (bold slashed rectangle) with L1 at a new genomic location. Chimeric pseudogenes are formed when the L1 RT switches templates to small non-coding RNAs, like the U6 snRNA, during TPRT. The L1 proteins also may be used to move non-autonomous retrotransposons, like *Alu* (black lines denote A and B boxes, speckled box represents A rich region), and cellular mRNAs to form pseudogenes. In all of these cases, L1-mediated insertions end in a poly (A) tail and are flanked by variable length target site duplications (arrows), which are hallmarks of TPRT.

L1 AS AN ARBITER OF GENOME DIVERSIFICATION

The sheer mass of L1s in mammalian genomes provides molecular scaffolds that sometimes can be coopted by the host as regulatory sequences for gene expression. For example, the polyadenylation signal of the mouse thymidylate synthetase resides within a L1 *(105)*. Similarly, *cis*-acting sequences that function in the regulation of the human apolipoprotein (A) gene, the human *C1D* gene, and the human *factor IX* gene are derived from L1s *(106–108)*. The over-representation of L1s on the X-chromosome has led to speculation that they might act as booster elements that function in X-inactivation *(109)*, though Boissinot et al. *(110)* have offered simpler interpretations to explain this phenomenon. Clearly, the analysis of whole genome sequences in conjunction with comparative genomic and functional studies should accelerate the discovery of retrotransposon sequences that function in host gene expression.

L1 also can serve as an agent of genomic diversification by facilitating the movement of non-L1 DNA sequences to new chromosomal locations (Fig. 6). For example, L1s can retrotranspose sequences from their 5' and 3' flanks to new genomic sites in *cis* by a process called "L1-mediated transduction." L1-mediated 5' transduction occurs when transcription is initiated from a cellular promoter that resides upstream of a retrotransposition-competent L1 *(1)*. L1-mediated 3' transduction occurs when the L1 poly (A) signal is bypassed in favor of a stronger downstream poly (A) signal present in flanking genomic DNA *(14,37)*. Retrotransposition of these transcripts allows the "duplication" of genomic DNA to a new chromosomal location. Because of the high frequency of 5' truncation, L1-mediated 5' transduction is relatively infrequent and only a few examples have been reported *in silico* and in vitro *(1,9,29,38)*. By comparison, 15–20% of Ta-subfamily L1s present in the HGWD contain 3' transductions, and it has been proposed that L1-mediated transduction is responsible for as much as 1% of human genomic DNA *(1,111,112)*.

The L1-encoded proteins also can mobilize non-autonomous retrotransposons (e.g., *Alu* and perhaps SVA elements), retrotransposition-defective L1s, cellular mRNAs, and partial mRNA transcripts (Fig. 6) *(7–9,113–115)*. The high copy number of *Alu* elements indicates that they have evolved a means to efficiently compete with L1 RNA for the L1 RT, perhaps by associating with ribosomes and commandeering the L1 RT during its translation *(116)*. Interestingly, only ORF2p is required for *Alu* retrotransposition *(8)*, whereas both ORF1p and ORF2p seemingly are required for processed pseudogene formation *(7,9)*. Thus, other proteins in *Alu* RNPs (SRP9 and SRP14) may compensate for ORF1p during retrotransposition (*see* Chapter 1) *(117)*.

Besides mobilizing RNA polymerase II transcripts *in trans* to generate processed pseudogenes, *in silico* analyses indicate that template switching between L1 RNA and some RNA polymerase III-derived transcripts can lead to the formation of chimeric pseudogenes (e.g., *U6/L1*, *U3/L1* and *7SL/L1*; Fig. 6). Indeed, these data suggest that a cohort of small uracil-rich nuclear RNAs can compete for the L1 retrotransposition machinery during TPRT and demonstrate that non-coding RNAs can be duplicated by retrotransposition *(118–120)*.

The mobilization of sequences by L1-mediated retrotransposition represents a potentially powerful mechanism to generate diversity in randomly mating sexual populations because: (1) the process does not depend on homologous DNA sequences; (2) the relative genomic locations of the "shuffled" sequences are not important; (3) the original donor sequence remains unchanged because the process occurs via an RNA intermediate; and (4) it provides a mechanism to exchange limited amounts of information between different chromosomes *(37,121)*.

Other than simply increasing the amount of "junk DNA" in the genome, L1-mediated retrotransposition occasionally can result in exon shuffling and the formation of new genes. For example, in mice the *Cdyl* gene produces two transcripts, one that is ubiquitously expressed and one that is testis specific. The human homologs of this gene (*CDYL* and *CDY*) are present on chromosome 13 and the Y chromosome, respectively. *CDY* is a processed pseudogene that is derived from *CDYL* and arose during primate evolution *(122)*. This duplication resulted in a partitioning of gene expression because *CDYL* is expressed ubiquitously, whereas *CDY* exhibits testis specific expression. Similarly, L1-mediated retrotransposition of a cyclophilin A mRNA into the *TRIM5* locus in owl monkeys led to the formation of a functional chimeric protein that acts to experimentally restrict HIV infection *(123)*.

Finally, L1 poly (A) tails tend to be unstable genetically and probably serve as seeding grounds for the generation of microsatellite repeats. Consistent with this hypothesis, microsatellites are more often found near the 3' ends of older L1 elements when compared to younger "human-specific" L1s *(124)*. A similar scenario has been observed for *Alu* elements *(125)* and is discussed further in Chapters 1 and 3.

INDIVIDUAL VARIATION IN L1 RETROTRANSPOSITION

The average human genome, as represented by the HGWD, contains approx 80–100 retrotransposition competent L1s and approx 10% of these elements are classified as highly active or "hot" *(35,126)*. The majority of these L1s, as well as 13/14 disease-producing L1 insertions, are members of the Ta (transcribed active) subfamily (Table 2). Many Ta-subset L1s are polymorphic with respect to presence, indicating that they have retrotransposed since the human-chimpanzee radiation *(39,43,98)*.

More recently, prospective assays have identified L1s that apparently are restricted to certain human populations or perhaps represent "private" polymorphisms in individual genomes *(42)*. Not surprisingly, there also appears to be an inverse correlation between the allele frequency of a given L1 and its inclusion in the HGWD. L1s present at low allele frequencies also tend to be more active for retrotransposition in cultured cells than those that are fixed in the population *(42,126)*. Thus, it is not unreasonable to assume that "recent" L1 retrotransposition events are systematically under-represented in the HGWD. Indeed, the notion that the average human genome only contains approx 80–100 retrotransposition-competent L1s, an extrapolation based on the estimated rate of new L1 insertions in the human population (ranging between 1/1000 spontaneous mutations to 1/10–1/100 new retrotransposition events in the male germ line) suggests that the actual number of retrotransposition-competent L1s in the extant population could, in principle, number in the thousands or perhaps millions.

Besides presence/absence variation (i.e., dimorphism), common L1 alleles also can vary widely in their retrotransposition potential as measured in cultured cells *(32)*. Thus, both L1 dimorphism and allelic heterogeneity have the potential to influence the L1 mutational load present in an individual genome. These findings raise interesting, albeit speculative, questions. Could differential retrotransposon activity affect human evolution? Are different geographic populations evolving at different rates? Clearly the answers to these questions will require further research.

NEXT IN LINE: REMAINING QUESTIONS

Recent technical advances will no doubt entice researchers to exploit L1s as tools for practical purposes. For example, engineered L1s have been proposed as transposon mutagens and gene delivery vehicles *(25,50,127,128)*, whereas dimorphic L1 insertions have applications as genetic markers in forensic and human population studies *(39,42–44)*. However, despite steady progress in recent years, we still know relatively little about the molecular mechanism of L1 retrotransposition and virtually nothing is known about host factors that interact with the L1 retrotransposition machinery. Similarly, we lack answers to the following basic science questions. What is the frequency of L1 retrotransposition in vivo? What types of cells accommodate L1 retrotransposition in vivo? How is L1 retrotransposition regulated?

Clearly, the cultured cell retrotransposition assay, biochemical studies, and whole genome analyses have been instrumental in increasing our knowledge of L1 biology. The recent development of transgenic animal models to study L1 retrotransposition also holds promise for future discoveries. However, the field is in dire need of robust biochemical systems to study L1 retrotransposition. Similarly, advanced computational algorithms to analyze whole genome sequences from closely related organisms are sorely needed and should allow an assessment of L1 catalyzed genome rearrangements that have occurred naturally during the course of genome evolution. Finally, mathematical modeling and the identification of L1s present in different geographical isolates should shed light on L1 population dynamics. In sum, though advancements have been made, we are just at the starting line and much progress is needed to fully understand L1 biology. Indeed, it is surprising how little we know about the molecular processes that have resulted in at least one billion of the three billion bases of our genome.

ACKNOWLEDGMENTS

The authors would like to thank Dr. John Goodier for helpful discussions. John V Moran is supported by a grant from the National Institutes of Health (NIH) (GM60518). Amy Hulme and Deanna A Kulpa were supported, in part, by an NIH Training Grant (GM07544). José Luis Garcia Perez is supported by a Ministerio Educacion y Ciencia (MEC)/Fulbright postdoctoral grant (EX-2003-0881, MEC, Spain).

REFERENCES

1. Lander ES, Linton LM, Birren B, et al. Initial sequencing and analysis of the human genome. Nature 2001;409:860–921.
2. Venter JC, Adams MD, Myers EW, et al. The sequence of the human genome. Science 2001;291:1304–1351.
3. Kleckner N. Regulation of transposition in bacteria. Annu Rev Cell Biol 1990;6:297–327.
4. Boeke JD, Garfinkel DJ, Styles CA, Fink GR. Ty elements transpose through an RNA intermediate. Cell 1985;40:491–500.
5. Mayer J, Meese E, Mueller-Lantzsch N. Multiple human endogenous retrovirus (HERV-K) loci with gag open reading frames in the human genome. Cytogenet Cell Genet 1997;78:1–5.
6. Mayer J. Status of HERV in human cells: expression and coding capacity of human proviruses. Dev Biol (Basel) 2001;106:439–441.
7. Esnault C, Maestre J, Heidmann J. Human LINE retrotransposons generate processed pseudogenes. Nat Genet 2000;24:363–367.
8. Dewannieux M, Esnault C, Heidmann T. LINE-mediated retrotransposition of marked Alu sequences. Nat Genet 2003;35:41–48.
9. Wei W, Gilbert N, Ooi SL, et al. Human L1 retrotransposition: cis preference versus trans complementation. Mol Cell Biol 2001;21:1429–1439.
10. Furano AV. The biological properties and evolutionary dynamics of mammalian LINE-1 retrotransposons. Prog Nucleic Acid Res Mol Biol 2000;64:255–294.
11. Deininger PL, Moran JV, Batzer MA, Kazazian HH Jr. Mobile elements and mammalian genome evolution. Curr Opin Genet Dev 2003;13:651–658.
12. Ostertag EM, Kazazian HH Jr. Biology of mammalian L1 retrotransposons. Annu Rev Genet 2001;35:501–538.
13. Dombroski BA, Mathias SL, Nanthakumar E, Scott AF, Kazazian HH Jr. Isolation of an active human transposable element. Science 1991;254:1805–1808.
14. Holmes SE, Dombroski BA, Krebs CM, Boehm CD, Kazazian HH Jr. A new retrotransposable human L1 element from the LRE2 locus on chromosome 1q produces a chimaeric insertion. Nat Genet 1994;7:143–148.
15. Dombroski BA, Scott AF, Kazazian HH Jr. Two additional potential retrotransposons isolated from a human L1 subfamily that contains an active retrotransposable element. Proc Natl Acad Sci USA 1993;90:6513–6517.
16. Swergold GD. Identification, characterization, and cell specificity of a human LINE-1 promoter. Mol Cell Biol 1990;10:6718–6729.
17. Scott AF, Schmeckpeper BJ, Abdelrazik M, et al. Origin of the human L1 elements: proposed progenitor genes deduced from a consensus DNA sequence. Genomics 1987;1:113–125.
18. Holmes SE, Singer MF, Swergold GD. Studies on p40, the leucine zipper motif-containing protein encoded by the first open reading frame of an active human LINE-1 transposable element. J Biol Chem 1992;267:19,765–19,768.
19. Hohjoh H, Singer MF. Cytoplasmic ribonucleoprotein complexes containing human LINE-1 protein and RNA. EMBO J 1996;15:630–639.

20. Ergun S, Buschmann C, Heukeshoven J, et al. Cell type-specific expression of LINE-1 open reading frames 1 and 2 in fetal and adult human tissues. J Biol Chem 2004;279:27,753–27,763.

21. Mathias SL, Scott AF, Kazazian HH Jr, Boeke JD, Gabriel A. Reverse transcriptase encoded by a human transposable element.. Science 1991;254:1808–1810.

22. Feng Q, Moran JV, Kazazian HH Jr, Boeke JD. Human L1 retrotransposon encodes a conserved endonuclease required for retrotransposition. Cell 1996;87:905–916.

23. Fanning T, Singer M. The LINE-1 DNA sequences in four mammalian orders predict proteins that conserve homologies to retrovirus proteins. Nucleic Acids Res 1987;15:2251–2260.

24. Hutchison CA, Hardies SC, Loeb DD, Sehee WR, Edgell MH. LINES and related retroposons: long inter-spersed sequences in the eucaryotic genome. In: *Mobile DNA* (Berg DE, Howe MM, eds.) Washington, DC: ASM Press, 1989.

25. Moran JV, Holmes SE, Naas TP, DeBerardinis RJ, Boeke JD, Kazazian HH Jr. High frequency retrotransposition in cultured mammalian cells. Cell 1996;87:917–927.

26. Freeman JD, Goodchild NL, Mager DL. A modified indicator gene for selection of retrotransposition events in mammalian cells. Biotechniques 1994;17:46–52.

27. Wei W, Morrish TA, Alisch RS, Moran JV. A transient assay reveals that cultured human cells can accommodate multiple LINE-1 retrotransposition events. Anal Biochem 2000;284:435–438.

28. Gilbert N, Lutz-Prigge S, Moran JV. Genomic deletions created on LINE-1 retrotransposition. Cell 2002;110:315–325.

29. Symer DE, Connelly C, Szak ST, et al. Human l1 retrotransposition is associated with genetic instability in vivo. Cell 2002;110:327–338.

30. Morrish TA, Gilbert N, Myers JS, et al., DNA repair mediated by endonuclease-independent LINE-1 retrotransposition. Nat Genet 2002;31:159–165.

31. Ostertag EM, Prak ET, DeBerardinis RJ, Moran JV, Kazazian HH Jr. Determination of L1 retrotransposition kinetics in cultured cells. Nucleic Acids Res 2000;28:1418–1423.

32. Lutz SM, Vincent BJ, Kazazian HH Jr, Batzer MA, Moran JV. Allelic heterogeneity in LINE-1 retrotransposition activity. Am J Hum Genet 2003;73:1431–1437.

33. DeBerardinis RJ, Goodier JL, Ostertag EM, Kazazian HH Jr. Rapid amplification of a retrotransposon subfamily is evolving the mouse genome. Nat Genet 1998;20:288–290.

34. Goodier JL, Ostertag EM, Du K, Kazazian HH Jr. A novel active L1 retrotransposon subfamily in the mouse. Genome Res 2001;11:1677–1685.

35. Sassaman DM, Dombroski BA, Moran JV, et al. Many human L1 elements are capable of retrotransposition. Nat Genet 1997;16:37–43.

36. Naas TP, DeBerardinis RJ, Moran JV, et al. An actively retrotransposing, novel subfamily of mouse L1 elements. EMBO J 1998;17:590–597.

37. Moran JV, DeBerardinis RJ, Kazazian HH Jr. Exon shuffling by L1 retrotransposition. Science 1999;283: 1530–1534.

38. Athanikar JN, Badge RM, Moran JV. A YY1-binding site is required for accurate human LINE-1 transcription initiation. Nucleic Acids Res 2004;32:3846–3855.

39. Boissinot S, Chevret P, Furano AV. L1 (LINE-1) retrotransposon evolution and amplification in recent human history. Mol Biol Evol 2000;17:915–928.

40. Waterston RH, Lindblad-Toh K, Birney E, et al. Initial sequencing and comparative analysis of the mouse genome. Nature 2002;420:520–562.

41. Gibbs RA, Weinstock GM, Metzker ML, et al. Genome sequence of the Brown Norway rat yields insights into mammalian evolution. Nature 2004;428:493–521.

42. Badge RM, Alisch RS, Moran JV. ATLAS: a system to selectively identify human-specific L1 insertions. Am J Hum Genet 2003;72:823–838.

43. Myers JS, Vincent BJ, Udall H, et al. A comprehensive analysis of recently integrated human Ta L1 elements. Am J Hum Genet 2002;71:312–326.

44. Boissinot S, Entezam A, Young L, Munson PJ, Furano AV. The insertional history of an active family of L1 retrotransposons in humans. Genome Res 2004;14:1221–1231.

45. Bennett EA, Coleman LE, Tsui C, Pittard WS, Devine SE. Natural genetic variation caused by transposable elements in humans. Genetics 2004;168:933–951.

46. Vincent BJ, Myers JS, Ho HJ, et al. Following the LINEs: an analysis of primate genomic variation at human-specific LINE-1 insertion sites. Mol Biol Evol 2003;20:1338–48.

47. Sheen FM, Sherry ST, Risch GM, et al. Reading between the LINEs: human genomic variation induced by LINE-1 retrotransposition. Genome Res 2000;10:1496–1508.

48. Trelogan SA, Martin SL. Tightly regulated, developmentally specific expression of the first open reading frame from LINE-1 during mouse embryogenesis. Proc Natl Acad Sci USA 1995;92:1520–1524.

49. Branciforte D, Martin SL. Developmental and cell type specificity of LINE-1 expression in mouse testis: implications for transposition. Mol Cell Biol 1994;14:2584–2592.

50. Ostertag EM, DeBerardinis RJ, Goodier JL, et al. A mouse model of human L1 retrotransposition. Nat Genet 2002;32:655–660.

51. Prak ET, Dodson AW, Farkash EA, Kazazian HH Jr. Tracking an embryonic L1 retrotransposition event. Proc Natl Acad Sci USA 2003;100:1832–1837.

52. Minakami R, Kurose K, Etoh K, Furuhata Y, Hattori M, Sakaki Y. Identification of an internal cis-element essential for the human L1 transcription and a nuclear factor(s) binding to the element. Nucleic Acids Res 1992;20:3139–3145.

53. Becker KG, Swergold GD, Ozato K, Thayer RE. Binding of the ubiquitous nuclear transcription factor YY1 to a cis regulatory sequence in the human LINE-1 transposable element. Hum Mol Genet 1993;2:1697–1702.

54. Tchenio T, Casella JF, Heidmann T. Members of the SRY family regulate the human LINE retrotransposons. Nucleic Acids Res 2000;28:411–415.

55. Yang N, Zhang L, Zhang Y, Kazazian HH Jr. An important role for RUNX3 in human L1 transcription and retrotransposition. Nucleic Acids Res 2003;31:4929–4940.

56. Nigumann P, Redik K, Matlik K, Speek M. Many human genes are transcribed from the antisense promoter of L1 retrotransposon. Genomics 2002;79:628–634.

57. Speek M. Antisense promoter of human L1 retrotransposon drives transcription of adjacent cellular genes. Mol Cell Biol 2001;21:1973–1985.

58. Kolosha VO, Martin SL. High-affinity, non-sequence-specific RNA binding by the open reading frame 1 (ORF1) protein from long interspersed nuclear element 1 (LINE-1). J Biol Chem 2003;278:8112–8117.

59. Kolosha VO, Martin SL. In vitro properties of the first ORF protein from mouse LINE-1 support its role in ribonucleoprotein particle formation during retrotransposition. Proc Natl Acad Sci USA 1997;94: 10,155–10,160.

60. Martin SL, Bushman FD. Nucleic acid chaperone activity of the ORF1 protein from the mouse LINE-1 retrotransposon. Mol Cell Biol 2001;21:467–475.

61. Martin SL, Branciforte D, Keller D, Bain DL. Trimeric structure for an essential protein in L1 retrotransposition. Proc Natl Acad Sci USA 2003;100:13,815–13,820.

62. Martin SL, Li J, Weisz JA. Deletion analysis defines distinct functional domains for protein-protein and nucleic acid interactions in the ORF1 protein of mouse LINE-1. J Mol Biol 2000;304:11–20.

63. Boissinot S, Furano AV. Adaptive evolution in LINE-1 retrotransposons. Mol Biol Evol 2001;18:2186–2194.

64. Martin F, Maranon C, Olivares M, Alonso C, Lopez MC. Characterization of a non-long terminal repeat retrotransposon cDNA (L1Tc) from Trypanosoma cruzi: homology of the first ORF with the ape family of DNA repair enzymes. J Mol Biol 1995;247:49–59.

65. Weichenrieder O, Repanas K, Perrakis A. Crystal structure of the targeting endonuclease of the human LINE-1 retrotransposon. Structure (Camb) 2004;12:975–986.

66. Feng Q, Schumann G, Boeke JD. Retrotransposon R1Bm endonuclease cleaves the target sequence. Proc Natl Acad Sci USA 1998;95:2083–2088.

67. Cost GJ, Boeke JD. Targeting of human retrotransposon integration is directed by the specificity of the L1 endonuclease for regions of unusual DNA structure. Biochemistry 1998;37:18,081–18,093.

68. Hattori, M., Hattori M, Kuhara S, Takenaka O, Sakaki Y. L1 family of repetitive DNA sequences in primates may be derived from a sequence encoding a reverse transcriptase-related protein. Nature 1986; 321:625–628.

69. Xiong Y, Eickbush TH. Origin and evolution of retroelements based on their reverse transcriptase sequences. EMBO J 1990;9:3353–3362.

70. Piskareva O, Denmukhametova S, Schmatchenko V. Functional reverse transcriptase encoded by the human LINE-1 from baculovirus-infected insect cells. Protein Expr Purif 2003;28:125–130.

71. Dombroski BA, Feng Q, Mathias SL, et al. An in vivo assay for the reverse transcriptase of human retrotransposon L1 in Saccharomyces cerevisiae. Mol Cell Biol 1994;14:4485–4492.

72. Usdin K, Furano AV. The structure of the guanine-rich polypurine:polypyrimidine sequence at the right end of the rat L1 (LINE) element. J Biol Chem 1989;264:15,681–15,687.73.

73. Lindtner S, Felber BK, Kjems J. An element in the 3' untranslated region of human LINE-1 retrotransposon mRNA binds NXF1(TAP) and can function as a nuclear export element. Rna 2002;8:345–356.

74. Moran JV, Gilbert N. Mammalian LINE-1 retrotransposons and related elements. In: *Mobile DNA II* (Craig N, Craggie R, Gellert M, Lambowitz AM, eds.). Washington, DC: ASM Press, 2002; pp 836–869.

75. Martin SL. Ribonucleoprotein particles with LINE-1 RNA in mouse embryonal carcinoma cells. Mol Cell Biol 1991;11:4804–4807.

76. Kinsey JA. Transnuclear retrotransposition of the Tad element of Neurospora. Proc Natl Acad Sci USA 1993;90:9384–9387.

77. Luan DD, Korman MH, Jakubczak JL, Eickbush TH. Reverse transcription of R2Bm RNA is primed by a nick at the chromosomal target site: a mechanism for non-LTR retrotransposition. Cell 1993;72:595–605.

78. Cost GJ, Feng Q, Jacquier A, Boeke JD. Human L1 element target-primed reverse transcription in vitro. EMBO J 2002;21:5899–5910.

79. Farley AH, Luning Prak ET, Kazazian Jr. HH. More active human L1 retrotransposons produce longer insertions. Nucleic Acids Res 2004;32:502–510.

80. Bibillo A, Eickbush TH. High processivity of the reverse transcriptase from a non-long terminal repeat retrotransposon. J Biol Chem 2002;277:34,836–34,845.

81. Ostertag EM, Kazazian Jr. HH. Twin priming: a proposed mechanism for the creation of inversions in L1 retrotransposition. Genome Res 2001;11:2059–2065.

82. Jurka J. Sequence patterns indicate an enzymatic involvement in integration of mammalian retroposons. Proc Natl Acad Sci USA 1997;94:1872–1877.

83. Salem AH, Kilroy GE, Watkins WS, Jorde LB, Batzer MA. Recently integrated Alu elements and human genomic diversity. Mol Biol Evol 2003;20:1349–1361.

84. Hayakawa T, Satta Y, Gagneux P, Varki A, Takahata N. Alu-mediated inactivation of the human CMP-N-acetylneuraminic acid hydroxylase gene. Proc Natl Acad Sci USA 2001;98:11,399–11,404.

85. Kojima T, Nakajima K, Mikoshiba K. The disabled 1 gene is disrupted by a replacement with L1 fragment in yotari mice. Brain Res Mol Brain Res 2000;75:121–127.

86. Garvey SM, Rajan C, Lerner AP, Frankel WN, Cox GA. The muscular dystrophy with myositis (mdm) mouse mutation disrupts a skeletal muscle-specific domain of titin. Genomics 2002;79:146–149.

87. Kazazian HH Jr. Goodier JL. LINE drive. Retrotransposition and genome instability. Cell 2002;110:277–280.

88. Voliva CF, Martin SL, Hutchison CA 3rd, Edgell MH. Dispersal process associated with the L1 family of interspersed repetitive DNA sequences. J Mol Biol 1984;178:795–813.

89. Kazazian HH Jr, Wong C, Youssoufian H, Scott AF, Phillips DG, Antonarakis SE. Haemophilia A resulting from de novo insertion of L1 sequences represents a novel mechanism for mutation in man. Nature 1988;332:164–166.

90. Kazazian HH Jr., Moran JV. The impact of L1 retrotransposons on the human genome. Nat Genet 1998;19:19–24.

91. Li X, Scaringe WA, Hill KA, et al. Frequency of recent retrotransposition events in the human factor IX gene. Hum Mutat 2001;17:511–519.

92. Kazazian HH Jr. An estimated frequency of endogenous insertional mutations in humans. Nat Genet 1999;22:130.

93. Miki Y. Retrotransposal integration of mobile genetic elements in human diseases. J Hum Genet 1998;43:77–84.

94. Alves G, Tatro A, Fanning T. Differential methylation of human LINE-1 retrotransposons in malignant cells. Gene 1996;176:39–44.

95. Asch HL, Eliacin E, Fanning TG, Connolly JL, Bratthauer G, Asch BB. Comparative expression of the LINE-1 p40 protein in human breast carcinomas and normal breast tissues. Oncol Res 1996;8:239–247.

96. Bratthauer GL, Fanning TG. LINE-1 retrotransposon expression in pediatric germ cell tumors. Cancer 1993;71:2383–2386.

97. Bratthauer GL, Fanning TG. Active LINE-1 retrotransposons in human testicular cancer. Oncogene 1992;7:507–510.

98. Skowronski J, Fanning TG, Singer MF. Unit-length line-1 transcripts in human teratocarcinoma cells. Mol Cell Biol 1988;8:1385–1397.

99. Perepelitsa-Belancio V, Deininger P. RNA truncation by premature polyadenylation attenuates human mobile element activity. Nat Genet 2003;35:363–366.

100. Han JS, Szak ST, Boeke JD. Transcriptional disruption by the L1 retrotransposon and implications for mammalian transcriptomes. Nature 2004;429:268–274.

101. Segal Y, Peissel B, Renieri A, et al. LINE-1 elements at the sites of molecular rearrangements in Alport syndrome-diffuse leiomyomatosis. Am J Hum Genet 1999;64:62–69.
102. Meischl C, Boer M, Ahlin A, Roos D. A new exon created by intronic insertion of a rearranged LINE-1 element as the cause of chronic granulomatous disease. Eur J Hum Genet 2000;8:697–703.
103. Tremblay A, Jasin M, Chartrand P. A double-strand break in a chromosomal LINE element can be repaired by gene conversion with various endogenous LINE elements in mouse cells. Mol Cell Biol 2000;20:54–60.
104. Kass DH, Batzer MA, Deininger PL. Gene conversion as a secondary mechanism of short interspersed element (SINE) evolution. Mol Cell Biol 1995;15:19–25.
105. Harendza CJ, Johnson LF. Polyadenylylation signal of the mouse thymidylate synthase gene was created by insertion of an L1 repetitive element downstream of the open reading frame. Proc Natl Acad Sci USA 1990;87:2531–2535.
106. Rothbarth K, Hunziker A, Stammer H, Werner D. Promoter of the gene encoding the 16 kDa DNA-binding and apoptosis-inducing C1D protein. Biochim Biophys Acta 2001;1518:271–275.
107. Yang Z, Boffelli D, Boonmark N, Schwartz K, Lawn R. Apolipoprotein(a) gene enhancer resides within a LINE element. J Biol Chem 1998;273:891–897.
108. Hsu W, Kawamura S, Fontaine JM, Kurachi K, Kurachi S. Organization and significance of LINE-1-derived sequences in the 5' flanking region of the factor IX gene. Thromb Haemost 1999;82:1782–1783.
109. Lyon MF. X-chromosome inactivation: a repeat hypothesis. Cytogenet Cell Genet 1998;80:133–137.
110. Boissinot S, Entezam A, Furano AV. Selection against deleterious LINE-1-containing loci in the human lineage. Mol Biol Evol 2001;18:926–935.
111. Goodier JL, Ostertag EM, Kazazian HH Jr. Transduction of 3'-flanking sequences is common in L1 retrotransposition. Hum Mol Genet 2000;9:653–657.
112. Pickeral OK, Makalowski W, Boguski MS, Boeke JD. Frequent human genomic DNA transduction driven by LINE-1 retrotransposition. Genome Res 2000;10:411–415.
113. Ostertag EM, Goodier JL, Zhang Y, Kazazian HH Jr. SVA elements are nonautonomous retrotransposons that cause disease in humans. Am J Hum Genet 2003;73:1444–1451.
114. Ejima Y, Yang L. Trans mobilization of genomic DNA as a mechanism for retrotransposon-mediated exon shuffling. Hum Mol Genet 2003;12:1321–1328.
115. Rozmahel R, Heng HH, Duncan AM, Shi XM, Rommens JM, Tsui LC. Amplification of CFTR exon 9 sequences to multiple locations in the human genome. Genomics 1997;45:554–561.
116. Boeke JD. LINEs and Alus–the polyA connection. Nat Genet 1997;16:6–7.
117. Sarrowa J, Chang DY, Maraia RJ. The decline in human Alu retroposition was accompanied by an asymmetric decrease in SRP9/14 binding to dimeric Alu RNA and increased expression of small cytoplasmic Alu RNA. Mol Cell Biol 1997;17:1144–1151.
118. Buzdin A, Ustyugova S, Gogvadze E, Vinogradova T, Lebedev Y, Sverdlov E. A new family of chimeric retrotranscripts formed by a full copy of U6 small nuclear RNA fused to the 3' terminus of l1. Genomics 2002;80:402–406.
119. Buzdin A, Ustyugova S, Gogvadze E, Lebedev Y, Hunsmann G, Sverdlov E. Genome-wide targeted search for human specific and polymorphic L1 integrations. Hum Genet, 2003. 112(5-6): p. 527-33.
120. Buzdin A, Gogvadze E, Kovalskaya E, et al. The human genome contains many types of chimeric retrogenes generated through in vivo RNA recombination. Nucleic Acids Res 2003;31:4385–4390.
121. Moran JV. Human L1 retrotransposition: insights and peculiarities learned from a cultured cell retrotransposition assay. Genetica 1999;107:39–51.
122. Lahn BT, Page DC. Retroposition of autosomal mRNA yielded testis-specific gene family on human Y chromosome. Nat Genet 1999;21:429–433.
123. Sayah DM, Sokolskaja E, Berthoux L, Luban J. Cyclophilin A retrotransposition into TRIM5 explains owl monkey resistance to HIV-1. Nature 2004;430:569–573.
124. Ovchinnikov I, Troxel AB, Swergold GD. Genomic characterization of recent human LINE-1 insertions: evidence supporting random insertion. Genome Res 2001;11:2050–2058.
125. Arcot SS, Wang Z, Weber JL, Deininger PL, Batzer MA. Alu repeats: a source for the genesis of primate microsatellites. Genomics 1995;29:136–144.
126. Brouha B, Schustak J, Badge RM, et al. Hot L1s account for the bulk of retrotransposition in the human population. Proc Natl Acad Sci USA 2003;100:5280–5285.
127. Soifer H, Higo C, Kazazian HH Jr, Moran JV, Mitani K, Kasahara N. Stable integration of transgenes delivered by a retrotransposon-adenovirus hybrid vector. Hum Gene Ther 2001;12:1417–1428.

128. Han JS, Boeke JD. A highly active synthetic mammalian retrotransposon. Nature 2004;429:314–318.
129. van den Hurk, J.A.J.M., et al. L1 retrotransposition during embryogenesis in the mother of a patient with choroideremia. In American Society of Human Genetics. Los Angeles, California: The University of Chicago Press 2003;73:58, abstract no. 2422.
130. Mukherjee S, Mukhopadhyay A, Banerjee D, Chandak GR, Ray K. Molecular pathology of haemophilia B: identification of five novel mutations including a LINE 1 insertion in Indian patients. Haemophilia 2004; 10:259–263.
131. Kumatori A, Faizunnessa NN, Suzuki S, Moriuchi T, Kurozumi H, Nakamura M. Nonhomologous recombination between the cytochrome b558 heavy chain gene (CYBB) and LINE-1 causes an X-linked chronic granulomatous disease. Genomics 1998;53:123–128.
132. Burwinkel B, Kilimann MW. Unequal homologous recombination between LINE-1 elements as a mutational mechanism in human genetic disease. J Mol Biol 1998;277:513–517.

4

Ancient Transposable Elements, Processed Pseudogenes, and Endogenous Retroviruses

Adam Pavlicek, PhD and Jerzy Jurka, PhD

BACKGROUND

The human genome contains a large number of repetitive elements derived from transposable elements (TEs). In addition to active *Alu* and long interspersed element (LINE or L1) interspersed repeats, the human genome comprises a large number of ancient TEs. These include fossil germ-line insertions of DNA transposons, fossil short interspersed elements (SINEs), L2, and L3 LINEs. Processed pseudogenes and human endogenous retroviruses (HERVs) have amplified more recently in evolutionary history and some of them are still well preserved. Copies of some of the recently extinct TEs continue to contribute to genomic rearrangements by homologous recombination. In this chapter, we review ancient SINE and LINE repeats, processed pseudogenes, HERVs, and DNA transposons. We briefly introduce the genomic structure and replication strategy of these elements, their expression competence, and focus on the contribution of these repeats to human diseases. We also discuss some of the TE-derived genes and regulatory elements.

INTRODUCTION

Repetitive elements or repeats are sequences present in multiple copies in the genome but, unlike multigene families, they do not have any clear function in the host. Low-copy repeats generated by large-scale genomic duplications represent a class by themselves, and are discussed in Chapter 5.

From: *Genomic Disorders: The Genomic Basis of Disease*
Edited by: J. R. Lupski and P. Stankiewicz © Humana Press, Totowa, NJ

Table 1
Repetitive Elements in the Human Genome

Type/class	Superfamily	Further division[a]	Family	Genome (%)[b]
Tandem repeats	Satellites			Approx 20?
	Telomeric and subtelomeric repeats			<0.01
	Microsatellites and minisatellites			1.4
Interspersed repeats	DNA transposons	Mariner/Tc1		11 families	2.8
		hAT		14 families	2.4
		PiggyBac		1 families	0.02
		MuDr		2 families	0.03
		Harbinger		*HARBI1* gene	—
		P		Single-copy genes	—
	Non-LTR retrotransposons	L1	LINE	L1	17
			SINE	*Alu*	10.5
				SVA (SINE-R)	0.13
			Retropseudogenes	—	0.1–0.3[c]
		CR1	LINE	L2	3.1
				L3	0.31
			SINE	MIR	1
				MIR3	0.29
	LTR retro-transposons	Copia (HERVs)	Class I (gamma retroviruses)	>90 families	2.5
			Class II (beta retroviruses)	11 families	0.5
			Class III (spumaviruses)	>30 families	6
		Gypsy		Single-copy genes	—

This table shows the basic division of human repetitive elements. *See* refs. *3,6,123,128*, and Repbase update *(4)*.
[a]For non-LTR transposons, we also included dependent nonautonomous elements (SINEs, retropseudogenes).
[b]The numbers represent the proportion of detectable repeats in the sequenced genome. Centromeric and heterochromatic satellites are underrepresented in the sequenced regions, but based on reassociation studies the proportion is estimated to be approx 20%.
[c]Depending on the detection method.

In general, repetitive elements are divided into tandem repeats and interspersed repeats (Table 1). Tandem repeats are head-to-tail repetitions of the same sequence motif. Interspersed repeats are active or inactive copies of TEs dispersed throughout the genome. Repetitive elements can be grouped into sets of similar copies, called families or subfamilies. Families of TEs that encode enzymes necessary for their replication are termed autonomous. Nonautonomous elements do not encode all necessary proteins, and their replication (amplification) depends on proteins provided by the autonomous elements. Nonautonomous elements can, thus, be viewed as parasitic elements competing for replication machinery with the autonomous copies. Amplification of both autonomous and nonautonomous elements depends also on additional factors provided by the host cell.

Based on their replication strategy, interspersed repeats are broadly divided into DNA transposons and retrotransposons. The DNA transposons amplify using the host DNA replication machinery, and their transcripts serve solely as mRNAs participating in translation of transposon-encoded proteins involved in the transposon insertions and excisions. The retrotransposons replicate via an RNA intermediate and, thus, their transcripts serve both as mRNAs for protein translation and as templates for DNA synthesis. Before integration into the genome, retrotransposon RNA must be copied into cDNA using RNA-dependent DNA polymerase, also known as reverse transcriptase (RT) *(1,2)*.

Recognizable copies of all repetitive elements constitute approx 50% of the human genome *(3)*. During the course of the human genome sequencing, more than 600 repeat families and subfamilies have been discovered. All are systematically organized in Repbase Update (RU) (http://www.girinst.org/Repbase_Update.html) *(4)*.

NON-LTR RETROTRANSPOSONS

Non-long terminal repeat (LTR) retrotransposons are the most abundant repetitive elements in human genomic DNA and represent approx one-third of the genome (Table 1). Their DNA copies are co-linear with the RNA transcripts and they lack LTRs present in retroviruses. Autonomous non-LTR retrotransposons are often referred to as LINEs and their nonautonomous counterparts as SINEs. The human genome contains two superfamilies of LINEs: active L1 (LINE1) elements, and extinct families of L2 and L3 elements (Table 1). The latter belong to the CR1 superfamily. Human SINEs are represented by the active *Alu* and SVA repeats retrotransposed by L1 elements, and by the extinct mammalian-wide interspersed repeat (MIR) and MIR3 SINEs that coamplified with L2 and L3 families, respectively. Active L1, *Alu* and SVA non-LTR retrotransposons are described in Chapters 2 and 3. Here, we concentrate on ancient LINE (*see* Ancient LINEs) and SINE (*see* Ancient SINEs) elements. We also review L1-retroposed copies of cellular transcripts known as processed pseudogenes (*see* Processed Pseudogenes).

Ancient LINEs

A typical structure of LINE elements is shown in Fig. 1A. LINEs usually contain two open reading frames referred to as *ORF1* and *ORF2*. The L3 ORF1 protein shares similarity with esterase domains *(5)*. L2 elements apparently lack *ORF1*, although it is possible that the very old age of L2 copies and frequent 5' truncation typical for LINEs prevented reconstruction of a full-length L2 element *(6)*. The ORF2 protein contains the RT and apurinic-apyrimidinic endonuclease enzymatic domains. The transcription of LINE elements starts from a poorly characterized internal promoter for RNA polymerase II (Fig. 1A). After translation, the complex of LINE RNA and protein(s) enters the nucleus, where an endonucleolytic nick at a DNA target serves to prime reverse transcription *(7)*. Target-primed reverse transcription is another feature distinguishing non-LTR from LTR retrotransposons, which normally use cellular tRNA as primers for reverse transcription (*see* Human Endogenous Retroviruses). Unlike in L1 and L1-dependent elements, no target site duplications are created during integration of L2 and L3 elements. Furthermore, L2 and L3 carry microsatellite-like 3' tails instead of the polyA tail found in L1 insertions *(6)*. Based on high sequence diversity, the age of L2 and L3 elements in the human genome is estimated to be approx 200–300 million years, corresponding to the early radiation of reptiles, birds, and mammals. Recognizable L2 and L3 copies, together with their nonautonomous counterparts MIR and MIR3, represent approx 5% of the human genome *(6)*.

The potential of L2 and L3 copies to stimulate genomic rearrangements is very limited owing to their ancient origin, and no such case has been identified in humans so far. The

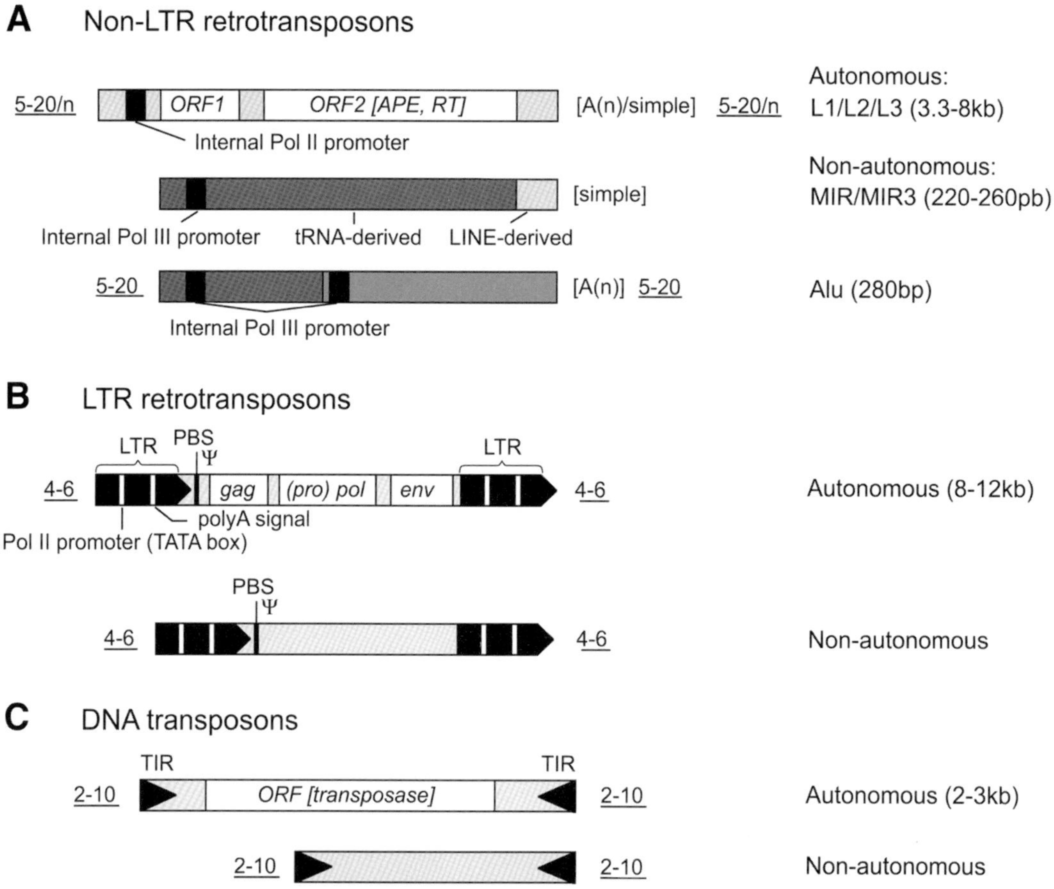

A   Non-LTR retrotransposons

	Autonomous:
	L1/L2/L3 (3.3-8kb)
	Non-autonomous:
	MIR/MIR3 (220-260pb)
	Alu (280bp)

B   LTR retrotransposons

Autonomous (8-12kb)

Non-autonomous

C   DNA transposons

Autonomous (2-3kb)

Non-autonomous

Fig. 1. Structure of human interspersed repeats. The figure shows typical structures of integrated interspersed repeats. (A) Structure of non-long terminal repeats (LTR) retrotransposons. The first bar shows a schematic organization of LINE elements. Human L1 and L3 elements contain two open reading frames (*ORFs*), L2 copies apparently lack *ORF1*. The function of the first *ORF1* is poorly understood. *ORF2* encodes a protein with the apurinic-apyrimidinic endonuclease and reverse transcriptase (RT) enzymatic domains. L1 insertions have a 3' polyA tail and are flanked by variable long target duplications, typically 5- to 20-bp long. L2 and L3 elements lack the target site duplications, and their 3' tails are composed of simple repeat sequences. The second and third schematic bars depict organization of SINEs. L2- and L3-dependent MIR and MIR3 SINEs (middle) consist of two parts. The 5' part (dark gray) is derived from a tRNA gene and harbors an internal pol III promoter. The 3' tails of MIRs are homologous to the 3' end of the corresponding LINE counterparts (light gray). *Alu* elements (bottom) derived from *7SL RNA* genes have a dimeric structure and contain a composite pol III promoter. SINEs share insertional characteristics with their LINE counterparts including the 3' end simple repeats in MIRs. L1-dependent *Alu* repeats contain 3' polyA tails and are flanked by 5- to 20-bp long direct repeats. (B) Structure of LTR retrotransposons. All LTR retrotransposons contain two LTRs, which include a pol II promoter and polyA signal. The internal part of autonomous elements comprises three main open reading frames: *gag*, *pol*, and *env*; in some HERV families *pro* can be separate from *pol*. The 5' part of the internal sequence contains a tRNA primer binding site (PBS) for initiation of reverse transcription and also an encapsidation sequence (Ψ) necessary for incorporation of retroviral RNA molecules into virions. Internal sequences of nonautonomous LTR retrotransposons may or may not share similarity with retroviral ORFs, but they contain all structures required for retroviral replication and reverse transcription such as LTRs, PBS, or the encapsidation signal. Both proliferation of L2 and L3 elements stopped long before the mammalian radiation, and recombination between highly diverged sequences is very unlikely. No protein-coding gene derived from L2 or L3 elements has been detected.

Ancient SINEs

Successful amplification of SINEs by the LINE machinery requires their transcription to be initiated by internal promoters. Typical SINEs are derived from cellular genes transcribed by RNA polymerase III, containing internal promoters. For example, L1-dependent *Alu* elements are derived from *7SL RNA* genes encoding the RNA scaffold of the signal recognition particle, whereas MIRs are derived from tRNA genes. The 5' parts of MIRs are homologous to tRNA genes, and the 3' terminal portions are homologous to the respective LINE elements on which their proliferation depends (Fig. 1A). MIR shares its 3' terminus with L2 elements, MIR3 with L3 elements *(6,8,9)*. MIR and MIR3 SINEs, like their LINE2 and LINE3 counterparts, are very old and their contribution to genomic rearrangements in the human genome seems to be minimal because no homologous recombination between ancient SINEs associated with human disease has been reported.

Processed Pseudogenes

Eukaryotic genomes contain a large number of pseudogenes *(10)*, which are homologous to known functional genes, but are apparently defective owing to the presence of various mutations, such as truncations, frameshifts, or missense changes. Pseudogenes are sometimes abbreviated using the Greek letter Ψ followed by the symbol of the original functional gene from which the pseudogene was derived. The human genome contains two types of pseudogenes: duplicated pseudogenes and processed pseudogenes generated in germ-line cells. Duplicated pseudogenes resemble normal cellular genes and are created by direct DNA duplications. Processed pseudogenes or retropseudogenes, on the other hand, are structurally distinct. Typically, they are characterized by the lack of both a promoter and introns, and by the acquisition of a polyA-like sequence at their 3' ends *(11,12)*. Because of co-linearity with spliced mRNAs, processed pseudogenes appear to originate by reverse transcription and integration of cellular mRNAs.

The mechanism of amplification of processed pseudogenes represented a long-standing puzzle. The presence of a polyA tail and lack of long terminal repeats indicated involvement of a non-retroviral enzymatic machinery *(12)*. Furthermore, processed pseudogenes share common insertion characteristics, such as the TTAAAA insertion motif shared with LINE-L1 and *Alu* repetitive sequences *(13)*, strongly pointing to active L1 elements as the donors of the RT. Indeed, a series of sophisticated experiments has demonstrated reverse transcription and integration of spliced reporter mRNA by the L1 enzymatic machinery with all hallmarks of processed pseudogenes *(14–18)*. Genomic studies of processed pseudogenes have disclosed additional characteristics of L1-mediated retroposition: integration independent of the chro-

---

the autonomous and nonautonomous elements are flanked by 4- to 6-bp long direct repeats. (C) Structure of DNA transposons. DNA transposons contain terminal inverted repeats (TIRs) of variable sizes (from approx 10 to several hundred nucleotides). Autonomous elements encode the replication enzyme transposase. Nonautonomous elements share TIRs with autonomous copies, which are recognized by transposase. DNA transposons are flanked by 2- to 10-bp long target site duplications, characteristic for each (super)family.

mosomal location of the parent gene *(19,20)*, preferential insertions into GC-poor DNA segments (isochores), dark Giemsa bands *(20–22)*, as well as frequent 5' truncations and inversions *(23–25)*. Therefore, it is generally accepted that human processed pseudogenes are copies of cellular RNA transcripts reverse transcribed and integrated into the genome by L1 machinery. Retroposition of cellular RNAs by other RT-encoding elements such as endogenous retroviruses appears to be rare *(26)*.

The number of processed pseudogenes derived from protein-coding mRNA is estimated to be somewhere between 10,000 and 30,000, depending on detection methods and stringency criteria *(20,27,28)*. Some may be misannoted as functional genes. Moreover, most pseudogenes are 5' truncated and contain only a partial 3' untranslated region and thus are not detectable by standard translated searches *(23)*. The majority of processed pseudogenes preserved in the human genome were created after the split between the rodent and primate lineages. The peak of their generation roughly corresponds to the main period of *Alu* amplification 60–40 million years ago, after which the frequency of retroposition has declined *(19,20,22)*.

The number of processed pseudogenes depends on several properties of mRNA. Short and GC-poor mRNAs tend to produce more pseudogenes *(27)*, although the significance of small size may be artificial *(23)*. The number of pseudogenes is positively correlated with the breadth of expression of the parental gene *(27)* and, as expected, with germline/embryonic cell expression *(20)*, because only germ-line retrotranspositions can be passed onto future generations. The contribution of functional gene groups to the human processed pseudogene population is not random either. Although the number of processed pseudogenes is comparable to the number of human genes, only approx 10% of human genes are represented among processed pseudogene(s), and 30 human genes account for 20% of all human processed pseudogenes *(20)*. Ribosomal protein genes, DNA/RNA binding proteins, receptors, kinases, metabolic enzymes, mitochondrial proteins, and housekeeping genes in general are represented by the highest number of processed pseudogenes *(19,20,22,25,29)*. In summary, it seems that genes expressed in germ-line cells, such as germ-line specific or housekeeping genes, have the highest chance of being retroposed by L1 elements.

In addition to typical transcripts of protein-coding genes, other RNAs can also be retroposed by L1 elements. Processed pseudogenes can be derived from alternatively spliced mRNAs *(24,25,30)*, antisense transcripts *(31)*, or mRNAs derived from other repetitive elements such as endogenous retroviruses *(30,32,33)*. It seems that virtually any RNA including non-coding RNAs can be potentially retroposed by L1 elements. The model of *Alu* and L1 retrotranspositions *(34)* implies two principal requirements for successful retroposition: (1) the RNAs should contain a polyA-like 3' terminal sequence and (2) they should be located close to the newly synthesized L1 proteins (e.g., cytoplasmic localization, close to ribosomes) owing to the L1 *cis* preference. This hints that both pol I and III transcripts may be transposed as well, if they meet the aforementioned conditions. *Alu* elements are a prominent example of polyA-terminated processed pseudogenes derived from a pol III transcribed gene (*7SL RNA*).

Retroposition of processed pseudogenes can serve as a mechanism of gene duplication *(35–37)*. However, unless they acquire a new promoter (most pol II genes have promoters upstream of the transcription start), typical processed pseudogenes cannot be expressed. Expression of recently integrated pseudogenes has been reported in several cases *(38–42)*, but it is not clear whether they encode functional proteins. Nevertheless, there are a few examples of retrogenes (i.e., functional and expressed intronless genes derived from retroposed mRNAs) in the human genome *(35,36)*. For example, retroposition can help to amplify X-linked genes, which have only one functional copy in somatic cells. X-linked mutations, thus, often result in loss of function and their transfer to autosomes or amplification on X can revert this phenotype. Several such examples of X-to-autosomes or X-to-X amplification of human as well as mouse genes have been reported *(43–54)*. Along the same lines, processed pseudogenes could also provide a new domain (exon) if they insert into introns of other genes. The only well-documented example of a successful exon shuffling in the human genome identified to date is SCAN domain-containing gene 2 *(SCAND2)*. This member of the SCAN nuclear protein family gene located on 15q25.2 harbors a C-terminal domain derived from the N-terminal part of *C1orf12/EGLN1* (egl nine homolog 1) located on 1q42.2 *(55)*. Despite the examples of functional retropseudogenes or exon shuffling, however, the vast majority of processed pseudogenes are clearly translationally incompetent (owing to truncations or stop codons), and they appear to follow mutation patterns consistent with neutral evolution *(20,27,28)*. Interestingly, such expressed processed pseudogenes without protein coding capacity can act as functional non-coding RNAs. For example, *Makorin1-p1* is an expressed processed pseudogene regulating the mRNA stability of its progenitor gene *Makorin1*. Disruption in the *Makorin1-p1* pseudogene results in polycystic kidneys and bone deformity in mice, demonstrating its importance for *Makorin1* function *(56)*. Searches for expressed pseudogenes in the human genome indicate that this type of regulation may be more common than previously anticipated *(42)*.

The potential contribution of processed pseudogenes to human diseases is far from being understood. Pseudogene integrations may cause insertional inactivation of genes, but, despite many reports of *Alu* and L1 insertion *(57)*, no processed pseudogene-related insertional mutation has been reported to date. Potential regulatory effects of pseudogene transcripts at the RNA level are intriguing, particularly in the light of early speculations on this subject *(58)*. Finally, it should be pointed out that processed pseudogenes (especially expressed copies) may interfere with the analysis of variation of human genes, because they can be misinterpreted as polymorphism or as mutated alleles of the functional genes.

HUMAN ENDOGENOUS RETROVIRUSES

Retroviruses belong to a broad class of (retro)elements that replicate via an RNA intermediate and include LTRs in their DNA copies. The retroviral life cycle is characterized by reverse transcription of the retroviral RNA genome followed by cDNA integration into the host nuclear DNA, where they can persist in the form of a stable integrated provirus. Retroviral infections of early embryonic and germ-line cells can be inherited by subsequent generations and such ancient proviral relics found in the genome are called ERVs. HERVs resemble well-known exogenous retroviruses and carry typical genes found in infectious retroviruses (reviewed in ref. *59*). The group-specific antigen *(gag)* open reading frame encodes internal structural proteins of the retroviral particle, whereas *pro* and *pol* genes encode enzymes necessary for retroviral amplification (Fig. 1B). Replication-competent retroviruses code these three enzymes: RT *(1,2)*, integrase, which inserts retroviral DNA into host chromosome, and protease, which posttranslationally cleaves Gag, Pol, and Env polyproteins into functional proteins. RT also performs an RNA degradation activity, encoded in a separate domain called RHase H. The last open reading frame *env* encodes surface (envelope) glycoproteins required for attachment of retroviral particles to the cellular receptor and penetration into the cell. The affinity for a particular receptor determines retroviral range of infectivity or tropism for cells and tissues expressing the given receptor. The transmembrane subunit of the Env proteins contains a so-called immunosuppressive domain, a conserved 17mer with effects on the proliferation and differentiation of lymphocytes *(60,61)*. Interestingly, the immunosuppressive domains of mammalian C-type retroviruses, including some HERV families, are similar to the analogous segments in the envelope glycoprotein of filoviruses (negative-strand RNA viruses) such as Ebola or Marburg viruses *(62)*. HERVs also may contain other auxiliary genes. Several class II and III families code deoxyuridine triphosphatase (dUTPase) *(63,64; RU)*. Some HERV-K elements encode a 105 aa functional homolog of the Rev/Rex proteins found in human immunodeficiency virus (HIV)-1 and human T-cell leukemia virus (HTLV), respectively. These proteins mediate nuclear transport of unspliced RNAs via the host factor CRM1 *(65,66)*.

The structure of an integrated DNA provirus is different from the structure of its RNA genome *(59)*. During the process of retroviral reverse transcription two identical copies of part of the retroviral sequence, known as long terminal repeats (LTRs), are generated. LTRs are located at both ends of the provirus and flank the protein-coding internal sequence. LTRs harbor the pol II promoter, enhancers, polyA signal, and other regulatory sequences. Typical HERV LTRs have conserved 5'-TG and 3'-CA termini. During integration, 4- to 6-bp target site duplications (TSDs) of the host DNA are created, which flank the integrated provirus. The length of TSDs is determined by the viral integrase and is characteristic of a given retrovirus or family of HERVs.

Since the discovery of the first human endogenous retrovirus in 1981 *(67)*, more than 400,000 HERV fragments have been found in the human genome, contributing approx 9% of human DNA (Table 1) *(3,6,68)*. HERV sequences were classified using several different systems and the nomenclature used in the literature is rather confusing *(69)*. The most frequently used classification is based on the binding site for the tRNA primer. For example, a recently active family of HERVs uses lysine (K) tRNA molecules to prime reverse transcription and is therefore known as HERVK. Although this classification was sufficient during the early years of HERV research, the system became obsolete after the discovery of many other HERV families in the human genome. Progress in classification based on primer binding sites is hampered by the fact that the same tRNA primer can be shared by unrelated families and further complicated by the existence of chimeric elements composed of segments derived from different families. Such chimeras probably arise by co-packaging of two different retroviral RNA into virion and subsequent template switching between the RNAs during reverse transcription *(70)*. Therefore, a different, more flexible classification system of HERVs is used in the RU database *(4)*. This classification uses a combination of traditional names and numbers. RU families are primarily defined based on a substantial DNA sequence divergence from other retroviral families. This classification together with a list of all known HERV families is extensively reviewed in ref. *6*.

Based on their similarity to exogenous retroviruses, HERV families are grouped into three classes. HERVs with homology to mammalian type C retroviruses (gamma retroviruses), such as murine leukemia virus (MLV), have been placed in class I. Class I represents a highly heterogeneous group of HERVs with many different families *(6)*. This class includes numerous nonautonomous families, some of which constitute a distinct subgroup called MER4. In addition, many class I elements are chimeras composed of segments derived from unrelated retroviruses. All class I families are flanked by 4–5 bp TSDs. Class II consists of HERVs related to mammalian type B and D retroviruses (beta retroviruses) represented by mouse mammary tumor virus. This class is often referred as the HERVK group, because most of the families use lysine (K) tRNA as the primer for reverse transcription. The HERVK elements are flanked by 6 bp target site duplications. In 1995, a new group (class III) of endogenous retroviruses similar to human foamy viruses (*Spumaviridae*) was discovered *(71)*. HERVL is a prototypic member of this group. With the exception of HERV18 and HERVL66, all other class III families lack *env*-like ORFs *(6)*. In addition to several families with similarity to retroviral proteins, this group contains a large number of nonautonomous elements known as mammalian apparent LTR retrotransposons (MaLRs) and THE1. All class III elements are flanked by 5 bp TSDs. No endogenous counterparts of exogenous lentiviruses such as HIV are known in the human genome. All retroviruses including HERVs belong to the *copia* superfamily of LTR-retrotransposons; no other superfamilies of LTR-retrotransposons have been detected in the human genome. Surprisingly, however, the human genome contains eight cellular genes with significant similarity to gypsy superfamily of LTR retrotransposons, probably derived from very old gypsy elements, whose remnants cannot be otherwise detected in genomic DNA *(6,72–74)*.

Endogenous retroviruses, although still active in mice *(75)*, are nearly extinct in the human genome. However, some class I elements contain potentially functional ORFs *(69,76–80*; RU). Class III elements are found in all placental mammals, and some lineages including simians and mice (but not rats) exhibit sustained activity of these elements *(63,71,81,82)*. In the human genome, on the other hand, class III elements lost their activity long ago and their age ranges from approx 20 to 150 million years *(6)*. Class II embraces the most recent retroviruses found in the human genome (HERVK10), many of which are human-specific *(83,84)*, and the youngest elements appear to be only approximately 1 million years old *(85)*. Only three elements in the human genome seem to harbor all full-length ORFs *(3)*. The most preserved HERVK element potentially capable of reinfections is known to be polymorphic in human populations *(86)*.

The genomic distribution of HERVs is a result of many factors including the integration preference, intensity of recombination, selection, and so on. Although there are no new HERV insertions reported, HERV integration preferences can be approximated from exogenous retroviruses such as HIV and MLV. HIV preferentially integrates into gene- and GC-rich regions *(87,88)*. MLV also targets genes, especially positions around transcription start sites *(89)*. In contrast to these exogenous retroviruses, HERVs are underrepresented in GC-rich regions and especially in genes, probably owing to interference of retroviral polyA signals with gene transcription if they are inserted in the sense orientation relative to transcription *(90)*. Recombination between two direct LTRs of a provirus leave a single copy of the LTR (solo LTR) in the genome *(91)*, and the remaining LTR with the internal sequence is discarded in the form of a circular episomal DNA. Approximately 90% of HERV genomic elements are such solo LTRs *(3)*. Full-length elements are mostly found in regions with low recombination rates, such as AT-rich regions or chromosome Y *(3,30,90,92,93)*. Thus, the HERV distribution is strikingly different from the insertional pattern of exogenous retroviruses and mostly reflects post-insertional processes.

The extent of HERV contribution to human diseases is a subject of considerable debate in the field. On the DNA level, HERV-mediated rearrangements are relatively rare as HERVs are essentially extinct in humans, and no HERV-related insertion is reported in mutational databases. Because of the ancient origin of most HERV copies and the existence of relatively low copy number families, the presence of highly similar, closely spaced HERV copies prone to recombination is infrequent. Indeed, recombination between two HERVs is a sporadic source of genomic instabilities *(6)*. One example involves recurrent deletions of Y-linked azoospermia factor a (*AZFa*) gene by homologous recombination between two HERV15 copies, associated with male infertility *(94–97)*. Recombination between solo LTRs has also contributed to allelic variation of the *HLA* locus in the human population *(98,99)*.

Expression of endogenous retroviruses has been implicated in the etiology of various human diseases including cancer and autoimmune disorders (reviewed in refs. *100–103*). We should stress, however, that the potential contribution of HERVs to these diseases is a highly controversial issue *(102,104–108)*, and despite two decades of research on the pathogenic potential of endogenous retroviruses, convincing evidence linking HERVs to diseases is still lacking.

Aside from the negative outcomes of retroviral insertions and recombinations on the host cell, retroviral regulatory elements and proteins could serve as a new source of material for evolutionary experiments. Indeed, there are several examples of HERV-derived promoters, polyA signals and other regulatory signals recruited by the host genome *(6,109–111)*. One famous example represents a HERVE insertion into the promoter of the amylase gene cluster during primate evolution, which stimulated rearrangements of this locus accompanied by the emergence of amylase expression in salivary glands *(112,113)*. Also, genes of protein-coding repetitive elements including HERVs may occasionally be recruited by the host genome as functional cellular genes. Notably, two *env* genes from the HERVW/HERV17 and HERV-FRD/MER50 families seem to serve as functional human genes coding for the syncytin proteins responsible for cell fusion during differentiation of the syncythiotrophoblast in the human placenta *(114–116)*. The extent of such contributions to cellular functions is unclear and the number of unequivocal cases of HERVs benefiting the host is very limited *(6)*.

DNA TRANSPOSONS

Approximately 5% of the human genome is derived from ancient copies of DNA transposons (Table 1) *(6)*. Preserved copies of DNA transposons are flanked by terminal inverted repeats (TIRs) of variable length (Fig. 1C). The main enzyme encoded by autonomous DNA transposons is called transposase. Trasposase has several activities: it specifically binds to TIRs, excises the integrated copy and pastes it to another place in the genome (cut-and-paste process). After insertion, 2- to 10-bp duplications of the target site are created. DNA transposons amplify by co-replicating with the host DNA as they preferentially excise from already replicated DNA and reinsert into nonreplicated segments. This asymmetric replication theoretically increases the number of DNA transposons by a factor of 1.5, though the real efficiency of this process is probably lower.

Human transposons represent ancient genomic fossils hardly recognizable at the DNA level. Consequently, the first evidence disclosing the presence of DNA transposons in the human genome was not obtained until large amounts of human genomic sequence became available *(117)*. To date, six transposon superfamilies have been found in humans: Mariner/Tc1, hAT, piggyBac, MuDR, Harbinger, and P-like elements (Table 1) *(6)*. Without exception, all these families became extinct in the past and no transposition-competent element is preserved in humans.

As in the case of other very old repeats, the pathogenic potential of human DNA transposons is probably very limited. Mariner elements were detected in a large number of genomic duplications including those linked to the Charcot-Marie-Tooth disease type 1A (CMT1A) duplication, and to hereditary neuropathy with liability to pressure palsies (HNPP) deletions *(118,119)*. However, the proposed involvement of the Mariner transposase in generating double stranded breaks stimulating the rearrangements *(118)* seems speculative given the fact that no translation-competent Mariner copy is found in the human genome. Yet, it should be noted that the human genome contains nearly 30 genes that were derived from DNA transposons and appear to be preserved between mammals and many vertebrates *(6)*. Well known recruited transposases include: RAG1, a part of V(D)J recombinase complex producing functional immunoglobulin and T-cell receptor genes in developing lymphocytes *(120)*, centromere protein CENP-B *(117)*, an the more recently described MER53 *(121)*, Jerky *(122)*, and HARBI1 *(123)*. Interestingly, the majority of known human genes derived from TEs evolved from DNA transposons. This is probably related to the fact that transposases are extremely diverged, as there is practically no detectable similarity between transposases from different superfamilies. Transposases, thus, provide a wide repertoire of sequence variants compared to more conserved retrotransposon proteins *(6)*. Although the function of the transposon-derived genes is mostly unknown, it is likely that they are involved in DNA recognition and rearrangements. Consequently, they may contribute to pathological genomic rearrangements. Notably, it has been shown that RAG1 nicking may stimulate homologous recombination *(124)* and also chromosomal translocation both in vivo and in vitro *(125)*. Finally, human cells seem to be in general permissive to DNA transposons *(126)* and these elements can, thus, be used as vectors for gene therapy *(127)*.

SUMMARY

The human genome has preserved a substantial fraction of ancient DNA transposons, MIR SINEs, L2, and L3 LINEs, that have limited potential to stimulate genomic rearrangements. Some HERVs have amplified more recently and sporadically stimulate genetic instabilities. Several processed pseudogenes, DNA transposons, as well as both ancient and recent LTR-retrotransposons were recruited by the host genome as new genes. Particularly intriguing is the presence of many genes derived from transposases of DNA transposons. Given the endonucleolytic activity of the transposases, it is possible that these recruited genes are involved in DNA processing.

REFERENCES

1. Temin HM, Mizutani S. RNA-dependent DNA polymerase in virions of Rous sarcoma virus. Nature 1970;226:1211–1213.
2. Baltimore D. RNA-dependent DNA polymerase in virions of RNA tumour viruses. Nature 1970;226: 1209–1211.
3. International Human Genome Sequencing Consortium. Initial sequencing and analysis of the human genome. Nature 2001;409:860–921.
4. Jurka J. Repbase update: a database and an electronic journal of repetitive elements. Trends Genet 2000;16:418–420.
5. Kapitonov VV, Jurka J. The esterase and PHD domains in CR1-like non-LTR retrotransposons. Mol Biol Evol 2003;20:38–46.
6. Kapitonov VV, Pavlicek A, Jurka J. Anthology of Human Repetitive DNA. In: *Encyclopedia of Molecular Cell Biology and Molecular Medicine, vol. 1* (Meyers RA, ed.). Weinheim, Germany: Wiley-VCH 2004; pp 251–306.
7. Luan DD, Korman MH, Jakubczak JL, Eickbush TH. Reverse transcription of R2Bm RNA is primed by a nick at the chromosomal target site: a mechanism for non-LTR retrotransposition. Cell 1993;72:595–605.
8. Smit AF, Riggs AD. MIRs are classic, tRNA-derived SINEs that amplified before the mammalian radiation. Nucleic Acids Res 1995;23:98–102.
9. Okada N, Hamada M, Ogiwara I, Ohshima K. SINEs and LINEs share common 3' sequences: a review. Gene 1997;205:229–243.

10. Jacq C, Miller JR, Brownlee GG. A pseudogene structure in 5S DNA of Xenopus laevis. Cell 1997;12:109–120.
11. Vanin EF. Processed pseudogenes: characteristics and evolution. Annu Rev Genet 1985;19:253–272.
12. Weiner AM, Deininger PL, Efstratiadis A. Nonviral retroposons: genes, pseudogenes, and transposable elements generated by the reverse flow of genetic information. Annu Rev Biochem 1986;55:631–661.
13. Jurka J. Sequence patterns indicate an enzymatic involvement in integration of mammalian retroposons. Proc Natl Acad Sci USA 1997;94:1872–1877.
14. Tchenio T, Segal-Bendirdjian E, Heidmann T. Generation of processed pseudogenes in murine cells. EMBO J 1993;12:1487–1497.
15. Maestre J, Tchenio T, Dhellin O, Heidmann T. mRNA retroposition in human cells: processed pseudogene formation. EMBO J 1995;14:6333–6338.
16. Dhellin O, Maestre J, Heidmann T. Functional differences between the human LINE retrotransposon and retroviral reverse transcriptases for in vivo mRNA reverse transcription. EMBO J 1997;16:6590–6602.
17. Esnault C, Maestre J, Heidmann T. Human LINE retrotransposons generate processed pseudogenes. Nat Genet 2000;24:363–367.
18. Wei W, Gilbert N, Ooi SL, et al. Human L1 retrotransposition: cis preference versus trans complementation. Mol Cell Biol 2001;21:1429–1439.
19. Ohshima K, Hattori M, Yada T, Gojobori T, Sakaki Y, Okada N. Whole-genome screening indicates a possible burst of formation of processed pseudogenes and Alu repeats by particular L1 subfamilies in ancestral primates. Genome Biol 2003;4:R74.
20. Zhang Z, Harrison PM, Liu Y, Gerstein M. Millions of years of evolution preserved: a comprehensive catalog of the processed pseudogenes in the human genome. Genome Res 2003;13:2541–2558.
21. Pavlicek A, Jabbari K, Paces J, Paces V, Hejnar J, Bernardi G. Similar integration but different stability of Alus and LINEs in the human genome. Gene 2001;276:39–45.
22. Zhang Z, Harrison P, Gerstein M. Identification and analysis of over 2000 ribosomal protein pseudogenes in the human genome. Genome Res 2002;12:1466–1482.
23. Pavlicek A, Paces J, Zika R, Hejnar J. Length distribution of long interspersed nucleotide elements (LINEs) and processed pseudogenes of human endogenous retroviruses: implications for retrotransposition and pseudogene detection. Gene 2002;300:189–194.
24. Zhang Z, Gerstein M. Identification and characterization of over 100 mitochondrial ribosomal protein pseudogenes in the human genome. Genomics 2003;81:468–480.
25. Strichman-Almashanu LZ, Bustin M, Landsman D. Retroposed copies of the HMG genes: a window to genome dynamics. Genome Res 2003;13:800–812.
26. Jamain S, Girondot M, Leroy P, et al. Transduction of the human gene FAM8A1 by endogenous retrovirus during primate evolution. Genomics 2001;78:38–45.
27. Goncalves I, Duret L, Mouchiroud D. Nature and structure of human genes that generate retropseudogenes. Genome Res 2000;10:672–678.
28. Torrents D, Suyama M, Zdobnov E, Bork P. A genome-wide survey of human pseudogenes. Genome Res 2003;13:2559–2567.
29. Harrison PM, Hegyi H, Balasubramanian S, et al. Molecular fossils in the human genome: identification and analysis of the pseudogenes in chromosomes 21 and 22. Genome Res 2002;12:272–280.
30. Pavlicek A, Paces J, EllederD, Hejnar J. Processed pseudogenes of human endogenous retroviruses generated by LINEs: their integration, stability, and distribution. Genome Res 2002;12:391–399.
31. Ejima Y, Yang L. Trans mobilization of genomic DNA as a mechanism for retrotransposon-mediated exon shuffling. Hum Mol Genet 2003;12:1321–1328.
32. Goodchild NL, Freeman JD, Mager DL. Spliced HERV-H endogenous retroviral sequences in human genomic DNA: evidence for amplification via retrotransposition. Virology 1995;206:164–173.
33. Costas J. Characterization of the intragenomic spread of the human endogenous retrovirus family HERV-W. Mol Biol Evol 2002;19:526–533.
34. Boeke JD. LINEs and Alus: the polyA connection. Nat Genet 1997;16:6–7.
35. Brosius J. RNAs from all categories generate retrosequences that may be exapted as novel genes or regulatory elements. Gene 1999;238:115–134.
36. Gentles AJ, Karlin S. Why are human G-protein-coupled receptors predominantly intronless? Trends Genet 1999;15:47–49.
37. Harrison PM, Gerstein M. Studying genomes through the aeons: protein families, pseudogenes and proteome evolution. J Mol Biol 2002;318:1155–1174.

38. McCarrey JR, Kumari M, Aivaliotis MJ, et al. Analysis of the cDNA and encoded protein of the human testis-specific PGK-2 gene. Dev Genet 1996;19:321–332.
39. Fujii GH, Morimoto AM, Berson AE, Bolen JB. Transcriptional analysis of the PTEN/MMAC1 pseudogene, psiPTEN. Oncogene 1999;18:1765–1769.
40. Olsen MA, Schechter LE. Cloning, mRNA localization and evolutionary conservation of a human 5-HT7 receptor pseudogene. Gene 1999;227:63–69.
41. Reyes A, Mezzina M, Gadaleta G. Human mitochondrial transcription factor A (mtTFA): gene structure and characterization of related pseudogenes. Gene 2002;291:223–232.
42. Yano Y, Saito R, Yoshida N, et al. A new role for expressed pseudogenes as ncRNA: regulation of mRNA stability of its homologous coding gene. J Mol Med 2004;82:414–422.
43. McCarrey JR, Thomas K. Human testis-specific PGK gene lacks introns and possesses characteristics of a processed gene. Nature 1987;326:501–505.
44. Ashworth A, Skene B, Swift S, Lovell-Badge R. Zfa is an expressed retroposon derived from an alternative transcript of the Zfx gene. EMBO J 1990;9:1529–1534.
45. Dahl HH, Brown RM, Hutchison WM, Maragos C, Brown GK. A testis-specific form of the human pyruvate dehydrogenase E1 alpha subunit is coded for by an intronless gene on chromosome 4. Genomics 1990;8:225–232.
46. Mardon G, Luoh SW, Simpson EM, Gill G, Brown LG, Page DC. Mouse Zfx protein is similar to Zfy-2: each contains an acidic activating domain and 13 zinc fingers. Mol Cell Biol 1990;10:681–688.
47. Sargent CA, Young C, Marsh S, Ferguson-Smith MA, Affara NA. The glycerol kinase gene family: structure of the Xp gene, and related intronless retroposons. Hum Mol Genet 1994;3:1317–1324.
48. Hendriksen PJ, Hoogerbrugge JW, Baarends WM, et al. Testis-specific expression of a functional retroposon encoding glucose-6-phosphate dehydrogenase in the mouse. Genomics 1997;41:350–359.
49. Sedlacek Z, Munstermann E, Dhorne-Pollet S, et al. Human and mouse XAP-5 and XAP-5-like (X5L) genes: identification of an ancient functional retroposon differentially expressed in testis. Genomics 1999;61:125–132.
50. Elliott DJ, Venables JP, Newton CS, et al. An evolutionarily conserved germ cell-specific hnRNP is encoded by a retrotransposed gene. Hum Mol Genet 2000;9:2117–2124.
51. Dass B, McMahon KW, Jenkins NA, Gilbert DJ, Copeland NG, MacDonald CC. The gene for a variant form of the polyadenylation protein CstF-64 is on chromosome 19 and is expressed in pachytene spermatocytes in mice. J Biol Chem 2001;276:8044–8050.
52. Wang PJ, Page DC. Functional substitution for TAF(II)250 by a retroposed homolog that is expressed in human spermatogenesis. Hum Mol Genet 2002;11:2341–2346.
53. Emerson JJ, Kaessmann H, Betran E, Long M. Extensive gene traffic on the mammalian X chromosome. Science 2004;303:537–540.
54. Bradley J, Baltus A, Skaletsky H, Royce-Tolland M, Dewar K, Page DC. An X-to-autosome retrogene is required for spermatogenesis in mice. Nat Genet 2004;36:872–876.
55. Dupuy D, Duperat VG, Arveiler B. SCAN domain-containing 2 gene (SCAND2) is a novel nuclear protein derived from the zinc finger family by exon shuffling. Gene 2002;289:1–6.
56. Hirotsune S, Yoshida N, Chen A, et al. An expressed pseudogene regulates the messenger-RNA stability of its homologous coding gene. Nature 2003;423:91–96.
57. Ostertag EM, Kazazian HH Jr. Biology of mammalian L1 retrotransposons. Annu Rev Genet 2001;35:501–538.
58. Scherrer K. Control of gene expression in animal cells: the cascade regulation hypothesis revisited. Adv Exp Med Biol 1974;44:169–219.
59. Coffin JM, Hughes SH, Varmus HE. *Retroviruses*. Cold Spring Harbor Laboratory Press, New York, NY, 1997.
60. Cianciolo GJ, Copeland TD, Oroszlan S, Snyderman R. Inhibition of lymphocyte proliferation by a synthetic peptide homologous to retroviral envelope proteins. Science 1985;230:453–455.
61. Sonigo P, Barker C, Hunter E, Wain-Hobson S. Nucleotide sequence of Mason-Pfizer monkey virus: an immunosuppressive D-type retrovirus. Cell 1986;45:375–385.
62. Bukreyev A, Volchkov VE, Blinov VM, Netesov SV. The GP-protein of Marburg virus contains the region similar to the 'immunosuppressive domain' of oncogenic retrovirus P15E proteins. FEBS Lett 1993;323:183–187.
63. Benit L, Lallemand JB, Casella JF, Philippe H, Heidmann T. ERV-L elements: a family of endogenous retrovirus-like elements active throughout the evolution of mammals. J Virol 1999;73:3301–3308.

64. Yin H, Medstrand P, Kristofferson A, Dietrich U, Aman P, Blomberg J. Characterization of human MMTV-like (HML) elements similar to a sequence that was highly expressed in a human breast cancer: further definition of the HML-6 group. Virology 1999;256:22–35.

65. Magin C, Lower R, Lower J. cORF and RcRE, the Rev/Rex and RRE/RxRE homologues of the human endogenous retrovirus family HTDV/HERV-K. J Virol 1999;73:9496–9507.

66. Yang J, Bogerd HP, Peng S, Wiegand H, Truant R, Cullen BR. An ancient family of human endogenous retroviruses encodes a functional homolog of the HIV-1 Rev protein. Proc Natl Acad Sci USA 1999;96:13,404–13,408.

67. Martin MA, Bryan T, Rasheed S, Khan AS. Identification and cloning of endogenous retroviral sequences present in human DNA. Proc Natl Acad Sci USA 1981;78:4892–4896.

68. Paces J, Pavlicek A, Zika R, Kapitonov VV, Jurka J, Paces V. HERVd: the Human Endogenous RetroViruses Database: update. Nucleic Acids Res 2004;32:D50.

69. Wilkinson DA, Mager DL, Leong JC. Endogenous human retroviruses. In: *The Retroviridae* (Levy, J. A., ed.). New York, NY: Plenum Press, 1994; pp 465–535.

70. Zhang J, Temin HM. Rate and mechanism of nonhomologous recombination during a single cycle of retroviral replication. Science 1993;259:234–238.

71. Cordonnier A, Casella JF, Heidmann T. Isolation of novel human endogenous retrovirus-like elements with foamy virus-related pol sequence. J Virol 1995;69:5890–5897.

72. Charlier C, Segers K, Wagenaar D, et al. Human-ovine comparative sequencing of a 250-kb imprinted domain encompassing the callipyge (clpg) locus and identification of six imprinted transcripts: DLK1, DAT, GTL2, PEG11, antiPEG11, and MEG8. Genome Res 2001;11:850–862.

73. Ono R, Kobayashi S, Wagatsuma H, et al. A retrotransposon-derived gene, PEG10, is a novel imprinted gene located on human chromosome 7q21. Genomics 2001;73:232–237.

74. Lynch C, Tristem M. A co-opted gypsy-type LTR-retrotransposon is conserved in the genomes of humans, sheep, mice, and rats. Curr Biol 2003;13:1518–1523.

75. Dewannieux M, Dupressoir A, Harper F, Pierron G, Heidmann T. Identification of autonomous IAP LTR retrotransposons mobile in mammalian cells. Nat Genet 2004;36:534–539.

76. Cohen M, Powers M, O'Connell C, Kato N. The nucleotide sequence of the env gene from the human provirus ERV3 and isolation and characterization of an ERV3-specific cDNA. Virology 1985;147:449–458.

77. Blond JL, Beseme F, Duret L, et al. Molecular characterization and placental expression of HERV-W, a new human endogenous retrovirus family. J Virol 1999;73:1175–1185.

78. Kjellman C, Sjogren HO, Salford LG, Widegren B. HERV-F (XA34) is a full-length human endogenous retrovirus expressed in placental and fetal tissues. Gene 1999;239:99–107.

79. Lindeskog M, Mager DL, Blomberg J. Isolation of a human endogenous retroviral HERV-H element with an open env reading frame. Virology 1999;258:441–450.

80. Benit L, Dessen P, Heidmann T. Identification, phylogeny, and evolution of retroviral elements based on their envelope genes. J Virol 2001;75:11,709–11,719.

81. Mouse Genome Sequencing Consortium. Initial sequencing and comparative analysis of the mouse genome. Nature 2002;420:520–562.

82. Rat Genome Sequencing Project Consortium. Genome sequence of the Brown Norway rat yields insights into mammalian evolution. Nature 2004;428:493–521.

83. Medstrand P, Mager DL. Human-specific integrations of the HERV-K endogenous retrovirus family. J Virol 1998;72:9782–9787.

84. Barbulescu M, Turner G, Seaman MI, Deinard AS, Kidd KK, Lenz J. Many human endogenous retrovirus K (HERV-K) proviruses are unique to humans. Curr Biol 1999;9:861–868.

85. Mayer J, Sauter M, Racz A, Scherer D, Mueller-Lantzsch N, Meese E. An almost-intact human endogenous retrovirus K on human chromosome 7. Nat Genet 1999;21:257–258.

86. Turner G, Barbulescu M, Su M, Jensen-Seaman MI, Kidd KK, Lenz J. Insertional polymorphisms of full-length endogenous retroviruses in humans. Curr Biol 2001;11:1531–1535.

87. Elleder D, Pavlicek A, Paces J, Hejnar J. Preferential integration of human immunodeficiency virus type 1 into genes, cytogenetic R bands and GC-rich DNA regions: insight from the human genome sequence. FEBS Lett 2002;517:285–286.

88. Schroder AR, Shinn P, Chen H, Berry C, Ecker JR, Bushman F. HIV-1 integration in the human genome favors active genes and local hotspots. Cell 2002;110:521–529.

89. Wu X, Li Y, Crise B, Burgess SM. Transcription start regions in the human genome are favored targets for MLV integration. Science 2003;300:1749–1751.

90. Smit AF. Interspersed repeats and other mementos of transposable elements in mammalian genomes. Curr Opin Genet Dev 1999;9:657–663.

91. Mager DL, Goodchild NL. Homologous recombination between the LTRs of a human retrovirus-like element causes a 5-kb deletion in two siblings. Am J Hum Genet 1989;45:848–854.

92. Erlandsson R, Wilson JF, Paabo S. Sex chromosomal transposable element accumulation and male-driven substitutional evolution in humans. Mol Biol Evol 2000;17:804–812.

93. Medstrand P, van de Lagemaat LN, Mager DL. Retroelement distributions in the human genome: variations associated with age and proximity to genes. Genome Res 2002;12:1483–1495.

94. Blanco P, Shlumukova M, Sargent CA, Jobling MA, Affara N, Hurles ME. Divergent outcomes of intrachromosomal recombination on the human Y chromosome: male infertility and recurrent polymorphism. J Med Genet 2000;37:752–758.

95. Sun C, Skaletsky H, Rozen S, et al. Deletion of azoospermia factor a (AZFa) region of human Y chromosome caused by recombination between HERV15 proviruses. Hum Mol Genet 2000;9:2291–2296.

96. Kamp C, Hirschmann P, Voss H, Huellen K, Vogt PH. Two long homologous retroviral sequence blocks in proximal Yq11 cause AZFa microdeletions as a result of intrachromosomal recombination events. Hum Mol Genet 2000;9:2563–2572.

97. Kamp C, Huellen K, Fernandes S, et al. High deletion frequency of the complete AZFa sequence in men with Sertoli-cell-only syndrome. Mol Hum Reprod 2001;7:987–994.

98. Kambhu S, Falldorf P, Lee JS. Endogenous retroviral long terminal repeats within the HLA-DQ locus. Proc Natl Acad Sci USA 1990;87:4927–4931.

99. Kulski JK, Gaudieri S, Martin A, Dawkins RL. Coevolution of PERB11 (MIC) and HLA class I genes with HERV-16 and retroelements by extended genomic duplication. J Mol Evol 1999;49:84–97.

100. Nakagawa K, Harrison LC. The potential roles of endogenous retroviruses in autoimmunity. Immunol Rev 1996;152:193–236.

101. Lower R. The pathogenic potential of endogenous retroviruses: facts and fantasies. Trends Microbiol 1999;7:350–356.

102. Nelson PN, Carnegie PR, Martin J, et al. Demystified. Human endogenous retroviruses. Mol Pathol 2003;56:11–18.

103. Perl A. Role of endogenous retroviruses in autoimmune diseases. Rheum Dis Clin North Am 2003;29:123–143.

104. Garson JA, Tuke PW, Giraud P, Paranhos-Baccala G, Perron H. Detection of virion-associated MSRV-RNA in serum of patients with multiple sclerosis. Lancet 1998;351:33.

105. Poser CM. Virion-associated MSRV-RNA in multiple sclerosis. Lancet 1998;351:755.

106. Lower R. Response from Lower. Trends Microbiol 1999;7:431–432.

107. Mager DL. Human endogenous retroviruses and pathogenicity: genomic considerations. Trends Microbiol 1999;7:431.

108. Stoye JP. The pathogenic potential of endogenous retroviruses: a sceptical view. Trends Microbiol 1999;7:430.

109. Sverdlov ED. Retroviruses and primate evolution. Bioessays 2000;22:161–171.

110. Landry JR, Mager DL, Wilhelm BT. Complex controls: the role of alternative promoters in mammalian genomes. Trends Genet 2003;19:640–648.

111. van de Lagemaat LN, Landry JR, Mager DL, Medstrand P. Transposable elements in mammals promote regulatory variation and diversification of genes with specialized functions. Trends Genet 2003;19:530–536.

112. Samuelson LC, Wiebauer K, Snow CM, Meisler MH. Retroviral and pseudogene insertion sites reveal the lineage of human salivary and pancreatic amylase genes from a single gene during primate evolution. Mol Cell Biol 1990;10:2513–2520.

113. Ting CN, Rosenberg MP, Snow CM, Samuelson LC, Meisler MH. Endogenous retroviral sequences are required for tissue-specific expression of a human salivary amylase gene. Genes Dev 1992;6:1457–1465.

114. Blond JL, Lavillette D, Cheynet V, et al. An envelope glycoprotein of the human endogenous retrovirus HERV-W is expressed in the human placenta and fuses cells expressing the type D mammalian retrovirus receptor. J Virol 2000;74:3321–3329.

115. Mi S, Lee X, Li X, et al. Syncytin is a captive retroviral envelope protein involved in human placental morphogenesis. Nature 2000;403:785–789.

116. Blaise S, de Parseval N, Benit L, Heidmann T. Genomewide screening for fusogenic human endogenous retrovirus envelopes identifies syncytin 2, a gene conserved on primate evolution. Proc Natl Acad Sci USA 2003;100:13,013–13,018.

117. Smit AF, Riggs AD. Tiggers and DNA transposon fossils in the human genome. Proc Natl Acad Sci USA 1996;93:1443–1448.

118. Reiter LT, Murakami T, Koeuth T, et al. A recombination hotspot responsible for two inherited peripheral neuropathies is located near a mariner transposon-like element. Nat Genet 1996;12:288–297.

119. Reiter LT, Liehr T, Rautenstrauss B, Robertson HM, Lupski JR. Localization of mariner DNA transposons in the human genome by PRINS. Genome Res 1999;9:839–843.

120. Kapitonov VV, Jurka J. RAG1 core and V(D)J recombination signal sequences were derived from Transib transposons. PLoS Biol 2005;3:e181.

121. Kapitonov VV, Jurka J. MER53, a non-autonomous DNA transposon associated with a variety of functionally related defense genes in the human genome. DNA Seq 1998;8:277–288.

122. Jurka J, Kapitonov VV. Sectorial mutagenesis by transposable elements. Genetica 1999;107:239–248.

123. Kapitonov VV, Jurka J. Harbinger transposons and an ancient HARBI1 gene derived from a transposase. DNA Cell Biol 2004;23:311–324.

124. Lee GS, Neiditch MB, Salus SS, Roth DB. RAG proteins shepherd double-strand breaks to a specific pathway, suppressing error-prone repair, but RAG nicking initiates homologous recombination. Cell 2004;117:171–184.

125. Raghavan SC, Swanson PC, Wu X, Hsieh CL, Lieber MR. A non-B-DNA structure at the Bcl-2 major breakpoint region is cleaved by the RAG complex. Nature 2004;428:88–93.

126. Ivics Z, Hackett PB, Plasterk RH, Izsvak Z. Molecular reconstruction of Sleeping Beauty, a Tc1-like transposon from fish, and its transposition in human cells. Cell 1997;91:501–510.

127. Yant SR, Meuse L, Chiu W, Ivics Z, Izsvak Z, Kay MA. Somatic integration and long-term transgene expression in normal and haemophilic mice using a DNA transposon system. Nat Genet 2000;25:35–41.

128. Jurka J. Repeats in genomic DNA: mining and meaning. Curr Opin Struct Biol 1998;8:333–337.

5 Segmental Duplications

Andrew J. Sharp, PhD and Evan E. Eichler, PhD

Contents

INTRODUCTION

Until recent times, the identification and characterization of segmental duplications has often been based purely on anecdotal reports. However, the completion of the Human Genome Project has now made possible the systematic analysis of the extent and distribution of duplicated sequences in humans. Both *in situ* hybridization and *in silico* approaches have shown that approx 5% of our genome is composed of highly homologous duplicated sequence *(1,2)*, with enrichments of six- to sevenfold in pericentromeric *(3)*, and two- to threefold in subtelomeric regions *(4)*, respectively. Not only does the presence of these paralogous segments represent a significant challenge to the correct assembly of the human genome, but there is also an increasing awareness of their role in human evolution, variation, and disease.

We present a review of segmental duplications in the mammalian genome. We describe their basic characteristics, distribution, and dynamic nature during recent evolutionary history. Based on these features, we discuss models to account for the proliferation of these sequences in the mammalian lineage, and also their contribution towards karyotypic evolution and phenotypic differences between primates. Finally, we highlight the role of segmental duplications as mediators of human variation at the genomic level.

FEATURES OF SEGMENTAL DUPLICATIONS

Human segmental duplications (also termed low-copy repeats) are blocks of DNA ranging from 1 to 200 kb in length that occur at more than one site within the genome and share a high level (often >90%) of sequence identity. They can include both genic sequences and high-copy repeats, such as long interspersed elements and short interspersed elements, and, unlike tandem duplications, are interspersed throughout the genome. This unique distribution pattern

From: *Genomic Disorders: The Genomic Basis of Disease*
Edited by: J. R. Lupski and P. Stankiewicz © Humana Press, Totowa, NJ

suggests that segmental duplications arise through a process termed duplicative transposition, whereby whole blocks of sequence are first duplicated and then transposed from one genomic location to another. Although they have been identified on every human chromosome, their distribution is nonuniform with some chromosomes and chromosomal regions showing peculiar enrichment. Segmental duplications tend to cluster within pericentromeric and, to a lesser extent, subtelomeric regions. Many human pericentromeric regions in particular contain high concentrations of duplicated sequence, often arranged in large blocks composed of complex modular structures of individual duplications *(3)*.

Segmental duplications may be further classified based on their chromosomal distribution. Although some blocks of sequence may be duplicated to multiple locations within a single chromosome (termed intrachromosomal duplication), others may be located on non-homologous chromosomes (inter- or transchromosomal duplication). Intriguingly, the distribution of these two types of duplication appears to be largely exclusive of one another *(2)*, suggesting mechanistic differences in their mode of propagation.

Intrachromosomal Duplications

Initial identification of chromosome-specific duplications often came about through the study of common microdeletion/micoduplication syndromes, such as Prader-Willi/Angelman syndromes, Williams-Beuren syndrome, Smith-Magenis syndrome, Charcot-Marie-Tooth disease type 1A, and DiGeorge/Velocardiofacial syndrome *(5)*. As more of these syndromes were analyzed, it became apparent that the presence of large and highly homologous segmental duplications flanking these sites of rearrangement was a recurring theme. Available evidence suggests that homology between these duplicated sequences acts as a substrate for unequal meiotic recombination, leading to the deletion, duplication, or inversion of the intervening sequence (Fig. 1). Review of known genomic disorders caused by chromosome-specific duplications shows that these usually involve duplications that are more than 95% similar and 10–500 kb in length, separated by 50 kb to 4 Mb of DNA *(5)*.

Although intrachromosomal duplications are found throughout the euchromatic portions of virtually every human chromosome, some chromosomes, such as 1, 9, 16, 17, and 22, show particularly high concentrations within their most proximal regions *(2)*. In these cases the density of duplication can be such that little or no unique sequence occurs across relatively large stretches (300 kb to 4 Mb) of DNA. The organization of these regions can be complex, with large duplication blocks often composed of smaller modules, which have been derived from different genomic locations. This feature has often led to difficulties in characterizing these regions, necessitating the development of specialized methods to allow these regions to be successfully mapped and sequenced.

Many intrachromosomal duplications also share very high levels of sequence identity, with the majority having more than 95% identity between paralogous copies. In extreme cases, this level of nucleotide identity approaches the frequency of allelic variation found in the genome as a whole (approx 1 base per kilobase) *(6)*. This property further confounds the mapping and identification of individual duplicated segments within the genome, and may also represent a significant impediment in the ability to distinguish true allelic polymorphism from paralogous genomic copies *(7–9)*. Indeed, both gene and single nucleotide polymorphism annotation show significant improvements in accuracy when duplicated sequences are correctly defined within a genome assembly *(10)*. Thus, the correct definition of segmental duplications is an important aspect of achieving high-quality genomic sequence *(11)*.

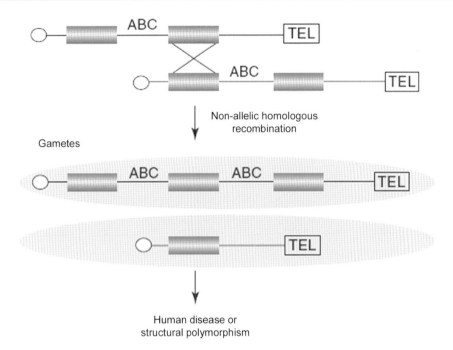

Fig. 1. Segmental duplications mediate structural rearrangement. Misalignment of paralogous blocks of sequence during meiosis leads to unequal recombination and the deletion or duplication of the intervening sequence. These events may create structural polymorphisms or, if the genes (A,B,C) flanked by the duplications are dosage sensitive, genomic disease. ○, centromere; TEL, telomere. (Reproduced with permission from ref. *95*.)

Based on the neutral mutation rate in primates of approx 1.5×10^{-9} substitutions per site per year *(12)*, the high levels of homology observed between many chromosome-specific duplications suggests they have emerged only recently during evolutionary history. Indeed, comparative analysis of different primate lineages has demonstrated that some are species-specific, confirming their dynamic nature *(13)*. In other cases, analysis of the levels of sequence divergence between pairs of duplication in different primates, such as those flanking the common Williams-Beuren syndrome deletion region in 7q11.23 and the large palindromic repeats on long arm of the Y chromosome, has provided evidence that they may also act as substrates for gene conversion *(14–16)*.

Although fluorescence *in situ* hybridization analysis shows the presence of these duplications in multiple primate species, thus, suggesting they originated before the separation of these lineages, estimates of their evolutionary age based on the rate of nucleotide divergence because of random mutation suggest a much more recent origin *(17,18)*. One explanation for this apparent contradiction is that the homology between pairs of repeats acts as a substrate for gene conversion events, thus, homogenizing their sequence and maintaining unexpectedly high levels of identity. Although less likely, an alternative explanation is that some segments of DNA have duplicated to the same genomic location independently in different primate lineages.

Interchromosomal Duplications

The most striking property of duplications that map to nonhomologous chromosomes is their propensity to accumulate adjacent to certain regions of the genome, particularly in pericentromeric and subtelomeric regions and in the short arms of the acrocentric chromosomes. *In silico* analysis has shown a six- to sevenfold enrichment of duplicated segments within 100 kb and 1 Mb of telomeres and centromeres, respectively *(3)*, and more than one-third of all interchromosomal duplications have a pericentromeric localization. Indeed, interchromosomal duplication has been one of the major forces involved in remodeling these chromosomal regions in recent primate evolution *(3)*.

As with chromosome-specific duplications, many of which have been implicated as mediators of recurrent microdeletion/microduplication syndromes, certain interchromosomal duplications have also been associated with recurrent chromosomal rearrangement *(19–21)*, albeit at much lower frequencies. In addition, certain pericentromeric and subtelomeric regions have been found to exhibit polymorphic variation within the human population, indicating that the process of interchromosomal duplication is ongoing *(22,23)*.

DISTRIBUTION OF SEGMENTAL DUPLICATIONS

One of the most remarkable features of segmental duplications is their tendency to often cluster in close proximity to one another, particularly within peri- and subtelomeric regions (Fig. 2). However, detailed mapping and sequencing studies show that the tendency for segmental duplications to accumulate within these regions is not a universal property of all human chromosomes. Although some human chromosomes (e.g., 7, 9, 15, 16, 17, 19, 22, and Y) are significantly enriched for duplications, certain pericentromeric regions, such as those on chromosomes 3, 4, and 19, are almost completely devoid of duplications *(2,3)*.

Study of other sequenced organisms shows that this propensity for duplications to accumulate in clusters within specific chromosomal regions is not unique to humans. Analysis of the working draft sequences of both *Rattus norvegicus* and *Mus musculus* shows that in both organisms, duplicated sequences are distributed nonrandomly, often occurring in large blocks with a distinct pericentromeric and subtelomeric bias *(24–26)*, suggesting that the genomic distribution of segmental duplications may be a general property of mammalian chromosomal architecture.

Pericentromeric Regions

Although the phenomenon of pericentromeric duplication is common to both men and mice, the properties of these duplicated regions differ. Typically, those found in mice are relatively small (<75 kb), whereas in humans they may be several 100 kb in length, and the degree of sequence identity between pairs of duplications are often much lower (<97% in mice compared with >97% in humans) *(8,28)*. Although this latter property may be, in part, because the higher neutral mutation rate in mice *(29)*, it suggests that many of the pericentromeric duplications in humans are evolutionary younger, and, therefore, more recently active, than those in mice.

This is supported by the fact that certain pericentromeric duplications are unique to the human lineage, and are either completely absent or occur at different chromosomal locations in other mammalian species. Indeed, the process of pericentromeric duplication appears to have occurred as punctuated events during primate evolution. Certain duplicated segments, such as those containing the genes *ALD* and *CTR*, are common to humans, chimpanzees, and

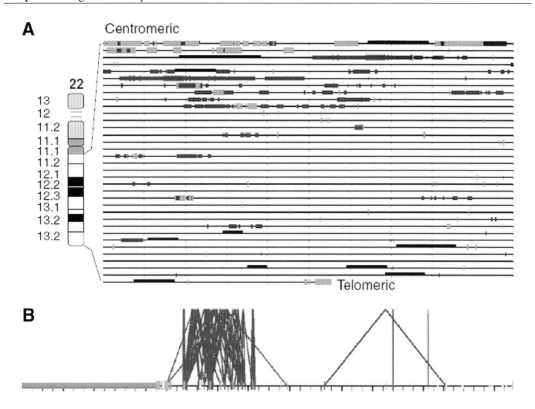

Fig. 2. Segmental duplications on chromosome 22. (A) An overview of duplicated sequence on the long arm of chromosome 22 *(27)*. A total of 715 duplications >1 kb in length and >90% sequence identity were identified. Each horizontal line represents 1 Mb. Top left-hand corner is the most centromeric sequence contig and at the bottom right is the most telomeric sequence. Gray bars, interchromosomal duplications between nonhomologous chromosomes; black bars, intrachromosomal duplications. Overall, 9.1% of the q arm is involved in large (>1 kb) duplications, with interchromosomal and intrachromosomal duplications constituting 3.9 and 6.4% of the total sequence, respectively. Note the preponderance of interchromosomal duplications near the centromere and telomere. (B) A reduced view of chromosome 22 (each tick mark represents 1 Mb) showing the relationship of intrachromosomal duplications (black joining lines). This region is enriched for a variety of genomic disorders (e.g., DiGeorge/velocardiofacial syndrome, cat-eye syndrome). (Reproduced with permission from ref. *95*.)

gorillas, but are absent in orangutans, indicating their emergence predates this speciation event approx 12 million years ago *(30–33)*. In contrast, analysis of duplications on chromosome 10 shows that these emerged at various times during primate evolution, ranging from 13 to 28 million years ago *(34)*. This suggests that, at least within the primate lineage, pericentromeric regions are evolutionarily malleable, able to diverge rapidly, and may underlie some of the phenotypic differences present between the great apes.

Analysis of certain pericentromeric regions, such as those on chromosomes 2 and 10, shows not only that these are composed almost exclusively of duplicated sequence, but also provides evidence that duplications often occur preferentially from one pericentromeric region to another *(6,35–39)*. Some duplicated segments, for example those containing *ALD* and *NF1*, occur at multiple different pericentromeric regions, with the most divergent, and therefore presumably progenitor, locus located outside the pericentromeric regions. In addition, complex modules

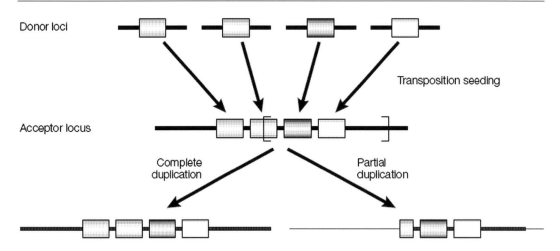

Fig. 3. A two-step model for the generation of pericentromeric duplication. An acceptor region acquires segments 1–200 kb in size from multiple independent regions of the genome (donor loci) by duplicative transposition. These events occur independently over time, creating large blocks of duplicated sequence with a mosaic structure. Secondary duplication events create copies of the initial module at new genomic locations. Because of the whole-scale nature of these latter events, the order and orientation of each constituent duplication is initially preserved within the transposed block. (Reproduced with permission from ref. *68.*)

of juxtaposed duplicated sequence are often found in the same order in multiple different pericentromeric regions. This conservation of both order and orientation of the constituent modules strongly suggests that these duplication blocks were transposed from one pericentromere to another, rather than originating from multiple independent transposition events.

These observations have led to a two-step model for the generation of pericentromeric duplications *(31,36)* (Fig. 3).

1. An initial series of seeding events in which one or more progenitor loci transpose material together to a pericentromeric acceptor location. This series of events creates a mosaic block of duplicated segments derived from different regions of the genome.
2. Subsequent inter- or intrachromosomal duplication events then transpose these large blocks of duplicated sequence and additional flanking material to create copies of the initial module at new genomic locations. Because of the whole-scale nature of these latter events, the order and orientation of each constituent duplication is preserved within the transposed block.

This model has since gained support from more recent studies *(34,40)*, providing an explanation for the complex paralogous structure of many pericentromeric regions of the primate genome.

Subtelomeric Regions

Like pericentromeres, subtelomeric regions appear to preferentially accumulate duplications, and as with pericentromeres, many of these regions also show differences between species and within the human population *(41,42)*. Olfactory receptor (OR) genes present a particularly striking example of this, and appear to have spread by recent subtelomeric duplication. As a species, nearly half of all human subtelomeres contain one or more OR gene copies, although their distribution and copy number shows wide variations both between and within different ethnic groups, attesting to their recent evolutionary origins *(23)*. Similarly, members of the zinc-finger and immunoglobulin heavy-chain gene families are also located within multiple human subtelomeres and, like the OR genes, show marked variations in their copy number and distribution. Indeed, greater than one-third of all subtelomeric regions show high levels of polymorphism (allelic frequency >10%) in their duplication content *(4)*. Such an abundance of gene families in subtelomeric regions is a common feature of most eukaryotes, and may reflect a generally increased recombination and tolerance of subtelomeric DNA for rapid evolutionary change.

Nonrandom Distribution of Duplicated Sequences

A number of different explanations have been put forward in an attempt to explain the propensity for duplications to accumulate within pericentromeric and subtelomeric regions of the genome. Some authors suggest that pericentromeric regions may be the only regions of the genome that are able to accept duplicated material without deleterious phenotypic conse-quence *(37)*. Perhaps owing to a reduced gene density, these regions may have a greater tolerance for duplicative transposition events. However, contrary to the predictions of this model, there are many large euchromatic "gene deserts" outside of the pericentromeres that do not show a similar accumulation of segmental duplications *(43,44)*. This suggests that if an absence of selective constraint is the basis for this pericentromeric bias, lowered gene density is not the cause. Alternatively, the observation that large tracts of duplicated sequence appear to transpose near centromeres and telomeres may simply be an artifact resulting from the fact that recombination is suppressed in these regions. Because of this reduced recombination rate, duplicated sequences may simply persist here for longer than in the rest of the genome, rather than being preferentially targeted to these regions. However, study of other sequenced organ-isms such as *Arabidopsis* and *Drosophila* shows no evidence for a similar accumulation of duplicated segments within pericentromeric regions, suggesting that this tendency may be a specific property of mammalian chromosomes.

Could specific sequences present in pericentromeric and subtelomeric regions of mamma-lian chromosomes actively target duplication events to these regions? Several authors have hypothesized the presence of hyper-recombinogenic sequences localized within peri-centromeric regions that preferentially attract segmental duplications, and analysis of dupli-cation breakpoints suggests that this is indeed the case. Unusual polypurine/pyrimidine minisatellite-like sequences, termed pericentromeric interspersed repeats, have been identified at the junctions of many duplication breakpoints *(30,31,35,45,46)*. Analysis of duplications of *NF1*, *ABCD1*, and several paralogous sequences on chromosome 10 reveals the presence of flanking arrays of CAGGG, GGGCAAAAAGCCG, GGAA, CATTT, and HSREP522 motifs located at their boundaries.

Although some of these sequences show homology to telomeric repeats and subtelomeric sequences *(30,31,45)*, others have similarity to known recombinogenic sequences, such as *Escherichia coli* Chi recombination signals, G4 DNA, which has been implicated in meiotic pairing of homologous chromosomes, and those found in the immunoglobulin heavy-chain recombination regions that promote nonhomologous sequence exchange events *(47,48)*. These similarities suggest a potential role in facilitating the integration and dispersal of duplicated sequences within pericentromeric regions during recent mammalian evolution. Furthermore, phylogenetic analysis of one of these sequences showed that the repeat was both restricted to the primate lineages in which the duplications arose, and was present within the pericentromeric region before the integration of the duplicated sequences, consistent with a potential role in promoting duplicative integration *(45)*.

A more recent genome-wide analysis of sequence features located at the junctions of duplications suggests that, in addition to certain types of satellite repeats, *Alu–Alu*-mediated recombination events also played a significant role in the recent proliferation of segmental duplications *(49)*. Approximately one-third of all human segmental duplications terminate within *Alu* repeats that were active during the last 45 million years of primate evolution. The primate-specific burst of *Alu* retrotransposition activity that occurred 35–40 million years ago *(50)* suggests a model in which numerous sites of *Alu–Alu* sequence identity were created within the primate genome, providing a substrate for homologous recombination and an increased predisposition to duplicative transposition events. This model provides a ready explanation for the several features of segmental duplications, including the disparity of segmental duplication between primates and other sequenced organisms, the timing of their proliferation within primates, and their bias towards gene-rich regions of the genome.

SEGMENTAL DUPLICATIONS AND EVOLUTION

The paradigm of segmental duplications as mediators of chromosomal rearrangement in a growing list of recurrent microdeletion/microduplication syndromes indicates their potential as catalysts of structural chromosome rearrangement. However, with the recent availability of DNA sequence from several mammalian species, it is now clear that segmental duplications are also a major driving force in karyotype evolution and speciation.

Comparative analysis of orthologous regions has provided strong evidence for a duplication-driven mechanism underlying chromosomal evolution. In several cases, analysis of evolutionary breakpoints of translocation or inversions between humans and other primates has revealed the presence of duplicated sequences at the sites of rearrangement *(51–54)*. Indeed, cross-species analysis using array comparative genomic hybridization (CGH) has shown a significant association of segmental duplications and sites of large scale rearrangement between the great apes, suggesting that the genomic architecture plays an important role in mediating evolutionary rearrangements *(55)*. Furthermore, recent comparative analyses of breaks in synteny between the genomes of humans and mice also show a highly significant enrichment of duplicated sequences at the sites of breakage *(56,57)*. Although definitive evidence showing that these duplicated sequences are the cause, and not a consequence, of the rearrangements, they strongly support a nonrandom model in which chromosomal evolution is driven by the duplication architecture of the genome.

However, segmental duplications may also play an important role in genome evolution in other ways besides mediating large-scale rearrangement (Fig. 4). Many duplications contain either partial or complete gene sequences, and their proliferation can, therefore, create additional copies of transcripts that have the potential to evolve independently from one another. It has been suggested that such duplication removes the pressure for conservation of function that would normally constrain translational change, and that gene duplication may, therefore, be one of the major forces involved in generating proteome diversity. Although it is true that the majority of such duplication events will create nonfunctional pseudogenes owing to the loss of crucial exons, regulatory elements, or the accumulation of deleterious mutations, several important examples exist of genes that have acquired novel functions following duplication events. These include the evolution of trichromatic color vision in the apes and monkeys

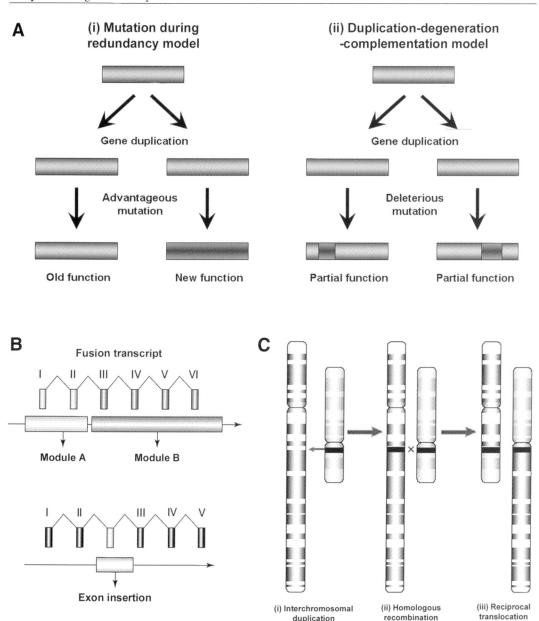

Fig. 4. Mechanisms of duplication-driven evolution: (A) gene evolution by complete duplication provides a period of relaxed selection, allowing the resultant copies to diverge and potentially acquire novel function. Two alternative models have been proposed: (1) the classical model of "mutation during redundancy" proposes that advantageous mutation in one duplicated copy leads to gain of function *(67)* and (2) an alternative model, termed "duplication–degeneration–complementation," that suggests deleterious mutations occur in both copies, leaving each with partial functions that complement one another *(67)*. (B) The creation of novel fusion transcripts by the juxtaposition of exons of independent origin, or alternatively insertion of novel exon(s) into an existing gene. (C) A hypothetical duplication-mediated chromosomal rearrangement that occurs as a result of an interchromosomal duplication followed by nonallelic homologous recombination. (Reproduced in part with permission from ref. *68*.)

(58,59) and novel immunological functions of the eosinophil proteins *ECP* and *EDN (60)*, demonstrating the ability of whole gene duplication to drive rapid phenotypic change. Similarly, gene duplication provides an opportunity for the daughter genes to achieve functional specialization in response to environmental pressures, acting as novel substrates for adaptive evolution *(61)*.

Segmental duplications may also lead to the modification or creation of new genes by a number of different mechanisms. Novel exons may be inserted into an existing gene, a mechanism termed exon shuffling, as has been reported for the fibrinolytic factors *(62)*. Alternatively, the juxtaposition of segmental duplications containing different exonic structures has the potential to join two independent transcriptional units, thereby creating novel fusion transcripts lacking in functional constraints and able to evolve rapidly. Examples of these include *POM-ZP3 (63)*, *PMCHL1-PMCHL2 (64)*, *CECR7 (46)*, *KIAA0187 (34)*, and *USP6 (65)*. Segmental duplications can also frequently lead to the creation of novel splice variants in existing genes. Indeed, analysis of alternatively spliced genes has shown that as many as 10% of all splice variants may have arisen from an initial intragenic duplication event *(66)*.

Finally, a recent survey of segmental duplications in the human genome found that approx 6% of transcribed exons are located in recently duplicated sequence *(2)*. Genes associated with immunity and defense, membrane surface interactions, drug detoxification, and growth and development were preferentially enriched, suggesting that gene duplication plays a major role in the evolution of these functions. Thus, in contrast to the popular conception in which single nucleotide polymorphisms and small mutations are the major method of evolutionary change, larger genomic rearrangements may instead represent the driving force behind much of recent primate evolution, facilitated by the presence of abundant highly homologous duplicated sequences throughout the genome *(68)*.

SEGMENTAL DUPLICATIONS AND GENOMIC VARIATION

The role of duplications as mediators of recurrent genomic disorders is well established, with more than 25 separate syndromes now recognized. However, there is a growing body of evidence that suggests segmental duplications may also play a significant role in normal variation. The existence of large genomic polymorphisms, originally termed heteromorphisms or euchromatic variants, has been recognized since the advent of high-resolution cytogenetic banding techniques *(69)* (summarized at http://www.som.soton.ac.uk/research/geneticsdiv/anomaly%20register/). Using more targeted molecular analyses, and more recently with the advent of high-throughput methodologies such as array CGH, large numbers of submicroscopic deletion/duplication and inversion polymorphisms have now been documented *(70,71)*. As with the recurrent genomic disorders, many of these similarly seem to be mediated by the presence of flanking duplicated sequences *(71,72)* (summarized in Table 1). In some instances these polymorphisms are associated with extreme divergences from one individual to another. For instance, copy number of *CYP2D6* has been found to vary from 0 to 13 per diploid genome *(73)*, while the olfactory receptor genes show enormous variation in their localization within subtelomeric regions of human chromosomes *(23)*. The majority of polymorphic duplication and deletion events identified to date involve genes with functions in metabolism and immunity. Alterations in copy number of these genes often have profound effects on an individual's metabolic rate or resistance to environmental pathogens, and as such may be significant susceptibility factors for many common human diseases.

Table 1

Summary of Polymorphic Deletions, Duplications, and Inversions Within the Human Genome[a]

Gene name(s)	Locus	Population frequency	Diploid copies	Size of variant segment	Associated phenotype	Refs.
(a) Deletions/duplications						
GSTM1	1p13.3	>3%	1–3	18 kb	Altered enzyme activity	74
RHD	1p36.11	15–20%	0–2	approx 50 kb	Rhesus blood group sensitivity	75
CYP21A2	6p21.32	1.6%	2–3	35 kb	Congenital adrenal hyperplasia	76
LPA	6q25.3	94%	2–38	5.5 kb	Altered coronary heart disease risk	77
β-Defensin gene cluster	8p23.1	Approx 90%	2–12	>240 kb	Immune system function?	78
IGHG1 region	14q32.33	12–74%	1–6	5–170 kb	Immune system function?	79,80
NF1/IGVH/GABRA5 pseudogenes	15q11.2-q13	80%	2–8	Approx 1 Mb	Unknown	81
CHRNA7/CHRFAM7A	15q13.3	10–80%	2–4	>270 kb	Unknown	82
IGVH/SLC6A8/CDM pseudogenes	16p11.2	Unknown	2–12	Undefined	Unknown	69
CCL3-L1/CCL4-L1	17q12	51/27%	0–6	>2 kb	Immune system function?	83
DNMT1	19p13.2	93%	2–5	>60 kb	Unknown	84
CYP2A6	19q13.2	1.7%	2–3	7 kb	Altered nicotine metabolism	85
IGL	22q11.22	28–85%	2–7	5.4 kb	Altered Igκ:Igλ in B lymphocytes	86
GSTT1	22q11.23	20%	0–2	>50 kb	Altered susceptibility to toxins and cancer	87
CYP2D6	22q13.1	1–29%	0–13	Undefined	Altered drug metabolism	73
Spermatogenesis genes	Yq11.2	3.2%	0–1	1.6 Mb	Low penetrance spermatogenic failure	88
OR genes	Multiple subtelomeres	Highly variable	7–11	>90 kb	Unknown	23
(b) Inversions						
NPHP1	2q13	21%		290 kb	Non-pathogenic	89
OR genes	4p16	12.5%		approx 6 Mb	Predisposition to t(4;8)(p16;p23) translocation	20
Williams-Beuren syndrome critical region	7q11.23	Unknown		1.6 Mb	Predisposition to deletion of WBS critical region (and atypical WBS phenotype?)	90
OR genes	8p23	26%		4.7 Mb	Predisposition to inv dup(8p), +der(8)(pter-p23.1:p23.2-pter) and del(8)(p23.1:p23.2)	19
EMD	Xq28	33%		48 kb	Non-pathogenic	91
Proximal Yp	Yp11.2	33%		approx 4 Mb	Predisposition to PRKX/PRKY translocation	92,93

[a]Adapted from ref. 72.

Although inversions are not usually associated with alterations in gene copy number and, thus, do not have a primary effect on phenotype, several of the polymorphic inversions identified to date confer a predisposition to further chromosomal rearrangement in subsequent generations. Clusters of olfactory receptor genes at 4p16 and 8p23 are both sites of large common inversions which occur in the heterozygous state at significantly higher frequencies in the transmitting parents of individuals with the recurrent t(4;8)(p16;p23) translocation (20), and inverted duplications, marker chromosomes and deletions of 8p23 (19), respectively. Similarly, a heterozygous inversion of the 1.6-Mb Williams-Beuren syndrome critical region at 7q11.23 is observed in one-third of the parents who transmit a deletion of this same region to their offspring, a frequency much higher than that observed in the normal population (90). Finally, an approx 4-Mb inversion in Yp11.2, present on one-third of normal Y chromosomes, is observed in nearly all cases of sex reversal with translocation between the X/Y homologous genes *PRKX* and *PRKY* (92,93). Presumably these inversions predispose to secondary rearrangement by switching the orientation of large homologous duplications on one chromosome homologue, allowing their subsequent alignment during synapsis, and, hence, facilitating unequal recombination. Given the difficulty of ascertaining these submicroscopic inversions, it seems likely that many other common inversion polymorphisms exist within the human genome.

SUMMARY

There is a growing recognition that the duplication architecture of the mammalian genome plays a fundamental role in shaping the processes of evolution, genomic diversity, and phenotype. Because of the limitations of available technologies, until recent times the major focus of genetic research has been on alterations at either the cytogenetic band or DNA sequence level. However, the availability of the complete genome sequence in combination with the advent of techniques such as pulsed-field gel electrophoresis, fluorescence *in situ* hybridization, and array CGH now allows the study of an additional level of human variation, one below that visualized with the light microscope but above that detected by most sequence-based methodologies (94). The prevalence of such variation is just beginning to be uncovered (70,71). Given the high gene content of duplicated sequences (2), it seems likely that many genomic polymorphisms may play a significant role in human phenotypic variation.

REFERENCES

1. Cheung VG, Nowak N, Jang W, et al. Integration of cytogenetic landmarks into the draft sequence of the human genome. Nature 2001;409:953–958.
2. Bailey JA, Gu Z, Clark RA, et al. Recent segmental duplications in the human genome. Science 2002;297:1003–1007.
3. She X, Horvath JE, Jiang Z, et al. The structure and evolution of centromeric transition regions within the human genome. Nature 2004;430:857–864.
4. Riethman H, Ambrosini A, Castaneda C, et al. Mapping and initial analysis of human subtelomeric sequence assemblies. Genome Res 2004;14:18–28.
5. Stankiewicz P, Lupski JR. Genome architecture, rearrangements and genomic disorders. Trends Genet 2002;18:74–82.
6. International Human Genome Sequencing Consortium. Initial sequencing and analysis of the human genome. Nature 2001;409:860–921.
7. Eichler EE. Segmental duplications: what's missing, misassigned, and misassembled—and should we care? Genome Res 2001;11:653–656.

8. Bailey JA, Yavor AM, Massa HF, Trask BJ, Eichler EE. Segmental duplications: organization and impact within the current human genome project assembly. Genome Res 2001;11:1005–1017.

9. Estivill X, Cheung J, Pujana MA, Nakabayashi K, Scherer SW, Tsui LC. Chromosomal regions containing high-density and ambiguously mapped putative single nucleotide polymorphisms (SNPs) correlate with segmental duplications in the human genome. Hum Mol Genet 2002;11:1987–1995.

10. Eichler EE. Masquerading repeats: paralogous pitfalls of the human genome. Genome Res 1998;8:758–762.

11. Eichler EE, Clark RA, She X. An assessment of the sequence gaps: unfinished business in a finished human genome. Nature Rev Genet 2004;5:345–354.

12. Liu G, Zhao S, Bailey JA, et al. Analysis of primate genomic variation reveals a repeat-driven expansion of the human genome. Genome Res 2003;13:358–368.

13. Keller MP, Seifried BA, Chance PF. Molecular evolution of the CMT1A-REP region: a human- and chimpanzee-specific repeat. Mol Biol Evol 1999;16:1019–1026.

14. DeSilva U, Massa H, Trask BJ, Green ED. Comparative mapping of the region of human chromosome 7 deleted in Williams syndrome. Genome Res 1999;9:428–436.

15. Rozen S, Skaletsky H, Marszalek JD, et al. Abundant gene conversion between arms of palindromes in human and ape Y chromosomes. Nature 2003;423:873–876.

16. Stankiewicz P, Shaw CJ, Withers M, Inoue K, Lupski JR. Serial segmental duplications during primate evolution result in complex human genome architecture. Genome Res 2004;14:2209–2220.

17. Shaikh TH, Kurahashi H, Saitta SC, et al. Chromosome 22-specific low copy repeats and the 22q11.2 deletion syndrome: genomic organization and deletion endpoint analysis. Hum Mol Genet 2000;9:489–501.

18. DeSilva U, Massa H, Trask BJ, Green ED. Comparative mapping of the region of human chromosome 7 deleted in Williams syndrome. Genome Res 1999;9:428–436.

19. Giglio S, Broman KW, Matsumoto N, et al. Olfactory receptor-gene clusters, genomic-inversion polymorphisms, and common chromosome rearrangements. Am J Hum Genet 2001;68:874–883.

20. Giglio S, Calvari V, Gregato G, et al. Heterozygous submicroscopic inversions involving olfactory receptor-gene clusters mediate the recurrent t(4;8)(p16;p23) translocation. Am J Hum Genet 2002;71:276–285.

21. Saglio G, Storlazzi CT, Giugliano E, et al. A 76-kb duplicon maps close to the BCR gene on chromosome 22 and the ABL gene on chromosome 9: possible involvement in the genesis of the Philadelphia chromosome translocation. Proc Natl Acad Sci USA 2002;99:9882–9887.

22. Ritchie RJ, Mattei MG, Lalande M. A large polymorphic repeat in the pericentromeric region of human chromosome 15q contains three partial gene duplications. Hum Mol Genet 1998;7:1253–1260.

23. Trask B, Friedman C, Martin-Gallardo A, et al. Members of the olfactory receptor gene family are contained in large blocks of DNA duplicated polymorphically near the ends of human chromosomes. Hum Molec Genet 1998;7:13–26.

24. Cheung J, Wilson MD, Zhang J, et al. Recent segmental and gene duplications in the mouse genome. Genome Biol 2003;4:R47.

25. Bailey JA, Church DM, Ventura M, Rocchi M, Eichler EE. Analysis of segmental duplications and genome assembly in the mouse. Genome Res 2004;14:789–801.

26. Tuzun E, Bailey JA, Eichler EE. Recent segmental duplications in the working draft assembly of the brown Norway rat. Genome Res 2004;14:493–506.

27. Bailey JA, Yavor AM, Viggiano L, et al. Human-specific duplication and mosaic transcripts: the recent paralogous structure of chromosome 22. Am J Hum Genet 2001;70:83–100.

28. Thomas JW, Schueler MG, Summers TJ, et al. Pericentromeric duplications in the laboratory mouse. Genome Res 2003;13:55–63.

29. Britten RJ. Rates of DNA sequence evolution differ between taxonomic groups. Science 1986;231:1393–1398.

30. Eichler EE, Lu F, Shen Y, et al. Duplication of a gene-rich cluster between 16p11.1 and Xq28: a novel pericentromeric-directed mechanism for paralogous genome evolution. Hum Molec Genet 1996;5:899–912.

31. Eichler EE, Budarf ML, Rocchi M, et al. Interchromosomal duplications of the adrenoleukodystrophy locus: a phenomenon of pericentromeric plasticity. Hum Molec Genet 1997;6:991–1002.

32. Orti R, Potier MC, Maunoury C, Prieur M, Creau N, Delabar JM. Conservation of pericentromeric duplications of a 200-kb part of the human 21q22.1 region in primates. Cytogenet. Cell Genet 1998;83:262–265.

33. Goodman M. The genomic record of Humankind's evolutionary roots. Am J Hum Genet 1999;64:31–39.

34. Crosier M, Viggiano L, Guy J, et al. Human paralogs of KIAA0187 were created through independent pericentromeric-directed and chromosome-specific duplication mechanisms. Genome Res 2002;12:67–80.

35. Guy J, Spalluto C, McMurray A, et al. Genomic sequence and transcriptional profile of the boundary between pericentromeric satellites and genes on human chromosome arm 10q. Hum Mol Genet 2000;9:2029–2042.
36. Horvath J, Viggiano L, Loftus B, Adams M, Rocchi M, Eichler EE. Molecular structure and evolution of an alpha/non-alpha satellite junction at 16p11. Hum Molec Genet 2000;9:113–123.
37. Jackson MS, Rocchi M, Thompson G, et al. Sequences flanking the centromere of human chromosome 10 are a complex patchwork of arm-specific sequences, stable duplications and unstable sequences with homologies to telomeric and other centromeric locations. Hum Mol Genet 1999;8:205–215.
38. Loftus B, Kim U, Sneddon VP, et al. Genome duplications and other features in 12 Mbp of DNA sequence from human chromosome 16p and 16q. Genomics 1999;60:295–308.
39. Ruault M, Trichet V, Gimenez S, et al. Juxta-centromeric region of human chromosome 21 is enriched for pseudogenes and gene fragments. Gene 1999;239:55–64.
40. Luijten M, Wang Y, Smith BT, et al. Mechanism of spreading of the highly related neurofibromatosis type 1 (NF1) pseudogenes on chromosomes 2, 14 and 22. Eur J Hum Genet 2000;8:209–214.
41. Monfouilloux S, Avet-Loiseau H, Amarger V, Balazs I, Pourcel C, Vergnaud G. Recent human-specific spreading of a subtelomeric domain. Genomics 1998;51:165–176.
42. Trask BJ, Massa H, Brand-Arpon V, et al. Large multi-chromosomal duplications encompass many members of the olfactory receptor gene family in the human genome. Hum Molec Genet 1998;7:2007–2020.
43. Hattori M, Fujiyama A, Taylor TD, et al. The DNA sequence of human chromosome 21. The chromosome 21 mapping and sequencing consortium. Nature 2000;405:311–319.
44. Caron H, van Schaik B, van der Mee M, et al. The human transcriptome map: clustering of highly expressed genes in chromosomal domains. Science 2001;291:1289–1292.
45. Eichler EE, Archidiacono N, Rocchi M. CAGGG repeats and the pericentromeric duplication of the hominoid genome. Genome Res 1999;9:1048–1058.
46. Footz TK, Brinkman-Mills P, Banting GS, et al. Analysis of the cat eye syndrome critical region in humans and the region of conserved synteny in mice: a search for candidate genes at or near the human chromosome 22 pericentromere. Genome Res 2001;11:1053–1070.
47. Davis M, Kim S, Hood L. DNA sequences mediating class switching in alpha-immunoglobulins. Science 1980;209:1360–1365.
48. Dempsey LA, Sun H, Hanakahi LA, Maizels N. G4 DNA binding by LR1 and its subunits, nucleolin and hnRNP D, A role for G-G pairing in immunoglobulin switch recombination. J Biol Chem 1999;274:1066–1071.
49. Bailey JA, Liu G, Eichler EE. An Alu transposition model for the origin and expansion of human segmental duplications. Am J Hum Genet 2003;73:823–834.
50. Shen MR, Batzer MA, Deininger PL. Evolution of the master Alu gene(s). J Mol Evol 1991;33:311–320.
51. Tunnacliffe A, Liu L, Moore JK, et al. Duplicated KOX zinc finger gene clusters flank the centromere of human chromosome 10: evidence for a pericentric inversion during primate evolution. Nucleic Acids Res 1993;21:1409–1417.
52. Nickerson E, Nelson DL. Molecular definition of pericentric inversion breakpoints occurring during the evolution of humans and chimpanzees. Genomics 1998;50:368–372.
53. Stankiewicz P, Park SS, Inoue K, Lupski JR. The evolutionary chromosome translocation 4;19 in Gorilla gorilla is associated with microduplication of the chromosome fragment syntenic to sequences surrounding the human proximal CMT1A-REP. Genome Res 2001;11:1205–1210.
54. Locke DP, Archidiacono N, Misceo D, et al. Refinement of a chimpanzee pericentric inversion breakpoint to a segmental duplication cluster. Genome Biol 2003;4:R50.
55. Locke DP, Segraves R, Carbone L, et al. Large-scale variation among human and great ape genomes determined by array comparative genomic hybridization. Genome Res 2003;13:347–357.
56. Armengol L, Pujana MA, Cheung J, Scherer SW, Estivill X. Enrichment of segmental duplications in regions of breaks of synteny between the human and mouse genomes suggest their involvement in evolutionary rearrangements. Hum Mol Genet 2003;12:2201–2208.
57. Bailey JA, Baertsch R, Kent WJ, Haussler D, Eichler EE. Hotspots of mammalian chromosomal evolution. Genome Biol 2004;5:R23.
58. Yokoyama S, Starmer WT, Yokoyama R. Paralogous origin of the red- and green-sensitive visual pigment genes in vertebrates. Mol Biol Evol 1993;10:527–538.
59. Nei M, Zhang J, Yokoyama S. Color vision of ancestral organisms of higher primates. Mol Biol Evol 1997;14:611–618.

60. Rosenberg HF, Dyer KD. Eosinophil cationic protein and eosinophil-derived neurotoxin. Evolution of novel function in a primate ribonuclease gene family. J Biol Chem 1995;270:21,539–21,544.
61. Zhang J, Zhang YP, Rosenberg HF. Adaptive evolution of a duplicated pancreatic ribonuclease gene in a leaf-eating monkey. Nature Genet 2002;30:411–415.
62. Patthy L. Evolution of the proteases of blood coagulation and fibrinolysis by assembly from modules. Cell 1985;41:657–663.
63. Kipersztok S, Osawa GA, Liang LF, Modi WS, Dean J. POM-ZP3, a bipartite transcript derived from human ZP3 and a POM121 homologue. Genomics 1995;25:354–359.
64. Courseaux A, Nahon JL. Birth of two chimeric genes in the Hominidae lineage. Science 2001;291:1293–1297.
65. Paulding CA, Ruvolo M, Haber DA. The Tre2 (USP6) oncogene is a hominoid-specific gene. Proc Natl Acad Sci USA 2003;100:2507–2511.
66. Kondrashov FA, Koonin EV. Origin of alternative splicing by tandem exon duplication. Hum Mol Genet 2001;10:2661–2669.
67. Force A, Lynch M, Pickett FB, Amores A, Yan YL, Postlethwait J. Preservation of duplicate genes by complementary, degenerative mutations. Genetics 1999;151:1531–1545.
68. Samonte RV, Eichler EE. Segmental duplications and the evolution of the primate genome. Nature Rev Genet 2002;3:65–72.
69. Barber JC, Reed CJ, Dahoun SP, Joyce CA. Amplification of a pseudogene cassette underlies euchromatic variation of 16p at the cytogenetic level. Hum Genet 1999;104:211–218.
70. Iafrate JA, Feuk L, Rivera MN, et al. Detection of large-scale variation in the human genome. Nat Genet 2004;36:949–951.
71. Sebat J, Lakshmi B, Troge J, et al. Large-scale copy number polymorphism in the human genome. Science 2004;305:525–528.
72. Buckland PR. Polymorphically duplicated genes: their relevance to phenotypic variation in humans. Ann Med 2003;35:308–315.
73. Dalen P, Dahl ML, Ruiz ML, Nordin J, Bertilsson L. 10-Hydroxylation of nortriptyline in white persons with 0, 1, 2, 3, and 13 functional CYP2D6 genes. Clin Pharmacol Ther 1998;63:444–452.
74. McLellan RA, Oscarson M, Alexandrie A, et al. Characterization of a Human Glutathione S-Transferase μ Cluster Containing a Duplicated GSTM1 Gene that Causes Ultrarapid Enzyme Activity. Mol Pharmacol 1997;52:958–965.
75. Colin Y, Cherif-Zahar B, Le Van Kim C, Raynal V, Van Huffel V, Cartron JP. Genetic basis of the RhD-positive and RhD-negative blood group polymorphism as determined by Southern analysis. Blood 1991;78:2747–2752.
76. Koppens PF, Hoogenboezem T, Degenhart HJ. Duplication of the CYP21A2 gene complicates mutation analysis of steroid 21-hydroxylase deficiency: characteristics of three unusual haplotypes. Hum Genet 2002;111:405–410.
77. Lackner C, Boerwinkle E, Leffert CC, Rahmig T, Hobbs HH. Molecular basis of apolipoprotein (a) isoform size heterogeneity as revealed by pulsed-field gel electrophoresis. J Clin Invest 1991;87:2153–2161.
78. Hollox EJ, Armour JA, Barber JC. Extensive normal copy number variation of a beta-defensin antimicrobial-gene cluster. Am J Hum Genet 2003;73:591–600.
79. Rabbani H, Pan Q, Kondo N, Smith CI, Hammarstrom L. Duplications and deletions of the human IGHC locus: evolutionary implications. Immunogenetics 1996;45:136–141.
80. Sasso EH, Buckner JH, Suzuki LA. Ethnic differences of polymorphism of an immunoglobulin VH3 gene. J Clin Invest 1995;96:1591–1600.
81. Fantes JA, Mewborn SK, Lese CM, et al. Organisation of the pericentromeric region of chromosome 15: at least four partial gene copies are amplified in patients with a proximal duplication of 15q. J Med Genet 2002;39:170–177.
82. Riley B, Williamson M, Collier D, Wilkie H, Makoff A. A 3-Mb map of a large segmental duplication overlapping the alpha7-nicotinic acetylcholine receptor gene (CHRNA7) at human 15q13-q14. Genomics 2002;79:197–209.
83. Townson JR, Barcellos LF, Nibbs RJB. Gene copy number regulates the production of the human chemokine CCL3-L1. Eur J Imm 2002;32:3016–3026.
84. Franchina M, Kay PH. Allele-specific variation in the gene copy number of human cytosine 5-methyltransferase. Hum Hered 2000;50:112–117.
85. Rao Y, Hoffmann E, Zia M, et al. Duplications and defects in the CYP2A6 gene: identification, genotyping, and in vivo effects on smoking. Mol Pharmacol 2000;58:747–755.

86. van der Burg M, Barendregt BH, van Gastel-Mol EJ, Tümkaya T, Langerak AW, van Dongen JJM. Unraveling of the polymorphic C2-C3 amplification and the Ke+Oz- polymorphism in the human Ig locus. J Immunol 2002;169:271–276.

87. Sprenger R, Schlagenhaufer R, Kerb R, et al. Characterization of the glutathione S-transferase GSTT1 deletion: discrimination of all genotypes by polymerase chain reaction indicates a trimodular genotype-phenotype correlation. Pharmacogenetics 2000;10:557–565.

88. Repping S, Skaletsky H, Brown L, et al. Polymorphism for a 1.6-Mb deletion of the human Y chromosome persists through balance between recurrent mutation and haploid selection. Nature Genet 2003;35:247–251.

89. Saunier S, Calado J, Benessy F, et al. Characterization of the NPHP1 locus: mutational mechanism involved in deletions in familial juvenile nephronophthisis. Am J Hum Genet 2000;66:778–789.

90. Osborne LR, Li M, Pober B, et al. A 1.5 million-base pair inversion polymorphism in families with Williams-Beuren syndrome. Nature Genet 2001;29:321–325.

91. Small K, Iber J, Warren ST. Emerin deletion reveals a common X-chromosome inversion mediated by inverted repeats. Nature Genet 1997;16:96–99.

92. Jobling MA, Williams GA, Schiebel GA, et al. A selective difference between human Y-chromosomal DNA haplotypes. Curr Biol 1998;8:1391–1394.

93. Sharp A, Kusz K, Jaruzelska J, et al. Variability of sexual phenotype in 46,XX(SRY+) patients: the influence of spreading X inactivation versus position effects. J Med Genet 2005;42:420–427.

94. Lupski JR. 2002 Curt Stern award address: genomic disorders: recombination-based disease resulting from genome architecture. Am J Hum Genet 2003;72:246–252.

95. Eichler EE. Recent duplication, domain accretion and the dynamic mutation of the human genome. Trends Genet 2001;17:661–669.

6 Non-B DNA and Chromosomal Rearrangements

Albino Bacolla, PhD and Robert D. Wells, PhD

CONTENTS

INTRODUCTION

Certain DNA sequences in the genome may exist either in the canonical right-handed B-duplex or in alternative non-B conformations, depending on conditions such as transcription, supercoil stress, protein binding, and so on. Analyses of breakpoint junctions at deletions, translocations, and inversions, where the sites of DNA breakage could be determined at the nucleotide level, revealed that most, if not all, of the breaks occurred within, or adjacent to, the predicted non-B conformations. These findings support a model whereby rearrangements are caused by recombination/repair processes between two distinct non-B conformations, which may reside either on the same chromosome or on two distinct chromosomes. This model was applicable to both *Escherichia coli* and humans, suggesting that the mechanisms involved are highly conserved.

The number of genomic disorders that are explicable in terms of non-B DNA conformation-mediated rearrangement is considerable (approx 30). Most involve recombination within (or between) chromosomal regions enriched in low-copy repeats (LCRs), whereas lymphoid-specific rearrangements depend on the recombination-activated gene (*RAG*) recombinase. However, considering the diseases associated with triplet repeat expansions, which are also believed to be mediated by non-B conformations, the total number of pathological conditions is around 50. This number may increase as further investigations are conducted on additional rearrangements.

The history of investigations on DNA conformations that differ from the canonical right-handed B-form, as related to genetic diseases, dates back to the mid-1960s. Early studies with high-molecular-weight DNA polymers of defined repeating nucleotide sequences demonstrated the role of DNA sequence in their properties and conformations *(1)*. Investigations with

From: *Genomic Disorders: The Genomic Basis of Disease*
Edited by: J. R. Lupski and P. Stankiewicz © Humana Press, Totowa, NJ

Name	Conformation	General Seq. Requirements	Sequence
Cruciform	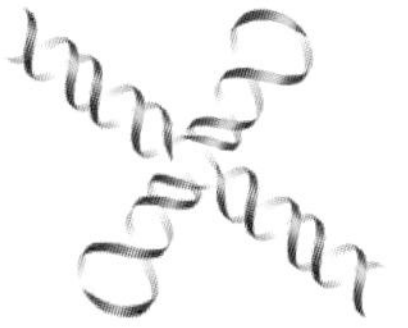	Inverted Repeats	TCGGTACCGA AGCCATGGCT
Triplex	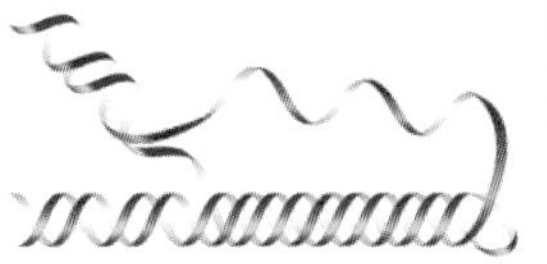	$(R \cdot Y)_n$ Mirror Repeats	AAGAGG GGAGAA TTCTCC CCTCTT
Slipped (Hairpin) Structure	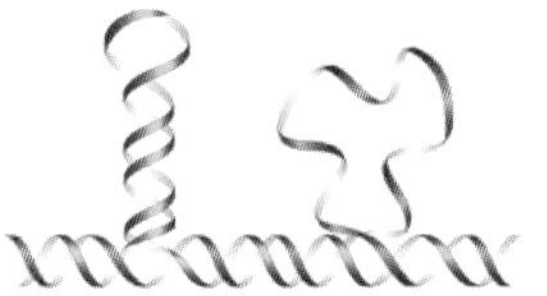	Direct Repeats	TCGGTTCGGT AGCCAAGCCA
Tetraplex	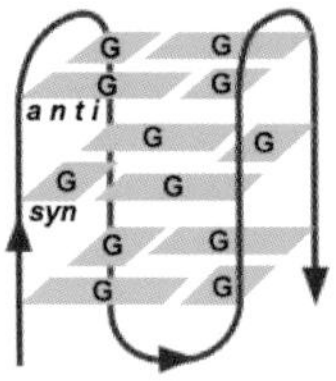	Oligo $(G)_n$ Tracts	$AG_3(T_2AG_3)_3$ single strand
Left-handed Z - DNA	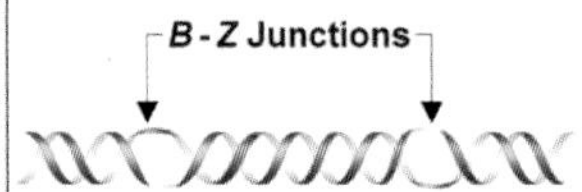	$(YR \cdot YR)_n$	CGCGTGCGTGTG GCGCACGCACAC

Fig. 1. Non-B DNA conformations involved in rearrangements.

repeating homo-, di-, tri-, and tetranucleotide motifs revealed the important role of DNA sequence in molecular behaviors. At that time, this concept was heretical because numerous prior physical and biochemical investigations with naturally occurring DNA sequences did not enable the realization of the effect of sequence (1). It should be noted that these biochemical/biophysical studies in the 1960s predated DNA sequencing by at least a decade.

Early studies were followed by a number of innovative discoveries on DNA conformational features in synthetic oligomers, restriction fragments, and recombinant DNAs. The DNA polymorphisms were shown to be a function of sequence, topology (supercoil density), ionic conditions, protein binding, methylation, carcinogen binding, and other factors (2). A number of non-B DNA structures have been discovered, approximately one new conformation every 3 years during the past 35 years, and include triplexes, left-handed DNA, bent DNA, cruciforms, nodule DNA, flexible and writhed DNA, G4 tetrad (tetraplexes), slipped structures, and sticky DNA (Fig. 1). From the outset, it has been realized (1,2) that these sequence effects probably have profound biological implications, and indeed their role in transcription (3) and in the maintenance of telomere ends (4) has been reviewed recently.

Moreover, in the past few years, dramatic advances in genomics, human genetics, physiology, and DNA structural biology have revealed the role of non-B conformations in the etiology of at least 46 human genetic diseases (Table 1) that involve genomic rearrangements, as well as other types of mutation events *(5)*.

NON-B DNA CONFORMATIONS

Segments of DNA are polymorphic. A large number of simple DNA repeat sequences can exist in at least two conformations that are interconvertible. All of these sequences adopt the orthodox right-handed B-form, probably for the majority of the time, with Watson-Crick (WC) A•T and G•C basepairs. However, perhaps transiently, at least 10 non-B conformations *(6–8)* are formed at specific sequence motifs as a function of negative supercoil density, generated in part by transcription, protein binding, or other factors.

Non-B DNA structures (Fig. 1) include cruciforms and left-handed Z-DNA, which have bp in the WC conformation, whereas triplexes, tetraplexes, and slipped structures rely in part, or exclusively, on non-WC interactions. Cruciform DNA occurs at inverted repeats (IR), which are defined as sequences of identical composition on the complementary strands. Each strand folds at the IR center of symmetry and reconstitutes an intramolecular B-helix capped by a single-stranded loop that may extend from a few basepairs to several kilobases. The term cruciform originates from the appearance of the duplex arms *(6,7)*, which at the four-way junction adopts either an "open" configuration that allows strand migration (Fig. 1) or a "stacked" (locked) arrangement, where the helices stack on each other. In both cases, the overall conformation and the intra-duplex angles mimic the Holliday junction *(9)*, and in fact these structures have been studied extensively as models of recombination intermediates. Cruciform DNA is often incorrectly referred to as a palindrome; a palindrome is a word or sentence that reads identically when spelled backwards, such as rotor or Hannah.

Triplex (triple-helix, H-DNA) DNA occurs at oligo(purine•pyrimidine) $[(R•Y)_n]$ tracts *(6,7,10,11)* and is favored by sequences containing a mirror repeat symmetry (*see* Fig. 1). The purine strand of the WC duplex engages the third strand through Hoogsteen hydrogen bonds in the major groove while maintaining the original duplex structure in a B-like conformation. Triplex DNA is polymorphic in the orientation and composition of the third strand; this may be either pyrimidine-rich and parallel to the complementary R-strand or purine-rich and anti-parallel to the complementary R-strand (the latter case is shown in Fig. 1). In addition, the participating third strand *(11)* may originate from within a single $(R•Y)_n$ tract (intramolecular triplex) or from a separate tract (intermolecular triplex).

Direct repeats (DR) aligning out of register give rise to slipped structures with looped-out bases (Fig. 1). When DR involve several repeating motifs, like the telomeric or triplet repeat sequences, the looped-out bases may form duplexes stabilized by unusual pairs, such as T•T in $(CTG)_n$ *(12)* or shared paired motifs (G•A and GC•AA), a specific arrangement characterized by interstrand, rather than intrastrand, stacking interactions *(13)*.

A guanine tetrad, as found in telomeric DNA, is a square coplanar array of four guanines *(4,8)*. Each base donates two Hoogsteen hydrogen bonds to one neighbor and receives two hydrogen bonds from the other neighbor in a cyclic arrangement involving N1, N2, O6, and N7. Four-stranded DNA (tetraplex DNA, G-quadruplex) is composed of guanine tetrads stacked on each other (Fig. 1), and, therefore, is favored by four runs of three or more guanines. This conformation is also endowed with a high degree of polymorphism in terms of strand

Table 1
Genetic Alterations, Diseases, and DNA Repeat Motifs

Genetic alteration	Syndrome or metabolic event	DNA motifs	Refs.
t(11;22)(q23;q11.2)	Supernumerary der(22) syndrome	IR	20,26,27
t(17;22)(q11.2;q11.2)	Neurofibromatosis type 1	IR	20
t(1;22)(p21.2;q11.2)	Ependymoma	IR	20
t(4;22)(q35.1;q11.2)	Velocardiofacial syndrome	IR	20
del(22)(q11.2q11.2)	DiGeorge, velocardiofacial, or conotruncal anomaly face syndrome	IR, DR	24,25
inv dup(22) (q11.2q11.2)	Cat-eye syndrome	IR, DR	24,25
del(Yq)	Spermatogenic failure	IR, DR	21,32,33
i(17q)	Hematologic malignances (chronic myeloid leukemia)	IR	22
del(17)(p11.2p11.2)	Smith-Magenis syndrome	IR, DR	31,35,37
dup(17)(p11.2p11.2)	dup(17)(p11.2p11.2) syndrome	IR, DR	34
dup(17)(p12p12)	Charcot-Marie-Tooth type 1	IR, DR	31
del(17)(p12p12)	Hereditary neuropathy with liability to pressure palsies	IR, DR	31
t(14;18)(q32.3;q21.3)	Follicular (B cells) lymphomas	(R•Y)-rich	42,43
del(7)(q11.23q11.23)	Williams-Beuren syndrome	IR, DR	52
inv(7)(q11.23q11.23)	Predisposition to Williams-Beuren syndrome	IR	52
del(15)(q11q13)	Prader-Willi and Angelman syndromes	IR, DR	53
t(X;22)(q27;q11)	Myeloschizis and lumbosacral spina bifida	IR	54
Expanded (CTG•CAG)n (coding)	Expanded polyglutamine diseases (Haw River, Huntington, Huntington's disease-like 2, spinobulbar muscular atrophy [Kennedy], spino-cerebellar ataxia [SCA] 1, SCA2, SCA3, SCA6, SCA7, SCA17)	DR	46,47
Expanded (CTG•CAG)n (non-coding)	Myotonic dystrophy type 1, SCA8, SCA12	DR	47
Expanded (CGG•CCG)n (coding)	Expanded polyalanine diseases (infantile spasm, cleidocranial dysplasia, blepharophimosis/ptosis/ epicanthus inversus type B, hand-foot-genital, synpolydactyly, oculopharyngeal muscular dystrophy, holoprosencephaly, oculopharyngeal muscular dystrophy)	DR	47,55
Expanded (CGG•CCG)n (non-coding)	Fragile XA, fragile XE, fragile XF, Jacobsen (FRA11B)	DR	46,47
Expanded (GAA•TTC)n	Friedreich's ataxia	DR with (R•Y)	46,47
Expanded (GAC•GTC)n	Pseudoachondroplasia, multiple epiphyseal dysplasia	DR	47
Expanded (CCTG•CAGG)n	Myotonic dystrophy type 2	DR	47
Expanded (ATTCT•AGAAT)n	SCA10	DR	47
Expanded (CCCCGCCCCGCG)n	Progressive myoclonus epilepsy type 1	DR	46,47
Expanded 24mer	Creutzfeldt-Jacob disease	DR	56
Contracted 3.3-kb D4Z4 repeat	Facioscapulohumeral muscular dystrophy	DR	57

DR, direct repeats; IR, inverted repeats; DR with (R•Y), direct repeats composed of $(R•Y)_n$ with mirror repeat symmetry.

stoichiometry and polarity, glycosidic torsion angles, groove size, and connecting loops. Pairing schemes with other bases have also been observed, such as a guanine tetrad sandwiched between two G•C and A•T WC pairs *(14)*.

Left-handed Z-DNA (Fig. 1) is adopted by alternating pyrimidine-purine $[(YR•YR)_n]$ sequences, such as $(CG•CG)_n$ and $(CA•TG)_n$. The transition from the right-handed B- to the left-handed Z-form is accomplished by a 180° flip (upside-down) of the basepair through the rotation of every other purine from the *anti* to the *syn* conformation and a corresponding change in the sugar puckering mode from the C2'- to the C3'-*endo* conformation. Contrary to the B-DNA, which possesses a major and a minor groove, Z-DNA contains only one groove *(3,7)*. Other architectures (sticky DNA, nodule DNA, bent DNA, i-motifs, and others *[6–8]*) are well known from a biochemical standpoint; their biological roles in genome instability are under current investigation.

CHROMOSOMAL REARRANGEMENTS

Non-B DNA Conformations Cause Rearrangements

The involvement of double-strand breaks (DSB) in genome instability is well-documented *(15)*, but the initiating events that lead to their formation are not fully understood. Recently, an increasing amount of information has revealed a major causative role for non-B DNA conformations. Indeed, analyses of large deletions stimulated by a 2.5 kb poly(R•Y) sequence from intron 21 of the polycystic kidney disease 1 gene *(PKD1)*, or by long $(CTG•CAG)_n$ repeats, in *E. coli* indicated that the breakpoints occurred invariably at nt abutting, or within, motifs capable of adopting non-B conformations *(16,17)*. Because the same *PKD1* tract also induced cell death in a supercoil-dependent manner *(18)*, we concluded that the large deletions were mediated by supercoil-dependent non-B conformations. In addition, the presence of short (direct or inverted) homologies at the breakpoint junctions suggested a model whereby two distantly located non-B DNA conformations induced DSB repair and, hence, demarcated the deletion endpoints. Similarly, a search of 222 rearrangement breakpoints from the human Gross Rearrangement Breakpoint Database (GRaBD) *(17)* revealed that both the frequency and the proximity of $(R•Y)_n$ and $(RY•RY)_n$ tracts to breakpoint junctions were significantly greater than expected by chance. A detailed analysis of the DNA sequences flanking the breakpoints in 11 deletions showed that, as in the bacterial cases, the events were explicable in terms of non-B DNA formation. Hence, non-B conformations appear to play a widespread role in rearrangement mutagenesis.

Site-Specific Non-Robertsonian Chromosome Translocations

A second line of evidence in establishing the role for DNA structural features in rearrangements was the recent identification of extremely large blocks of repeated sequences termed LCRs (duplicons, segmental duplications) *(19)*. Such blocks constitute a fertile substrate for recurrent rearrangements associated with more than 30 human genomic disorders (Table 1) *(20–23)* because they may adopt conformations of unprecedented complexity and size. Chromosome 22q11 is characterized by four large LCRs (LCR-A to D) that encompass approx 350 kb of DNA over an approx 3-Mb region *(24,25)*. Sequence analyses of constitutional translocation breakpoints between chromosomes 22 and 1, 4, 11, or 17 have shown the hallmarks of cruciform DNA structures. For example, the breakpoints on LCR-B clustered in a narrow IR A/T-rich region that, in conjunction with flanking nuclear factor-1-like sequences *(20,26)*, is predicted to form an approx 600 bp-long cruciform. Furthermore, the clustering of breakpoints occurred within 15 bp from the IR center and involved the symmetric deletion of a few basepair on either side of the IR apex *(27)*, consistent with the prediction that cruciform loops are susceptible to cleavage, and, hence, to repair *(28)*. The breakpoints on chromosomes 1p21.2, 4q35.1, 11q23, and 17q11.2, also occurred at, or near, the centers of IR A/T-rich sequences *(20)*. Sperm analyses *(29)* confirm that the t(11;22) translocation recurs at high frequency (approx $1–9 \times 10^{-5}$) in the cell population as a *de novo* mutation and, concurrently, in vitro studies provide direct evidence that the chromosome 11 IR has the capacity to fold into stable cruciform conformations *(30)*. These data support the strong destabilizing role for the sequences/structures involved. Interestingly, a case of ependymoma associated with the t(1;22) translocation revealed that the breakpoint on chromosome 1 was flanked by six copies of a 33 bp-long motif with IR symmetry *(20)*. Conversely, the human genome assembly sequenced clone indicated the presence of only two such repeats; if the number of repeats is indeed polymorphic in the general population, this finding suggests that expansion may predispose to DNA instability, possibly by increasing the propensity (and/or stability) for cruciform formation. Recombination events between highly homologous (97–98%) sequences within LCR-A to D are associated with recurrent deletions and duplications (approx 1:3000 live births), leading to the DiGeorge, velocardiofacial, conotruncal anomaly face and cat-eye syndromes *(24,25,31)* (Table 1), suggesting that non-B DNA conformations may also be involved in these conditions.

Interstitial Deletions and Male Infertility

Interstitial deletions in male-specific regions on chromosome Yq are a major source of infertility (AZF) *(32,33)* (Table 1). Of the commonly affected regions (AZFa, AZFb and AZFc), AZFb and AZFc are located within an approx 8-Mb interval and are mostly comprised of five large IR (P1–P5), each consisting of a complex array of direct and inverted blocks harboring male-specific genes. Large (>90 kb) regions of near-perfect identity exist among these IRs; nevertheless, the breakpoints strongly cluster toward the IR spacers (i.e., the regions that separate the two inverted repeat sequences) where, in some cases, they took place between sequences that shared no homology. These features are consistent with a cruciform-mediated mechanism for the deletions *(21,33)*.

Chromosomal Region-Specific Rearrangements Causing Multiple Disorders and Cancer

Isochromosomes are abnormal chromosomes that contain a duplication of a single chromosome arm *(31)*. Isochromosome 17q [i(17q)] is the most common isochromosome associated with human neoplasia, including neuroectodermal tumors and medullablastomas, representing approx 3% of single or additional chromosomal abnormalities in carcinomas and hematologic malignancies, and occur in approx 21% of such cases during chronic myeloid leukemia disease progression *(22)*. The i(17q) breakpoints cluster within 17p11.2, either in the very pericentromeric section or within the approx 4-Mb Smith-Magenis Syndrome common deletion region. An approx 240-kb interval (RNU3) encompassing the i(17q) breakpoint cluster region contains two LCRs, REPA and REPB, whereby two inverted copies of REPA (REPA1 and REPA2, approx 38 kb) separated by a single copy of REPB (REPB3, approx 48 kb), are followed by two inverted copies of REPB (REPB2, approx 43 kb, and REPB1, approx 49 kb). This arrangement provides the structural basis for the formation of large cruciform structures.

The i(17q) is consistent with a recombination mechanism between sister-chromatids mediated by a REPB1-REPB2 cruciform, which predicts formation of the dicentric i(17q) and an acentric chromosome that is expected to be lost (22). The i(17q) RNU3 LCRs are part of a complex array of LCRs involved in deletions and duplications leading to the Smith-Magenis Syndrome *(31)*, the dup(17)(p11.2p11.2) syndrome *(34)*, hereditary neuropathy with liability to pressure palsies (HNPP), and the Charcot-Marie-Tooth type 1 disease (CMT1A) *(35,36)* (Table 1). Also in these cases, the presence of strand exchange hotspots *(37)* strongly favors the concept of the formation of non-B DNA conformations as the molecular trigger for the rearrangements.

RAG-Dependent Recombination and Lymphoid Malignancy

During V(D)J recombination, V, D, and J coding segments are fused in varying permutations to create antigen receptor variable region exons with diverse antigen-binding potentials *(38,39)*. The V, D, and J coding segments are flanked by recombination signal sequences (RSS), which consist of conserved heptamer and nonamer motifs separated by a spacer region of either 12 or 23 bp. The RSS are specifically recognized by the RAG complex, which binds to two separated sequences to effect a DSB-dependent recombination reaction *(38,39)*. Nonauthentic RSS may also be targeted for recombination, and specific chromosomal rearrangements involving Ig/TCR antigen receptor genes and proto-oncogenes, such as *LMO2*, *Ttg-1*, and *SIL* are caused by such a promiscuous RAG activity *(40)*. These chromosomal abnormalities are a major feature of lymphoid neoplasms *(41)*. The t(14;18)(q32.3;q21.3) translocation is the most common translocation in cancer and accounts for almost all follicular lymphomas *(40)*. This chromosomal aberration, which is also owing to RAG activity, does not rely on degenerate RSS motifs. The gene involved on chr18 is the proto-oncogene *bcl-2*, which is generally fused to one of the J_H gene segments from the immunoglobulin heavy chain IgH locus on chr14 to generate the derivative chromosome 14. Der(18) is generated by the joining of a D_H gene segment from the IgH locus on chr14 with the remaining 3' bcl-2 untranslated region exon on chr18 *(40)*. Despite the size of the *bcl-2* gene (>200 kb), 75% of translocations occur within 150 bp located in the untranslated portion of the exon three major breakpoint region (Mbr). Within these 150 bp, three peaks of breakage take place, each 15–20 bp in size, whose sequence adopt a non-B DNA conformation *(42)*. The nature of the non-B conformation(s), which is under investigation, consists of Hoogsteen hydrogen bonding and one or more single-stranded regions that generate a structure recognized by the RAG complex *(43)*. Additional diseases believed to be mediated by non-B conformations are listed in Table 1.

We should emphasize that, whereas rigorous proof exists for the structural properties of non-B DNA conformations (Fig. 1) as well as for the genome rearrangements and their involvement in human disease (Table 1), direct biophysical determinations to definitively demonstrate the involvement of these non-B elements remain to be performed in most cases. Obviously, the most compelling evidence would be derived from in vivo conformational determinations; however, these analyses are extremely difficult and hence have only been performed in limited cases *(6,44,45)*. Nonetheless, even the more facile in vitro studies are lacking in most cases.

Triplet Repeat Diseases

At least 20 hereditary neurological diseases (Table 1) are caused by the expansion of simple triplet repeat sequences in either coding or non-coding regions. These expansions are mediated by DNA replication, repair, and recombination *(44–47)*. DNA slipped structures (Fig. 1) play a prominent role in all of these mechanisms and the preferential formation of hairpin loops with long repeating CTG, GGC, and GAA strands, compared to their complementary strands, are critical to the expansion and deletion behaviors (genetic instabilities). Furthermore, the flexible and writhed conformations *(48)* adopted by long CTG•CAG and CCG•CGG tracts promote these behaviors.

Friedreich's ataxia (FRDA) (Table 1) is the only hereditary neurological disease caused by an expanded GAA•TTC sequence. This tract, which occurs in intron 1, is well known to adopt the triplex conformation (Fig. 1) as well as the more complex sticky DNA structure between two long GAA•TTC tracts at distant locations of the same molecule *(49,50)*. All workers in this field agree *(46)* that the triplex and/or sticky DNA conformation adopted by this repeating sequence is involved in the inhibition of transcription of the FRDA gene to give a reduction in the amount of the frataxin protein. Accordingly, the in vivo discovery of sticky DNA along with its molecular biological implications *(50,51)* may be one of the more convincing cases of a non-B DNA structure involved in disease pathology.

FUTURE CHALLENGES

Dramatic advances were realized from the combined efforts of biophysics, human genetics, genomics, and molecular biological studies in our comprehension of the role of non-B DNA conformations in mutagenesis involved in genetic diseases. The thesis of this chapter is that, in general, all segments of DNA are usually in the orthodox right-handed B-conformation; however, certain repeat tracts occasionally adopt a non-B structure as a function of supercoil density or protein binding, and so on. These non-B conformations (cruciforms, triplexes, tetraplexes, and others) are recognized by DNA repair systems and serve as breakpoints for several types of genome rearrangements, which are the genetic basis for a number of diseases. Future emphases will attempt to fine-tune the adoption of the non-B conformations at specific loci in order to correlate more rigorously this behavior with the generation of rearrangement endpoints. In addition, analyses may be performed to identify the types of non-B DNA structures that elicit certain kinds of mutations and the enzyme systems involved. Many more diseases probably will be recognized as owing to mutations at non-B DNA structures.

SUMMARY

Specific DNA sequences adopt a number of alternative conformations (cruciforms, triplexes, slipped structures, tetraplexes, Z-DNA), also called non-B DNA, which determine the breakpoints responsible for chromosomal rearrangements and other mutations at sites of homology. The non-B DNA structures, rather than the sequences *per se*, are the likely triggers for these recombination/repair functions. More than 40 human genetic disorders may be initiated by these processes.

ACKNOWLEDGMENTS

This research was supported by Grants from the National Institutes of Health (NS37554 and ES11347), the Robert A. Welch Foundation, the Muscular Dystrophy Association, the Friedreich's Ataxia Research Alliance, and the Seek-a-Miracle Foundation. A portion of this chapter was published previously *(5)* and is expanded herein with the permission of the American Society for Biochemistry and Molecular Biology.

REFERENCES

1. Wells RD, Wartell RM. The influence of nucleotide sequence on DNA properties. In: *Biochemistry of Nucleic Acids, vol. 6* (Burton K, ed.), Stoneham, MA: Butterworth Publishing Co., 1974, pp 41–64.
2. Wells RD, Blakesley RW, Hardies SC, et al. The role of DNA structure in genetic regulation. CRC Crit Rev Biochem 1977;4:305–340.
3. Rich A, Zhang S. Timeline: Z-DNA: the long road to biological function. Nat Rev Genet 2003;4:566–572.
4. Neidle S, Parkinson GN. The structure of telomeric DNA. Curr Opin Struct Biol 2003;13:275–283.
5. Bacolla A, Wells RD. Non-B DNA conformations, genomic rearrangements, and human disease. J Biol Chem 2004;279:47,411–47,414.
6. Wells RD. Unusual DNA structures. J Biol Chem 1988;263:1095–1098.
7. Sinden RR. DNA Structure and Function. San Diego, CA: Academic, 1994.
8. Majumdar A, Patel DJ. Identifying hydrogen bond alignments in multistranded DNA architectures by NMR. Acc Chem Res 2002;35:1–11.
9. Watson J, Hays FA, Ho PS. Definitions and analysis of DNA Holliday junction geometry. Nucleic Acids Res 2004;32:3017–3027.
10. Soyfer VN, Potaman VN. *Triple-Helical Nucleic Acids.* New York, NY: Springer-Verlag, 1996.
11. Zain R, Sun JS. Do natural DNA triple-helical structures occur and function in vivo? Cell Mol Life Sci 2003;60:862–870.
12. Gao X, Huang X, Smith GK, Zheng M. Structure and dynamics of single-stranded nucleic acids containing trinucleotide repeats. In: *Genetic Instabilities and Hereditary Neurological Diseases* (Wells RD, Warren ST, eds.). San Diego, CA: Academic, pp. 623–646.
13. Chou SH, Chin KH, Wang AH. Unusual DNA duplex and hairpin motifs. Nucleic Acids Res 2003;31:2461–2474.
14. Zhang N, Gorin A, Majumdar A, et al. Dimeric DNA quadruplex containing major groove-aligned A-T-A-T and G-C- G-C tetrads stabilized by inter-subunit Watson-Crick A-T and G-C pairs. J Mol Biol 2001;312:1073–1088.
15. Elliott B, Jasin M. Double-strand breaks and translocations in cancer. Cell Mol Life Sci 2002;59:373–385.
16. Wojciechowska M, Bacolla A, Larson JE, Wells RD. The myotonic dystrophy type 1 triplet repeat sequence induces gross deletions and inversions. J Biol Chem 2005;280:941–952.
17. Bacolla A, Jaworski A, Larson JE, et al. Breakpoints of gross deletions coincide with non-B DNA conformations. Proc Natl Acad Sci USA 2004;101:14,162–14,167.
18. Bacolla A, Jaworski A, Connors TD, Wells RD. PKD1 unusual DNA conformations are recognized by nucleotide excision repair. J Biol Chem 2001;276:18,597–18,604.
19. Stankiewicz P, Lupski JR. Genome architecture, rearrangements and genomic disorders. Trends Genet 2002;18:74–82.
20. Gotter AL, Shaikh TH, Budarf ML, Rhodes CH, Emanuel BS. A palindrome-mediated mechanism distinguishes translocations involving LCR-B of chromosome 22q11.2. Hum Mol Genet 2004;13:103–115.
21. Repping S, Skaletsky H, Lange J, et al. Recombination between palindromes P5 and P1 on the human Y chromosome causes massive deletions and spermatogenic failure. Am J Hum Genet 2002;71:906–922.
22. Barbouti A, Stankiewicz P, Nusbaum C, et al. The breakpoint region of the most common isochromosome, i(17q), in human neoplasia is characterized by a complex genomic architecture with large, palindromic, low-copy repeats. Am J Hum Genet 2004;74:1–10.
23. Lupski JR. Genomic disorders: structural features of the genome can lead to DNA rearrangements and human disease traits. Trends Genet 1998;14:417–422.
24. Saitta SC, Harris SE, Gaeth AP, Det al. Aberrant interchromosomal exchanges are the predominant cause of the 22q11.2 deletion. Hum Mol Genet 2004;13:417–428.
25. Shaikh TH, Kurahashi H, Saitta SC, et al. Chromosome 22-specific low copy repeats and the 22q11.2 deletion syndrome: genomic organization and deletion endpoint analysis. Hum Mol Genet 2000;9:489–501.
26. Edelmann L, Spiteri E, Koren K, et al. AT-rich palindromes mediate the constitutional t(11;22) translocation. Am J Hum Genet 2001;68:1–13.
27. Kurahashi H, Emanuel BS. Long AT-rich palindromes and the constitutional t(11;22) breakpoint. Hum Mol Genet 2001;10:2605–2617.

28. Richardson C, Jasin M. Frequent chromosomal translocations induced by double-strand breaks. Nature 2000;405:697–700.
29. Kurahashi H, Emanuel BS. Unexpectedly high rate of de novo constitutional t(11;22) translocations in sperm from normal males. Nat Genet 2001;29:139–140.
30. Kurahashi H, Inagaki H, Yamada K, et al. Cruciform DNA structure underlies the etiology for palindrome-mediated human chromosomal translocations. J Biol Chem 2004;279,:35,377–35,383.
31. Shaffer LG, Lupski JR. Molecular mechanisms for constitutional chromosomal rearrangements in humans. Annu Rev Genet 2000;34:297–329.
32. Rozen S, Skaletsky H, Marszalek JD, et al. Abundant gene conversion between arms of palindromes in human and ape Y chromosomes. Nature 2003;423:873–876.
33. Kuroda-Kawaguchi T, Skaletsky H, Brown LG, et al. The AZFc region of the Y chromosome features massive palindromes and uniform recurrent deletions in infertile men. Nat Genet 2001;29:279–286.
34. Potocki L, Chen KS, Park SS, et al. Molecular mechanism for duplication 17p11.2- the homologous recombination reciprocal of the Smith-Magenis microdeletion. Nat Genet 2000;24:84–87.
35. Stankiewicz P, Shaw CJ, Dapper JD, et al. Genome architecture catalyzes nonrecurrent chromosomal rearrangements. Am J Hum Genet 2003;72:1101–1116.
36. Shaw CJ, Withers MA, Lupski JR. Uncommon deletions of the Smith-Magenis syndrome region can be recurrent when alternate low-copy repeats act as homologous recombination substrates. Am J Hum Genet 2004;75:75–81.
37. Bi W, Park SS, Shaw CJ, Withers MA, Patel PI, Lupski JR. Reciprocal crossovers and a positional preference for strand exchange in recombination events resulting in deletion or duplication of chromosome 17p11.2. Am J Hum Genet 2003;73:1302–1315.
38. Fugmann SD, Lee AI, Shockett PE, Villey IJ, Schatz DG. The RAG proteins and V(D)J recombination: complexes, ends, and transposition. Annu Rev Immunol 2000;18:495–527.
39. Jung D, Alt FW. Unraveling V(D)J recombination; insights into gene regulation. Cell 2004;116:299–311.
40. Raghavan SC, Lieber MR. Chromosomal translocations and non-B DNA structures in the human genome. Cell Cycle 2004;3:762–768.
41. Kuppers R, Dalla-Favera R. Mechanisms of chromosomal translocations in B cell lymphomas. Oncogene 2001;20:5580–5594.
42. Raghavan SC, Houston S, Hegde BG, Langen R, Haworth IS, Lieber MR. Stability and strand asymmetry in the non-B DNA structure at the Bcl-2 major breakpoint region. J Biol Chem 2004;279:46,213–46,225.
43. Raghavan SC, Swanson PC, Wu X, Hsieh CL, Lieber MR. A non-B-DNA structure at the Bcl-2 major breakpoint region is cleaved by the RAG complex. Nature 2004;428:88–93.
44. Bowater RP, Wells RD. The intrinsically unstable life of DNA triplet repeats associated with human hereditary disorders. Prog Nucleic Acid Res Mol Biol 2000;66:159–202.
45. Wells RD. Molecular basis of genetic instability of triplet repeats. J Biol Chem 1996;271:2875–2878.
46. Wells RD, Warren ST. Genetic Instabilities and Hereditary Neurological Diseases. San Diego, CA: Academic, 1998.
47. Cleary JD, Pearson CE. The contribution of cis-elements to disease-associated repeat instability: clinical and experimental evidence. Cytogenet Genome Res 2003;100:25–55.
48. Bacolla A, Gellibolian R, Shimizu M, et al. Flexible DNA: genetically unstable CTG•CAG and CGG•CCG from human hereditary neuromuscular disease genes. J Biol Chem 1997;272:16,783–16,792.
49. Napierala M, Dere R, Vetcher A, Wells RD. Structure-dependent recombination hot spot activity of GAA•TTC sequences from intron 1 of the Friedreich's ataxia gene. J Biol Chem 2004;279:6444–6454.
50. Vetcher AA, Napierala M, Iyer RR, Chastain PD, Griffith JD, Wells RD. Sticky DNA, a long GAA•GAA•TTC triplex that is formed intramolecularly, in the sequence of intron 1 of the frataxin gene. J Biol Chem 2002;277:39,217–39,227.
51. Vetcher AA, Wells RD. Sticky DNA formation in vivo alters the plasmid dimer/monomer ratio. J Biol Chem 2004;279:6434–6443.
52. Bayes M, Magano LF, Rivera N, Flores R, Perez Jurado LA. Mutational mechanisms of Williams-Beuren syndrome deletions. Am J Hum Genet 2003;73:131–151.
53. Nicholls RD, Knepper JL. Genome organization, function, and imprinting in Prader-Willi and Angelman syndromes. Annu Rev Genomics Hum Genet 2001;2:153–175.
54. Debeer P, Mols R, Huysmans C, Devriendt K, Van de Ven WJ, Fryns JP. Involvement of a palindromic chromosome 22-specific low-copy repeat in a constitutional t(X; 22)(q27;q11). Clin Genet 2002;62:410–414.

55. Brais B, Bouchard JP, Xie YG, et al. Short GCG expansions in the PABP2 gene cause oculopharyngeal muscular dystrophy. Nat Genet 1998;18:164–167.
56. Goldfarb LG, Brown P, McCombie WR, et al. Transmissible familial Creutzfeldt-Jakob disease associated with five, seven, and eight extra octapeptide coding repeats in the PRNP gene. Proc Natl Acad Sci USA 1991;88:10,926–10,930.
57. Lemmers RJ, Van Overveld PG, Sandkuijl LA, et al. Mechanism and timing of mitotic rearrangements in the subtelomeric D4Z4 repeat involved in facioscapulohumeral muscular dystrophy. Am J Hum Genet 2004;75: 44–53.

7

Genetic Basis of Olfactory Deficits

Idan Menashe, MSc, Ester Feldmesser, MSc and Doron Lancet, PhD

CONTENTS

INTRODUCTION

The completion of the human genome sequencing has opened new opportunities to better understand complex biological systems. In this realm, the human sense of smell is an excellent example of how genome analysis provides new information on genome organization and on deficits. Before the advent of genomic tools, the understanding of this highly sophisticated sensory neuronal pathway has been rather sketchy. In this chapter we summarize the relevant progress made in the last decade, and highlight the initial elucidation of two classes of olfactory deficits and their possible underlying genetic mechanisms.

THE SENSE OF SMELL

Olfaction, the sense of smell, is a versatile and sensitive mechanism for detecting volatile odorous molecules (odorants). Many organisms rely on olfactory cues for a wide range of activities such as food acquisition, reproduction, migration, and predator alarming. For that, the olfactory system is characterized by a remarkable ability to detect and discriminate thousands of low-molecular-mass compounds. This sophisticated chemical detection apparatus, which has evolved over approx 1 billion years, has long intrigued scientists attempting to understand its molecular facets.

From: *Genomic Disorders: The Genomic Basis of Disease*
Edited by: J. R. Lupski and P. Stankiewicz © Humana Press, Totowa, NJ

OLFACTORY PERCEPTION

Olfactory perception is a result of a cascade of biochemical and electrophysiological processes, in which the intrinsic information in the molecular structure of an odorant is converted into the perception of a characteristic odor quality. Odorants of various chemical configurations are inhaled and reach the olfactory epithelium, situated at the posterior region of the nasal cavity. This is the interface where odorants are bound and recognized, and where from axonal electrical messages are transmitted to the olfactory bulb of the brain. The human olfactory epithelium accommodates approx 10 million olfactory sensory neurons, each extending a single dendrite to the surface of the epithelium. The mucus-bathed dendritic ends bear specialized cilia, which expand the receptive membrane surface. Odorants, carried by a stream of inhaled air, dissolve in mucus, and then interact with receptor proteins within the ciliary membrane. The binding of odorants to one or more of a repertoire of hundreds of specific receptor proteins initiates a cascade of signal transduction events, involving the G protein-dependent elevation of cyclic adenosine monophosphate (cAMP), opening of cation channels, and membrane depolarization (Fig. 1). This process triggers action potential in the unmyelinated axons of the olfactory sensory neurons, leading to the olfactory bulb. There, the axons form synapses with apical dendrites of mitral cells within structures called glomeruli. Mitral axons leaving the olfactory bulb project widely to other brain structures, such as the olfactory cortex, where further information processing occurs.

It is generally accepted that the olfactory system employs a combinatorial strategy to discriminate among the millions of odorous compounds and their mixtures. Odor perception appears to be a multidimensional task, whereby every olfactory receptor (OR) binds numerous types of odorants with different affinities and vice versa *(1–3)*. Consequently, a unique combinatorial code is generated for every odor stimulus, suggesting that olfactory discrimination is a polygenic trait. However, based on the receptor affinity distribution model *(4)*, most of the odorant binding affinities of an OR are weak, and only few have biological significance. Of these, the strongest affinity receptor determines the detection and recognition thresholds, which may, therefore, be treated as a single gene trait *(2)*.

OLFACTORY RECEPTORS

OR proteins, of which the Nobel-awarded discovery took place 13 years ago *(5)*, belong to the G protein-coupled receptors (GPCRs) superfamily, transducers of a wide array of extracellular signaling molecules that constitute important targets in the pharmaceutical industry *(6)*. Members of this protein superfamily share features of sequence and structure, including seven hydrophobic transmembrane helices, as well as three intracellular and three extracellular loops that link these helices. ORs belong to GPCR family A, or rhodopsin-like GPCRs, which is the largest and most well-studied. Although the overall sequence similarity between the various members of this family is very low, with mean amino acid pairwise identity of 17% *(6)*, they share several highly conserved sequence motifs that are thought to play an essential role in either maintaining the structure and functional conformational transitions of these proteins, or in interacting with upstream and downstream partners *(7)*.

In most mammals, the olfactory repertoire has 1000–1400 OR genes, constituting the largest gene family within their genomes *(8–10)*. The OR coding region spans approx 1 kb, almost always without introns, a property that facilitates their identification and cloning from genomic DNA. OR genes are divided into two classes containing 17 families, which further divided into

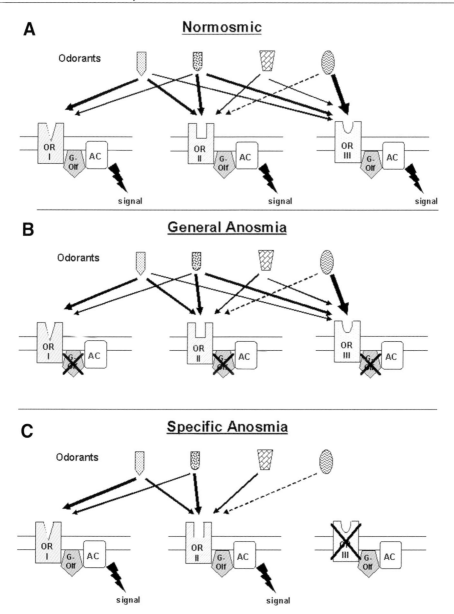

Fig. 1. A schematic drawing of olfactory perception and potential underlying mechanisms of olfactory deficits. The three principal olfactory traits in human beings are depicted. (A) Normosmic—both the olfactory receptors (ORs) and the subsequent signaling cascade molecules are intact, allowing the perception of all available odorous volatile molecules (odorants). (B) General anosmia—damaging mutation in one or more of the olfactory signal transduction proteins would extinguish the olfactory signal stemming from all OR types. (C) Specific anosmia—inactivation of one OR would eliminate the response or significant decrease the threshold toward one or a few particular odorants. Such specific OR inactivation would likely not affect perception of other odorants.

subfamilies, all based on sequence similarity scores. ORs with more than 40% protein sequence identity are considered within the same family and if they share more than 60%—as belonging to the same subfamily *(11)*. It was suggested that ORs of the same subfamily might recognize

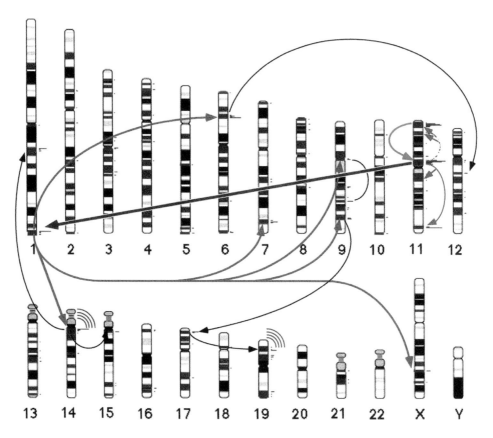

Fig. 2. A tentative schematic view of olfactory receptor (OR) genes genomic expansion. The proposed steps, in rough chronological order, are: (1) a duplication on chromosome 11 that resulted in the formation of the first class II cluster out of an original class I cluster (thick cyan). (2) A duplication that led to the formation of a cluster on chromosome 1, most likely in the framework of a whole genome diploidization (thick magenta). (3) Internal duplications within chromosome 11 (thin green), and expansion from chromosome 1 onto a number of other chromosomes (thick green). (4) Additional isolated duplications (thin black), gene scattering of family 4 (red "radio waves") and family 7 (blue "radio waves"). Only the generation of clusters larger than five members is explicitly shown. The small red histograms to the right of the chromosomal bands indicate OR gene cluster locations, with the area proportional to cluster size (*see* http://bip.weizmann.ac.il/HORDE for details). (Reproduced with permission from ref. *8*.)

molecules with similar chemical and/or physical characteristics *(3,12,13)*. However, more experimental evidences are needed to fully confirm this assumption *(14,15)*.

Vertebrate OR genes are organized in genomic clusters and are distributed on almost all chromosomes. As an example, in humans they are absent only on chromosomes 20 and Y. This wide genomic distribution is believed to have evolved from a single OR gene cluster on human chromosome 11 (11 at 4.96) that contains only OR genes of class I. An intrachromosomal duplication may have originated the first class II OR gene cluster. This cluster is inferred to have further duplicated to the q-telomeric region of human chromosome 1 and from there to have expanded to many other genomic loci (Fig. 2). This evolutionary process of OR genes migration was favored by strong selective pressure toward expanding and diversifying the OR gene repertoire, as increased OR count likely enhances both sensitivity and selectivity *(4)*. Interestingly, this repertoire augmentation process appears to have been reversed in primates in the last 20 million years, probably because they became less dependent on olfactory cues *(16–18)*. This is manifested in the observation that in such species OR genes underwent a massive accumulation of pseudogenizing mutations, generating in-frame stop codons. This process of OR gene loss has remarkably accelerated in the human lineage leaving less than half of the OR genes intact *(8,16,17,19,20)*. The high prevalence of defective human OR coding regions is a wide evolutionary deterioration, and its phenotypic impact awaits elucidation. Each such pseudogene may be regarded as a natural knockout, potentially affecting the human ability to detect and discriminate odorants.

HUMAN OLFACTORY PHENOTYPE VARIABILITY

Human beings are considered microsmatic organisms (organisms with a more feeble sense of smell). Although we are less dependent on olfactory cues for survival, we utilize them extensively in enjoying perfumes, food, and beverage, avoiding poisons and stale food, as well as in subtle social interactions. It stands to reason that the relative small number of OR genes in the human genome, as opposed to other macrosmatic mammals (animals with enhanced sense of smell, e.g., mouse and dog) *(8–10,20)*, is the reason for our somewhat poor olfactory sensitivity. Nevertheless, a recent study demonstrated that in human and other primates, typical detection thresholds toward various odorants are comparable to those of rodents *(21)*. It appears that the massive OR gene loss in human could underlie more subtle olfactory deficits.

It has indeed been known for decades that human beings are highly variable in their olfactory sensitivities. This inter-individual variability is in the form of cases of significant threshold deficiencies toward particular odorants, termed specific anosmia or "smell blindness" *(1,22–24)*. Such human deficiencies have been studied for dozens of odorous chemicals *(24)*. An ambitious study in this field was carried out under the auspices of the *National Geographic* magazine, examining six distinct odorants in nearly 1.5 million of its readers *(25)*. Pronounced variability was observed, with the most notable cases (approx 30% prevalence) of specific anosmia being toward Androstenone and Galaxolide (musk). This survey as well as other olfactory studies also demonstrated that olfactory sensitivity toward particular odorants may vary significantly according to age, gender, geographical location, and various environmental factors suggesting a complex trait *(26–29)*.

CONGENITAL GENERAL ANOSMIA

In addition to the human inter-individual diversity in perceiving specific odorants, humans also vary in their general olfactory capabilities. This covers a wide range of phenomena, from general anosmia through hyposmia (diminished sensitivity to smell). At the other end of the scale is general hyperosmia (enhanced smell sensitivity) *(30)*. Moreover, during aging, a general olfactory loss occurs, which is also a feature of several neurodegenerative diseases such as Alzheimer's and Parkinson's diseases *(31)*.

It is estimated that approx 1% of the Western world population suffers from chemosensory disorders. Most of the people suffering from smell disorders have an acquired condition, which develops during life, owing to allergy, viral upper respiratory tract infection, nasal sinus diseases, head trauma, inhalation of noxious chemicals, or medicinal drug intake *(32,33)*. A much smaller minority is born without a sense of smell, an affliction referred to here as congenital general anosmia (CGA). Two broad categories of CGA can be considered: CGA occurring with other anomalies (syndromic) and CGA seen as an isolated condition. Prevalence for isolated CGA is roughly estimated to be between 1:5000 and 1:20,000. Several past reports have described the condition, including a few familial cases. One of them shows 22 patients with 8 being familial *(34)*. On examination by biopsy of the olfactory region in several anosmic patients, their respiratory epithelium was found to be normal, but not their olfactory epithelium, some of them lacking it totally. In all cases, axonal abnormalities and the absence of mature olfactory sensory neurons were observed. It has been proposed that the olfactory epithelium may degenerate because of functional failure in olfaction *(34,35)*. Another study found a large four-generation family with 27 CGA-affected individuals *(36)*, and recently, two Iranian families with isolated CGA have been reported with a suggested 46-cm linkage interval on chromosome 18 *(37)*. A parallel study *(38)* has collected 27 individuals in 10 families and 56 sporadic cases of CGA. The three major candidate genes (*ADCY3, GNCA2, GNAL*) were screened in these individuals, but no causative mutations for CGA could be found. Although the number of affected families and individuals is small, all familial cases described are consistent with an autosomal dominant mode of inheritance with partial penetrance.

The most well studied group of syndromic CGA is related to the Kallmann syndrome. Such patients exhibit hypogonadotropic hypogonadism and anosmia, secondary to failure of gonadotropin-releasing hormone (GnRH)-producing neurons to migrate from the olfactory placode to the brain, and to agenesis of the olfactory bulbs. The prevalence of the disease has been estimated at 1 in 10,000 in males and five to seven times lower in females. Three different modes of inheritance have been reported in familial cases of Kallmann Syndrome, X chromosome-linked, autosomal dominant, and autosomal recessive *(39)*. The X-linked form of the Kallmann Syndrome has been well characterized, being caused by mutations in the gene *KAL1* (chromosome Xp22.3) *(40–42)*. The *KAL1* protein, anosmin-1, is a locally restricted component of basement membranes and/or extracellular matrices during the organogenesis period *(39)*. It has been found to enhance axonal branching from olfactory bulb output neurons *(43)* and to affect the migratory activity of GnRH-producing neurons *(44)*.

To date, no causative genes have been described for isolated human CGA. However in mouse, three transduction genes have revealed behavioral phenotypes consistent with general anosmia when they are inactivated. Mice generated by homologous recombination, lacking the functional olfactory cyclic nucleotide-gated channel (Cnga2) *(45)*, the stimulatory olfactory G-protein (Gnal), *(46)* or enzyme adenylyl cyclase III (Adcy3) *(47)*, display profound reductions or even absence of physiological responses to odorants. Most of the homozygously deficient mice die within a few days after birth owing to an apparent inability to locate their mother's nipple and suckle.

Congenital and progressive blindness have been studied much more extensively. Inherited forms of blindness can be caused by anomalies in the central nervous system *(48)* or in different parts of the eye: cornea, iris, lens, retina, and the optic nerve. About 140 genomic loci have been associated with retinal dystrophies and more than 60 genes have been identified. The partial similarity in the transduction processes between olfaction and vision may facilitate the future identification of some of the causative genes of CGA and its mode of genetic transmission.

SPECIFIC ANOSMIA

Specific anosmia is defined as incapacity of an individual with an otherwise normal smell sensitivity to detect particular odorants. Specific anosmia is seldom absolute, and most often a person has a 10- to 100-fold diminished sensitivity to a given odorant, hence, the more exact term is specific hyposmia. In contrast, specific hyperosmia, is described as enhanced sensitivity toward a specific odorant *(24)*. Both hyper- and hyposensitivity toward specific odorants are likely driven by the same molecular mechanism, yet despite the wide variety of reports of specific anosmia, no comparable evidence has been reported for specific hyperosmia.

Considerable evidence indicates that specific anosmia is genetically determined. For example, various studies showed that anosmia to Androstenone (16-Androsten-3-one), a steroid of gonadal origin that serves as a boar pheromone, is highly concordant in monozygotic twins *(22,49)*. Whissell-Buechy et al. *(50)* demonstrated that anosmia to the odorant Pentadecalactone behaves as a recessive trait in human beings. A similar Mendelian recessive inheritance was observed in mice with specific deficiency to detect Isovaleric acid *(51)*. A subsequent linkage analysis study has associated this phenotype with two distinct genomic loci, on mouse chromosomes 4 and 6 *(52)*. Interestingly, a small fraction in the human population is also incapable to specifically detect Isovaleric acid *(23)*. A comparable linkage analysis in human, potentially focusing on the human syntenic regions would be advisable.

Although specific anosmia has a strong genetic element, other confounding factors contribute to the overall olfactory variability of a human individual. For example, olfactory faculties are age dependent, reaching a maximum in the late teenage and then declining gradually *(26)*. This deterioration accelerates and becomes significant during the sixth decade. Similarly olfactory sensitivity may be influenced by the gender, whereby women have been reported to perform better than men in certain olfactory tests *(26)*. Other environmental and behavioral factors were also suggested to affect olfactory performance, whereby subjects allegedly anosmic to Androstenone became capable of smelling it following repeated exposure *(53)*. This phenomenon of "olfactory plasticity" could explain part of the variability in Androstenone perception, and in general, incomplete penetrance has to be taken into account for this odorant and its functional homologs. Overall, this evidence illustrates that human response to odorous molecules is a complex trait, regulated by genetic, developmental, and environmental factors.

The molecular basis of "odor blindness" (specific anosmia) is believed to be analogous to color blindness and specific taste deficits. Color vision is controlled by three genes encoding cone opsin receptors for long (red) and medium (green) wavelength (on chromosome X) and for short (blue) wavelengths (autosomal). Mutations that inactivate one of these genes abolishes significantly our color discrimination ability and resulting in a different form of color blindness *(54)*. A similar phenomenon was recently observed in the more complex system of taste perception. A member of the taste receptors class II (*T2R38*) gene was associated with the gustatory capability to detect phenylthiocarbamide (PTC) *(55)*. Like many cases of specific anosmia, the ability to taste the bitter taste of PTC was subject to various psychophysical studies that indicated a Mendelian recessive trait *(56)* with possible genetic and environmental confounding factors *(57)*. Indeed, the two haplotypes of the *T2R38* gene that segregated significantly between tasters and the nontasters of PTC could not explain the entire diversity in the study. Thus, it was suggested that PTC detection is a complex trait with a major quantitative trait locus, with relatively high phenotypic effect. In this aspect, smell perception is more closely related to gustation than to color vision, because it also employs a group of chemoreceptors to distinguish between large varieties of chemicals. Still, as all these three sensory pathways utilize the same operating principles that are based on GPCRs it may be suggested that their inter-individual phenotypic variability is driven by broadly similar genetic mechanisms.

THE POTENTIAL GENETIC MECHANISMS
OF HUMAN OLFACTORY DEFICITS

The potential underlying genetic mechanisms of human olfactory deficits may be deduced from the biochemical pathways of olfactory perception. The binding of an odorant to an OR initiates a cascade of events leading to olfactory signaling (Fig. 1), and damage in different steps of the transduction chain may lead to a deficient phenotype. The first group of candidate genes includes genes that participating in the olfactory signal transduction and its termination. Among these, the three main components of the olfactory transduction chain are the human orthologs of the mouse transduction genes previously described. Olfactory marker protein (OMP), a well-established marker of olfactory tissues (58) is another candidate gene, as it has been also shown to modulate the kinetics of olfactory electrophysiological responses. In addition, there are two kinds of phosphodiesterases (PDEs): calmodulin-PDE (PDE1C) and cAMP-PDE (PDE4E), and various protein kinases (59) that were implicated in the termination of the olfactory signal transduction. A second group of candidate genes for CGA are biotransformation enzymes proposed to play a role in the post-signaling processing of the odorant molecules themselves, thus eliminating them from the vicinity of ORs. These include cytochrome P-450 (CYP2G1) and uridine diphospho (UDP) glucoronosyl transferase (UGT2A1) (60,61). The third group consists of transcription factors that are crucial for the development and functionality of the olfactory system. These proteins are members of the Olf/Early B-cell factor and nuclear factor I transcription factor families, which mainly expressed in postmitotic olfactory neurons (62,63) and control the expression of several genes (ADCY3, CNGA2, and OMP). Finally, odorant-binding proteins (OBP2A), lipocalins that may mediate the binding of odorants to the olfactory receptors or prevent saturation of olfactory receptors by excessive odorant concentration (64), have a potential to underlie CGA. It should be noted that some of these candidate genes are functionally expressed in other non-olfactory tissues, and mutations in these components may result in more compound disorders or syndromic anosmia.

In contrast to the diverse genetic mechanisms that could underlie CGA, the main obvious candidate genetic determinants to be associated with specific anosmia are OR genes. Moreover, odorant-specific threshold deficits are significantly more prevalent than general anosmia (24,65) and, hence, are likely caused by more frequent genetic variations. Single nucleotide polymorphisms (SNPs) sites at which two alternative bases occur at appreciable frequency, are the most common genetic variation in the human genome. Consequently, they are believed to constitute the genetic component of most multifactorial human traits. In the case of specific anosmia, SNPs that damage a particular OR function could lead to significant threshold sensitivity differences toward a particular odorant. This could be rationalized by the "threshold hypothesis" (2). According to this premise, the highest-affinity receptor toward a certain odorant is the one that determines the odorant's threshold sensitivity. If this OR is being inactivated, the threshold will be defined by the next highest-affinity receptor. In the case of a larger OR repertoire, as in rodents, a higher level of functional redundancy will obtain, and the loss of the highest-affinity receptor will have a diminished probability to generate a recognizable olfactory deficit. In contrast, in humans, where the OR repertoire has diminished significantly, affinity values would tend to be more widely spaced, and threshold variations could become more prevalent. In these cases, an inactivating polymorphism in an OR encodes the best receptor for a certain odorant, is expected to cause significant threshold difference between individuals who carry the functional OR to those in whom it is deleted.

Various types of SNPs in OR genes might underlie odorant-specific olfactory deficits. The most obvious ones are the approx 600 nonsynonymous SNPs that may change a crucial residue to the protein function *(66)*. For example, changing the arginine (R) in the highly conserved MAYDRY motif that is believed to participate in the coupling of the G protein to the receptor was demonstrated to terminate the protein function *(67)*. Despite the relatively high conservation of this residue, it has been found to display polymorphisms in 15 different OR genes, which is significantly more than the average of the polymorphism count per residue along the protein sequence. Other types of candidate polymorphisms are those that change amino acids in the complementarity-determining region for odorant recognition in a functional OR *(12,13)*. These might not inactivate the receptor but rather change the affinity spectrum of its corresponding odorants. In addition, polymorphisms in the promoter or other regulatory regions of OR genes might also cause OR inactivation *(68)*. The present partial knowledge about the genomic disposition and control mechanisms of ORs renders the detection of such important deleterious polymorphisms less straightforward.

The most promising candidates for underlying odorant-specific olfactory deficits are recently discovered SNPs of a highly unusual disposition. These generate a premature stop codon in the OR gene sequence and consequently segregate between an intact gene and an inactive one (pseudogene). Several dozens such segregating pseudogenes have been discovered in the human OR subgenome *(69)*. These define a remarkable genetic variability, whereby almost every human being possesses a unique assortment of intact and disrupted ORs. Furthermore, significant differences were observed between various ethnic groups in the degree to which certain polymorphic pseudogenes are conserved in their intact forms. Although these ethnic differences in functional OR repertoires could be explained in terms of geographic isolation and bottleneck events, an alternative evolutionary mechanism is related selection, suggesting that different intact ORs tend to be conserved more effectively depending on geography or lifestyle. These OR segregating pseudogenes introduce a remarkable genetic diversity to the human genome, whose phenotypic correlates awaits elucidation.

Another type of potential causative genetic polymorphisms in human OR genes are the observed variations in copy number of several OR genes, mainly on chromosomal telomeric regions *(70)*. These polymorphisms are believed to have emerged via meiotic nonallelic homologous recombination (NAHR) events that are associated with genomic segmental duplication in the human genome. In rare meioses, these segmental duplications are mistaken for allelic sequences, with the result that chromosomes are incorrectly spliced. Consequently, NAHR could account for various types of genomic rearrangement in OR clusters, such as deletions, duplication, and inversions. Similarly, it may account for gene conversion events that may underlie disruptive mutations, by introducing nonfunctional sequences from a pseudogene into a functional gene *(16,71)*.

Although ORs are the best candidates, the potential involvement of nonreceptor genes in specific anosmia cannot be ruled out. A well-known example is the involvement of Acj6, a POU-domain transcription factor, in specific anosmia to a subset of odorants in the fruit fly *Drosophila melanogaster (72)*.

FUTURE PROSPECTS IN OLFACTORY GENETICS

The significance of olfaction to human's life quality is often underestimated. This sensory pathway plays a key role in food and beverage recognition and enjoyment, it enables people to avoid dangers such as smoke, spoiled food, and poison, and it affects human social interactions. The realization of the underlying genetic mechanisms of human olfactory diversity would open new opportunities to both the food and fragrance industry. For example, human panels for the testing of new products would be selected such that their genetic profiles will fit those of the targeted consumers in an optimal way. Similarly, products could be directed to certain segments of the population according to their predictable olfactory capabilities. Alternatively, specific anosmia or hyperosmia could be artificially induced to eliminate or enhance specific odors. This could be done both in the genomic level where specific OR gene would be silenced or overexpressed, and at the protein level, using agonists and antagonist. Thus, much of the future of olfactory research and development might depend on deciphering the genetic basis of human-specific deficiencies.

Pseudogenes, nonfunctional copies of genes, have been considered always as molecular relics with no effect on human traits. Therefore, they have been attributed always to the neglected genomic majority of non-coding "junk" DNA. With the completion of the human genome sequencing, it became clear that pseudogenes are comparably distributed in our genome as coding genes *(73,74)*. Consequently, there is a higher interest in improving the pseudogene annotation in the human genome and in studying their functional roles *(75)*. In this realm, the special evolutionary state of the human OR gene family where many members exist at the border between functional genes and nonfunctional pseudogenes provides an unusual opportunity to explore the effect of pseudogene accumulation to human fitness. Finding the phenotypic correlates of segregating pseudogenes in the human olfactory system could shed new light on the function of pseudogenes in the human genome.

Finally, in the post-genome era, considerable efforts are devoted to decipher the genetic basis of human multi-factorial traits, attempting to correlate between phenotypes and genotypes. In this realm, genetic research of olfactory deficits could be an excellent model system for understanding the genetics of human variation in gene families in general. As in olfaction, there are many biological systems where genes families subserve a particular functional role in identification and processing various ligand libraries. We propose, therefore, that a better understanding, through genetic studies, of odorant-OR relations would significantly help to form a better picture of similar complex systems.

SUMMARY

The sense of smell, a discriminator of millions of volatile compounds, is crucial for survival and well being. Mutations in the olfactory G protein transduction pathway result in complete olfactory deficiency in mouse. Owing to the rarity of the human counterpart deficit, CGA, only a few affected families have been described, and no causative mutations have been identified as of yet. In contrast, genetic polymorphisms in OR genes are prevalent and amply documented. Some of these genetic variants exchange between a functional and nonfunctional forms of the coded OR protein (segregating pseudogenes), whereas others segregate between gene existence and absence. These genetic polymorphisms are promising candidate to underlie the abundant human olfactory threshold variations—the specific anosmia phenotypes. Future studies of human olfactory deficits would shed further light on the molecular mechanism of odor perception, as well as on the genetics of analogous biological systems.

REFERENCES

1. Amoore JE. Specific anosmia: a clue to the olfactory code. Nature 1967;214:1095–1098.

2. Lancet D, Ben-Arie N, Cohen S, et al. Olfactory receptors: transduction, diversity, human psychophysics and genome analysis. Ciba Found Symp 1993;179:131–141.
3. Malnic B, Hirono J, Sato T, Buck L. Combinatorial receptor codes for odors. Cell 1999;96:1–20.
4. Lancet D, Sadovsky E, Seidemann E. Probability model for molecular recognition in biological receptor repertoires: significance to the olfactory system. Proc Natl Acad Sci USA 1993;90:3715–3719.
5. Buck L, Axel R. A novel multigene family may encode odorant receptors: a molecular basis for odor recognition. Cell 1991;65:175–187.
6. Schoneberg T, Schulz A, Gudermann T. The structural basis of G-protein-coupled receptor function and dysfunction in human diseases. Rev Physiol Biochem Pharmacol 2002;144:143–227.
7. Gether U. Uncovering molecular mechanisms involved in activation of G protein-coupled receptors. Endocr Rev 2000;21:90–113.
8. Glusman G, Yanai I, Rubin I, Lancet D. The complete human olfactory subgenome. Genome Res 2001;11: 685–702.
9. Zhang X, Firestein S. The olfactory receptor gene superfamily of the mouse. Nat Neurosci 2002;5:124–133.
10. Olender T, Fuchs T, Linhart C, et al. The canine olfactory subgenome. Genomics 2004;83:361–372.
11. Glusman G, Sosinsky A, Ben-Asher E, et al. Sequence, structure and evolution of complete human olfactory receptor gene cluster. Genomics 2000;63:227–245.
12. Pilpel Y, Lancet D. The variable and conserved interfaces of modeled olfactory receptor proteins. Protein Science 1999;8:969–977.
13. Man O, Gilad Y, Lancet D. Prediction of the odorant binding site of olfactory receptor proteins by human-mouse comparisons. Protein Sci 2004;13:240–254.
14. Zhao H, Ivic L, Otaki JM, Hashimoto M, Mikoshiba K, Firestein S. Functional expression of a mammalian odorant receptor. Science 1998;279:237–242.
15. Krautwurst D, Yau KW, Reed RR. Identification of ligands for olfactory receptors by functional expression of a receptor library. Cell 1998;97:917–926.
16. Sharon D, Glusman G, Pilpel Y, et al. Primate evolution of an olfactory receptor cluster: diversification by gene conversion and recent emergence of pseudogenes. Genomics 1999;1:24–36.
17. Gilad Y, Man O, Paabo S, Lancet D. Human specific loss of olfactory receptor genes. Proc Natl Acad Sci USA 2003;100:3324–3327.
18. Gilad Y, Wiebe V, Przeworski M, Lancet D, Paabo S. Loss of olfactory receptor genes coincide with aquisition of full trichromatic vision in primates. PLoS Biol 2004;2:E5.
19. Zozulya S, Echeverri F, Nguyen T. The human olfactory receptor repertoire. Genome Biol 2001;2, RESEARCH0018.
20. Young JM, Friedman C, Williams EM, Ross JA, Tonnes-Priddy L, Trask BJ. Different evolutionary processes shaped the mouse and human olfactory receptor gene families. Hum Mol Genet 2002;11:1683.
21. Laska M, Seibt A, Weber A. 'Microsmatic' primates revisited: olfactory sensitivity in the squirrel monkey. Chem Senses 2000;25:47–53.
22. Gross-Isseroff R, Ophir D, Bartana A, Voet H, Lancet D. Evidence for genetic determination in human twins of olfactory thresholds for a standard odorant. Neurosci Lett 1992;141:115–118.
23. Amoore JE, Venstrom D, Davis AR. Measurments of specific anosmia. Percep Motor Skills 1968;26:143–164.
24. Amoore JE, Steinle S. A graphic history of specific anosmia. Chem Senses 1991;3:331–351.
25. Gibbons B. Smell survey. National Geographic. 1986;170:3.
26. Russell MJ, Cummings BJ, Profitt BF, Wysocki CJ, Gilbert AN, Cotman CW. Life span changes in the verbal categorization of odors. J Gerontol 1993;48:P49–P53.
27. Corwin J, Loury M, Gilbert AN. Workplace, age, and sex as mediators of olfactory function: data from the National Geographic Smell Survey. J Gerontol B Psychol Sci Soc Sci 1995;50:P179–P186.
28. Wysocki CJ, Gilbert AN. National Geographic Smell Survey. Effects of age are heterogenous. Ann NY Acad Sci 1989;561:12–28.
29. Schiffman SS, Nagle HT. Effect of environmental pollutants on taste and smell. Otolaryngol Head Neck Surg 1992;106:693–700.
30. Henkin RI. Hyperosmia and depression following exposure to toxic vapors. JAMA 1990;264:2803.
31. Kovacs T. Mechanisms of olfactory dysfunction in aging and neurodegenerative disorders. Ageing Res Rev 2004;3:215–232.
32. Apter AJ, Gent JF, Frank ME. Fluctuating olfactory sensitivity and distorted odor perception in allergic rhinitis. Arch Otolaryngol Head Neck Surg 1999;125:1005–1010.

33. Zusho H. Posttraumatic anosmia. Arch Otolaryngol 1982;108:90–92.
34. Leopold DA, Hornung DE, Schwob JE. Congenital lack of olfactory ability. Ann Otol Rhinol Laryngol 1992;101:229–236.
35. Jafek BW, Gordon AS, Moran DT, Eller PM. Congenital anosmia. Ear Nose Throat J 1990;69:331–337.
36. Lygonis CS. Familiar absence of olfaction. Hereditas 1969;61:413–416.
37. Ghadami M, Morovvati S, Majidzadeh AK, et al. Isolated congenital anosmia locus maps to 18p11.23-q12.2. J Med Genet 2004;41:299–303.
38. Feldmesser E, Halbertal S, Frydman M, Gross-Iseroff R, Lancet D. List of Abstracts from AChemS XXIII: The molecular genetics of human congenital general anosmia. Chem Senses 2002;27:663.
39. Hardelin JP, Soussi-Yanicostas N, Ardouin O, Levilliers J, Petit C. Kallmann syndrome. Adv Otorhinolaryngol 2000;56:268–274.
40. del Castillo I, Cohen-Salmon M, Blanchard S, Lutfalla G, Petit C. Structure of the X-linked Kallmann syndrome gene and its homologous pseudogene on the Y chromosome. Nat Genet 1992;2:305–310.
41. Ballabio A, Parenti G, Tippett P, et al. X-linked ichthyosis, due to steroid sulphatase deficiency, associated with Kallmann syndrome (hypogonadotropic hypogonadism and anosmia): linkage relationships with Xg and cloned DNA sequences from the distal short arm of the X chromosome. Hum Genet 1986;72:237–240.
42. Franco B, Guioli S, Pragliola A, et al. A gene deleted in Kallmann's syndrome shares homology with neural cell adhesion and axonal path-finding molecules. Nature 1991;353:529–536.
43. Soussi-Yanicostas N, de Castro F, Julliard AK, Perfettini I, Chedotal A, Petit C. Anosmin-1, defective in the X-linked form of Kallmann syndrome, promotes axonal branch formation from olfactory bulb output neurons. Cell 2002;109:217–228.
44. Cariboni A, Pimpinelli F, Colamarino S, et al. The product of X-linked Kallmann's syndrome gene (KAL1) affects the migratory activity of gonadotropin-releasing hormone (GnRH)-producing neurons. Hum Mol Genet 2004;13:2781–2791.
45. Brunet LJ, Gold GH, Ngai J. General anosmia caused by a targeted disruption of the mouse olfactory cyclic nucleotide-gated cation channel. Neuron 1996;17:1–20.
46. Belluscio L, Gold GH, Nemes A, Axel R. Mice deficient in G(olf) are anosmic. Neuron 1998;20:69–81.
47. Wong ST, Trinh K, Hacker B, et al. Disruption of the type III adenylyl cyclase gene leads to peripheral and behavioral anosmia in transgenic mice. Neuron 2000;27:487–497.
48. Pietrobon D. Calcium channels and channelopathies of the central nervous system. Mol Neurobiol 2002;25:31–50.
49. Wysocki CJ, Beauchamp GK. Ability to smell androstenone is genetically determined. Proc Natl Acad Sci USA 1984;81:4899–4902.
50. Whissell-Buechy D, Amoore JE. Odour-blindness to musk: simple recessive inheritance. Nature 1973;242: 271–273.
51. Wysocki CJ, Whitney G, Tucker D. Specific anosmia in the laboratory mouse. Behav Genet 1977;7:171–188.
52. Griff IC, Reed RR. The genetic basis for specific anosmia to isovaleric acid in the mouse. Cell 1995;83: 407–414.
53. Wysocki CJ, Dorries KM, Beauchamp GK. Ability to perceive androstenone can be acquired by ostensibly anosmic people. Proc Natl Acad Sci USA 1989;86:7976–7978.
54. Nathans J. The evolution and physiology of human color vision: insights from molecular genetic studies of visual pigments. Neuron 1999;24:299–312.
55. Kim UK, Jorgenson E, Coon H, Leppert M, Risch N, Drayna D. Positional cloning of the human quantitative trait locus underlying taste sensitivity to phenylthiocarbamide. Science 2003;299:1221–1225.
56. Guo SW, Reed DR. The genetics of phenylthiocarbamide perception. Ann Hum Biol 2001;28:111–142.
57. Olson JM, Boehnke M, Neiswanger K, Roche AF, Siervogel RM. Alternative genetic models for the inheritance of the phenylthiocarbamide taste deficiency. Genet Epidemiol 1989;6:423–434.
58. Ivic L, Pyrski MM, Margolis JW, Richards LJ, Firestein S, Margolis FL. Adenoviral vector-mediated rescue of the OMP-null phenotype in vivo. Nat Neurosci 2000;3:1113–1120.
59. Nakamura T. Cellular and molecular constituents of olfactory sensation in vertebrates. Comp Biochem Physiol A Mol Integr Physiol 2000;126:17–32.
60. Lazard D, Tal N, Rubinstein M, Khen M, Lancet D, Zupko K. Identification and biochemical analysis of novel olfactory-specific cytochrome P-450IIA and UDP-glucuronosyl transferase. Biochemistry 1990;29: 7433–7440.
61. Nef P, Heldman J, Lazard D, et al. Olfactory-specific cytochrome P-450. cDNA cloning of a novel neuroepithelial enzyme possibly involved in chemoreception. J Biol Chem 1989;264:6780–6785.

62. Behrens M, Venkatraman G, Gronostajski RM, Reed RR, Margolis FL. NFI in the development of the olfactory neuroepithelium and the regulation of olfactory marker protein gene expression. Eur J Neurosci 2000;12: 1372–1384.

63. Wang SS, Tsai RY, Reed RR. The characterization of the Olf-1/EBF-like HLH transcription factor family: implications in olfactory gene regulation and neuronal development. J Neurosci 1997;17:4149–4158.

64. Pelosi P. The role of perireceptor events in vertebrate olfaction. Cell Mol Life Sci 2001;58:503–509.

65. Gilbert AN, Wysocki CJ. Results of the Smell Survey. National Geographic 1987;172:514–525.

66. Olender T, Feldmesser E, Atarot T, Eisenstein M, Lancet D. The olfactory receptor universe – from whole genome analysis to structure and evolution. Genet Mol Res 2004;3:545–553.

67. Gaillard I, Rouquier S, Chavanieu A, Mollard P, Giorgi D. Amino-acid changes acquired during evolution by olfactory receptor 912-93 modify the specificity of odorant recognition. Hum Mol Genet 2004;13:771–780.

68. Serizawa S, Miyamichi K, Sakano H. One neuron-one receptor rule in the mouse olfactory system. Trends Genet 2004;20:648–653.

69. Menashe I, Man O, Lancet D, Gilad Y. Different noses for different people. Nat Genet 2003;34:143–144.

70. Trask BJ, Friedman C, Martin-Gallardo A, et al. Members of the olfactory receptor gene family are contained in large blocks of DNA duplicated polymorphically near the ends of human chromosomes. Hum Mol Genet 1998;7:13–26.

71. Nagawa F, Yoshihara S, Tsuboi A, Serizawa S, Itoh K, Sakano H. Genomic analysis of the murine odorant receptor MOR28 cluster: a possible role of gene conversion in maintaining the olfactory map. Gene 2002;292:73–80.

72. Clyne P, Warr C, Freeman M, Lessing D, Kim J, Carlson J. A novel family of divergent seven-transmembrane proteins: candidate odorant receptors in Drosophila. Neuron 1999;22:327–338.

73. Harrison PM, Gerstein M. Studying genomes through the aeons: protein families, pseudogenes and proteome evolution. J Mol Biol 2002;318:1155–1174.

74. Torrents D, Suyama M, Zdobnov E, Bork P. A genome-wide survey of human pseudogenes. Genome Res 2003;13:2559–2567.

75. Hirotsune S, Yoshida N, Chen A, et al. An expressed pseudogene regulates the messenger-RNA stability of its homologous coding gene. Nature 2003;423:91–96.

8

Genomic Organization and Function of Human Centromeres

Huntington F. Willard, PhD
and M. Katharine Rudd, PhD

CONTENTS

BACKGROUND

Centromeres are required for normal chromosome segregation in mitosis and meiosis, and a substantial proportion of human pathology stems from abnormalities of chromosome segregation, the underlying genomic basis and mechanism(s) of which are largely unknown. Human centromeres consist of megabases of α-satellite DNA, a tandemly repeated DNA family whose genomic organization, evolution, and function is increasingly well understood. The study of normal, abnormal, and engineered human chromosomes is providing insights into the nature of human centromeres and their mechanism of action, as well as enabling comparison with centromeres of other eukaryotic organisms and the identification of genomic elements required for normal centromere function.

INTRODUCTION

The centromere in all eukaryotic organisms including humans plays a critical role in each step of chromosome segregation in mitosis and meiosis. As the site of the proteinaceous kinetochore, the centromere is responsible for attaching chromosomes to spindle microtubules that then align the chromosomes at the metaphase plate *(1)*. Proteins localized to the centromere are also involved in the metaphase to anaphase checkpoint and signal the attachment of all chromosomes to spindle microtubules before allowing the cell to progress into anaphase

From: *Genomic Disorders: The Genomic Basis of Disease*
Edited by: J. R. Lupski and P. Stankiewicz © Humana Press, Totowa, NJ

(2). Finally, sister chromatid cohesion must be resolved at the centromere, and proper timing of the removal of cohesion is of vital importance for segregating chromatids *(3)*.

The centromere is defined by specific genomic DNA sequences, as well as by a specialized chromatin structure. Although centromere proteins are highly conserved among a number of eukaryotic organisms, DNA sequences at the centromere are not well conserved *(4,5)*. In fact, centromeres range in size and complexity from the 125-bp centromere found in budding yeast to the human centromere that spans several megabases. Like centromeres in most complex organisms, the human centromere is made up of repetitive DNA. α-satellite DNA, a tandemly repeated DNA family based on a fundamental unit length of approx 171 bp, has been found at all human centromeres *(6–8)* and has served as a model to study the genomics, evolutionary dynamics, and general potential function(s) of satellite DNAs.

The focus of this chapter is the structure and function of centromeric regions in the human genome. We discuss the genomic organization and evolution of α-satellite DNA, current concepts of centromeric chromatin, and efforts to assess normal centromere function in human chromosomes, utilizing both structurally abnormal chromosomes derived from patient material and engineered human artificial chromosomes.

CENTROMERE ORGANIZATION

Eukaryotic Centromere Organization

The sequences that make up the centromeres of diverse organisms are extremely variable. Most well-characterized centromeres contain repetitive DNA with an AT-richness greater than that of the genome average *(9,10)*. However, individual organisms have evolved different genomic structures to create a locus capable of chromosome segregation *(11)*.

The simplest centromere organization is found in the chromosomes of the yeast, *Saccharomyces cerevisiae*. Only approx 125 bp is required for centromere function in the budding yeast, and this sequence motif is shared among the centromeres of all 16 chromosomes. Unlike other characterized centromeres, the budding yeast centromere consists of largely unique DNA *(12)*.

In contrast to the simple centromere of the budding yeast, the fission yeast centromere is more similar to the centromeres of higher eukaryotes in its size and complexity. *Schizosaccharomyces pombe* centromeres are made up of inner and outer inverted repeats flanking a nonrepetitive central core *(12)*, and each of these regions is AT-rich. Among the three *S. pombe* chromosomes, the centromeres are similar, but not identical in organization (Fig. 1). Overall, *S. pombe* centromeres are 35–110 kb in size *(12)*, spanning a few percent of the linear length of each chromosome. The inner repeats and central core are necessary for centromere function and bind spindle microtubules *(13,14)*, whereas the outer repeats recruit heterochromatin proteins and are more likely responsible for functions such as heterochromatin formation and sister chromatid cohesion *(15,16)*.

Centromeres in several other organisms are characterized by long stretches of so-called "satellite DNA." The *Drosophila* centromere has been defined by a 420-kb region of a minichromosome that is required for chromosome transmission. The fly centromeric region consists of two adjacent blocks of short microsatellites, based on AATAT and AAGAG repeats, that are interspersed with transposons as well as AT-rich DNA *(11,17,18)*. Normal fly centromeres have not been fully sequenced, owing to the difficulty of sequencing and assembling highly heterochromatic regions of the genome *(19)*. However, the chromatin environment of endogenous *Drosophila* centromeres has been very well characterized *(20–22)*.

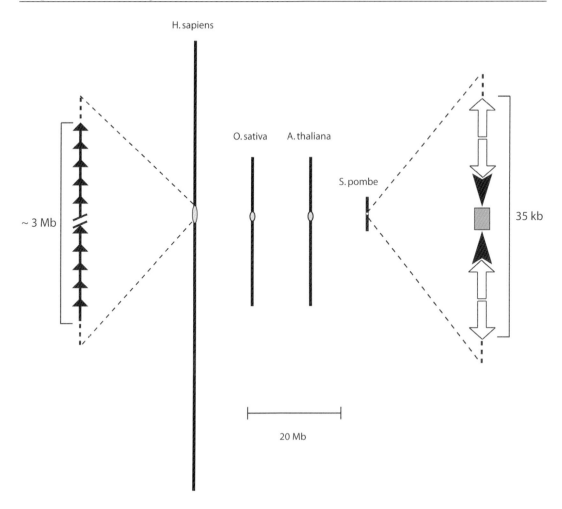

Fig. 1. Schematic representation of genomic organization of centromeres. In the center of the figure are representative chromosomes drawn to scale from the human (*Homo sapiens*), rice (*Oryza sativa*), Arabidopsis (*Arabidopsis thaliana*), and fission yeast (*Schizosaccharomyces pombe*) genomes. For each, the extent of the centromere region is indicated by the gray oval and comprises a few percent of each chromosome. At the right is an expanded view of a centromere from *S. pombe*. Each *S. pombe* centromere contains an approx 4-kb central core (gray box), bordered by approx 6 kb of imperfect repeats on the chromosome arms. The organization of the outer repeats is more variable among chromosomes, but all belong to the same subfamilies of repeats. At the left is an expanded view of a centromere from a human chromosome. A typical centromere region spans several megabases and consists of 1000 or more tandem copies of α-satellite higher-order repeats (indicated by arrows). Higher-resolution views are available from refs. *33* and *34* and in Fig. 2.

Plant centromeres are very similar to the satellite- and transposon-rich fly centromeres *(23)*. The major component of the *Arabidopsis thaliana* centromere is an AT-rich 180-bp repeat unit, spanning 400 kb to 1.4 Mb among chromosomes *(24)*. The *Arabidopsis* centromere is also enriched for retrotransposons not usually found on chromosome arms. A similar picture has emerged for the rice (*Oryza sativa*) centromere, which is comprised predominantly of a 155-bp tandem repeat unit arranged in arrays ranging from 65 kb to 2 Mb among the 12 rice chromosomes *(25)* (Fig. 1). These arrays are interspersed with gypsy-class retrotransposons. The *Arabidopsis* and rice centromeres have recently been defined at the level of chromatin, and chromatin immunoprecipitation experiments using antibodies to proteins required for centromere function have been conducted in both species. As expected, centromere proteins are associated with satellite repeats in both *Arabidopsis (26)* and rice *(27)*. However, within the functional domain of the smallest rice centromere, there are also four expressed genes. This finding is surprising because centromeres are classically thought of as heterochromatic regions resistant to gene expression *(28,29)*.

As opposed to all other normal centromeres described, the centromeres of *Caenorhabditis elegans* appear to be completely sequence-independent. *C. elegans* chromosomes are holocentric, meaning that many sites along the chromosome act as a centromere, capable of recruiting centromere proteins necessary for segregation *(30–32)*. Holocentric chromosomes are a curious contrast to the monocentric chromosomes found in most other species typically containing repetitive AT-rich DNA at the centromeres.

Human Centromere Organization

The human centromere is made up of highly repetitive DNA known as α-satellite, which together comprise an estimated 2–3% of the human genome *(7,33)*. All normal human centromeres are comprised of α-satellite DNA, although the organization of α-satellite varies from centromere to centromere *(8)*. The most basic unit of α-satellite DNA is an approx 171-bp monomer, and monomers may be arranged in one of two configurations of α-satellite, designated "higher-order" or "monomeric" *(6,33,34)*. Higher-order α-satellite is made up of monomers organized in highly homogeneous higher-order repeat units *(8,34)*. For example, the higher-order α-satellite array found on chromosome 17, D17Z1, is made up of 16 monomers arranged head to tail to form a 2.7-kb higher-order repeat unit that is in turn repeated in tandem over a thousand times at the chromosome 17 centromere *(7)*. Higher-order α-satellite has been found at all human centromeres, and higher-order arrays on individual chromosomes in the population range from a few hundred kilobases on some Y chromosomes to nearly 5 Mb in size for some autosomes (Fig. 1).

α-Satellite with a less homogeneous monomeric organization is also found at most, if not all, human centromeric regions, and this type of α-satellite by definition lacks any higher-order periodicity *(33,34)*. Where monomeric α-satellite has been described, it has been found adjacent to higher-order α-satellite and is less abundant than the megabase-sized arrays of higher-order α-satellite. Unlike higher-order α-satellite, monomeric α-satellite is regularly interspersed with other repeat elements and with duplicated sequences, as well as some unique sequences *(34,35)*.

Although higher-order α-satellite has been linked to centromere function, there is no evidence for monomeric α-satellite contributing to proper chromosome segregation. Thus, higher-order and monomeric α-satellites occupy physically and functionally distinct regions of each chromosome (Fig. 2A). To reflect these distinctions, the arrays of higher-order α-satellite and adjacent regions including monomeric α-satellite and other sequences are most clearly termed the "centromere" and "pericentromere," respectively *(36,37)*.

α-SATELLITE EVOLUTION

The organization of α-satellite is a product of concerted evolutionary processes *(7)*, and, thus, these sequences typically exhibit higher sequence identity within a species than between

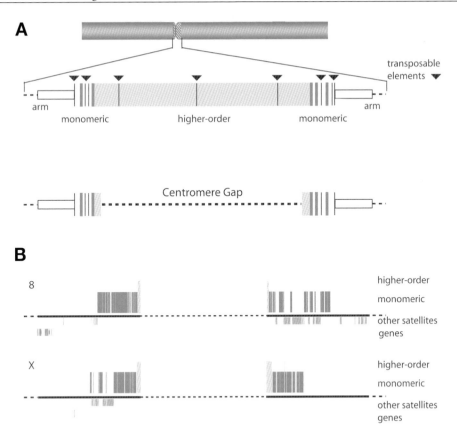

Fig. 2. Genomic organization and annotation of human centromeres. (A) General model of centromeric region. The centromere itself is contained within a large array of higher-order α-satellite (light gray) that spans several megabases and is only rarely interrupted by nonsatellite sequences such as transposable elements. The array is flanked by shorter segments of monomeric α-satellite, which is interspersed with other satellite sequences, duplicated sequence, a high frequency of transposable elements, and occasional single-copy sequences before transitioning into the euchromatin of the chromosome arms. (B) Because the human genome sequence covers mostly euchromatic sequence, the available contigs do not contain much (and in most cases, any) of the higher-order repeat arrays *(34)* on individual chromosomes. Thus, by comparison to the model in (A), the current map and sequence of each chromosome has a large centromere gap, whose size can only be approximated. Two of the most complete annotated maps are shown for chromosomes 8 and the X, indicating the location of known higher-order repeat α-satellite, monomeric α-satellite, other satellite sequences, and genes close to the centromere.

species *(38)*. Although α-satellite has been found at all primate centromeres studied, the organization and types of α-satellite vary among species *(6,7)* and have begun to inform hypotheses about centromere evolution.

Higher-order α-satellite has been found at some of the centromeres of chimpanzees, gorillas, and orangutans *(7)*. Notably, higher-order α-satellite has not been found in more distant primates; indeed, only monomeric α-satellite has been found in Old World monkeys, New World monkeys, and prosimians. As the centromeres from these monkeys have not been fully analyzed, however, the apparent absence of higher-order α-satellite should be interpreted with caution. Nonetheless, these findings are consistent with a model of α-satellite evolution in which higher-order evolved relatively recently from monomeric α-satellite *(6,39,40)*.

Although a number of processes, collectively referred to as "molecular drive" *(38)* and including mechanisms such as unequal crossover, gene conversion, and transposition, may be participating in α-satellite evolution to some extent, the homogenization of α-satellite can largely be accounted for by unequal crossover. Recurring rounds of crossovers will homogenize tandem repeats, leading to nearly identical repeat units. This process can explain not only the emergence of α-satellite DNA approx 30–50 millions of years ago, but also the initial homogenization of subsets of monomeric α-satellite to form the higher-order repeat units that subsequently expanded to make up the megabase-sized arrays currently present on human centromeres.

The relationships among α-satellite on different chromosomes, homologs of the same chromosome, and sister chromatids are very informative for determining the relative rates of unequal crossover events predicted to occur in α-satellite evolution. With the exception of the centromeres on the acrocentric chromosomes, higher-order α-satellite in the human genome is chromosome-specific, meaning that higher-order α-satellite on one chromosome may be distinguished from that on another chromosome *(8)*. This can best be explained by unequal crossover events limited to homologous chromosomes that homogenized α-satellite into a chromosome-specific higher-order array *(40–42)*. The high sequence identity among thousands of higher-order repeat units on a given chromosome argues that *intra*chromosomal exchange (i.e., within and between homologs) is an efficient mechanism for homogenizing α-satellite *(7,38)*.

However, there is also evidence of ancient *inter*chromosomal exchanges involving α-satellite. Higher-order repeats from different chromosomes have related organizations and fall into suprachromosomal families *(7,43)*. Although the related higher-order arrays on different chromosomes provides evidence for ancient interchromosomal exchanges, the overall sequence variation among higher-order repeats within a suprachromosomal family suggests that this type of exchange event occurs much less frequently than intrachromosomal exchanges between homologous chromosomes *(42)*.

GENOMIC ANALYSIS OF HUMAN CENTROMERES

To better understand the organization, evolution and function of α-satellite, it would ideally be possible to fully sequence and analyze at least some human centromeres *(33)*. However, assembling the extremely identical repeat units that make up arrays of higher-order α-satellite is a daunting task. The euchromatic portion of the human genome has now been sequenced and assembled *(44)*, yet, the centromere regions were intentionally omitted from the human genome project, and thus no human centromere has been completely assembled *(34)*.

Notwithstanding the incomplete nature of centromere sequences, several of the contigs of chromosome arms in the now-completed sequence of the eukaryotic portion of the human genome extend into higher-order arrays of α-satellite *(34,35,40)* (Fig. 2B). The next step in sequencing human centromeric regions would logically focus on further connecting existing chromosome arm contigs to higher-order α-satellite and then developing a strategy to sequence across the highly homogeneous arrays of higher-order α-satellite.

The most challenging part of sequencing across megabases of higher-order α-satellite is not the sequencing *per se*, but the assembly process. The assembly of sequences within genomic clones from these arrays is expected to be far more complicated than assembling typical genomic DNA, as higher-order repeat units are up to 100% identical *(40,41)*. Although the merits of attempting to sequence across several megabases of nearly identical repeats are open to debate, in the meantime it is important to recognize and acknowledge that the existing chromosome arm contigs end some distance—substantial for some chromosomes—from the functional centromere itself *(34)*. Thus, from a practical standpoint, analysis and especially interpretation of human chromosome defects involving the centromere or pericentromeric region on the basis of the available genome sequences and resources must necessarily be made with caution.

CENTROMERIC CHROMATIN AND CENTROMERE FUNCTION

Although, as outlined above, the organization of centromeric DNA varies widely among eukaryotic organisms, the chromatin modifications and proteins involved in centromere function are very well conserved from yeast to humans *(21,22,45,46)*.

The likely primary epigenetic mark of the functional centromere is the histone H3 variant CENP-A, also known as CenH3 *(47)*. CENP-A is found at active centromeres in every organism studied *(11)*. Depleting CENP-A causes chromosome segregation defects and also has downstream effects on the localization of other centromere proteins, supporting its role as the primary epigenetic mark. CENP-A and histone H3 nucleosomes are interspersed at the centromeres of flies and humans *(21)*, and CENP-A can substitute for histone H3 in reconstituted nucleosomes in vitro *(48)*. Given the fact that CENP-A is a histone variant, it is tempting to posit that it sets up the centromere-specific chromatin conformation that then recruits other centromere proteins.

Such proteins include a number of DNA-binding proteins, as well as motor proteins, that are part of the kinetochore. Centromere protein B (CENP-B) is a DNA-binding protein found at the centromeres of diverse organisms, and it recognizes a 17 bp sequence known as the "CENP-B box" in mouse minor satellite and human higher-order α-satellite *(49)*. The CENP-B box sequence has also been found at the centromeres of the great apes, but not in Old World monkeys, New World monkeys, or prosimians. Despite its evolutionary conservation, the role of this protein in centromere function is questionable. Another DNA-binding protein, however, CENP-C, which localizes only to active centromeres *(50)*, is clearly directly involved in centromere function, as its depletion causes chromosome segregation defects. Other proteins such as dynein, MCAK, and CENP-E are also members of the kinetochore, playing a role in chromosome movement along the microtubules *(1)*. Also, spindle checkpoint proteins such as Mad2 and Bub1 are critical for chromosome segregation as they signal the start of anaphase once all kinetochores are attached to the spindle *(2)*.

Proper resolution of sister chromatid cohesion is also required for chromosome segregation. After proceeding into mitotic anaphase, sister chromatids completely lose cohesion and separate to opposite poles of the cell. Loss of sister chromatid cohesion is a two-step process in meiosis; in the first meiotic division, cohesion is removed from chromosome arms but maintained at the centromere, and then in the second meiotic division cohesion is completely removed *(51)*. In the absence of cohesins, chromosomes missegregate, exhibiting chromosome lag and premature sister chromatid separation *(3)*.

The relationships among centromeric chromatin, kinetochore formation, spindle checkpoints, and resolution of sister chromatid cohesion have been best described in model organisms. Although the role of specific genomic elements in the various functions previously summarized and associated with proper chromosome segregation is unknown, the general picture to emerge from genetic and molecular studies of the fission yeast or fly centromere is that each can be divided into centromeric and pericentromeric chromatin domains, each of which is characterized by a distinct set of chromatin (and heterochromatin) proteins *(11,15,21)*, but both of which are required for proper chromosome segregation.

It is tempting to apply this domain model to the organization of the human centromere *(9,11,22,52)*. It may be that, although monomeric α-satellite cannot nucleate the site of the kinetochore on its own *(53)*, it is required for setting up the pericentromeric chromatin state, similar to the kinetochore flanking sequences in *S. pombe* and *D. melanogaster*. Future studies carefully dissecting the locations of centromere proteins, chromatin modifications, heterochromatin proteins, and cohesins at the human centromere will determine the unique nature of centromeric chromatin, its distinction from euchromatin and heterochromatin, and likely differences between the centromeric and pericentromeric domains *(22,54)*.

ASSESSING CENTROMERE FUNCTION IN HUMAN CHROMOSOMES

Although the requirements for centromeric and pericentromeric functions have been well-defined in model organisms, similar analyses of the human centromere lack the tractable genetic systems found in other organisms, making it difficult to test specific regions functionally for centromere activity. The respective roles of genomic sequence and epigenetic modifications in specifying human centromere function are a topic of substantial debate *(1,11,55–57)* and have been much informed by two lines of investigation: first, the analysis of abnormal human chromosomes derived from patient material; second, the development of approaches to generate and analyze engineered human chromosomes suitable for testing specific hypotheses.

Dicentric Chromosomes

Dicentric human chromosomes have been known about for 30 years *(58)* and contain two distinct arrays of α-satellite on the same chromosome, formed by chromosome breakage and fusion events. To maintain chromosome stability, there must be only one active centromere, because if the chromosome attaches to spindle microtubules at two sites it could be pulled to opposite poles of the cell, causing chromosome breakage or anaphase bridging *(59)*. The stability of dicentric human chromosomes can be achieved either by inactivating one centromere *(50,58)* or by coordinating the activity of the two centromeres such that they orient to the same pole *(60)*.

Centromere inactivation involves the loss of the ability of that centromere to bind proteins involved in spindle microtubule attachment *(50,60)*, most likely involving reversal of the epigenetic modifications that mark functional centromeric chromatin. The fact that a region of otherwise functionally competent α-satellite can exist on a chromosome without conferring centromeric activity has led some to argue that α-satellite must not be sufficient for centromere function and that centromere function, therefore, must be sequence independent *(1,55–57)*. However, this argument seems misleading *sensu stricto*; notwithstanding the effects of epigenetic silencing, an inactive centromere is no less a "centromere" than an inactive gene (i.e., as a result of imprinting, X inactivation, or tissue differentiation) is still a "gene."

Neocentromeres

The existence of neocentromeres also provides an argument for the sequence independence of centromere function. Neocentromeres are regions of chromosomes that do not contain typical centromeric DNA, but that have been modified epigenetically to act as a centromere and segregate the chromosome faithfully. Neocentromeres were first described in maize and have also been engineered in flies *(9,56,61)*.

At least several dozen human neocentromeres are found on marker chromosomes detected in patient material and appear to derive from chromosome breakage events in which a previously acentric fragment acquires centromere activity *(62,63)*. Neocentromeres have been extensively characterized to determine the molecular structure and epigenetic modifications responsible for centromere activity. There appear to be "hotspots" for neocentromere formation as certain regions of the genome have been involved in neocentromere formation multiple times. The simplest model that such regions share particular sequence characteristics has been challenged by a finding that three marker chromosomes derived from the same region of chromosome 13 all have different CENP-A binding domains *(64)*. Thus, the regions of the genome from which marker chromosomes are derived may be hotspots for chromosome breakage events; however, based on current evidence, the acquisition of centromeric activity by neocentromeres is not obviously strictly sequence-dependent.

Other epigenetic parameters such as centromere protein deposition, replication timing, and histone acetylation status have been implicated in neocentromere function *(62–65)*. These data clearly establish that α-satellite DNA is not always necessary for centromere function, although it should be emphasized both that neocentromere formation is an extremely rare event and that the existence of neocentromeres on abnormal chromosomes need not impugn the now well-established role of α-satellite in determining centromere identity in normal chromosomes.

Normal Human Centromeres

To complement the analysis of abnormal chromosomes, requirements for human centromere function can be addressed using normal human chromosomes. In one approach, antibodies to centromere proteins known to be present at functional centromeres are used to determine which DNA sequences colocalize with the active centromere. Such colocalization of centromere proteins and α-satellite DNA has been demonstrated in a number of studies. For example, antibodies to CENP-A bind to a portion of the α-satellite at human centromeres, at the site of the inner kinetochore *(66)*. Most recently, extended chromatin fiber experiments have demonstrated directly that both centromere proteins like CENP-A, as well as centromere-specific chromatin modifications, only characterize a portion of the α-satellite at human centromeres *(21,22)*. Although, together, these data suggest that only a subset of α-satellite DNA is part of the functional centromere, they do not define the particular type of α-satellite participating in centromere function.

Chromatin immunoprecipitation experiments with antibodies to centromere proteins directly support a functional role for α-satellite DNA and identify the specific genomic DNA sequences involved in centromeric chromatin. Vafa and Sullivan first showed that α-satellite does in fact immunoprecipitate with antibodies to CENP-A and proposed a specialized phasing for CENP-A-containing nucleosomes *(67)*. In another study, antibodies to CENP-B and CENP-C as well as CENP-A were found to immunoprecipitate α-satellite-containing chromatin *(68)*. After cloning and sequencing the chromatin immunoprecipitated DNA, the only type of α-satellite associated with centromere proteins contained CENP-B boxes. As CENP-B recognition sites are found only in higher-order α-satellite and not monomeric α-satellite, these findings suggest that only higher-order α-satellite is part of the kinetochore complex at human centromeres. These two chromatin immunoprecipitation studies are consistent with numerous cytological centromere protein colocalization experiments and strongly support a role for higher-order α-satellite in normal centromere function.

Chromosome Engineering

In addition to strategies that examine the DNA and protein composition at normal centromeres of endogenous chromosomes, studies of engineered chromosomes have explored the minimal requirements for centromere function. Telomere sequences can be introduced into human cell lines to truncate existing chromosomes into smaller "minichromosomes" *(69,70)*. Such minichromosomes can be mapped subsequently to determine the sequences that are present and responsible for centromere function on this minimal chromosome *(71)*. In contrast, human artificial chromosomes are derived from naked DNA transfected into tissue culture cells *(53,72)*. Artificial chromosomes may be used as an assay to determine the types of sequences capable of forming a *de novo* centromere and are a promising tool for determining the sequence requirements for centromere function.

MINICHROMOSOMES

Farr et al. *(69)* engineered telomere truncation chromosomes by introducing telomere repeats in a nontargeted fashion to truncate the human X chromosome at a number of locations along the q arm. These chromosomes were further truncated along the p arm to generate centric minichromosomes less than 2.4 Mb in size *(73,74)*. The minimal chromosome that retained mitotic stability was 1.4 Mb overall (compared to the approx 150 Mb normal X) with a 670 kb array of DXZ1 higher-order α-satellite (about a quarter of a typical DXZ1 array). Below this threshold, chromosomes with less DXZ1 or less flanking sequence on the p side of DXZ1 were mitotically unstable, suggesting that both higher-order α-satellite and neighboring pericentromeric sequence may be required for proper centromere function *(75)*.

Similar chromosome truncation studies have been conducted on the human Y chromosome *(71)*. The smallest Y chromosome-based minichromosome exhibiting faithful segregation was 1.8 Mb overall, with an approx 100 kb array of DYZ3 higher-order α-satellite *(76)*. These data from X- and Y-based minichromosomes demonstrate that higher-order α-satellite is capable of maintaining centromere function after the original chromosome has been significantly truncated and/or rearranged. The fact that the smallest minichromosomes are larger than just the higher-order α-satellite array may reflect a requirement for other flanking sequences for proper chromosome segregation, as also suggested by studies in model organisms.

HUMAN ARTIFICIAL CHROMOSOMES

Human artificial chromosome studies address the requirements for centromere establishment as well as maintenance. Candidate DNA sequences are transfected into human tissue culture cells to test them for the ability to form an artificial chromosome with a *de novo* centromere derived from the input DNA *(53,72)*. Numerous artificial chromosome studies in the 7 years since development of this technology have tested α-satellite sequences, non-α-satellite sequences, and different types of α-satellite for centromere competence.

The first human artificial chromosome study combined the principal components of chromosomes—centromeres, telomeres, and genomic DNA (presumably containing origins of replication)—to generate small linear artificial chromosomes *(72)*. In an alternate approach, others engineered a yeast artificial chromosome construct containing α-satellite and telomere sequences on a single molecule *(53)*. In both approaches, artificial chromosomes were mitotically stable in the absence of drug selection and bound antibodies to centromere proteins, demonstrating the assembly of fully functional human centromeres.

Since these two original studies, a number of constructs containing well-characterized higher-order α-satellite *(40,54,77–82)* have been successful in generating artificial chromosomes. Conversely, constructs containing monomeric α-satellite *(53)*, the sequences comprising a neocentromere *(83)*, as well as other non-α-satellite sequences *(78,79)* have failed to form artificial chromosomes, thus clearly implicating higher-order α-satellite as a major genomic determinant of human centromere function.

Higher-order α-satellite containing CENP-B boxes provides a functional capability that is absent from monomeric α-satellite. So what characteristic of higher-order α-satellite is responsible for conferring centromere function? Is it the extremely homogeneous organization of higher-order repeats? Or the presence of CENP-B boxes in higher-order but not monomeric α-satellite? Or are specific basepairs present in higher-order repeats besides the CENP-B box responsible for centromere function?

Expanding on the earlier study involving α-satellite from chromosome 21 *(53)*, Ohzeki et al. generated a number of constructs to begin to address the specific characteristics of higher-order α-satellite that nucleate centromere function *(84)*. A mutation was introduced into the CENP-B boxes in the higher-order repeat unit, eliminating the ability to bind CENP-B protein in a gel shift assay. Importantly, the mutated higher-order α-satellite was incapable of artificial chromosome formation. These data suggest that the mutations in this construct are responsible for the absence of centromere function, but it remains to be determined if centromere function was abolished by the mutation specifically in the CENP-B box or if any mutation in higher-order α-satellite might similarly hinder centromere function. This remains an important area for future inquiry.

SUMMARY

Although still substantially incomplete at the sequence level, the genomic organization of human centromeric regions is, nonetheless, increasingly well-defined on many chromosomes as a combined result of the now-completed human genome sequencing effort, which has provided the sequence of the euchromatic chromosome arms and targeted efforts to map and characterize the various satellite DNAs that comprise the centromeric region of each chromosome. Combined with the availability of a variety of chromosome-specific α-satellite probes and immunocytochemical reagents that have revolutionized cytogenetic analysis of centromeres over the past two decades, new genomic resources can be evaluated for their suitability to contribute to our understanding of both normal and abnormal centromere structure and behavior. Increasingly relevant will be studies of centromeric and pericentromeric chromatin, characterization of transition zones between the euchromatin of chromosome arms and pericentric heterochromatin, identification of gene content near centromeres, and determination of genomic mechanisms that involve centromeric and pericentromeric sequences, such as isochromosomes and isodicentric chromosomes or pericentromeric duplications and deletions.

ACKNOWLEDGMENTS

Work in the Willard lab on centromeres has been supported by research awards from the National Institutes of Health and the March of Dimes Birth Defects Foundation. This work has benefited enormously from helpful discussions among those in the centromere group over the past 20 years.

REFERENCES

1. Cleveland DW, Mao Y, Sullivan KF. Centromeres and kinetochores. From epigenetics to mitotic checkpoint signaling. Cell 2003;112:407–421.
2. Shah JV, Cleveland DW. Waiting for anaphase: Mad2 and the spindle assembly checkpoint. Cell 2000;103: 997–1000.
3. Lee JY, Orr-Weaver TL. The molecular basis of sister-chromatid cohesion. Annu Rev Cell Dev Biol 2001;17:753–777.
4. Malik HS, Henikoff S. Conflict begets complexity: the evolution of centromeres. Curr Opin Genet Dev 2002;12:711–718.
5. Willard HF. Centromeres: the missing link in the development of human artificial chromosomes. Curr Opin Genet Dev 1998;8:219–225.
6. Alexandrov I, Kazakov A, Tumeneva I, Shepelev V, Yurov Y. Alpha-satellite DNA of primates: old and new families. Chromosoma 2001;110:253–266.
7. Warburton P, Willard HF. Evolution of centromeric alpha satellite DNA: molecular organization within and between human and primate chromosomes. In: *Human Genome Evolution* (Jackson M, Dover G, eds.), Oxford: BIOS Scientific Publishers, 1996, pp. 121–145.
8. Willard HF, Waye JS. Hierarchical order in chromosome-specific human alpha satellite DNA. Trends Genet 1987;3:192–198.
9. Choo KH. Domain organization at the centromere and neocentromere. Dev Cell 2001;1:165–177.
10. Koch J. Neocentromeres and alpha satellite: a proposed structural code for functional human centromere DNA. Hum Mol Genet 2000;9:149–154.
11. Sullivan BA, Blower MD, Karpen GH. Determining centromere identity: cyclical stories and forking paths. Nat Rev Genet 2001;2:584–596.
12. Clarke L. Centromeres of budding and fission yeasts. Trends Genet 1990;6:150–154.
13. Baum M, Nagan VK, Clarke L. The centromeric K-type repeat and the central core are together sufficient to establish a functional Schizosaccaromyces pombe centromere. Mol Biol Cell 1994;5:747–761.
14. Hahnenberger KM, Carbon J, Clarke L. Identification of DNA regions required for mitotic and meiotic functions within the centromere of Schizosaccaromyces pombe chromosome 1. Mol Cell Biol 1991;11:2206–2215.
15. Partridge JF, Borgstrom B, Allshire RC. Distinct protein interaction domains and protein spreading in a complex centromere. Genes Dev 2000;14:783–791.
16. Partridge JF, Scott KC, Bannister AJ, Kouzarides T, Allshire RC. cis-acting DNA from fission yeast centromeres mediates histone H3 methylation and recruitment of silencing factors and cohesin to an ectopic site. Curr Biol 2002;12:1652–1660.
17. Sun X, Wahlstrom J, Karpen G. Molecular structure of a functional Drosophila centromere. Cell 1997;91: 1007–1019.
18. Sun X, Le HD, Wahlstrom JM, Karpen GH. Sequence analysis of a functional Drosophila centromere. Genome Res 2003;13:182–194.
19. Hoskins RA, Smith CD, Carlson JW, et al. Heterochromatic sequences in a Drosophila whole-genome shotgun assembly. Genome Biol 2002;3:85.1-85.14.
20. Blower MD, Karpen GH. The role of Drosophila CID in kinetochore formation, cell-cycle progression and heterochromatin interactions. Nat Cell Biol 2001;3:730–739.
21. Blower MD, Sullivan BA, Karpen GH. Conserved organization of centromeric chromatin in flies and humans. Dev Cell 2002;2:319–330.
22. Sullivan BA, Karpen GH. Centromeric chromatin displays a pattern of histone modifications that is distinct from both euchromatin and heterochromatin. Nat Struct Mol Biol 2004;11:1076–1083.
23. Hall AE, Keith KC, Hall SE, Copenhaver GP, Preuss D. The rapidly evolving field of plant centromeres. Curr Opin Plant Biol 2004;7:108–114.
24. Copenhaver GP, Nickel K, Kuromori T, et al. Genetic definition and sequence analysis of Arabidopsis centromeres. Science 1999;286:2468–2474.
25. Cheng Z, Dong F, Langdon T, et al. Functional rice centromeres are marked by a satellite repeat and a centromere-specific retrotransposon. Plant Cell 2002;14:1691–1704.
26. Nagaki K, Cheng Z, Ouyang S, et al. Sequencing of a rice centromere uncovers active genes. Nat Genet 2004;36:138–145.

27. Nagaki K, Talbert PB, Zhong CX, Dawe RK, Henikoff S, Jiang J. Chromatin immunoprecipitation reveals that the 180-bp satellite repeat is the key functional DNA element of Arabidopsis thaliana centromeres. Genetics 2003;163:1221–1225.
28. Dillon N, Festenstein R. Unravelling heterochromatin: competition between positive and negative factors regulates accessibility. Trends Genet 2002;18:252– 258.
29. Cooke HJ. Silence of the centromeres—not. Trends Biotechnol 2004;22:319–321.
30. Buchwitz BJ, Ahmad K, Moore LL, Roth MB, Henikoff S. A histone-H3-like protein in C. elegans. Nature 1999;401:547–548.
31. Moore LL, Morrison M, Roth MB. HCP-1, a protein involved in chromosome segregation, is localized to the centromere of mitotic chromosomes in Caenorhabditis elegans. J Cell Biol 1999;147:471–480.
32. Oegema K, Desai A, Rybina S, Kirkham M, Hyman AA. Functional analysis of kinetochore assembly in Caenorhabditis elegans. J Cell Biol 2001;153:1209–1226.
33. Rudd MK, Schueler MG, Willard HF. Sequence organization and functional annotation of human centromeres. Cold Spring Harbor Symp Quant Biol 2004;68:141–≠149.
34. Rudd MK, Willard HF. Analysis of the centromeric regions of the human genome assembly. Trends Genet 2004;20:529–533.
35. She X, Horvath JE, Jiang Z, et al. The structure and evolution of centromeric transition regions within the human genome. Nature 2004;430:857–864.
36. Horvath JE, Bailey JA, Locke DP, Eichler E. Lessons from the human genome: transitions between euchromatin and heterochromatin. Hum Mol Genet 2001;10:2215–2223.
37. Jackson M. Duplicate, decouple, disperse: the evolutionary transience of human centromeric regions. Curr Opin Genet Dev 2003;13:629–635.
38. Dover G. Molecular drive: a cohesive mode of species evolution. Nature 1982;299:111–117.
39. Ventura M, Archidiacono N, Rocchi M. Centromere emergence in evolution. Genome Res 2001;11:595–599.
40. Schueler MG, Higgins AW, Rudd MK, Gustashaw K, Willard HF. Genomic and genetic definition of a functional human centromere. Science 2001;294:109–115.
41. Schindelhauer D, Schwarz T. Evidence for a fast, intrachromosomal conversion mechanism from mapping of nucleotide variants within a homogeneous alpha-satellite DNA array. Genome Res 2002;12:1815–1826.
42. Warburton PE, Willard HF. Interhomologue sequence variation of alpha satellite DNA from human chromosome 17: evidence for concerted evolution along haplotypic lineages. J Mol Evol 1995;41:1006–1015.
43. Alexandrov IA, Mitkevich SP, Yurov YB. The phylogeny of human chromosome specific alpha satellites. Chromosoma 1988;96:443–453.
44. International Human Genome Sequencing Consortium. Finishing the euchromatic sequence of the human genome. Nature 2004;431:931–945.
45. Henikoff S, Ahmad K, Malik HS. The centromere paradox: stable inheritance with rapidly evolving DNA. Science 2001;293:1098–1102.
46. Talbert PB, Bryson TD, Henikoff S. Adaptive evolution of centromere proteins in plants and animals. J Biol 2004;3:1–17.
47. Ahmad K, Henikoff S. Histone H3 variants specify modes of chromatin assembly. Proc Natl Acad Sci USA 2002;99:16,477–16,484.
48. Yoda K, Ando S, Morishita S,et al. Human centromere protein A (CENP-A) can replace histone H3 in nucleosome reconstitution in vitro. Proc Natl Acad Sci USA 2000;97:7266–7271.
49. Masumoto H, Masukata H, Muro Y, Nozaki N, Okazaki T. A human centromere antigen (CENP-B) interacts with a short specific sequence in alphoid DNA, a human centromeric satellite. J Cell Biol 1989;109:1963–1973.
50. Sullivan BA, Schwartz S. Identification of centromeric antigens in dicentric Robertsonian translocations: CENP-C and CENP-E are necessary components of functional centromeres. Hum Mol Genet 1995;5:2189–2198.
51. Dej KJ, Orr-Weaver TL. Separation anxiety at the centromere. Trends Cell Biol 2000;10:392–399.
52. Sullivan BA. Centromere round-up at the heterochromatin corral. Trends Biotechnol 2002;20:89–92.
53. Ikeno M, Grimes B, Okazaki T, et al. Construction of YAC-based mammalian artificial chromosomes. Nat Biotechnol 1998;16:431–439.
54. Grimes BR, Babcock J, Rudd MK, Chadwick B, Willard HF. Assembly and characterization of heterochromatin and euchromatin on human artificial chromosomes. Genome Biol 2004;5:R89.
55. Choo KH. Centromerization. Trends Cell Bio 2000;10:182–188.

56. Karpen GH, Allshire RC. The case for epigenetic effects on centromere identity and function. Trends Genet 1997;13:489–496.
57. Murphy TD, Karpen GH. Centromeres take flight: alpha satellite and the quest for the human centromere. Cell 1998;93:317–320.
58. Therman E, Sarto GE, Patau K. Apparently isodicentric but functionally monocentric X chromosome in man. Am J Hum Genet 1974;26:83–92.
59. McClintock B. The behavior in successive nuclear divisions of a chromosome broken in meiosis. Proc Natl Acad Sci USA 1939;25:405–416.
60. Sullivan BA, Willard HF. Stable dicentric X chromosomes with two functional centromeres. Nat Genet 1998;20:227–228.
61. Maggert KA, Karpen GH. The activation of a neocentromere in Drosophila requires proximity to an endogenous centromere. Genetics 2001;158:1615–1628.
62. Amor DJ, Choo KH. Neocentromeres: role in human disease, evolution and centromere study. Am J Hum Genet 2002;71:695–714.
63. Warburton PE. Epigenetic analysis of kinetochore assembly on variant human centromeres. Trends Genet 2001;17:243–247.
64. Alonso A, Mahmood R, Li S, Cheung F, Yoda K, Warburton PE. Genomic microarray analysis reveals distinct locations for the CENP-A binding domains in three human chromosome 13q32 neocentromeres. Hum Mol Genet 2003;12:2711–2721.
65. Craig JM, Wong LH, Lo AW, Earle E, Choo KH. Centromeric chromatin pliability and memory at a human neocentromere. Embo J 2003;22:2495–2504.
66. Warburton PE, Cooke CA, Bourassa S, et al. Immunolocalization of CENP-A suggests a distinct nucleosome structure at the inner kinetochore plate of active centromeres. Curr Biol 1997;7:901–904.
67. Vafa O, Sullivan KF. Chromatin containing CENP-A and alpha satellite DNA is a major component of the inner kinetochore plate. Current Biology 1997;7:897–900.
68. Ando S, Yang H, Nozaki N, Okazaki T, Yoda K. CENP-A, -B, and -C chromatin complex that contains the I-type alpha-satellite array constitutes the prekinetochore in HeLa cells. Mol Cell Biol 2002;22:2229–2241.
69. Farr CJ, Stevanovic M, Thomson EJ, Goodfellow PN, Cooke HJ. Telomere-associated chromosome fragmentation: applications in genome manipulation analysis. Nature Genetics 1992;2:275–282.
70. Barnett MA, Buckle VJ, Evans EP, et al. Telomere-directed fragmentation of mammalian chromosomes. Nucl Acids Res 1993;21:27–36.
71. Heller R, Brown KE, Burtgorf C, Brown WRA. Mini-chromosomes derived from the human Y chromosome by telomere directed chromosome breakage. Proc Natl Acad Sci USA 1996;93:7125–7130.
72. Harrington JJ, Van Bokkelen G, Mays RW, Gustashaw K, Willard HF. Formation of de novo centromeres and construction of first-generation human artificial microchromosomes. Nat Genet 1997;15:345–355.
73. Farr CJ, Bayne RAL, Kipling D, Mills W, Critcher R, Cooke HJ. Generation of a human X-derived minichromosome using telomere-associated chromosome fragmentation. EMBO J 1995;14:5444–5454.
74. Mills W, Critcher R, Lee C, Farr CJ. Generation of an approximately 2.4 Mb human X centromere-based minichromosome by targeted telomere-associated chromosome fragmentation in DT40. Hum Mol Genet 1999;8:751–761.
75. Spence JM, Critcher R, Ebersole TA, et al. Co-localization of centromere activity, proteins and topoisomerase II within a subdomain of the major human X alpha-satellite array. Embo J 2002;21:5269–5280.
76. Yang JW, Pendon C, Yang J, Haywood N, Chand A, Brown WR. Human mini-chromosomes with minimal centromeres. Hum Mol Genet 2000;9:1891–1902.
77. Larin Z, Mejia JE. Advances in human artificial chromosome technology. Trends Genet 2002;18:313–319.
78. Ebersole TA, Ross A, Clark E, et al. Mammalian artificial chromosome formation from circular alphoid input DNA does not require telomere repeats. Hum Mol Genet 2000;9:1623–1631.
79. Grimes BR, Rhoades AA, Willard HF. Alpha-satellite DNA and vector composition influence rates of human artificial chromosome formation. Mol Ther 2002;5:798–805.
80. Mejia JE, Alazami A, Willmott A, et al. Efficiency of de novo centromere formation in human artificial chromosomes. Genomics 2002;79:297–304.
81. Kouprina N, Ebersole T, Koriabine M, et al. Cloning of human centromeres by transformation-associated recombination in yeast and generation of functional human artificial chromosomes. Nucl Acids Res 2003;31:922–934.

82. Rudd MK, Mays RW, Schwartz S, Willard HF. Human artificial chromosomes with alpha satellite-based de novo centromeres show increased frequency of nondisjunction and anaphase lag. Mol Cell Biol 2003;23: 7689–7697.
83. Saffery R, Wong LH, Irvine DV, et al. Construction of neocentromere-based human minichromosomes by telomere-associated chromosomal truncation. Proc Natl Acad Sci USA 2001;98:5705–5710.
84. Ohzeki J, Nakano M, Okada T, Masumoto H. CENP-B box is required for de novo centromere chromatin assembly on human alphoid DNA. J Cell Biol 2002;159:765–775.

III   GENOME EVOLUTION

9 Primate Chromosome Evolution

Stefan Müller, PhD

BACKGROUND

During the last two decades, comparative cytogenetics and genomics has evolved from a specialized discipline to a highly dynamic field of research. This development was driven by major technological advancements as well as emergence of the deeper insight that many aspects of human genome function can be better understood when information about its evolutionary changes is taken into account. Whole-genome sequencing projects of biomedical model species and domesticated animals provided important clues to the molecular mechanisms that shaped the human genome. These strategies were complemented by the launch of the chimpanzee genome project, leading to the recent publication of the first chimpanzee draft sequence and its alignment with the human reference sequence.

The objective of this chapter is to (1) review recent technical developments in the field of comparative cytogenetics and genomics provide knowledge about ancestral primate chromosomal traits and on evolutionary landmark rearrangements; (2) recapitulate the molecular cytogenetic evidence for the evolutionary history of human chromosomes with special emphasis on great apes; and (3) summarize the present data about the genomic environment of evolutionary chromosomal breakpoints in human and great apes.

Rates and the direction of evolutionary rearrangements are discussed in the context of the emerging patterns of evolutionary genomic changes and future perspectives including whole genome sequencing and microarray based approaches are addressed.

From: *Genomic Disorders: The Genomic Basis of Disease*
Edited by: J. R. Lupski and P. Stankiewicz © Humana Press, Totowa, NJ

INTRODUCTION

The introduction of fluorescence *in situ* hybridization (FISH) to comparative karyotype analysis *(1)* marked a paradigm shift from the analysis of chromosome morphology toward chromosomal DNA content. The use of human chromosome-specific probes in cross-species chromosome painting experiments for the first time allowed the secure identification of chromosomal homologies between species at a resolution of 3–5 Mb within primates and 5–10 Mb when comparing human with nonprimate mammals. A second landmark was the establishment of a reproducible Zoo-FISH protocol *(2)* for the analysis of any mammalian species with human probes. In addition, chromosome-specific "painting" probes were established from several nonhuman primates as well as from other mammalian and vertebrate species by fluorescence-activated chromosome sorting and subsequent degenerate oligonucleotide-primed polymerase chain reaction amplification *(3)*, for example, from lemurs *(4)*, mouse *(5)*, and chicken *(6)*. The availability of chromosome paint probes from nonhuman species for Zoo-FISH experiments allowed the assembly of comparative chromosome maps in a reciprocal way *(7)* (Fig. 1). This approach is particularly helpful when analyzing distantly related species in which the hybridization efficiency is low. Moreover, when performing reverse painting to human chromosomes, evolutionary breakpoints can be localized on the human sequence map for a subsequent detailed characterization of evolutionary breakpoints. Further development of this strategy led to the concept of multidirectional chromosome painting *(8)*, where members of a species group of interest are systematically analyzed with human paint probes and in addition with paint probes of a species from the targeted species group.

Cross-species chromosome painting certainly has a number of limitations: apart from the limited resolution, intrachromosomal rearrangements usually escape detection. For the construction of more detailed comparative genome maps, several complementary methods have been established, among others Zoo-FISH employing chromosome bar codes and subregional DNA probes, comparative radiation hybrid mapping and, ultimately, whole genome sequencing.

In order to obtain high-resolution comparative chromosome maps, Zoo-FISH with vector-cloned DNA probes can be performed. Bacterial artificial chromosome (BAC) libraries from numerous species are publicly available (http://bacpac.chori.org), among them human, chicken, mouse, rat, cat, pig, and cow, and several nonhuman primates (chimpanzee, orangutan, gibbon, macaque, squirrel monkey, lemur, and others). Because human, mouse, and rat genome projects are essentially complete, "tile path" BAC probes from these species provide an excellent source for comparative FISH mapping studies with a direct link to the genome sequence (www.ensembl.org). For FISH analysis of distantly related species, human BAC probes can be selected from genomic regions with high evolutionary sequence conservation between human and mouse *(9)*.

Alternatively, somatic cell hybrid panels may serve a template for physical mapping studies in order to assemble interspecies homology maps. High-resolution radiation hybrid panels have been established, for example, for the rhesus macaque *(10)*. For chimpanzee, gorilla, and orangutan, lower resolution panels are available *(11)*.

The rapid progress of the human, mouse, and rat genome projects already provides a detailed and comprehensive insight into the ancestral mammalian genome organization. Although the major mammalian evolutionary breakpoints are hidden among the noise that stems from the extreme genome reshuffling in rodents, it is increasingly possible to read the human/mouse sequence alignment like cross-species chromosome painting data. With other more recently

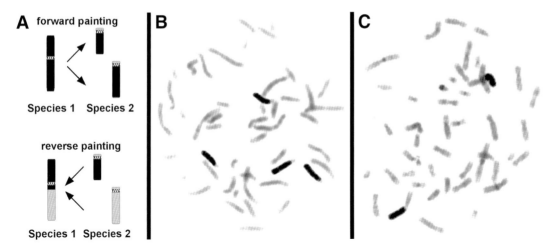

Fig. 1. (A) The principle of reciprocal chromosome painting. (B,C) Reciprocal chromosome painting between human and orangutan: (B) *in situ* hybridization of human chromosome 2 probe to an orangutan metaphase delineates two homologs. (C) Reverse painting of the orangutan 2q homolog to human chromosomes hybridizes to the 2q13-qter segment.

launched genome projects (i.e., chicken, dog, and chimpanzee *[12]*) advancing even faster, the view becomes increasingly clear. For example, the fusion point of human chromosome 2 in 2q13 can readily be identified on the human/chimpanzee comparative sequence map (www.ensembl.org) at the junction of chimpanzee chromosome 12 and 13 homologous sequences.

RECONSTRUCTION OF PRIMATE KARYOTYPE EVOLUTION

The Ancestral Primate Karyotype

Because chromosomal homology maps between human and approx 30 nonprimate mammals and more than 50 primates have been established, the data set available provides a firm basis on which proposals for common ancestral mammalian chromosomal traits and shared derived primate-specific chromosome forms can be made. For the sake of clarity and simplicity, in the following sections chromosomes are always numbered according to their human homologous counterparts.

When comparing the karyotypes of species from different placental mammalian orders, a surprisingly high degree of conservation can be observed for the majority of species. The homologs of human autosomes 1, 5, 6, 9, 11, 13, 17, 18, and 20 are found conserved as separate entities in several different orders and are therefore assumed to represent ancestral mammalian chromosome forms. In addition, human chromosome 3, 4, 14, 15, and 21 homologs are entirely conserved in other mammalian orders, however, translocated. Syntenic associations of human homologous chromosomes 3/21, 4/8p, and 14/15 are, therefore, also considered to be ancestral for placental mammals. Human chromosome 2, 7, 8, 10, 16, and 19 homologs are found split in two separate syntenic segments, some of them are associated with further chromosomal material. Human chromosome 2 is a fusion product of two separate ancestral homologs 2pter-q13 (2a) and 2q13-qter (2b). Human chromosome 7 is a complex fusion product of

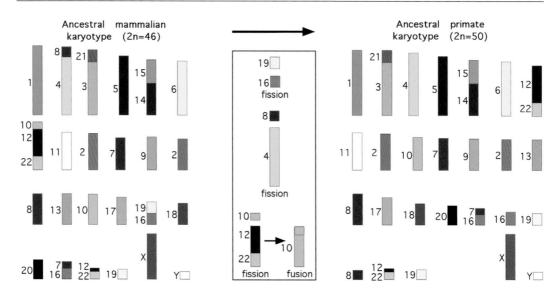

Fig. 2. Inferred ancestral mammalian and ancestral primate karyotypes with the assignment of human homologies to the left, based on multidirectional chromosome painting data. The primate karyotype is derived by fissions of 10p and 12pter-q23.3, 16q and 19q, and 4 and 8p, followed by fusion of 10p/10q.

ancestral chromosome forms (7p21-q11.21, 7q11.23-21.3, 7q22.1-qter) and (7pter-p22, 7q11.21-11.23, 7q21.3-22.1)/16p. Human chromosomes 12 and 22 resulted from a reciprocal translocation t(12;22)(q23.3;q12.3) of the two ancestral homologs 10p/12pter-q23.3/22q12.3-qter and 22q11.2-22q12.3/12q23.3-qter. Chromosome 16q and 19q homologs are associated on a single chromosome, whereas 8q, 10q and 19p are found as separate entities (13) (Fig. 2). The ancestral karyotype of placental mammals may therefore have comprised of 2n = 46 chromosomes.

The putative ancestral primate karyotype shows only a very few differences when compared to the ancestral mammalian karyotype. In the inferred primate ancestor presumably fissions of 10p and 12pter-q23.3, 16q and 19q, and 4 and 8p occurred, followed by fusion of 10p/10q, resulting in a karyotype of 2n = 50 chromosomes with conserved human homologous chromosome (segments) 1, 2pter-q13, 2q13-qter, 4, 5, 6, (7p21-q11.21, 7q11.23-21.3, 7q22.1-qter), 8p, 8q, 9, 10, 11, 13, 16q, 17, 18, 19p, 19q, 20, X, Y, and the association of 3/21, (7pter-p22, 7q11.21-11.23, 7q21.3-22.1)/16p, 12pter-q23.3/22q12.3-qter, 22q11.2-22q12.3/12q23.3-qter, 14/15 (Fig. 2).

The following section provides an overview of the current knowledge on karyotype evolution in prosimians and higher primates (anthropoidea), the latter being subdivided in New World monkeys (platyrrhini), Old World monkeys (cercopithecoidea), and apes (hominoidea, gibbons, and great apes).

Prosimians

Prosimians are comprised of lorises, bush-babies, and lemurs. Only five species were fully analyzed using human chromosome painting probes: brown, black, and ring-tailed lemur (4,9), and two bush-babies (14). In addition, black lemur chromosome-specific probes were characterized by reverse painting to human chromosomes (4). The results so far revealed that these prosimians retained ancestral primate chromosome forms 12/22, 3/21, 14/15, and probably

7/16, but showed common derived fissions of chromosome 1 (two fissions), 4, 5, 6, 8, and 15. In addition, the investigated lemurs share four derived fissions and five translocations, the two bush-babies five fissions, and six translocations *(14)*. Numerous further rearrangements were noticed, for example eight fusions only found in the black lemur *(4)*. By conclusion, none of the prosimians analyzed to date has conserved a primitive primate karyotype, instead prosimians have highly derived karyotypes.

New World Monkeys

The 16 genera and over 100 recognized species of New World monkeys (platyrrhini) show a high degree of karyotypic diversity with chromosome numbers ranging from 2n = 16 in *Callicebus lugens* to 2n = 62 in *Lagothrix lagotricha*. With established comparative genome maps between human and more than 20 species by cross-species chromosome painting with human probes, New World monkeys represent the most comprehensively studied group of species among mammals altogether. In addition, several species have been analyzed by multi-directional chromosome painting employing tamarin (*Saguinus oedipus*) *(15)* and woolly monkey (*L. lagothricha*) *(16)* chromosome-specific probes.

In the inferred ancestral New World monkey karyotype of 2n = 54 chromosomes *(17)*, human chromosomes 4, 6, 9, 11, 12, 13, 17, 19, 20, 22, X, and Y homologs are found entirely conserved as separate chromosomes. Chromosome 5, 14, 18, and 21 homologs show conserved synteny, are however associated with other homologs (5/7a, 14/15a, 8a/18, and 3a/21). The remaining human homologs are fragmented: 1a, 1b, 1c, 2a, 2b/16b, 3b, 3c, 7b, 8b, 10a/16a, 10b, and 15b.

Among the family callitrichidae, two tamarins (*S. oedipus* and *Leontopithecus chrysomelas*), three marmoset species (*Callithrix jacchus*, *Cebuella pygmaea*, and *Callithrix argentata*), and *Callimico goeldii* were analyzed by multidirectional chromosome painting *(17–19)*. The data showed that *C. goeldii* exclusively shares derived syntenic associations 13/9/22 and 13/17/20 with all callithrichids. A study on an interspecies hybrid between a female Common marmoset (*C. jacchus*, 2n = 46) and a male Pygmy marmoset (*C. pygmaea*, 2n = 44) with a diploid chromosome number of 2n = 45 gave further support for the inclusion of *Cebuella* within genus *Callithrix (20)*. Genomic imbalances between this interspecies hybrid and other callithrichidae, visualized by interspecies Comparative genomic hybridization (iCGH), were confined to centromeric and subtelomeric heterochromatin. Cross-species FISH with a micro-dissection derived *C. pygmaea* repetitive probe revealed species-specificity of several 50 Mb and larger blocks of heterochromatin, thus providing a dramatic example for amplification of noncentromeric repetitive sequences within approximately 5 million years of evolution *(20)*.

Zoo-FISH data are also available from the squirrel monkey, capucin monkeys, and three species of titi monkey (family cebidae). The squirrel monkey shares the derived syntenic association 2/15 with callithrichidae *(17)*. Capuchin monkeys have conserved almost completely the ancestral New World monkey karyotype *(21–23)*. Titi monkeys *Callicebus moloch*, *Callicebus donacophilus* (both 2n = 50), and *C. lugens* (2n = 16), are phylogenetically linked by common derived associations 10/11, 22/2/22, and 15/7 *(24–26)*. The low chromosome number of *C. lugens* is the result of at least 22 fusions and 6 fissions.

The diploid chromosome numbers of atelidae (Howler monkeys, genus *Alouatta*, Spider monkeys, genus *Ateles*, Wooly monkeys, genus *Lagothrix,* and Wooly spider monkeys, genus *Brachyteles*) range from 2n = 32 in *Ateles* to 2n = 62 in *Brachyteles* and *Lagothrix*. Species from all four genera have been analyzed by multi-directional chromosome painting *(16,27,28)*. All atelidae analyzed share the derived fissions of human chromosome 1, 4, and 5 homologs, inversion of the 10/16 and 5/7 homologs, and a translocation 4/15. The ancestral atelidae karyotype is comprised of 2n = 62 chromosomes and is conserved in *Lagothrix* and *Brachyteles*. Howler monkeys represent the genus with the most extensive karyotype diversity within platyrrhini with high levels of intra-specific chromosomal variability *(29,30,27)*. Molecular cytogenetic studies in Spider monkeys (genus *Ateles*) revealed that at least 17 fusions and three fissions are necessary to derive the putative ancestral *Ateles* karyotype conserved in *A. b. marginatus* (2n = 34) *(23,28,31)*.

Old World Monkeys

Macaques and baboons have strongly conserved and uniform karyotypes with 2n = 42 chromosomes. Compared to the human karyotype all chromosomes show conserved synteny, except for two human chromosome 2 (two homologs) *(32)*. The reduced chromosome number is the result of two fusions, leading to syntenic association of chromosome 7/21 and 20/22 homologs. They further conserved the primate ancestral association of 14/15 homologs. Among guenons, fissions are the main mechanism driving the evolutionary trend toward higher chromosome numbers of 2n = 60 in the African green monkey (*Chlorocebus aethiops*) *(33)* and to 2n = 72 in *Cercopithecus wolfi*.

Leaf-eating monkeys have fairly conserved karyotypes, compared with human with chromosome numbers of 2n = 44 in the black and white colobus (*Colobus guereza*) *(34)* and 2n = 48 in the proboscis monkey (*Nasalis larvatus*) *(35)*. These Colobines share the derived association of human chromosomes 21/22. The Asian members further share a reciprocal translocation of the human chromosome 1 and 19 homolog that was followed by a pericentric inversion.

Hominoids

The four gibbon subgenera show distinct karyomorphs with 2n = 38 in *Bunopithecus*, 2n = 44 in *Hylobates*, 2n = 50 in *Symphalangus,* and 2n = 52 in *Nomascus*. During the last decade all four subgenera were studied by Zoo-FISH, which revealed extensive chromosome reshuffling in all gibbons. First studies employed human chromosome paint probes *(36–39)*. More recently, gibbons were reanalyzed by multidirectional painting *(40–42)*.

The inferred ancestral karyotype of all extant gibbons differed from the putative ancestral hominoid karyotype by at least five reciprocal translocations, eight inversions, 10 fissions, and one fusion *(42)*. It included homologs to human chromosomes 7, 9, 13, 14, 15, 20, 21, 22, X, and Y with conserved synteny and homologous segments of human chromosome 1 (three segments), 2, 3, 4, 5, 6 (two segments each), 8, 11, 12, and 17, respectively. Finally, syntenic associations of segments homologous to human chromosomes were included: 3/8, 3/12/19, 5/16, 5/16/5/16, 19/12/19, 10/4 (twice), 12/3/8, 17/2/17/2, and 18/11. The White-cheeked gibbon, Siamang and White-handed gibbon further share at least five common derived chromosome forms: associations 2/7, 8/3/11/18, 4/5, 22/5/16, and an inversion. In the last common ancestor of the White-cheeked gibbon and the Siamang, one fusion and four fissions may have occurred. In addition, each gibbon accumulated a large number of species-specific rearrangements (between 10 in the White-handed gibbon and 28 in the Hoolock).

Comparative high resolution G-banding analysis of human and great apes indicated, that the only interchromosomal changes are species-specific: a fusion of chromosome 2 in the human lineage, a reciprocal translocation t(5;17) in the gorilla and a band insertion ins(8;20) in the orangutan *(44)*. Chromosome painting of great ape genomes with human probes confirmed the

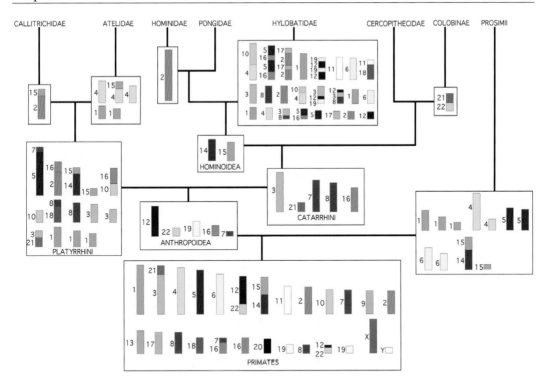

Fig. 3. Superimposition of primate evolutionary landmark rearrangements onto the consensus phylogenetic tree.

fusion of human chromosome 2 and the translocation t(5;17) in the gorilla, but not the insertion ins(8;20) in the orangutan *(1,36,43)*. Further, G-banding indicated that human and great ape genomes would differ by the presence and chromosomal location of constitutive heterochromatin, in the number of nucleolar organizer region-bearing chromosomes, and by several inversions *(44)*. For example, chimpanzee and human chromosome 1, 4, 5, 9, 12, 15, 16, 17, and 18 homologs would differ by pericentric inversions and chromosome 7 homologs of chimpanzee and gorilla by a paracentric inversion. Human and gorilla chromosome 16 homologs as well as human and orangutan chromosome 3 and 17 homologs would have diverged by both peri- and paracentric inversions.

Primate Evolutionary Landmark Rearrangements

On the basis of molecular cytogenetic evidence it is possible to draw increasingly accurate conclusions on landmark rearrangements that occurred during primate evolution (Fig. 3). These landmarks are shared by defined subgroups of primates and thus provide fundamental phylogenetic links between members of these species groups. They can further be superimposed onto the consensus primate phylogenetic tree, which permits an estimate of the timing of these events. The putative ancestor of all primates most probably acquired separate chromosomes 4 and 10 homologs by fission/fusion events and lost the association of 16/19 homologs by fission about 60 million years ago (Fig. 2). The inferred ancestor of higher primates only retained ancestral primate syntenic associations 14/15 and 3/21, but acquired separate chromosome 12 and 22 homologs by reciprocal translocation, a single chromosome 19 homolog by

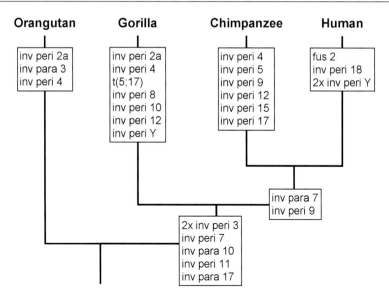

Fig. 4. Overview on chromosome rearrangements that occurred in orangutan, gorilla, chimpanzee and human (*see* The Evolutionary History of Human Chromosomes for details).

a fusion, and lost the association of human 7/16 homologs by fission. These events can be dated before the emergence of New and Old World monkeys (approx 30–40 million years ago). After the New/Old World monkey split, platyrrhini acquired common derived associations 5/7, 2/16, 10/16, 8/18, and several fissions, whereas in the catarrhini ancestor (about 25 million years ago) a fission led to separate chromosomes 3 and 21, whereas fusions resulted in single chromosome 7, 8, and 16 homologs. Approximately 18 million years ago, in the common ancestor of hominoids fission of the association 14/15 took place, leading to separate chromosomes 14 and 15. Finally, less than 6 million years ago and after the divergence of human and chimpanzee, the fusion of human chromosome 2 occurred (Fig. 3).

THE EVOLUTIONARY HISTORY OF HUMAN CHROMOSOMES

This section recapitulates the evolutionary history of selected chromosomes, which are rearranged in human and great apes and for which molecular cytogenetic evidence is available. Figure 4 summarizes all hominoid evolutionary rearrangements.

Chromosome 2

The ancestral condition for all mammals is two separate chromosome 2 homologs. One is homologous to human 2pter-q13, the other to the remaining 2q13-qter segment. Comparative studies with a human chromosome 2q arm-specific paint probe, cosmid clones derived from the human V κ gene cluster, and yeast artificial chromosomes (YACs) indicated that the chimpanzee and the macaque 2pter-q13 homologs may be ancestral, whereas in gorilla and orangutan, independent and probably convergent inversions involving the pericentromeric region of the 2p homolog may have occurred *(45–47)*. More recently, a detailed FISH study with 2q12-14 cosmids revealed the same clone order in human and chimpanzee, which differed from that in the macaque *(48)*.

Chromosome 3

According to one study, the putative ancestral primate chromosome 3 homolog is conserved in the Brown lemur, from which a pericentric inversion led to the ancestral Old World primate homolog conserved in the Bornean orangutan *(49)*. Human/African ape homologs would differ from this chromosome form by two inversions. An even more complex scenario involving several recurrent sites of new centromere seeding was proposed by Ventura et al. *(50)*, according to which human and Bornean orangutan would differ by three inversions. A third hypothesis suggested that from the ancestral simian homolog a common derived and two independent inversions would lead to Bornean orangutan and human chromosome 3 homologs *(51)*. In conclusion, the evolutionary history of human chromosome 3 is probably the most dynamic and complex of all human chromosomes studied in detail so far.

Chromosome 4

Detailed comparative studies on the evolution of human chromosome 4 homologs of great apes and the macaque *(52)* indicated that the human homolog would represent the ancestral hominoid chromosome form. A minimum of seven different breakpoints were observed, some of them were located in the 4p pericentromeric region *(52)*. For three of these inversions breakpoint spanning YAC clones were identified, of which one was confirmative for a previous analysis *(53)*. Interestingly, one clone showed a split signal in chimpanzee and macaque, indicating two independent evolutionary breakpoints in close proximity to each other.

Chromosome 5

Both chromosome bar codes and detailed Zoo-FISH studies with YACs and subregional paint probes identified the chromosome forms shared by macaque, orangutan, and human to be ancestral for hominoids *(54,55)*. From this, the homolog of the chimpanzee is directly derived by a pericentric inversion, those of the gorilla by a reciprocal translocation t(5;17) *(1)*.

Chromosome 6

In a recent FISH study *(56)*, it was shown that the remarkable conservation of chromosome 6 is also present at the subchromosomal level. Despite this, evolutionary centromere relocation events were observed. One of these events may have occurred in the ancestor of great apes, where the centromere moved from 6p22.1 to the present day location. This hypothesis gained support from the observation that in the assumed ancestral location in a cluster of intrachromosomal segmental duplications was found, which the authors explained as remnants of duplicons that flanked the ancestral inactivated centromere *(56)*.

Chromosome 7

A FISH study on evolutionary changes of human chromosome 7 revealed that the ancestral mammalian homologs were comprised of two chromosomes (7a and 7b/16p) as observed in carnivores *(57)*. The ancestral primate segment 7a shared by a lemur and higher Old World monkeys is the result of a paracentric inversion. The ancestral higher primate chromosome form was derived by a fission of 7b and 16p, followed by a centric fusion of 7a/7b in higher Old World primates as observed in the orangutan. In hominoids two further inversions with four distinct breakpoints occurred: the pericentric inversion in the human/African ape ancestor and the paracentric inversion in the common ancestor of human and chimpanzees (Fig. 5) *(57)*.

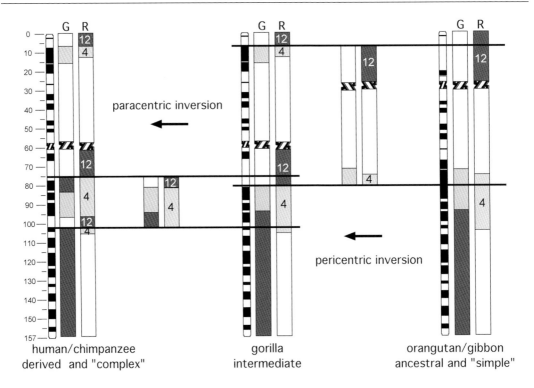

Fig. 5. Hominoid chromosome 7 evolutionary rearrangements delineated by comparative sequence maps of human and rat (R) and cross-species fluorescence *in situ* hybridization with gibbon painting probes (G). Both data sets visualize the inversion breakpoints and their evolutionary direction by an increasingly simple pattern when tracking the rearrangements in the evolutionary reverse direction. Horizontal bars indicate inversion breakpoints.

Chromosome 9

Zoo-FISH with 12 evenly spaced YAC clones *(58)* revealed an identical marker order in Old and New World monkeys, which may therefore represent the ancestral chromosome form for higher primates. A paracentric inversion would derive the ancestral hominoid chromosome form, which was conserved in orangutan and gorilla. A further pericentric inversion would lead to the chromosome form of the last common ancestor of human and chimpanzee. Human conserved this evolutionary intermediate chromosome form, from which the homolog of chimpanzees differs by another pericentric inversion. One of the inversion breakpoints in the chimpanzee homolog was previously identified *(53)*. As for the evolution of human chromosomes 3 and 6, this reconstruction takes into account the evolutionary emergence of neocentromeres.

Chromosome 10

The evolutionary history of human chromosome 10 was tracked by Zoo-FISH with a panel of partial chromosome paint probes, YACs, and BACs *(59)*. These results suggest that in the inferred primate ancestor chromosome 10 homologs were organized as two separate syntenic units, whereas the observation of a single chromosome 10 homolog in two galago species (prosimians) *(14)* would argue for a single chromosome 10 in the ancestral primate. Additional data on other prosimian species may be required to clarify this issue. Among hominoid primates, the ancestral chromosome form is conserved by orangutan, from which the ancestor of human and African apes is derived by a paracentric inversion. A further species-specific pericentric inversion occurred in the gorilla homolog *(55,59)*.

Y Chromosome

The mammalian Y chromosome shows a broad spectrum of species-specific rearrangements *(60)*. To explain the morphology of the human Y chromosome in comparison to those of the great apes, at least a pericentric and a paracentric inversion specific for the human lineage have to be assumed. Another pericentric inversion was observed in the gorilla homolog. Further, a translocation from chromosome 1 to the Y chromosome took place in a common ancestor of humans and chimpanzees. In addition, submicroscopic deletions and duplications occurred in human, chimpanzee, and orangutan *(60)*.

EVOLUTIONARY BREAKPOINT ANALYSIS

This section provides an overview on the current knowledge about the genomic context of evolutionary chromosomal breakpoints in human and great apes. By analogy to the functional importance of genomic alterations related with acquired chromosomal aberrations in cancers, it was anticipated that changes of the genomic environment caused by evolutionary chromosome rearrangements might hold the key for a better understanding of the origins of our own species.

The Fusion of Human Chromosome 2

Two head-to-head arrays of degenerate telomere repeats are found directly at the fusion site in 2q13 *(61)*. Their inverted orientation indicates a telomeric fusion. Subsequently, the inactivation of one of the two ancestral centromeres must have occurred. Indeed, close to the fusion point in band 2q21 a degenerate alphoid domain was found by low stringency FISH of a satellite DNA probe *(62)*.

Like in other subtelomeric regions, large blocks surrounding the fusion point are comprised of duplicated sequences *(63)*. Chromosome 2q13 paralogs of 96–99% identity were identified on chromosome 9pter, 9p11.2, 9q13, 22qter, and 2q11.2. The emergence of some of these segmental duplications could be dated back prior to hominid divergence, whereas others appeared to be of more recent origin. It can be speculated that these duplicons may have been the cause for the fusion and that human chromosome 2 is the product of paralogous recombination between two different chromosomes using a duplicated segment as recombination substrate *(63)*.

The fusion point is located in a gene-rich region, with at least 24 potentially functional genes and 16 pseudogenes located within less than 1 Mb distance or in paralogous regions elsewhere in the genome *(64)*. At least 18 of these genes are transcriptionally active, for example members of the cobalamin synthetase W domain (*CBWD*) and forkhead domain *FOXD4* gene families, thus providing an example of genomic innovation connected with duplication and evolutionary rearrangement of subtelomeric and pericentromeric regions.

Inversions of Chromosome 3 in Hominoids

A detailed molecular cytogenetic characterization of evolutionary inversion breakpoints in hominoid chromosome 3 homologs revealed that the ancestral pericentromeric region is associated with both large-scale and micro-rearrangements *(51)*. Small segments homologous to human 3q11.2 and 3q21.2 were repositioned intrachromosomally in the orangutan lineage. The breakpoint in the human 3p12.3 homologous region of the orangutan is associated with extensive transchromosomal duplications observed in multiple subtelomeric regions. A second breakpoint in the same region, but with a distinctly different location, is flanked by sequences present in all subtelomeric regions of the Siamang (gibbon) genome.

Reciprocal Translocation t(4;19) in the Gorilla

The breakpoints of the reciprocal translocation t(4;19) in the gorilla are located in regions syntenic to human 5q14.1 between *HMGCR* and *RASA1* genes, and in 17p12 with an approx 383-kb region-specific low-copy repeat (LCR)17pA *(65,66)*. The 17p12 region is also susceptible to constitutional rearrangements in human. The authors proposed a series of consecutive evoloutionary segmental duplications involving LCR17pA and approx 191-kb LCR17pB copies that resulted in complex genome architecture in the rearrangements. Detailed comparative analysis of the corresponding region identified remnants of DNA-transposable element MER1-Charlie3 and retroviral ERVL elements at the translocation breakpoint in a pre-gorilla individual *(66)*. In addition, genomic rearrangements involving LCR17pA and LCR17pB resulted in the creation of novel genes at the breakpoint junctions *(66)*.

Inversions of Chromosome 7 in Great Apes

Comparative FISH analysis with BAC clones that were derived from the Williams-Beuren syndrome region in 7q11.23 and which contained LCRs including *NCF1* (p47-phox) sequences revealed duplicated segments in the 7q11.23 homologous region of chimpanzee, gorilla, orangutan, and a gibbon *(67)*. As in human, cross-hybridization was observed in the inversion breakpoint regions at 7q22 and 7p22 in African apes, but not in the homologous chromosome regions in orangutan and gibbon.

Zoo-FISH analysis employing BAC probes confined the 7p22.1 breakpoint of the pericentric inversion in the human/African ape ancestor to 6,8 Mb on the human reference sequence map and the 7q22.1 breakpoint to 97,1 Mb *(57)* in regions with predominantly inter-chromosomal duplications with paralogs on human chromosomes 2–4 and 8–15. These duplicons were already present in the orangutan, but spread to a variety of additional chromosomes in the gorilla. The paracentric inversion breakpoints in the common ancestor of human and chimpanzees were found in 7q11.23 between 76,1 Mb and 76,3 Mb and in 7q22.1 at 101,9 Mb, respectively. Intrachromosomal duplicons mark an at least 110-kb stretch of nearly identical DNA sequence, which is most probably directly flanking both breakpoints. The 7q11.23 breakpoint is further located in close proximity to a 200-kb or larger insertion of chromosome 1 material, which could be dated back to the African ape ancestor *(57)*. Considering that the duplicated sequences flanking the four inversion breakpoints as well as the chromosome 1 transposition were already present in the evolutionary ancestral state prior to the inversions, segmental duplications may have been the cause rather than the result of both rearrangements.

Inversions of Chromosome 12 in Chimpanzee and Gorilla

Both chimpanzee and gorilla show derived pericentric inversions of the chromosome 12 homologs. In a first comparative FISH study, the 12p12 breakpoints in both species were mapped to the same YAC clone, whereas the 12q15 breakpoints were shown to be located in distinctly different regions *(53)*. In addition, a chimpanzee BAC clone was identified, which also spanned the 12p12 breakpoint *(68)*. Recently it could be demonstrated that this clone did not span the 12p12 breakpoint in the gorilla, thus, demonstrating that both the 12q and 12p inversion breakpoints differ in chimpanzee and gorilla *(69)*. Sequence analysis of the breakpoints in the chimpanzee genome revealed two large duplications in both breakpoint regions, which probably emerged in concert with the inversion because they were shown to be chimpanzee-specific *(69)*.

Fission of the Ancestral Chromosome 14/15 Synteny in the Great Ape Ancestor

The fission that separated human chromosome 14 and 15 homologs led to the inactivation of the ancestral centromere in 15q25 and to the formation of two new centromeres in the locations where they can be found in human. Detailed comparative molecular cytogenetic analysis of the region 15q24-26 revealed 500 kb of duplicons, which flank both sides of the single ancestral centromere in Old World monkeys *(70)*. Notably, the same duplicons are associated with neocentromeres in 15q24-26 in two clinical cases. This suggests that neocentromere formation in human pathology in a region of an evolutionary inactivated centromere may be triggered by the persistence of recombinogenic pericentromeric duplications.

Inversion of Chromosome 15 in Chimpanzee

Chimpanzee and bonobo share a derived pericentric inversion of their chromosome 15 homologs. A comparative FISH and *in silico* approach was used to narrow down the breakpoint interval of this pericentric inversion to the 15q11-q13 homologous region *(71)*. The breakpoint mapped to a 600-kb segmental duplication cluster. Sequence analysis indicated that this region comprises a duplication of the *CHRNA7* gene and several Golgin-linked-to-PML duplications. Notably, this evolutionary breakpoint did not colocalize with one of the three major common disease rearrangement breakpoints in 15q11-q13.

Inversion of Chromosome 17 in Chimpanzee

FISH was used to investigate the derived pericentric inversion with breakpoints in 17p13 and 17q21.3 homologous regions, by which chimpanzee chromosome 19 differs from human chromosome 17. Breakpoint-spanning BACs were subsequently used to clone and sequence the junction fragments *(72)*. Both breakpoints were localized in intergenic regions rich in *Alu* and LTR elements, but were not associated with LCRs, duplicated regions, or deletions. The findings suggest that repetitive sequence mediated nonhomologous recombination has facilitated inversion formation. In close proximity of the breakpoints, *NGFR* and *NXPH3* genes are located in 17q21.3 and *GUC2D* and *ALOX15B* in 17p13. Most likely, the genomic structure, the expression level or the replication timing of these genes was not affected by the inversion *(72)*.

Inversion of Chromosome 18 in Human

Human chromosome 18 differs from its great ape homologues by a pericentric inversion, which can be assigned to the human lineage. Recently, chimpanzee BAC clones that span one of the breakpoint regions where were identified by FISH, because in human split signals were observed on 18p11.3 and 18q11 *(73,74)*. Interspecies sequence comparisons indicated that the ancestral break occurred between the *ROCK1* and *USP14* gene. In human, the inversion translocated *ROCK1* near centromeric heterochromatin and *USP14* into proximity of 18p subtelomeric repeats. *USP14* is differentially expressed in human and chimpanzee cortex as well as fibroblast cell lines. Further, a 19-kb segmental duplication with paralogs in pericentromeric regions of chromosomes 1, 9 and the acrocentric chromosomes is also flanking both 18p11.3 and 18q11 regions in inverted orientation. The authors propose a model, according to which the 19-kb 18q segment containing part of the *ROCK1* gene was first locally duplicated and then transposed to the pericentromeric region of the ancestral 18p. Subsequently, the segmental duplication may have mediated an intrachromosomal crossover, resulting in modern human chromosome 18.

CONCLUSION

Rates and Direction of Evolutionary Chromosomal Changes

Primates, like mammals in general, show strikingly divergent diploid chromosome numbers ranging from 2n = 16 in the New World monkey *C. lugens* to 2n = 72 in the Old World monkey *C. wolfi*. Interestingly, several examples provide evidence against a certain trend toward higher or lower chromosome numbers. In New World monkeys, for example, the ancestor of the monophyletic group atelidae has 2n = 62 chromosomes, compared to the ancestor of all platyrrhini with 2n = 54 chromosomes. More recently in atelidae evolution, the chromosome number in the common ancestor of genus *Ateles* was reduced to 2n = 34.

On average, extant species differ from the inferred ancestral eutherian karyotype by 32 chromosome breaks (*13* and references therein for review). The rate of chromosomal exchange, however, varies greatly. The cat and the mink conserved the ancestral mammalian chromosome forms almost unchanged (11–16 breaks) *(75)*, whereas in the dog genome at least 66 breaks occurred *(76)*. Rodents show even greater differences between evolutionary conserved and extremely reshuffled genomes. A recent summary on the current state of the rat genome project listed 278 disrupted chromosomal syntenies between human and rat and 280 between human and mouse as a consequence of 353 rearrangements *(77)*. The vast majority of these rearrangements can be assigned to the muridae lineage because squirrels, which also belong to the order rodentia, show a highly conserved genome organization (21 breaks) *(78)*. A similar situation is found in primates: human chromosomes differ by only 21 breaks from the eutherian ancestor, whereas gibbon genomes accumulated at least 90 breaks. In summary, a "chromosomal evolutionary clock" does certainly not exist. Instead, the rate of chromosomal evolution may change over time in a phylogenetic lineage and could be interrelated with changing environmental impacts and population dynamics.

Patterns of Evolutionary Genomic Changes

Together with retroposon integrations, indels (insertions and deletions), changes of the mitochondrial gene order, gene duplications, and genetic code changes, evolutionary chromosome rearrangements can be classified as rare genomic changes. A bioinformatics approach to reconstruct the succession human/mouse chromosome rearrangements revealed a surprisingly large number of breakpoint hotspots: 190 of the 245 breaks analyzed reused a genomic region, although the authors emphasized that they were not necessarily located in exactly the same nucleotide position *(79)*. The existence of breakpoint clusters would argue against random breakage *(80)* and in favor of a fragile breakage model. Some other reports support this non-random breakage model. On human chromosome 1 and its homologs in placental mammals, evolutionary fissions cluster in two breakpoint hotspots on the long arm *(81)*. Further, at the resolution of chromosome banding, in the macaque 9 out of 17 evolutionary breakpoints correspond to evolutionary conserved fragile sites *(82)*. Because the vast majority of the rearrangements analyzed *(79)* are confined to the muridae lineage, a careful inspection of breakpoints in other mammals is required in order to determine whether this model applies to mammalian genome evolution in general.

In the majority of mammalian species, Robertsonian (centromeric) and tandem fusions or fissions appear to be the predominant type of evolutionary rearrangements. For example, in all New World primates that were analyzed by Zoo-FISH, 64% of the 149 recorded rearrangements were fissions, 24% fusions, and 10% intra-chromosomal rearrangements. Only two rearrangements were identified as reciprocal translocations. Notably, some of the whole chromosome fusions were not simple centromeric head-to-head fusions, but head-to-tail fusions between centromeric and telomeric regions *(see* ref. *17).* The majority of the evolutionary rearrangements appear to be mediated by highly repetitive regions of the genome and are accompanied by gain or loss of centromeric or telomeric function.

A second group of repetitive sequences, which came into the focus of attention as cause for genomic disorders and evolutionary genome instability, are segmental duplications or LCRs *(83–86).* So far, they have been found to be associated with almost every evolutionary chromosomal rearrangement in hominoid primates that was characterized in detail. Among these were the fusion of human chromosome 2, the reciprocal translocation t(5;17) in the gorilla, several inversions and the formation of neocentromeres. Within the primate lineage, the explosive expansion of the majority of these elements can be correlated with the burst of primate *Alu* retroposition activity approx 35 million years ago *(87).* At least for some of the rearrangements in hominoid primates it was demonstrated that the associated segmental duplications were present prior to the rearrangement and may have been a cause for it rather than a consequence. In addition, segmental duplications are statistically significantly enriched in genomic regions, which are differentially expressed in the human and chimpanzee brain *(88).* It would certainly be interesting to know to which degree the chromosomal distribution of duplicated segments in rat and mouse genomes *(89,90)* corresponds with sites of genome reshuffling in these two species.

FUTURE PERSPECTIVES

Sequencing whole genomes of a large number of mammalian species would obviously provide the most comprehensive information on the molecular mechanisms of genome organization and evolution. Recently eight nonprimate mammals (among them the African elephant, the European common shrew, the European hedgehog, guinea pig, the nine-banded armadillo, the rabbit, and the domestic cat) and the orangutan were added to the National Human Genome Research Institute sequencing pipeline (www.nhgri.nih.gov). These species will complement sequence data from other species, which are already available (*Drosophila, Fugu, Caenorhabditis elegans,* mouse, and rat) or rapidly emerging (cow, dog, chicken, zebrafish, chimpanzee, and rhesus macaque). Despite these efforts, whole genome sequencing projects will always be limited to key species from different phylogenetic lineages. For an in depth study of primate genome evolution, genomic sequence from at least two species from each major evolutionary branching point would be desirable to reduce species-specific noise. An alternative scenario could be that comparative molecular cytogenetic- and array-based screening technologies will guide the way to relevant genomic regions, which will then be targeted by genome sequencing projects.

A key technology with great promise for evolutionary studies employs genomic clone-based microarrays. In the past, iCGH to metaphase chromosomes provided only limited information about genomic imbalances between species owing to a low resolution of approx 10 Mb *(20,91)*. The introduction of comparative genomic hybridization to microarrays with almost 2500 human BAC clones evenly spaced in approx 1-Mb distance (array CGH) lead to a 10-fold increase in resolution *(92)*. A first evolutionary array CGH study *(93)* identified 63 sites of DNA copy-number variation between human and the great apes. Most of these copy number changes affected interstitial euchromatic chromosome regions suggesting that such large-scale events are not restricted to subtelomeric or pericentromeric regions.

Another recently introduced genomic microarray based technique was termed "array painting" *(94)*. It involves a BAC microarray as the target for reverse painting of aberrant chromosomes for the analysis of chromosomal breakpoints. The complete composition and the breakpoints of aberrant chromosomes can be analyzed at the same resolution as mentioned above for array CGH. Initial experiments with gibbon chromosome paint probes successfully demonstrated that this technology has the potential to significantly speed up the molecular characterization of evolutionary breakpoints *(95)*.

The impact of the higher order nuclear architecture on the complex epigenetic mechanisms responsible for cell type specific gene expression patterns in multi-cellular organisms has become an important field of genome research. Initial studies on the gene-density correlated radial arrangement of chromatin revealed a remarkable evolutionary conservation over a period of at least 30 million years *(96)*. As in certain human cell types, in a variety of higher primate species gene-dense chromatin is preferentially located in the nuclear center, whereas gene-poor chromatin shows an orientation toward the nuclear periphery. This probabilistic but highly nonrandom arrangement is still strictly maintained in species like gibbons with extremely reshuffled genomes. This evolutionary conservation argues for a still unknown functional significance of distinct radial higher-order chromatin arrangements. It may also be hypothesized that evolutionary chromosome rearrangements are triggered by certain nonrandom chromatin arrangements. Alternatively, such events may lead to the dislocation of chromosomal material to a different nuclear environment, which in turn may have consequences for the transcriptional activity of the affected loci.

SUMMARY

The current knowledge about genome organization in a large number of mammalian species, based on molecular cytogenetic and whole genome sequence data, already enables a number of fundamental conclusions about the evolutionary forces that shaped the human genome, whereas some other evolutionary aspects of genome organization still remain speculative. For the future, it may be expected that comparative cytogenetics, gene mapping, and genomics will become even more integrated methodolocical approaches in evolutionary studies, which enhance and complement each other concerning resolution and applicability to a wide range of species.

REFERENCES

1. Wienberg J, Jauch A, Stanyon R, Cremer T. Molecular cytotaxonomy of primates by chromosomal in situ suppression hybridization. Genomics 1990;8:347–350.
2. Scherthan H, Cremer T, Arnason U, Weier HU, Lima-de-Faria A, Froenicke L. Comparative chromosome painting discloses homologous segments in distantly related mammals. Nat Genet 1994;6:342–347.
3. Telenius H, Pelmear AH, Tunnacliffe A, et al. Cytogenetic analysis by chromosome painting using DOP-PCR amplified flow-sorted chromosomes. Genes Chromosomes Cancer 1992;4:257–263.

4. Müller S, O'Brien PC, Ferguson-Smith MA, Wienberg J. Reciprocal chromosome painting between human and prosimians (Eulemur macaco macaco and E. fulvus mayottensis). Cytogenet Cell Genet 1997;78:260–271.

5. Rabbitts P, Impey H, Heppell-Parton A, et al. Chromosome specific paints from a high resolution flow karyotype of the mouse. Nat Genet 1995;9:369–375.

6. Griffin DK, Haberman F, Masabanda J, et al. Micro- and macrochromosome paints generated by flow cytometry and microdissection: tools for mapping the chicken genome. Cytogenet Cell Genet 1999;87:278–281.

7. Arnold N, Stanyon R, Jauch A, O'Brien P, Wienberg J. Identification of complex chromosome rearrangements in the gibbon by fluorescent in situ hybridization (FISH) of a human chromosome 2q specific microlibrary, yeast artificial chromosomes, and reciprocal chromosome painting. Cytogenet Cell Genet 1996;74:80–85.

8. Müller S, Stanyon R, O'Brien PC, Ferguson-Smith MA, Plesker R, Wienberg J. Defining the ancestral karyotype of all primates by multidirectional chromosome painting between tree shrews, lemurs and humans. Chromosoma 1999;108:393–400.

9. Cardone MF, Ventura M, Tempesta S, Rocchi M, Archidiacono N. Analysis of chromosome conservation in Lemur catta studied by chromosome paints and BAC/PAC probes. Chromosoma 2002;111:348–356.

10. Murphy WJ, Page JE, Smith C, Jr., Desrosiers RC, O'Brien SJ. A radiation hybrid mapping panel for the rhesus macaque. J Hered 2001;92:516–519.

11. Marzella R, Carrozzo C, Chiarappa P, Miolla V, Rocchi M. Panels of somatic cell hybrids specific for chimpanzee, gorilla, orangutan, and baboon. Cytogenet Genome Res 2005;108:223–228.

12. Pennisi E. Evolution. Chimp genome draft online. Science 2003;302:1876.

13. Froenicke L. Origins of primate chromsomes-as delineated by Zoo-FISH and alignments of human and mouse draft genome sequences. Cytogenet Genome Res 2005;108:122–138.

14. Stanyon R, Kochler U, Consigliere S. Chromosome painting reveals that galagos have highly derived karyotypes. Am J Phys Anthropol 2002;117:319–326.

15. Müller S, Neusser M, O'Brien PC, Wienberg J. Molecular cytogenetic characterization of the EBV-producing cell line B95-8 (Saguinus oedipus, Platyrrhini) by chromosome sorting and painting. Chromosome Res 2001;9:689–693.

16. Stanyon R, Consigliere S, Bigoni F, Ferguson-Smith M, O'Brien PC, Wienberg J. Reciprocal chromosome painting between a New World primate, the woolly monkey, and humans. Chromosome Res 2001;9:97–106.

17. Neusser M, Stanyon R, Bigoni F, Wienberg J, Müller S. Molecular cytotaxonomy of New World monkeys (Platyrrhini): comparative analysis of five species by multi-color chromosome painting gives evidence for a classification of Callimico goeldii within the family of Callitrichidae. Cytogenet Cell Genet 2001;94:206–215.

18. Sherlock JK, Griffin DK, Delhanty JD, Parrington JM. Homologies between human and marmoset (Callithrix jacchus) chromosomes revealed by comparative chromosome painting. Genomics 1996;33:214–219.

19. Gerbault-Serreau M, Bonnet-Garnier A, Richard F, Dutrillaux B. Chromosome painting comparison of Leontopithecus chrysomelas (Callitrichine, Platyrrhini) with man and its phylogenetic position. Chromosome Res 2004;12:691–701.

20. Neusser M, Münch M, Anzenberger G, Müller S. Investigation of marmoset hybrids (Cebuella pygmaea x Callithrix jacchus) and related Callitrichinae (Platyrrhini) by cross-species chromosome painting and comparative genomic hybridization. Cytogenet Genome Res 2005;108:191–196.

21. Richard F, Lombard M, Dutrillaux B. ZOO-FISH suggests a complete homology between human and capuchin monkey (Platyrrhini) euchromatin. Genomics 1996;36:417–423.

22. Garcia F, Nogues C, Ponsa M, Ruiz-Herrera A, Egozcue J, Garcia Caldes M. Chromosomal homologies between humans and Cebus apella (Primates) revealed by ZOO-FISH. Mamm Genome 2000;11:399–401.

23. Garcia F, Ruiz-Herrera A, Egozcue J, Ponsa M, Garcia M. Chromosomal homologies between Cebus and Ateles (primates) based on ZOO-FISH and G-banding comparisons. Am J Primatol 2002;57:177–188.

24. Stanyon R, Consigliere S, Muller S, Morescalchi A, Neusser M, Wienberg J. Fluorescence in situ hybridization (FISH) maps chromosomal homologies between the dusky titi and squirrel monkey. Am J Primatol 2000;50:95–107.

25. Barros RM, Nagamachi CY, Pieczarka JC, et al. Chromosomal studies in Callicebus donacophilus pallescens, with classic and molecular cytogenetic approaches: multicolour FISH using human and Saguinus oedipus painting probes. Chromosome Res 2003;11:327–334.

26. Stanyon R, Bonvicino CR, Svartman M, Seuanez HN. Chromosome painting in Callicebus lugens, the species with the lowest diploid number (2 n=16) known in primates. Chromosoma 2003;112:201–206.

27. de Oliveira EH, Neusser M, Figueiredo WB, et al. The phylogeny of howler monkeys (Alouatta, Platyrrhini): reconstruction by multicolor cross-species chromosome painting. Chromosome Res 2002;10:669–683.

28. de Oliveira EH, Neusser M, Pieczarka JC, Nagamachi C, Sbalqueiro IJ, Müller S. Phylogenetic inferences of Atelinae (Platyrrhini) based on multi-directional chromosome painting in Brachyteles arachnoides, Ateles paniscus paniscus and Ateles b. marginatus. Cytogenet Genome Res 2005;108:183–190.
29. Consigliere S, Stanyon R, Koehler U, Agoramoorthy G, Wienberg J. Chromosome painting defines genomic rearrangements between red howler monkey subspecies. Chromosome Res 1996;4:264–270.
30. Consigliere S, Stanyon R, Koehler U, Arnold N, Wienberg J. In situ hybridization (FISH) maps chromosomal homologies between Alouatta belzebul (Platyrrhini, Cebidae) and other primates and reveals extensive inter-chromosomal rearrangements between howler monkey genomes. Am J Primatol 1998;46:119–133.
31. Morescalchi MA, Schempp W, Consigliere S, Bigoni F, Wienberg J, Stanyon R. Mapping chromosomal homology between humans and the black-handed spider monkey by fluorescence in situ hybridization. Chromosome Res 1997;5:527–536.
32. Wienberg J, Stanyon R, Jauch A, Cremer T. Homologies in human and Macaca fuscata chromosomes revealed by in situ suppression hybridization with human chromosome specific DNA libraries. Chromosoma 1992;101:265–270.
33. Finelli P, Stanyon R, Plesker R, Ferguson-Smith MA, O'Brien PC, Wienberg J. Reciprocal chromosome painting shows that the great difference in diploid number between human and African green monkey is mostly due to non-Robertsonian fissions. Mamm Genome 1999;10:713–718.
34. Bigoni F, Koehler U, Stanyon R, Ishida T, Wienberg J. Fluorescene in situ hybridization establishes homology between human and silvered leaf monkey chromosomes, reveals reciprocal translocations between chromosomes homologous to human Y/5, 1/9, and 6/16, and delineates an X1X2Y1Y2/X1X1X2X2 sex-chromosome system. Am J Phys Anthropol 1997;102:315–327.
35. Bigoni F, Stanyon R, Wimmer R, Schempp W. Chromosome painting shows that the proboscis monkey (Nasalis larvatus) has a derived karyotype and is phylogenetically nested within Asian Colobines. Am J Primatol 2003;60:85–93.
36. Jauch A, Wienberg J, Stanyon R, et al. Reconstruction of genomic rearrangements in great apes and gibbons by chromosome painting. Proc Natl Acad Sci USA 1992;89:8611–8615.
37. Koehler U, Arnold N, Wienberg J, Tofanelli S, Stanyon R. Genomic reorganization and disrupted chromosomal synteny in the siamang (Hylobates syndactylus) revealed by fluorescence in situ hybridization. Am J Phys Anthropol 1995;97:37–47.
38. Koehler U, Bigoni F, Wienberg J, Stanyon R. Genomic reorganization in the concolor gibbon (Hylobates concolor) revealed by chromosome painting. Genomics 1995;30:287–292.
39. Yu D, Yang F, Liu R. [A comparative chromosome map between human and Hylobates hoolock built by chromosome painting]. Yi Chuan Xue Bao 1997;24:417–423.
40. Nie W, Rens W, Wang J, Yang F. Conserved chromosome segments in Hylobates hoolock revealed by human and H. leucogenys paint probes. Cytogenet Cell Genet 2001;92:248–253.
41. Müller S, Neusser M, Wienberg J. Towards unlimited colors for fluorescence in-situ hybridization (FISH). Chromosome Res 2002;10:223–232.
42. Müller S, Hollatz M, Wienberg J. Chromosomal phylogeny and evolution of gibbons (Hylobatidae). Hum Genet 2003;113:493–501.
43. Stanyon R, Wienberg J, Romagno D, Bigoni F, Jauch A, Cremer T. Molecular and classical cytogenetic analyses demonstrate an apomorphic reciprocal chromosomal translocation in Gorilla gorilla. Am J Phys Anthropol 1992;88:245–250.
44. Yunis JJ, Prakash O. The origin of man: a chromosomal pictorial legacy. Science 1982;215:1525–1530.
45. Wienberg J, Jauch A, Ludecke HJ, et al. The origin of human chromosome 2 analyzed by comparative chromosome mapping with a DNA microlibrary. Chromosome Res 1994;2:405–410.
46. Arnold N, Wienberg J, Ermert K, Zachau HG. Comparative mapping of DNA probes derived from the V kappa immunoglobulin gene regions on human and great ape chromosomes by fluorescence in situ hybridization. Genomics 1995;26:147–150.
47. Haaf T, Bray-Ward P. Region-specific YAC banding and painting probes for comparative genome mapping: implications for the evolution of human chromosome 2. Chromosoma 1996;104:537–544.
48. Kasai F, Takahashi E, Koyama K, et al. Comparative FISH mapping of the ancestral fusion point of human chromosome 2. Chromosome Res 2000;8:727–735.
49. Müller S, Stanyon R, Finelli P, Archidiacono N, Wienberg J. Molecular cytogenetic dissection of human chromosomes 3 and 21 evolution. Proc Natl Acad Sci USA 2000;97:206–211.

50. Ventura M, Weigl S, Carbone L, et al. Recurrent sites for new centromere seeding. Genome Res 2004;14: 1696–1703.

51. Tsend-Ayush E, Grutzner F, Yue Y, et al. Plasticity of human chromosome 3 during primate evolution. Genomics 2004;83:193–202.

52. Marzella R, Viggiano L, Miolla V, et al. Molecular cytogenetic resources for chromosome 4 and comparative analysis of phylogenetic chromosome IV in great apes. Genomics 2000;63:307–313.

53. Nickerson E, Nelson DL. Molecular definition of pericentric inversion breakpoints occurring during the evolution of humans and chimpanzees. Genomics 1998;50:368–372.

54. Marzella R, Viggiano L, Ricco AS, et al. A panel of radiation hybrids and YAC clones specific for human chromosome 5. Cytogenet Cell Genet 1997;77:232–237.

55. Müller S, Wienberg J. "Bar-coding" primate chromosomes: molecular cytogenetic screening for the ancestral hominoid karyotype. Hum Genet 2001;109:85–94.

56. Eder V, Ventura M, Ianigro M, Teti M, Rocchi M, Archidiacono N. Chromosome 6 phylogeny in primates and centromere repositioning. Mol Biol Evol 2003;20:1506–1512.

57. Müller S, Finelli P, Neusser M, Wienberg J. The evolutionary history of human chromosome 7. Genomics 2004;84:458–467.

58. Montefalcone G, Tempesta S, Rocchi M, Archidiacono N. Centromere repositioning. Genome Res 1999;9:1184–1188.

59. Carbone L, Ventura M, Tempesta S, Rocchi M, Archidiacono N. Evolutionary history of chromosome 10 in primates. Chromosoma 2002;111:267–272.

60. Wimmer R, Kirsch S, Rappold GA, Schempp W. Evolutionary breakpoint analysis on Y chromosomes of higher primates provides insight into human Y evolution. Cytogenet Genome Res 2005;108:204–210.

61. Ijdo J, Baldini A, Ward DC, Reeders ST, Wells RA. Origin of human chromosome 2: an ancestral telomere-telomere fusion. Proc Natl Acad Sci USA 1991;88:9051–9055.

62. Avarello R, Pedicini A, Caiulo A, Zuffardi O, Fraccaro M. Evidence for an ancestral alphoid domain on the long arm of human chromosome 2. Hum Genet 1992;89:247–249.

63. Fan Y, Linardopoulou E, Friedman C, Williams E, Trask BJ. Genomic structure and evolution of the ancestral chromosome fusion site in 2q13-2q14.1 and paralogous regions on other human chromosomes. Genome Res 2002;12:1651–1662.

64. Fan Y, Newman T, Linardopoulou E, Trask BJ. Gene content and function of the ancestral chromosome fusion site in human chromosome 2q13-2q14.1 and paralogous regions. Genome Res 2002;12:1663–1672.

65. Stankiewicz P, Park SS, Inoue K, Lupski JR. The evolutionary chromosome translocation 4;19 in Gorilla gorilla is associated with microduplication of the chromosome fragment syntenic to sequences surrounding the human proximal CMT1A-REP. Genome Res 2001;11:1205–1210.

66. Stankiewicz P, Shaw CJ, Withers M, Inoue K, Lupski JR. Serial segmental duplications during primate evolution result in complex human genome architecture. Genome Res 2004;14:2209–2220.

67. DeSilva U, Massa H, Trask BJ, Green ED. Comparative mapping of the region of human chromosome 7 deleted in williams syndrome. Genome Res 1999;9:428–436.

68. Fujiyama A, Watanabe H, Toyoda A, et al. Construction and analysis of a human-chimpanzee comparative clone map. Science 2002;295:131–134.

69. Kehrer-Sawatzki H, Sandig H, Goidts V, Hameister H. Breakpoint analysis of the pericentric inversion between chimpanzee chromosome 10 and the homologous chromosome 12 in humans. Cytogenet Genome Res 2005;108:91–97.

70. Ventura M, Mudge JM, Palumbo V, et al. Neocentromeres in 15q24-26 map to duplicons which flanked an ancestral centromere in 15q25. Genome Res 2003;13:2059–2068.

71. Locke DP, Archidiacono N, Misceo D, et al. Refinement of a chimpanzee pericentric inversion breakpoint to a segmental duplication cluster. Genome Biol 2003;4:R50.

72. Kehrer-Sawatzki H, Schreiner B, Tanzer S, Platzer M, Müller S, Hameister H. Molecular characterization of the pericentric inversion that causes differences between chimpanzee chromosome 19 and human chromosome 17. Am J Hum Genet 2002;71:375–388.

73. Dennehey BK, Gutches DG, McConkey EH, Krauter KS. Inversion, duplication, and changes in gene context are associated with human chromosome 18 evolution. Genomics 2004;83:493–501.

74. Goidts V, Szamalek JM, Hameister H, Kehrer-Sawatzki H. Segmental duplication associated with the human-specific inversion of chromosome 18: a further example of the impact of segmental duplications on karyotype and genome evolution in primates. Hum Genet 2004;115:116–122.

75. Dixkens C, Klett C, Bruch J, et al. ZOO-FISH analysis in insectivores: "evolution extols the virtue of the status quo." Cytogenet Cell Genet 1998;80:61–67.

76. Breen M, Thomas R, Binns MM, Carter NP, Langford CF. Reciprocal chromosome painting reveals detailed regions of conserved synteny between the karyotypes of the domestic dog (Canis familiaris) and human. Genomics 1999;61:145–155.

77. Gibbs RA, Weinstock GM, Metzker ML, et al. Genome sequence of the Brown Norway rat yields insights into mammalian evolution. Nature 2004;428:493–521.

78. Stanyon R, Stone G, Garcia M, Froenicke L. Reciprocal chromosome painting shows that squirrels, unlike murid rodents, have a highly conserved genome organization. Genomics 2003;82:245–249.

79. Pevzner P, Tesler G. Human and mouse genomic sequences reveal extensive breakpoint reuse in mammalian evolution. Proc Natl Acad Sci USA 2003;100:7672–7677.

80. Nadeau JH, Taylor BA. Lengths of chromosomal segments conserved since divergence of man and mouse. Proc Natl Acad Sci USA 1984;81:814–818.

81. Murphy WJ, Froenicke L, O'Brien SJ, Stanyon R. The origin of human chromosome 1 and its homologs in placental mammals. Genome Res 2003;13:1880–1888.

82. Ruiz-Herrera A, Ponsa M, Garcia F, Egozcue J, Garcia M. Fragile sites in human and Macaca fascicularis chromosomes are breakpoints in chromosome evolution. Chromosome Res 2002;10:33–44.

83. Lupski JR. Genomic disorders: structural features of the genome can lead to DNA rearrangements and human disease traits. Trends Genet 1998;14:417–422.

84. Stankiewicz P, Lupski JR. Molecular-evolutionary mechanisms for genomic disorders. Curr Opin Genet Dev 2002;12:312–319.

85. Samonte RV, Eichler EE. Segmental duplications and the evolution of the primate genome. Nat Rev Genet 2002;3:65–72.

86. Eichler EE, Sankoff D. Structural dynamics of eukaryotic chromosome evolution. Science 2003;301:793–797.

87. Bailey JA, Liu G, Eichler EE. An Alu transposition model for the origin and expansion of human segmental duplications. Am J Hum Genet 2003;73:823–834.

88. Khaitovich P, Muetzel B, She X, et al. Regional patterns of gene expression in human and chimpanzee brains. Genome Res 2004;14:1462–1473.

89. Tuzun E, Bailey JA, Eichler EE. Recent segmental duplications in the working draft assembly of the brown Norway rat. Genome Res 2004;14:493–506.

90. Bailey JA, Church DM, Ventura M, Rocchi M, Eichler EE. Analysis of segmental duplications and genome assembly in the mouse. Genome Res 2004;14:789–801.

91. Toder R, Xia Y, Bausch E. Interspecies comparative genome hybridization and interspecies representational difference analysis reveal gross DNA differences between humans and great apes. Chromosome Res 1998;6:487–494.

92. Snijders AM, Nowak N, Segraves R, et al. Assembly of microarrays for genome-wide measurement of DNA copy number. Nat Genet 2001;29:263–264.

93. Locke DP, Segraves R, Carbone L, et al. Large-scale variation among human and great ape genomes determined by array comparative genomic hybridization. Genome Res 2003;13:347–357.

94. Fiegler H, Gribble SM, Burford DC, et al. Array painting: a method for the rapid analysis of aberrant chromosomes using DNA microarrays. J Med Genet 2003;40:664–670.

95. Gribble SM, Fiegler H, Burford DC, et al. Applications of combined DNA microarray and chromosome sorting technologies. Chromosome Res 2004;12:35–43.

96. Tanabe H, Müller S, Neusser M, et al. Evolutionary conservation of chromosome territory arrangements in cell nuclei from higher primates. Proc Natl Acad Sci USA 2002;99:4424–4429.

10 Genome Plasticity in Evolution

The Centromere Repositioning

Mariano Rocchi, PhD and Nicoletta Archidiacono, PhD

BACKGROUND

The centromere repositioning phenomenon consists in the move of the centromere along the chromosome during evolution. This phenomenon is relatively frequent, and has been documented in primates, nonprimate mammals, and birds. It implies the inactivation of the old centromere and the rapid progression of the newly seeded centromere toward the complex organization that probably stabilizes its activity. Both events have a huge impact on chromosomal architecture. The segmental duplicon clusters at 6p22.1 and 15q24-26 are clear examples of remains of inactivated ancestral centromeres. These duplicons are dispersed in a relatively large area (approx 10 Mb), and contribute to the bulk of nonpericentromeric segmental duplications that constitute approx 5% of the human genome.

Human neocentromeres are rare newly created centromeres formed in a previously noncentromeric location and devoid of alphoid sequences. Two human neocentromeres emerged in the same 15q24-26 chromosomal region where an ancestral centromere inactivated, establishing an intriguing connection between neocentromeres and inactivated ancestral centromeres. An other human neocentromere was found to be located in the same 3q26.1 region where an evolutionary centromere was seeded and fixed in Old World monkey (OWM) ancestor, indicating that the 3q26.1 region conserved a centromeric competence that was present before hominoids/OWM splitting. These findings further support the idea that some chromosomal domains have inherent centromeric capability.

From: *Genomic Disorders: The Genomic Basis of Disease*
Edited by: J. R. Lupski and P. Stankiewicz © Humana Press, Totowa, NJ

Two peculiar neocentromere cases, on chromosome 3 and on chromosome 4, have been recently reported in literature. Both arose in otherwise normal chromosomes of normal individuals, and were transmitted to the subsequent generation. They can be considered as living examples of centromere repositioning events at their very early stages.

INTRODUCTION

The centromere is a specialized structure responsible for chromosome segregation at mitosis and meiosis, and is conserved throughout evolution. Unexpectedly, sequences underlying the centromere function are not evolutionary conserved, and show variations even among closely related species *(1,2)*. Pericentromeric regions also show a high degree of evolutionary plasticity. They accumulate large amount of segmental duplications, which appear intrinsically more unstable than the bulk of euchromatic DNA *(3–7)*. A detailed analysis of pericentromeric segmental duplications and their role in evolution can be found in Chapter 5.

Evolutionary studies aimed at tracking chromosomal marker order conservation in primates unveiled an additional peculiar feature of centromeres: the centromere repositioning, consisting in the evolutionary movement of the centromere along the chromosome in the absence of any pericentric inversion that would account for the discrepancy in centromere location between two species. In this chapter, we focus on this biological phenomenon that is relatively frequent during the evolution of mammals.

CENTROMERE REPOSITIONING

We discovered this phenomenon while studying the evolutionary history of human chromosome 9 in primates *(8)*. Figure 1 summarizes the results obtained using a panel of yeast artificial chromosome clones used to establish marker order along this chromosome in 9 different primate species. If the position of the centromere is not taken into account, a relatively small number of rearrangements can be invoked to reconstruct the marker order in the studied species. Conversely, if the centromere is included in the analysis, a paradox emerges: the centromere appears to have undergone an independent evolutionary history. We hypothesized that the movement of the centromere toward the new location was not owing to classical chromosomal rearrangements (essentially inversions), but, rather, to the inactivation of the old centromere and the simultaneous appearance of a new centromere in a different location. The complexity of the evolutionary history of chromosome 9 did not allow certain alternative hypotheses to be discarded, such as two successive inversions, the first involving the centromere and the second restoring the previous marker order with the exception of the centromere.

For these reasons we undertook similar studies on other chromosomes. According to Ohno's law, the gene content of the chromosome X has barely changed throughout mammalian development in the last 125 million years *(9)*. The X chromosome was, therefore, an ideal chromosome in this respect. The position of the centromere of this chromosome is substantially unchanged in primates, with two exceptions in prosimians: the black lemur (*Eulemur macaco* [EMA]), and the ring-tailed lemur (*Lemur catta* [LCA]). The chromosome X appears acrocentric in black lemur and almost metacentric in ring-tailed lemur (Fig. 2). We investigated the marker order organization using a variety of different molecular cytogenetic tools, but no variation in marker order was found *(10)*. We concluded that the move of the centromere in EMA and LCA was because of the centromere repositioning event.

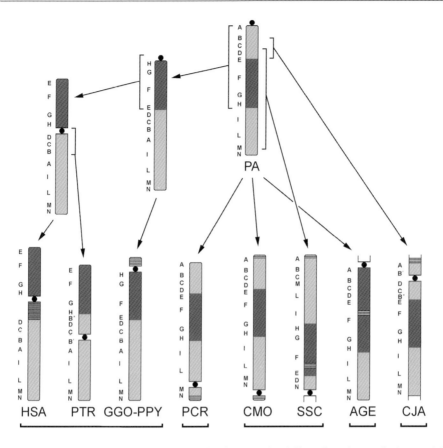

Fig. 1. Summary of fluorescence *in situ* hybridization results delineating the evolutionary history of human chromosome 9 in primates. The hypothesized pericentric or paracentric inversions are indicated by brackets spanning the inverted segment. The brackets at the bottom of the figure groups species in which the difference in centromere position cannot be explained on the basic of classical rearrangements. Species studied: common chimpanzee (*Pan troglodytes*, PTR), gorilla (*Gorilla gorilla*, GGO), and orangutan (*Pongo pygmaeus*, PPY). Old World monkeys, silvered leaf-monkey (*Presbytis cristata*, PCR). New World monkeys, dusky titi (*Callicebus molloch*, CMO), spider monkey (*Ateles geoffroyi*); common marmoset (*Callithrix jacchus*, CJA), and squirrel monkey (*Saimiri sciureus*, SSC). (Adapted with permission from ref. *8*.)

A centromere repositioning implies the inactivation of an ancestral centromere and the seeding of a new centromere. Neocentromere appearance is not a rare event in human. Human neocentromeres are defined as "rare human chromosomal aberrations where a new centromere has formed in a previously non-centromeric location" *(11)*. The first well-documented case of a human neocentromere was reported by du Sart et al. *(12)*. Since then, more than 50 neo-centromere cases have been described *(13)*. Some neocentromeres are clustered in "hotspots" for neocentromere formation, which include 3q26-qter, 8p, 13q21-q32, and 15q24-q26 regions. Most of the neocentromeres arise in acentric fragments because of a cytogenetic rearrange-ment. Acentric chromosomal fragments are usually lost. However, in some cases, their mitotic survival is rescued by neocentromere appearance, which is always an accidental event with respect to the rearrangement. In two cases, the neocentromere that emerged on chromosome

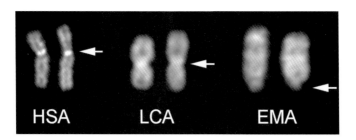

Fig. 2. DAPI-banded chromosome X in humans (HSA), ring-tailed lemur (LCA), and black lemur (EMA), showing a completely different position of the centromere, indicated by arrows. EMA chromosome X is upside down to match marker order in humans and LCA.

Y was not accompanied by a rearrangement *(14,15)*. In one of these cases, the chromosome was segregating in the family *(15)*.

Remains of Inactivated Centromeres

Human chromosome 2 is the result of a telomere–telomere fusion between two ancestral acrocentric chromosomes that occurred after human–chimpanzee divergence *(16)*, with one of the two centromeres becoming inactive. Indeed, stretches of alphoid sequences and clusters of segmental duplications, as remains of the inactivated centromere, are apparent at 2q21 *(17,18)*. We have hypothesized that the evolutionary appearance of new centromeres, as part of a centromere-repositioning event, implies the inactivation of a functioning centromere. Studies on the evolutionary history of chromosome 6 provided evidence that remains of an inactivated centromere, which resulted from a centromere repositioning, are present in the human genome *(19)*. Figure 3 summarizes the evolutionary history of chromosome 6, which is substantially conserved in evolution. Marker order analysis strongly suggested that the arrangement of the two New World monkeys (NWM), common marmoset (*Callithrix jacchus* [CJA]), and wooly monkey (*Lagothrix lagothricha* [LLA]) maintained the primate ancestral form. The marker arrangement of cat, chosen as the outgroup, supported this hypothesis. The centromeres of OWM and great apes, therefore, are evolutionary new centromeres. The major point of this analysis was the finding, in humans, of a duplicon cluster at 6p22.1 exactly corresponding to the region where the ancestral centromere was inactivated (Fig. 4). No remains of alphoid centromeric sequences, however, were detected. It can be hypothesized that, following the centromere inactivation, the pericentromeric duplicons dispersed in a relatively wide area (approx 10 Mb), whereas the large alphoid block, typical of active primate centromeres, completely disappeared. A second example of remains of an ancestral inactivated centromere is presented next.

Ancestral Centromeres and Neocentromeres

Centromeres are visible cytogenetically as the primary constriction and in primates are always associated with the presence of an array of α-satellite DNA *(20)*. α-satellite, however, it is not an absolute requirement for centromere function, as evident in neocentromeres, which are devoid of satellite DNA.

The mechanisms underpinning neocentromere emergence is obscure. du Sart et al. *(12)* have hypothesized the existence of latent centromeres with a finite capacity for neocentromerization.

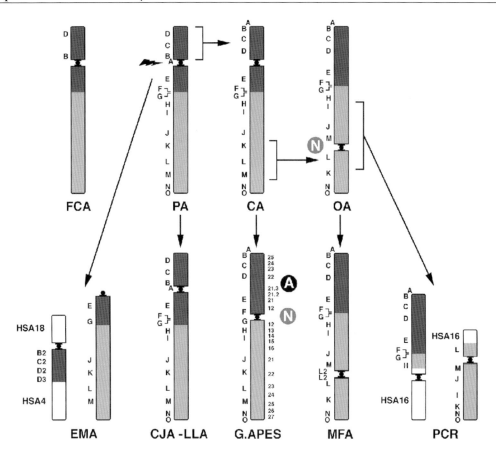

Fig. 3. Evolutionary history of human chromosome 6 established on the bases of marker order comparison among the orthologous chromosomes in great apes, Old World monkeys, New World monkeys, and prosimians. MFA, long-tailed macaque, *Macaca fascicularis*; PCR, silvered leaf-monkey, *Presbytis cristata*; CJA, common marmoset, *Callithrix jacchus*; LLA, wooly monkey, *Lagothrix lagothricha*; EMA, black lemur, *Eulemur macaco*; FCA, cat, *Felis catus*. N in a gray circle stands for a new centromere; A in the black circle stands for an ancestral centromere. PA, primate ancestor; CA, catarrhini ancestor; OA, OWM ancestor. (Adapted with permission from ref. *19*.)

Our investigations of chromosome 15 evolution provided evidence of an obscure but intriguing relationship between neocentromeres and ancestral inactivated centromeres.

Chromosomes 14 and 15 in humans and in great apes are separate chromosomes. In OWM, they form a unique chromosome (chromosome 7 in macaque) *(21)*. We used a panel of bacterial artificial chromosome (BAC) clones to track the evolutionary history of the 14/15 association in macaque (*Macaca mulatta* [MMU]), sacred baboon (*Papio hamadryas* [PHA]), long-tailed macaque (*Macaca fascicularis* [MFA]), and silvered-leaf monkey (*Presbytis cristata* [PCR]). All these species were found to share the 14/15 association, corresponding to chromosomes MMU7, PHA7, MFA7, and PCR5 *(22)*. The results are summarized in Fig. 5. In all species these chromosomes appeared consistent with human chromosome14 and 15 being fused head–tail and retaining colinearity. The 14/15 association has been reported as ancestral to mammals *(23)*. It can be deduced that in the ancestor to great apes, a noncentromeric fission event occurred between markers F and G, disrupting the 14/15 association and generating the present-day human

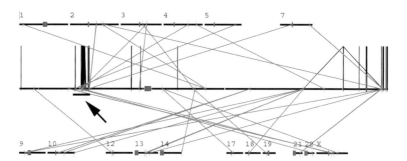

Fig. 4. Distribution of segmental duplications between chromosome 6 and other human chromosomes. Lines represent interchromosomal (*gray*) and intrachromosomal (*black*) alignments. Arrow indicates the cluster of intrachromosomal duplications at 6p22.1, which are the remains of an inactivated ancestral centromere. Note also that the pericentromeric region is relatively devoid of segmental duplications. This is in agreement with the finding that human the chromosome 6 centromere is an evolutionary neocentromere. (Courtesy of Dr. E. E. Eichler.)

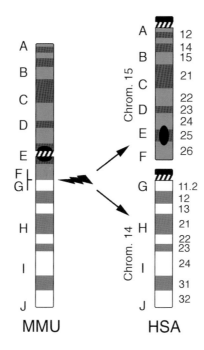

Fig. 5. The diagram shows the organization of human chromosomes 14/15 association in macaque (MMU, *Macaca mulatta*). A fission event gave rise to chromosomes 14 and 15. The fission was followed by the emergence of two new centromeres and by the inactivation of the old centromere at 15q25. (Adapted with permission from ref. *22*.)

chromosomes 14 and 15. The ancestral centromere at 15q25 was inactivated and two new centromeres were generated in regions corresponding to their present-day locations in humans. Segmental duplication analysis showed a large cluster of intrachromosomal segmental duplications at 15q24-q26 (data not shown). This cluster very likely derives from the inactivated ances-

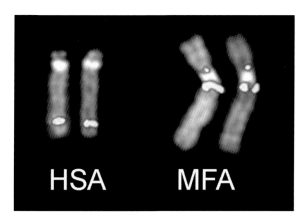

Fig. 6. Partial metaphases showing fluorescence *in situ* hybridization experiments using the human bacterial artificial chromosome clone RP11-182J1 (chr15:82,764,242-82,935,727; 15q25.2) on human chromosome 15 (left) and on macaque chromosome X.

tral centromere. Fluorescence *in situ* hybridization (FISH) experiments using BAC probes containing duplicons of this region flanked the centromere in macaque (Fig. 6), strongly indicating that they are dispersed remains of the ancestral inactivated centromere. The region encompassed by duplicons that flanked the ancestral centromere is approx 11 Mb in size. Similarly to the inactivated ancestral centromere at 6p22.1, no remains of alphoid sequences were found.

The structural organization of the centromeres of the present-day human chromosomes 14 and 15 are indistinguishable from any other human centromere. The conclusion is that the evolutionary new centromeres progressively acquired the complexity of a normal centromere, which very likely stabilize the centromere function.

Interestingly, one of the hotspot site of neocentromeres appearance in clinical cases is at 15q24-q26. We studied two of these neocentromeres that were found several megabases apart but inside the region encompassed by duplicons of the ancestral centromere.

Alonso et al. *(24)* have reported that neocentromeres mapping at the 13q32 hotspot span a 6.5-Mb region. Both sets of data disproved the hypothesis that the neocentromere hotspots refer to a single specific locus. Interestingly, however, both 15q25 neocentromeres mapped to duplicons that are the remains of the ancestral centromere, therefore establishing an intriguing but unclear correlation between duplicon dispersal and neocentromere emergence. If this correlation is correct, one would expect the appearance of neocentromeres at 6p22.1 and at 2q21, where abundant duplicon remains of an inactivated centromere are present. We think, however, that other important factors are involved in neocentromere appearance. It is worth noting that most of the acentric fragments are small in size and associated with phenotypes compatible with embryo development. It could be hypothesized that aneuploidies generated by other latent centromeres are incompatible with life and will never be detected among liveborn.

EVOLUTION OF CHROMOSOME 3: RECURRENT SITES FOR NEW CENTROMERE SEEDING

Because the evolutionary history of the neocentromere hotspot at 15q25 revealed a connection to an ancestral inactivated centromere, we undertook a comprehensive study of the evolutionary history of chromosome 3, harboring an additional neocentromere hotspot at 3q25-q26

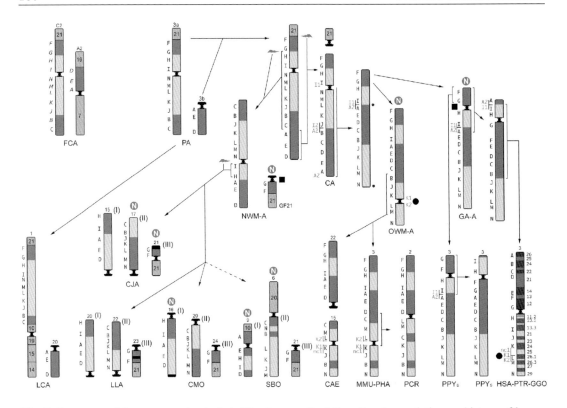

Fig. 7. Summary of fluorescence *in situ* hybridization results delineating the evolutionary history of human chromosome 3 in primates. The hypothesized pericentric or paracentric inversions are indicated by square parentheses spanning the inverted segment. Some chromosomes are upside down to facilitate comparison. PA, primate ancestor; CA, catarrhini ancestor; OWM-A, Old World monkeys ancestor; NWM-A, New World monkeys ancestor; GA-A, great ape ancestor; N (in a gray circle), new centromere. The number that identifies the chromosome in each species is reported on top of the chromosome. Arrows with hatched lines point to species for which an intermediate ancestor has not been drawn. A white N in a gray circle indicates the chromosomes where new centromeres appeared during evolution. The black circles (HSA and OWM-A) and the black squares (GA-A and NWM-A) are positioned at loci where seeding of an evolutionary new centromere was detected. Cat (FCA) probes were identified using the following strategy. The sequence encompassed by each human bacterial artificial chromosome (BAC) was searched for conservation against mouse and rat genome. "Overgo" probes were designed on the most conserved region of each BAC and were then used to screen the cat BAC library RPCI-86. Cat probes, therefore, map to loci orthologous the loci encompassed by the corresponding human BACs. Species analyzed: great ape: common chimpanzee (*Pan troglodytes*, PTR), gorilla (*Gorilla gorilla*, GGO), Borneo (*Pongo pygmaeus pygmaeus,* PPY-B) and Sumatra (*Pongo pygmaeus abelii,* PPY-S) orangutan; Old World monkeys (OWM): rhesus monkey (*Macaca mulatta*, MMU, Cercopithecinae), sacred baboon (*Papio hamadryas*, PHA, Cercopithecinae), African green monkey (*Cercopithecus aethiops*, CAE, Cercopithecinae), silvered leaf-monkey (*Presbytis cristata,* PCR, Colobinae); New World monkeys (NWM): wooly monkey (*Lagothrix lagothricha*, LLA, Atelinae), common marmoset (*Callithrix jacchus*, CJA, Callitrichinae), dusky titi (*Callicebus moloch*, CMO, Callicebinae), squirrel monkey (*Saimiri boliviensis*, SBO); prosimians: ring-tailed lemur (*Lemur catta*, LCA). (Adapted with permission from ref. *25*.)

(25). A panel of human BAC clones was used to reconstruct the order of chromosome 3 markers in representative extant primates (Fig. 7). The analysis clearly showed the emergence of new centromeres in OWM and great ape ancestors. Two human neocentromere cases at 3q25-26 were investigated. These two cases were found to have distinct but important implications

toward a better understanding of new centromere emergence phenomenon both in evolution and in clinical cases. In the first case, the neocentromere emergence occurred at 3q26.1 as part of a complex rearrangement. The functional centromere was excised, and a neocentromere seeded in the acentric derivative chromosome. Human BAC clone RP11-498P15 was identified to be the closest to the neocentromere. This same clone (nc1 in Fig. 7) was found a few kilobases apart from the evolutionary new centromere that appeared in OWM ancestor. This coincidence suggested that the region at 3q26.1 maintained a latent centromere competence that was present before OWM/Hominidae divergence that occurred approx 25 million years ago *(26)*. Furthermore, the new centromere that appeared in the great ape ancestor was seeded very close to marker G (Fig. 7). Interestingly, a new centromere was also seeded in this region in NWM ancestor (chromosome GF21 in Fig. 7) suggesting, again, that the same latent centromeric region was activated twice, in great ape and NWM ancestors. Pevzner and Tesler *(27)*, comparing mouse and human evolutionary breakpoints, have suggested the "reuse" of breakpoint regions in evolution. Similarly, the examples of neocentromeres we have discovered, both in evolution and in clinical cases, seem to extend the "reuse" concept to centromeres.

Evolution of Chromosome 3: Centromeres and Telomeres

In four NWM species examined, human chromosome 3 is split into three chromosomes annotated as (I), (II), and (III) in the Fig. 7. Chromosomes (I) and (II) have an identical marker order in common marmoset (CJA), wooly monkey (LLA), and dusky titi (*Callicebus moloch* [CMO]), if centromeres are not considered. The position of the centromeres, on the contrary, appears peculiar: the centromere is located at the opposite telomere in both (I) and (II) chromosomes in CMO with respect to the ancestral form of CJA and LLA. We have found similar examples of telomere–centromere functional exchanges in the evolution of other chromosomes, for instance, chromosome 20 *(28)*, and chromosomes 11 and 13 (Rocchi, unpublished results, 2005). Low-copy repeat-mediated exchanges may be responsible for centromere jumping between telomeres.

Evolutionary New Centromere Progression

A new centromere was seeded in OWM chromosome 6 during evolution (*see* Remains of Inactivated Centromeres; Fig. 3). The human BAC clone RP11-474A9 (L2 in Fig. 3), mapping at 6q24.3, yielded clear signals on both sides of the MFA6 centromere. Apparently, the new centromere recruited the huge amount of centromeric/pericentromeric sequences without affecting the displaced flanking sequences. The scenario accompanying the progression of the OWM new centromere that appeared on OWM chromosome 3 was different. We found that this centromere is encompassed by human K1 and K2 markers (BAC clones RP11-355I21 and RP11-418B12, respectively), located 436 kb apart in human. BAC clones spanning this gap did not yield any appreciable FISH signal in macaque, African green monkey (CAE), and PCR, whereas giving normal FISH signals in all great apes. Thus the 436-kb region appears lost in OWMs as a consequence of the neocentromerization event. This chromosomal trait was investigated for gene content. The human region (UCSC chr3:163,941,067-164,377,941) appears devoid of genes, harboring only two transcribed but not translated spliced RNAs (UCSC, July 2003 release). It can be hypothesized that the absence of functional constraint made possible the loss (or complete restructuring) of the region. On the contrary, the functional elements around the new centromere insertion on chromosome 6 in OWM (*see* above) behaved as a strong selective barrier to the degenerative activity of the evolving centromeric region.

Gene expression around the neocentromere that emerged at 10q25 *(12,29)* was investigated by Saffery et al. *(30)*. The authors concluded that the neocentromere formation did not affect underlying gene expression. The likely scenario of the progression of an evolutionary new centromere appears as a competition between the degenerative activity of the centromere in the seeding area, and the selection acting against disturbance of functional elements present in the region. Nagaki et al. *(31)* have reported recently the organization of rice chromosome 8 centromere featuring an unusual organization, with genes embedded in the centromeric heterochromatin, as if the centromere were at an intermediate stage between new centromere seeding and a final stage in which all genes are excluded from the completely heterochromatized centromere, as occurs in the remaining rice centromeres.

Additional Euchromatic Duplicon Clusters of Pericentromeric Origin

Segmental duplications accumulate at greater density in pericentromeric and telomeric regions *(6)*. However, large blocks of duplicons exist also in euchromatic locations. We have previously shown that duplicon clusters located, in humans, at euchromatic regions 6p22.1 and 15q25 are the remains of inactivated centromeres. Other chromosomal rearrangements can relocate pericentromeric duplicons in noncentromeric areas. One of the two breakpoints of both pericentric and paracentric evolutionary inversions falls, rather frequently, in pericentromeric regions *(8,28,32)*. In these cases part of a pericentromeric duplicated region can be repositioned far apart from the centromere. Two nonpericentromeric olfactory receptor clusters lying on chromosome 3 are precisely located at domains identified by A2 and I1 markers (Fig. 7). The evolutionary history of chromosome 3 we have reconstructed indicated that these two clusters are examples of duplicons that were pericentromerically located during evolution (*see* marker organization in the primate ancestor [PA] in Fig. 7).

Most mutations of the *CYP21* locus (steroid 21-hydroxylase gene) are owing to a close pseudogene (*CYP21P*) that triggers gene conversions during unequal crossovers *(33)*. Both *CYP21* and *CYP21P* are located inside the duplicon cluster at 6p22.1 that represents the remains of an evolutionary inactivated centromere (*see* above). Gene conversion, therefore, is an additional, indirect mechanism by which duplicon cluster contribute to human genome morbidity.

CENTROMERE REPOSITIONING "IN PROGRESS"

Most of human neocentromere cases arise as a consequence of a rearrangement that generated an acentric fragment. The presence of the acentric fragment as a supernumerary chromosome results in phenotypic abnormalities, which indirectly prevent the transmission of the neocentromere-bearing chromosome to successive generations. They, therefore, have no evolutionary relevance. Very recently, however, Amor et al. *(34)* and Ventura et al. *(25)* have documented two unprecedented neocentromere cases, at 4q21.3 and 3q24, respectively, that arose in an otherwise normal and mitotically stable chromosomes that were transmitted to subsequent generations. These individuals had normal phenotypes. They can be regarded as present-day episodes equivalent to new centromere appearance that occurred during the course of evolution and that were fixed in the population. Individuals with chromosomal changes not accompanied by clinical signs or reproductive problems usually escape detection. It can be reasonably supposed that the "normal" cases reported so far are only a minimal fraction of the existing ones.

In individuals heterozygous for the neocentromere, an odd number of meiotic exchanges internal to the chromosomal region encompassed by the two active centromeres leads to the formation of dicentric and acentric chromosomes. These problems could affect the fitness of heterozygous individuals and act as a negative selective pressure. Meiotic drive in females in favor of the repositioned chromosome is among the possible mechanisms favoring the fixation of the neocentromere. Meiotic drive favoring Robertsonian translocations has been reported by Pardo-Manuel de Villenna and Sapienza *(35)*.

NEOCENTROMERES IN NONPRIMATE MAMMALS

One of the first steps in a sequencing project is the construction of detailed genetic and physical maps obtained using linkage analysis and radiation hybrids studies, respectively. Radiation hybrid maps have been constructed, i.e., for cattle *(36)*, cat *(37)*, horse *(38)*, and pig *(39)*. These studies could represent, in theory, an efficient tool to pinpoint centromere-repositioning events when maps of different species are compared. However, most of these studies were not focused on evolutionary aspect of genome organization. The paper on the bovine radiation hybrids map published by Band et al. *(40)*, on the contrary, took into account the position of the cattle centromeres with respect to humans. The authors concluded that "the comparative map suggests that 41 translocation events, a minimum of 54 internal rearrangements, and repositioning of all but one centromere can account for the observed organizations of the cattle and human genomes." Most likely, they have overestimated the centromere-repositioning phenomenon in cattle. However, it indicates that the repositioning phenomenon may be much more widespread than expected.

Horse and donkey (equidae) diverged about 2 million years ago *(41)*. They produce hybrids (mule and hinny) that are mostly sterile owing to the several chromosomal rearrangements that differentiate horse and donkey chromosomes *(42)*. Yang et al. *(43)*, using a combination of classical G-banding and whole chromosome paints, have noticed the discordant position of the centromere in four orthologous chromosomes, i.e., four distinct centromere repositioning events occurred in a relatively short evolutionary time.

CONCLUDING REMARKS

Centromere repositioning is a newly discovered, unprecedented phenomenon that has a substantial impact on chromosomal architecture. Indeed, the newly seeded centromere rapidly acquires the large size and the complex organization of a normal centromere, whereas the inactivated one disperses in the area large blocks of segmental duplications that were recruited around it when active. In addition, these remainings can contribute to the instability of the human genome *(44)*. Segmental duplicons, indeed, have been shown to play a crucial role in triggering genomic disorders (*see* Chapters 2–23).

It can be reasonably assumed that only a few new centromere events have been fixed in the population during evolution. Therefore, the baseline rate of new centromere occurrence could be relatively high. The two healthy human individuals with a repositioned but otherwise "normal" chromosomes, recently reported in the literature, provide living examples of centromere repositioning events at the very early stages, further supporting the centromere repositioning hypothesis.

ACKNOWLEDGMENTS

Centro di Eccellenza Geni in campo Biosanitario e Agroalimentare (CEGBA), Ministero Italiano della Universita' e della Ricerca (MIUR), Cluster C03, Prog. L.488/92, and European

Commission (INPRIMAT, QLRI-CT-2002-01325) are gratefully acknowledged for financial support. Critical reading of Dr. R. Stanyon is also acknowledged.

REFERENCES

1. Archidiacono N, Antonacci R, Marzella R, Finelli P, Lonoce A, Rocchi M. Comparative mapping of human alphoid sequences in great apes using fluorescence in situ hybridization. Genomics 1995;25:477–484.
2. Henikoff S, Ahmad K, Malik HS. The centromere paradox: stable inheritance with rapidly evolving DNA. Science 2001;293:1098–1102.
3. Jackson MS, Rocchi M, Thompson G, et al. Sequences flanking the centromere of human chromosome 10 are a complex patchwork of arm-specific sequences, stable duplications and unstable sequences with homologies to telomeric and other centromeric locations. Hum Mol Genet 1999;8:205–215.
4. Eichler EE, Archidiacono N, Rocchi M. CAGGG repeats and the pericentromeric duplication of the hominoid genome. Genome Res 1999;9:1048–1058.
5. Horvath JE, Gulden CL, Bailey JA, et al. Using a pericentromeric interspersed repeat to recapitulate the phylogeny and expansion of human centromeric segmental duplications. Mol Biol Evol 2003;20:1463–1479.
6. She X, Horvath JE, Jiang Z, et al. The structure and evolution of centromeric transition regions within the human genome. Nature 2004;430:857–864.
7. Bailey JA, Yavor AM, Viggiano L, et al. Human-specific duplication and mosaic transcripts: the recent paralogous structure of chromosome 22. Am J Hum Genet 2002;70:83–100.
8. Montefalcone G, Tempesta S, Rocchi M, Archidiacono N. Centromere repositioning. Genome Res 1999;9:1184–1188.
9. Ohno S. *Monographs on Endocrinology. Sex Chromosomes and Sex-Linked Genes.* Heidelberg: Springer-Verlag, 1967.
10. Ventura M, Archidiacono N, Rocchi M. Centromere emergence in evolution. Genome Res 2001;11:595–599.
11. Warburton PE. Chromosomal dynamics of human neocentromere formation. Chromosome Res 2004;12: 617–626.
12. du Sart D, Cancilla MR, Earle E, et al. A functional neo centromere formed through activation of a latent human centromere and consisting of non-alpha-satellite DNA. Nat Genet 1997;16:144–153.
13. Amor DJ, Choo KH. Neocentromeres: role in human disease, evolution, and centromere study. Am J Hum Genet 2002;71:695–714.
14. Bukvic N, Susca F, Gentile M, Tangari E, Ianniruberto A, Guanti G. An unusual dicentric Y chromosome with a functional centromere with no detectable alpha-satellite. Hum Genet 1996;97:453–456.
15. Tyler-Smith C, Gimelli G, Giglio S, et al. Transmission of a fully functional human neocentromere through three generations. Am J Hum Genet 1999;64:1440–1444.
16. Ijdo JW, Baldini A, Ward DC, Reeders ST, Wells RA. Origin of human chromosome 2: an ancestral telomere-telomere fusion. Proc Natl Acad Sci USA 1991;88:9051–9055.
17. Baldini A, Ried T, Shridhar V, et al. An alphoid DNA sequence conserved in all human and great ape chromosomes: evidence for ancient centromeric sequences at human chromosomal regions 2q21 and 9q13. Hum Genet 1993;90:577–583.
18. Bailey JA, Gu Z, Clark RA, et al. Recent segmental duplications in the human genome. Science 2002;297: 1003–1007.
19. Eder V, Ventura M, Ianigro M, Teti M, Rocchi M, Archidiacono N. Chromosome 6 phylogeny in primates and centromere repositioning. Mol Biol Evol 2003;20:1506–1512.
20. Willard HF, Waye JS. Hierarchical order in chromosome-specific human alpha satellite DNA. Trends Genet 1987;3:192–198.
21. Wienberg J, Stanyon R, Jauch A, Cremer T. Homologies in human and Macaca fuscata chromosomes revealed by in situ suppression hybridization with human chromosome specific libraries. Chromosoma 1992;101: 265–270.
22. Ventura M, Mudge JM, Palumbo V, et al. Neocentromeres in 15q24-26 map to duplicons which flanked an ancestral centromere in 15q25. Genome Res 2003;13:2059–2068.
23. Murphy WJ, Stanyon R, O'Brien SJ. Evolution of mammalian genome organization inferred from comparative gene mapping. Genome Biol 2001;2:REVIEWS0005.

24. Alonso A, Mahmood R, Li S, Cheung F, Yoda K, Warburton PE. Genomic microarray analysis reveals distinct locations for the CENP-A binding domains in three human chromosome 13q32 neocentromeres. Hum Mol Genet 2003;12:2711–2721.
25. Ventura M, Weigl S, Carbone L, et al. Recurrent sites for new centromere seeding. Genome Res 2004;14: 1696–1703.
26. Goodman M. The genomic record of humankind's evolutionary roots. Am J Hum Genet 1999;64:31–39.
27. Pevzner P, Tesler G. Human and mouse genomic sequences reveal extensive breakpoint reuse in mammalian evolution. Proc Natl Acad Sci USA 2003;100:7672–7677.
28. Misceo D, Cardone MF, Carbone L, et al. Evolutionary history of chromosome 20. Mol Biol Evol 2005;22: 360–366.
29. Lo AW, Craig JM, Saffery R, et al. A 330 kb CENP-A binding domain and altered replication timing at a human neocentromere. EMBO J 2001;20:2087–2096.
30. Saffery R, Sumer H, Hassan S, et al. Transcription within a functional human centromere. Mol Cell 2003;12:509–516.
31. Nagaki K, Cheng Z, Ouyang S, et al. Sequencing of a rice centromere uncovers active genes. Nat Genet 2004;36:138–145.
32. Goidts V, Szamalek JM, Hameister H, Kehrer-Sawatzki H. Segmental duplication associated with the human-specific inversion of chromosome 18: a further example of the impact of segmental duplications on karyotype and genome evolution in primates. Hum Genet 2004;115:116–122.
33. Tusie-Luna MT, White PC. Gene conversions and unequal crossovers between CYP21 (steroid 21-hydroxylase gene) and CYP21P involve different mechanisms. Proc Natl Acad Sci USA 1995;92:10,796–10,800.
34. Amor DJ, Bentley K, Ryan J, et al. Human centromere repositioning "in progress". Proc Natl Acad Sci USA 2004;101:6542–6547.
35. Pardo-Manuel de Villena F, Sapienza C. Transmission ratio distortion in offspring of heterozygous female carriers of Robertsonian translocations. Hum Genet 2001;108:31–36.
36. Williams JL, Eggen A, Ferretti L, et al. A bovine whole-genome radiation hybrid panel and outline map. Mamm Genome 2002;13:469–474.
37. Menotti-Raymond M, David VA, Chen ZQ, et al. Second-generation integrated genetic linkage/radiation hybrid maps of the domestic cat (Felis catus). J Hered 2003;94:95–106.
38. Chowdhary BP, Raudsepp T, Kata SR, et al. The first-generation whole-genome radiation hybrid map in the horse identifies conserved segments in human and mouse genomes. Genome Res 2003;13:742–751.
39. Yerle M, Pinton P, Delcros C, Arnal N, Milan D, Robic A. Generation and characterization of a 12,000-rad radiation hybrid panel for fine mapping in pig. Cytogenet. Genome Res 2002;97:219–228.
40. Band MR, Larson JH, Rebeiz M, et al. An ordered comparative map of the cattle and human genomes. Genome Res 2000;10:1359–1368.
41. Oakenfull E, Lim H, Ryder O. A survey of equid mitochondrial DNA: Implications for the evolution, genetic diversity and conservation of Equus. Conservation Genet 2000;1:341–355.
42. Raudsepp T, Chowdhary BP. Construction of chromosome-specific paints for meta- and submetacentric autosomes and the sex chromosomes in the horse and their use to detect homologous chromosomal segments in the donkey. Chromosome Res 1999;7:103–114.
43. Yang F, Fu B, O'Brien PCM, Nie W, Ryder OA, Ferguson-Smith MA. Refined genome-wide comparative map of the domestic horse, donkey and human based on cross-species chromosome painting: insight into the occasional fertility of mules. Chromosome Res 2004;12:65–76.
44. Jackson M. Duplicate, decouple, disperse: the evolutionary transience of human centromeric regions. Curr Opin Genet Dev 2003;13:629–635.

IV Genomic Rearrangements and Disease Traits

11 The CMT1A Duplication and HNPP Deletion

Vincent Timmerman, PhD and
James R. Lupski, MD, PhD

CONTENTS

INTRODUCTION

The Charcot-Marie-Tooth type 1A (CMT1A) duplication was the first recurrent, large (>1 Mb), submicroscopic DNA duplication rearrangement found to be associated with a common autosomal dominant trait. Mechanistic studies of the CMT1A duplication have set the paradigm for genomic disorders. The CMT1A-REP low-copy repeats (LCRs) were among the first identified nongenic genomic architectural features that could act as substrates for nonallelic homologous recombination (NAHR). Identification of the predicted reciprocal recombination product, the hereditary neuropathy with liability to pressure palsies (HNPP) deletion, resulted in a model for reciprocal duplication/deletion genomic disorders.

From: *Genomic Disorders: The Genomic Basis of Disease*
Edited by: J. R. Lupski and P. Stankiewicz © Humana Press, Totowa, NJ

CLINICAL ENTITIES

CMT disease is a common inherited neuropathy with two major forms distinguished by whether the myelin (type 1 [CMT1]) or the axon (type 2 [CMT2]) is primarily affected. Both CMT1 and CMT2 are genetically heterogeneous with some 35 linked loci, and 25 of the corresponding genes having been identified (http://www.molgen.ua.ac.be/CMTMutations). CMT is characterized by symmetric slowly progressive length-dependent neuropathy, which manifests as a distal weakness of the legs progressing proximally. CMT1 can be distinguished from CMT2 by electrophysiological studies that reveal slowed nerve conduction velocities (NCVs) and neuropathology showing "onion bulbs." The most common form of CMT1 is that associated with the CMT1A locus mapping to 17p12. HNPP is an episodic, asymmetric neuropathy, which may be preceded by an antecedent event, such as motor nerve compression or trauma. Presentations may include pressure palsies or focal neuropathy and sometimes carpal tunnel syndrome. The electrophysiology may show conduction blocks, whereas the neuropathology reveals tomacula—sausage-like thickening of the nerve myelin sheath. CMT1A and HNPP are, therefore, both myelinopathies, but clinically distinguishable entities *(1,2)*.

THE CMT1A DUPLICATION

The CMT1A duplication was identified independently in Europe *(3)* and in the United States *(4)*. Multiple molecular methods including: (1) the presence of three informative alleles revealed by polymorphic simple sequence repeats and restriction fragment length polymorphism (RFLP) analysis in affected individuals; (2) the identification of a 500-kb patient-specific junction fragment by pulsed-field gel electrophoresis (PFGE); and (3) duplication of probes detected by interphase fluorescence *in situ* hybridization (FISH) revealed the duplication (Fig. 1).

The CMT1A duplication was identified as a prominent cause for CMT1A and confirmed in many world populations *(5–13)*. In population-based studies, the CMT1A duplication was shown to be responsible for about 70% of CMT1 *(13,14)*.

DE NOVO DUPLICATION

Remarkably, the CMT1A duplication was also shown to frequently occur *de novo (14–18)* and, in fact, causes 76–90% of sporadic CMT1 *(13,15)*. Intriguingly, the *de novo* duplication occurs preferentially during male meiosis *(19)*. The first molecular demonstration of a *de novo* duplication was shown by informative polymorphic alleles in an European family wherein the segregation of marker genotypes revealed evidence for unequal crossing over during meiosis *(3)*. This finding stimulated a search for genomic architectural features, such as LCRs that might act as recombination substrates. Recombination mediated by paralogous copies (i.e., NAHR) could result in duplication or deletion of the unique sequence located between the LCRs.

CMT1A-REP: AN LCR-MEDIATING NAHR

Physical analysis revealed proximal 17p region-specific LCR (CMT1A-REP) that flank the genomic region duplicated in the CMT1A duplication *(20)*. The CMT1A-REP LCR was not found in early mammals (mouse and hamster) *(20)*, but instead shown to have evolved during primate speciation. CMT1A-REP segmental duplication occurred after the divergence of gorilla and chimpanzee because there were two copies noted in the chimpanzee genome, whereas only

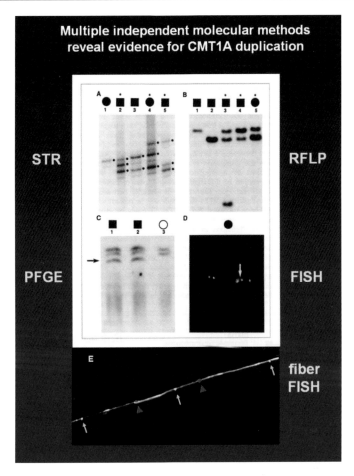

Fig. 1. Multiple methods reveal evidence for duplication. Shown are four separate methods (A–D) that originally enabled visualization of the duplication *(74)*. Simple sequence repeat or short tandem repeat analysis showed three alleles in informative affected individuals. Restriction fragment length polymorphism (RFLP) analysis showed a dosage difference in heterozygous affected individuals, whereas some patients with the CMT1A duplication were fully informative with three different RFLP alleles observed. Pulsed-field gel electrophoresis identified a patient-specific junction fragment of approx 500 kb in size. Fluorescence *in situ* hybridization (FISH) showed the duplicated segment (two adjacent red dots) only in interphase (this is not resolved in metaphase nuclei) where the control probe (green dots) was not replicated enabling one to distinguish duplication from replication. Note the duplicated chromosome has two red signals and one green signal compared to the normal (one red and one green) control chromosome 17 homolog. (E) Fiber FISH (bottom) reveals the predicted three copies of CMT1A-REP (green) and two copies of *PMP22* (red) in the CMT1A duplication bearing chromosome *(75)*.

one copy was present in the gorilla genome *(21–23)*. Segmental duplications occurring during primate genome evolution are a recurrent theme in genome architectural features associated with rearrangements causing genomic disorders *(24)*. The proximal CMT1A-REP and distal CMT1A-REP share about 24,000 bp of approx 99% DNA sequence identity *(23)*. The proximal (centromeric) copy of CMT1A-REP derived from the distal (telomeric) copy. The *COX10* gene, encoding the hemeA:farnesyltransferase that farnesylates the hemeA group that is incorporated into cytochrome oxidase, spans the distal CMT1-REP. Proximal CMT1A-REP represents a segmental

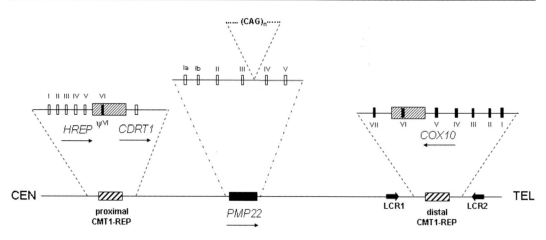

Fig. 2. Partial genome structure of the 1.4-Mb region duplicated in CMT1A and deleted in HNPP. The genomic region is flanked by proximal and distal CMT1A-REP low copy repeats (hatched rectangles). The *COX10* gene (exons depicted as filled boxes) spans the distal CMT1A-REP. Proximal CMT1A-REP was generated by segmental duplication of *COX10* exon VI and surrounding intronic sequences. This insertional event created two new genes, *HREP* through exon accretion (its exon VI is formed from the complementary strand of the segmentally duplicated *COX10* pseudoexon (Ψ)VI) and *CDRT1*, that are transcribed in different tissues. Distal CMT1A-REP is flanked by low-copy repeats (LCR)1 and LCR2. The dosage sensitive *PMP22* gene, with exons shown as open boxes, is located within the genomic interval that is rearranged. It contains an intronic polymorphic CAG trinucleotide repeat between exons III and IV.

duplication of *COX10* exon VI plus 24 kb of surrounding intronic sequences (i.e., distal CMT1A-REP) *(23,25)* (Fig. 2). After the segmental duplication event, the complementary strand of the duplicated *COX10* exon VI ("pseudoexon VI") is transcribed *(23,26)* as part of a new gene created through exon accretion *(27)*. In fact, the segmental duplication that created proximal CMT1A-REP from the distal copy actually created two new genes, *HREP* and *CDRT1*; (Fig. 2), with differing expression profiles *(27,28)*. Exon accretion and the creation of new genes associated with segmental duplication appears to be a common occurrence *(29)*.

MECHANISM FOR THE CMT1A DUPLICATION

The approx 3.0-Mb CMT1A duplication, consisting of two tandem 1.4-Mb copies, results from NAHR, whereby the proximal CMT1A-REP and distal CMT1A-REP, that are separated by 1.4 Mb of genomic DNA *(27)*, recombine resulting in a duplication (Fig. 3). This mechanism was supported by genetic evidence that showed the *de novo* duplication was accompanied by unequal crossover of flanking markers *(3)*. Interestingly, as anticipated, the duplication chromosome has three copies of CMT1A-REP *(20)* (Fig. 1). Moreover, the CMT1A duplication was shown to be a tandem or direct duplication, and not inverted, by both PFGE and FISH *(20,30)*. The mechanism of NAHR using flanking CMT1A-REP repeats as substrates for recombination predicted the existence of a reciprocal recombination product that would result in a deletion of the same genomic region that is duplicated in the CMT1A duplication *(20)*.

THE RECIPROCAL HNPP DELETION

HNPP mapped to the same region as CMT1A and all 17p12 genetic markers known to be duplicated in CMT1A were shown to be deleted in HNPP *(31)*. The HNPP deletion breakpoints

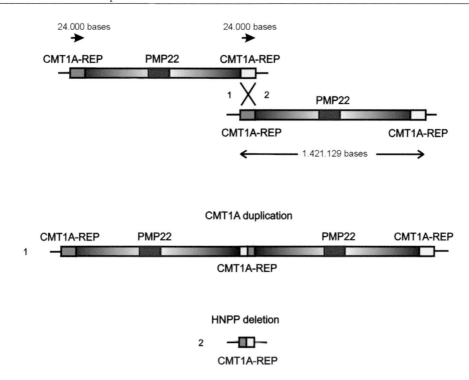

Fig. 3. Nonallelic homologous recombination (NAHR) generates the reciprocal CMT1A duplication and HNPP deletion. Schematic representation of the unequal crossover resulting from misalignment of the low-copy repeat elements, the proximal CMT1A-REP (green) and the distal CMT1A-REP (yellow) sizes of the CMT1A region and CMT1A-REPs are indicated in number of nucleotides or bases. The CMT1A-REPs share 99% of DNA sequence identity. The CMT1A-REP copies can act as substrates for homologous recombination with reciprocal crossovers (numbered 1 and 2) resulting in either the CMT1A tandem duplication or the reciprocal HNPP deletion as alternate products of NAHR.

mapped to the same intervals as those in the CMT1A duplication. The 1.4-Mb HNPP deletion was demonstrated to be the reciprocal recombination product to the CMT1A duplication by the identification of predicted PFGE junction fragments and by showing the expected one copy of CMT1A-REP on the recombinant deleted chromosome (Fig. 3) (32,33). Thus, the HNPP deletion and CMT1A duplication represent the products of a reciprocal NAHR involving CMT1A-REP.

RECOMBINATION HOTSPOT IN CMT1A-REP

Observations regarding the dosage of CMT1A-REP-specific restriction fragments suggested that the CMT1A duplication and HNPP deletion arose from recombination events within a limited region of CMT1A-REP (33). The CMT1A-REP copies are approx 99% identical. The sequence differences between the two paralogous copies, which resulted in different restriction endonuclease recognition sites, were exploited for the mapping of the strand exchanges (i.e., crossovers) within CMT1A-REP. Such paralogous sequence variations, or differences between the two copies located on the same chromosome homolog, are referred to as *cis*-morphisms to distinguish them from polymorphisms-variations of allelic copies on homologous chromosomes (34). The majority of crossovers occurred within a limited region of CMT1A-REP defining a recombination hotspot. This was the first NAHR hotspot defined-initially in a US cohort *(35,36)* and confirmed in a European cohort *(37)*. The CMT1A-REP recombination hotspot was also found in the French *(38)*, Japanese *(39)*, and Chinese *(40)* populations. Such NAHR recombination hotspots have been identified in all genomic disorders in which the strand exchanges have been studied at the nucleotide sequence level *(41)*.

Examination of the products of recombination in the recombinant CMT1A-REP from both patients with the HNPP deletion *(42)* and the CMT1A duplication *(43)* revealed evidence for gene conversion. The products of recombination are best explained by the double-strand break model for homologous recombination. Although *cis* acting recombinogenic sequences that might stimulate double strand breaks have been postulated *(41–43)* none have been either verified experimentally or shown to be common among different hotspots.

CONSEQUENCES OF DUPLICATION/DELETION MUTATIONS ON SEGREGATION OF MARKER GENOTYPES AND LINKAGE ANALYSIS

The failure to recognize a molecular duplication can lead to misinterpretation of marker genotypes for affected individuals, the identification of false recombinants, and incorrect localization of the disease locus *(4,44)*. This occurs because the usual biallelic locus is now triallelic as a result of the duplication *(34)*. By contrast, the deletion results in a lack of transmission of alleles to affected offspring such that the failure to recognize the deletion may lead to an erroneous exclusion of paternity or maternity *(31)*.

PERIPHERAL MYELIN PROTEIN 22 (*PMP22*) GENE DOSAGE ABNORMALITIES CAUSE NEUROPATHY

The initial hypothesis that gene dosage may be mechanistically important with respect to the CMT disease phenotype came from the observation of a more severe neuropathy phenotype in a patient homozygous for the CMT1A duplication *(4)*. Subsequent studies of patients with cytogenetically visible duplications of 17p revealed that as long as the 17p12 region containing the CMT1A locus was duplicated, then part of the complex phenotype observed in the patient would include the decreased NCV diagnostic of CMT1 *(1,45)* consistent with a gene dosage effect causing the disease.

After the identification of the CMT1A duplication in the majority of CMT1 families the peripheral myelin protein 22 (*PMP22*) gene was mapped in the middle of the CMT1A region *(30,46–48)*. Important is that the rare smaller duplications and deletions that cause neuropathy still contained the *PMP22* gene within the rearrangement interval *(19,49,50)*, supporting a *PMP22* gene dosage effect as the disease mechanism *(51)*.

The fact that the phenotype in CMT1A duplication and HNPP deletion patients results from abnormal *PMP22* gene dosage was supported by multiple lines of independent experimental evidence including: (1) quantitative *PMP22* mRNA and (2) PMP22 protein studies in the peripheral nerves from patients with the duplication and deletion rearrangement *(52–59)*. Moreover, rodent models that overexpress *PMP22*, or disrupt it by gene targeting or antisense, recapitulated the respective CMT1A and HNPP phenotypes *(60–65)*. Strategies aimed at normalizing the *PMP22* gene dosage may provide therapeutic approaches as recently demonstrated in rodent models *(66–68)*.

STRUCTURE OF THE 1.4-MB CMT1A DUPLICATION/HNPP DELETION GENOMIC REGION

The genomic interval that is duplicated in the CMT1A duplication and deleted in the HNPP deletion spans 1.4 Mb and is flanked by the 24-kb CMT1A-REP copies (Fig. 2). This interval contains 21 genes and 6 pseudogenes *(27)*. Additional architectural features include two copies of an 11-kb LCR (LCR1 and LCR2), that are inverted with respect to one another and flank the distal CMT1A-REP *(27)*. No evidence could be found for inversion of the intervening sequences using LCR1 and LCR2 as NAHR substrates after evaluating dozens of Caucasian individuals (data not shown) *(27)*. The 1.4 Mb interval also contains 53 simple sequence repeats with more than 11 repeating units *(27,69)*. Interestingly, one of these is a CAG trinucleotide repeat located within the largest (20 kb) intron of *PMP22* between exons III and IV (Fig. 2). We hypothesized that in rare families with CMT accompanied by anticipation, the anticipation may be related to an expanded allele of this triplet repeat. We could not find any data to support this hypothesis in one CMT1A family manifesting anticipation that was examined for expansion of this allele *(27,70)*. It is possible that variation at this *PMP22* intronic polymorphic trinucleotide repeat may affect *PMP22* expression and severity of disease in patients with the CMT1A duplication or HNPP deletion. With the exception of a few rare cases, the CMT1A duplication and HNPP deletion appear to almost always have the same size (i.e., 1.4 Mb), suggesting that a precise recurrent recombination mediated by the CMT1A-REP repeat sequences in this region is the predominant cause for DNA rearrangement. A patient, mosaic for the CMT1A duplication was reported to have a reversion of the 1.4-Mb CMT1A duplication in several somatic tissues *(71)*.

SUMMARY

CMT1A and HNPP are common autosomal dominant traits that result from a 1.4 Mb reciprocal duplication/deletion. The CMT1A duplication and HNPP deletion rearrangements occur via NAHR using flanking LCRs (LCRs termed proximal and distal CMT1A-REP) as the recombination substrates, setting the paradigm for genomic disorders *(72,73)*. A hotspot for strand exchanges, that is associated with the unequal crossover, is located within CMT1A-REP. The CMT1A-REP evolved by segmental duplication of *COX10* exon VI and surrounding intronic sequences during primate genome evolution and speciation. This segmental duplication created two new genes with different tissue expression profiles. The CMT1A duplication has consequences for the interpretation of marker genotypes because it creates a triallelic locus. Finally, the phenotype associated with CMT1A duplication and HNPP deletion results because of an abnormal *PMP22* gene dosage effect. Therapeutic strategies should be directed at correcting the dosage of *PMP22* or ameliorating the consequences of its abnormal expression.

REFERENCES

1. Lupski JR, Garcia A. Charcot-Marie-Tooth peripheral neuropathies and related disorders. In: *The Metabolic and Molecular Bases of Inherited Diseases* (Scriver CR, Beaudet AL, Sly WS, Valle D, Vogelstein B, Childs B, eds.) New York, NY: McGraw-Hill, 2001; pp. 5759–5788.
2. Shy ME, Lupski JR, Chance PF, Klein CJ, Dyck PJ. Hereditary motor and sensory neuropathies. In: *Peripheral Neuropathy* (Dyck PJ, Thomas PK, eds.) Philadelphia, PA: Eliesevier Science, 2005; pp. 1623–1658.

3. Raeymaekers P, Timmerman V, Nelis E, et al. Duplication in chromosome 17p11.2 in Charcot-Marie-Tooth neuropathy type 1a (CMT 1a). The HMSN Collaborative Research Group. Neuromuscul Disord 1991;1:93–97.

4. Lupski JR, de Oca-Luna RM, Slaugenhaupt S, et al. DNA duplication associated with Charcot-Marie-Tooth disease type 1A. Cell 1991;66:219–232.

5. Nicholson GA, Kennerson ML, Keats BJ, et al. Charcot-Marie-Tooth neuropathy type 1A mutation: apparent crossovers with D17S122 are due to a duplication. Am J Med Genet 1992;44:455–460.

6. Hallam PJ, Harding AE, Berciano J, Barker DF, Malcolm S. Duplication of part of chromosome 17 is commonly associated with hereditary motor and sensory neuropathy type I (Charcot-Marie-Tooth disease type 1). Ann Neurol 1992;31:570–572.

7. Hertz JM, Borglum AD, Brandt CA, Flint T, Bisgaard C. Charcot-Marie-Tooth disease type 1A: the parental origin of a *de novo* 17p11.2-p12 duplication. Clin Genet 1994;46:291–294.

8. Brice A, Ravise N, Stevanin G, et al. Duplication within chromosome 17p11.2 in 12 families of French ancestry with Charcot-Marie-Tooth disease type 1a. The French CMT Research Group. J Med Genet 1992;29:807–812.

9. Bellone E, Mandich P, Mancardi GL, et al. Charcot-Marie-Tooth (CMT) 1a duplication at 17p11.2 in Italian families. J Med Genet 1992;29:492–493.

10. Guzzetta V, Santoro L, Gasparo-Rippa P, et al. Charcot-Marie-Tooth disease: molecular characterization of patients from central and southern Italy. Clin Genet 1995;47:27–32.

11. Holmberg BH, Holmgren G, Nelis E, van Broeckhoven C, Westerberg B. Charcot-Marie-Tooth disease in northern Sweden: pedigree analysis and the presence of the duplication in chromosome 17p11.2. J Med Genet 1994;31:435–441.

12. Ohnishi A, Li LY, Fukushima Y, et al. Asian hereditary neuropathy patients with peripheral myelin protein-22 gene aneuploidy. Am J Med Genet 1995;59:51–58.

13. Nelis E, Van Broeckhoven C, De Jonghe P, et al. Estimation of the mutation frequencies in Charcot-Marie-Tooth disease type 1 and hereditary neuropathy with liability to pressure palsies: a European collaborative study. Eur J Hum Genet 1996;4:25–33.

14. Wise CA, Garcia CA, Davis SN, et al. Molecular analyses of unrelated Charcot-Marie-Tooth (CMT) disease patients suggest a high frequency of the CMTIA duplication. Am J Hum Genet 1993;53:853–863.

15. Hoogendijk JE, Hensels GW, Gabreels-Festen AA, et al. *De-novo* mutation in hereditary motor and sensory neuropathy type I. Lancet 1992;339:1081–1082.

16. Mancardi GL, Uccelli A, Bellone E, et al. 17p11.2 duplication is a common finding in sporadic cases of Charcot-Marie-Tooth type 1. Eur Neurol 1994;34:135–139.

17. Blair IP, Nash J, Gordon MJ, Nicholson GA. Prevalence and origin of *de novo* duplications in Charcot-Marie-Tooth disease type 1A: first report of a *de novo* duplication with a maternal origin. Am J Hum Genet 1996;58:472–476.

18. Bort S, Martinez F, Palau F. Prevalence and parental origin of de novo 1.5-Mb duplication in Charcot-Marie-Tooth disease type 1A. Am J Hum Genet 1997;60:230–233.

19. Palau F, Lofgren A, De Jonghe P, et al. Origin of the *de novo* duplication in Charcot-Marie-Tooth disease type 1A: unequal nonsister chromatid exchange during spermatogenesis. Hum Mol Genet 1993;2:2031–2035.

20. Pentao L, Wise CA, Chinault AC, Patel PI, Lupski JR. Charcot-Marie-Tooth type 1A duplication appears to arise from recombination at repeat sequences flanking the 1.5 Mb monomer unit. Nat Genet 1992;2:292–300.

21. Kiyosawa H, Chance PF. Primate origin of the CMT1A-REP repeat and analysis of a putative transposon-associated recombinational hotspot. Hum Mol Genet 1996;5:745–753.

22. Boerkoel CF, Inoue K, Reiter LT, Warner LE, Lupski JR. Molecular mechanisms for CMT1A duplication and HNPP deletion. Ann N Y Acad Sci 1999;883:22–35.

23. Reiter LT, Murakami T, Koeuth T, Gibbs RA, Lupski JR. The human *COX10* gene is disrupted during homologous recombination between the 24 kb proximal and distal CMT1A-REPs. Hum Mol Genet 1997;6:1595–1603.

24. Stankiewicz P, Lupski JR. Molecular-evolutionary mechanisms for genomic disorders. Curr Opin Genet Dev 2002;12:312–319.

25. Murakami T, Reiter LT, Lupski JR. Genomic structure and expression of the human heme A:farnesyltransferase (COX10) gene. Genomics 1997;42:161–164.

26. Kennerson ML, Nassif NT, Dawkins JL, DeKroon RM, Yang JG, Nicholson GA. The Charcot-Marie-Tooth binary repeat contains a gene transcribed from the opposite strand of a partially duplicated region of the *COX10* gene. Genomics 1997;46:61–69.

27. Inoue K, Dewar K, Katsanis N, et al. The 1.4-Mb CMT1A duplication/HNPP deletion genomic region reveals unique genome architectural features and provides insights into the recent evolution of new genes. Genome Res 2001;11:1018–1033.
28. Inoue K, Lupski JR. Molecular mechanisms for genomic disorders. Annu Rev Genomics Hum Genet 2002;3:199–242.
29. Eichler EE. Recent duplication, domain accretion and the dynamic mutation of the human genome. Trends Genet 2001;17:661–669.
30. Valentijn LJ, Bolhuis PA, Zorn I, et al. The peripheral myelin gene *PMP-22/GAS-3* is duplicated in Charcot-Marie-Tooth disease type 1A. Nat Genet 1992;1:166–170.
31. Chance PF, Alderson MK, Leppig KA, et al. DNA deletion associated with hereditary neuropathy with liability to pressure palsies. Cell 1993;72:143–151.
32. Roa BB, Garcia CA, Pentao L, et al. Evidence for a recessive *PMP22* point mutation in Charcot-Marie-Tooth disease type 1A. Nat Genet 1993;5:189–194.
33. Chance PF, Abbas N, Lensch MW, et al. Two autosomal dominant neuropathies result from reciprocal DNA duplication/deletion of a region on chromosome 17. Hum Mol Genet 1994;3:223–228.
34. Lupski JR. 2002 Curt Stern Award Address. Genomic disorders recombination-based disease resulting from genomic architecture. Am J Hum Genet 2003;72:246–252.
35. Reiter LT, Murakami T, Koeuth T, et al. A recombination hotspot responsible for two inherited peripheral neuropathies is located near a mariner transposon-like element. Nat Genet 1996;12:288–297.
36. Kiyosawa H, Lensch MW, Chance PF. Analysis of the CMT1A-REP repeat: mapping crossover breakpoints in CMT1A and HNPP. Hum Mol Genet 1995;4:2327–2334.
37. Timmerman V, Rautenstrauss B, Reiter LT, et al. Detection of the CMT1A/HNPP recombination hotspot in unrelated patients of European descent. J Med Genet 1997;34:43–49.
38. Lopes J, LeGuern E, Gouider R, et al. Recombination hot spot in a 3.2-kb region of the Charcot-Marie-Tooth type 1A repeat sequences: new tools for molecular diagnosis of hereditary neuropathy with liability to pressure palsies and of Charcot-Marie-Tooth type 1A. French CMT Collaborative Research Group. Am J Hum Genet 1996;58:1223–1230.
39. Yamamoto M, Yasuda T, Hayasaka K, et al. Locations of crossover breakpoints within the CMT1A-REP repeat in Japanese patients with CMT1A and HNPP. Hum Genet 1997;99:151–154.
40. Chang JG, Jong YJ, Wang WP, et al. Rapid detection of a recombinant hotspot associated with Charcot-Marie-Tooth disease type IA duplication by a PCR-based DNA test. Clin Chem 1998;44:270–274.
41. Lupski JR. Homologous recombination hotspots in the human genome - not all homolgous sequences are equal. Genome Biology 2004;5:242.
42. Reiter LT, Hastings PJ, Nelis E, De Jonghe P, Van Broeckhoven C, Lupski JR. Human meiotic recombination products revealed by sequencing a hotspot for homologous strand exchange in multiple HNPP deletion patients. Am J Hum Genet 1998;62:1023–1033.
43. Lopes J, Tardieu S, Silander K, et al. Homologous DNA exchanges in humans can be explained by the yeast double-strand break repair model: a study of 17p11.2 rearrangements associated with CMT1A and HNPP. Hum Mol Genet 1999;8:2285–2292.
44. Matise TC, Chakravarti A, Patel PI, et al. Detection of tandem duplications and implications for linkage analysis. Am J Hum Genet 1994;54:1110–1121.
45. Lupski JR, Wise CA, Kuwano A, et al. Gene dosage is a mechanism for Charcot-Marie-Tooth disease type 1A. Nat Genet 1992;1:29–33.
46. Matsunami N, Smith B, Ballard L, et al. *Peripheral myelin protein-22* gene maps in the duplication in chromosome 17p11.2 associated with Charcot-Marie-Tooth 1A. Nat Genet 1992;1:176–179.
47. Patel PI, Roa BB, Welcher AA, et al. The gene for the peripheral myelin protein *PMP-22* is a candidate for Charcot-Marie-Tooth disease type 1A. Nat Genet 1992;1:159–165.
48. Timmerman V, Nelis E, Van Hul W, et al. The peripheral myelin protein gene *PMP-22* is contained within the Charcot-Marie-Tooth disease type 1A duplication. Nat Genet 1992;1:171–175.
49. Valentijn LJ, Baas F, Zorn I, Hensels GW, de Visser M, Bolhuis PA. Alternatively sized duplication in Charcot-Marie-Tooth disease type 1A. Hum Mol Genet 1993;2:2143–2146.
50. van de Wetering RA, Gabreels-Festen AA, Timmerman V, Padberg GM, Gabreels FJ, Mariman EC. Hereditary neuropathy with liability to pressure palsies with a small deletion interrupting the *PMP22* gene. Neuromuscul Disord 2002;12:651–655.

51. Lupski JR. Charcot-Marie-Tooth disease: a gene-dosage effect. Hosp Pract (Off Ed) 1997:32–85.
52. Yoshikawa H, Nishimura T, Nakatsuji Y,et al. Elevated expression of messenger RNA for peripheral myelin protein 22 in biopsied peripheral nerves of patients with Charcot-Marie-Tooth disease type 1A. Ann Neurol 1994;35:445–450.
53. Hanemann CO, Stoll G, D'Urso D, et al. Peripheral myelin protein-22 expression in Charcot-Marie-Tooth disease type 1a sural nerve biopsies. J Neurosci Res 1994;37:654–659.
54. Hanemann CO, Stoll G, Muller HW. *PMP22* expression in CMT1a neuropathy. Ann Neurol 1995;37:136.
55. Kamholz J, Shy M, Scherer S. Elevated expression of messenger RNA for peripheral myelin protein 22 in biopsied peripheral nerves of patients with Charcot-Marie-Tooth disease type 1A. Ann Neurol 1994;36: 451–452.
56. Schenone A, Nobbio L, Mandich P, et al. Underexpression of messenger RNA for peripheral myelin protein 22 in hereditary neuropathy with liability to pressure palsies. Neurology 1997;48:445–449.
57. Schenone A, Nobbio L, Caponnetto C, et al. Correlation between *PMP-22* messenger RNA expression and phenotype in hereditary neuropathy with liability to pressure palsies. Ann Neurol 1997;42:866–872.
58. Gabriel JM, Erne B, Pareyson D, Sghirlanzoni A, Taroni F, Steck AJ. Gene dosage effects in hereditary peripheral neuropathy. Expression of peripheral myelin protein 22 in Charcot-Marie-Tooth disease type 1A and hereditary neuropathy with liability to pressure palsies nerve biopsies. Neurology 1997;49:1635–1640.
59. Vallat JM, Sindou P, Preux PM, et al. Ultrastructural PMP22 expression in inherited demyelinating neuropathies. Ann Neurol 1996;39:813–817.
60. Huxley C, Passage E, Manson A, et al. Construction of a mouse model of Charcot-Marie-Tooth disease type 1A by pronuclear injection of human YAC DNA. Hum Mol Genet 1996;5:563–569.
61. Magyar JP, Martini R, Ruelicke T, et al. Impaired differentiation of Schwann cells in transgenic mice with increased PMP22 gene dosage. J Neurosci 1996;16:5351–5360.
62. Sereda M, Griffiths I, Puhlhofer A, et al. A transgenic rat model of Charcot-Marie-Tooth disease. Neuron 1996;16:1049–1060.
63. Huxley C, Passage E, Robertson AM, et al. Correlation between varying levels of *PMP22* expression and the degree of demyelination and reduction in nerve conduction velocity in transgenic mice. Hum Mol Genet 1998;7:449–458.
64. Adlkofer K, Frei R, Neuberg DH, Zielasek J, Toyka KV, Suter U. Heterozygous peripheral myelin protein 22-deficient mice are affected by a progressive demyelinating tomaculous neuropathy. J Neurosci 1997;17: 4662–4671.
65. Maycox PR, Ortuno D, Burrola P, et al. A transgenic mouse model for human hereditary neuropathy with liability to pressure palsies. Mol Cell Neurosci 1997;8:405–416.
66. Sereda MW, Meyer zu Horste G, Suter U, Uzma N, Nave KA. Therapeutic administration of progesterone antagonist in a model of Charcot-Marie-Tooth disease (CMT-1A). Nat Med 2003;9:1533–1537.
67. Passage E, Norreel JC, Noack-Fraissignes P, et al. Ascorbic acid treatment corrects the phenotype of a mouse model of Charcot-Marie-Tooth disease. Nat Med 2004;10:396–401.
68. De Jonghe P, Timmerman V. Anti-steroid takes aim at neuropathy. Nat Med 2003;9:1457–1458.
69. Badano JL, Inoue K, Katsanis N, Lupski JR. New polymorphic short tandem repeats for PCR-based Charcot-Marie-Tooth disease type 1A duplication diagnosis. Clin Chem 2001;47:838–843.
70. Kovach MJ, Lin JP, Boyadjiev S, et al. A unique point mutation in the *PMP22* gene is associated with Charcot-Marie-Tooth disease and deafness. Am J Hum Genet 1999;64:1580–1593.
71. Liehr T, Rautenstrauss B, Grehl H, et al. Mosaicism for the Charcot-Marie-Tooth disease type 1A duplication suggests somatic reversion. Hum Genet 1996;98:22–28.
72. Lupski JR. Genomic disorders: structural features of the genome can lead to DNA rearrangements and human disease traits. Trends Genet 1998;14:417–422.
73. Stankiewicz P, Lupski JR. Genome architecture, rearrangements and genomic disorders. Trends Genet 2002;18:74–82.
74. Patel PI, Lupski JR. Charcot-Marie-Tooth disease: a new paradigm for the mechanism of inherited disease. Trends Genet 1994;10:128–133.
75. Rautenstrauss B, Fuchs C, Liehr T, Grehl H, Murakami T, Lupski JR. Visualization of the CMT1A duplication and HNPP deletion by FISH on stretched chromosome fibers. J Peripher Nerv Syst 1997;2:319–322.

12

Smith-Magenis Syndrome Deletion, Reciprocal Duplication dup(17)(p11.2p11.2), and Other Proximal 17p Rearrangements

Paweł Stankiewicz, MD, PhD, Weimin Bi, PhD, and James R. Lupski, MD, PhD

CONTENTS

INTRODUCTION

An approx 4-Mb genomic segment on chromosome 17p11.2 commonly deleted in 70–80% of patients with the Smith-Magenis syndrome (SMS) is flanked by large, complex, highly identical (approx 98.7%), and directly oriented, proximal (approx 256 kb) and distal (approx 176 kb) low-copy repeats (LCRs), termed SMS-REPs. These LCR copies mediate nonallelic homologous recombination (NAHR), resulting in both SMS deletion and the reciprocal duplication dup(17)(p11.2p11.2). A third copy, the middle SMS-REP (approx 241 kb) is inverted and located between them. Several additional large LCR17ps have been identified fomented by breakpoint mapping in patients with deletions ascertained because of an SMS phenotype. LCRs in proximal 17p constitute more than 23% of the analyzed genome sequence, approx fourfold higher than predictions based on virtual analysis of the entire human genome. LCRs appear to play a significant role not only in common recurrent deletions and duplications, but also in other rearrangements including unusual sized (i.e., uncommon, recurrent and nonrecurrent) chromosomal deletions, reciprocal translocations, and marker chromosomes. DNA sequence analysis from both common and unusual sized recurrent SMS deletions and common dup(17)(p11.2p11.2) reveals "recombination hotspots" or a remarkable positional preference for strand exchange in NAHR events. Large palindromic LCRs, mapping between proximal and middle SMS-REPs, are responsible for the origin of a recurrent somatic isochromosome

From: *Genomic Disorders: The Genomic Basis of Disease*
Edited by: J. R. Lupski and P. Stankiewicz © Humana Press, Totowa, NJ

i(17q), one of the most common recurrent structural abnormalities observed in human neoplasms, suggesting genome architecture may play a role in mitotic as well as meiotic rearrangements. LCRs in proximal 17p are also prominent features in the genome evolution of this region whereby several serial segmental duplications have played an important role in chromosome evolution accompanying primate speciation.

The gene- and LCR-rich, human genomic region 17p11.2-p12 is rearranged in a variety of different constitutional, evolutionary, and cancer-associated structural chromosome aberrations, and thus is an excellent model to investigate the role of genome architecture in DNA rearrangements *(1–9)*.

CONSTITUTIONAL RECURRENT GENOMIC DISORDERS IN PROXIMAL 17p

Similar to Charcot-Marie-Tooth disease type 1A (CMT1A) and hereditary neuronopathy with pressure palsies (HNPP), the LCR-mediated NAHR mechanism is responsible for two other constitutional genomic disorders in proximal chromosome 17p: SMS and the dup(17)(p11.2p11.2) syndrome.

Smith-Magenis Syndrome

SMS (MIM 182290) is a multiple congenital anomalies and mental retardation disorder associated with an interstitial deletion within chromosome 17p11.2 *(10–13)*. Clinical characteristics include minor craniofacial and skeletal anomalies such as brachycephaly, frontal bossing, synophrys, midfacial hypoplasia, short stature, and brachydactyly, neurobehavioral abnormalities such as aggressive and self-injurious behavior and sleep disturbances, ophthalmic, otolaryngological, cardiac, and renal anomalies *(13,14)*.

As defined by fluorescence *in situ* hybridization (FISH) and by a unique *de novo* junction fragment identified in pulsed-field gel electrophoresis, 70–80% of SMS patients harbor a common approx 4-Mb deletion within 17p11.2 *(3,12,15,16)*. Approximately 20–25% SMS patients have either smaller or larger sized deletions *(16–19)*. Recently, premature termination codon mutations in the retinoic acid inducible-1 gene, *RAI1*, which maps within the SMS critical region, have been found in five SMS-like patients without deletion *(20–21)*, suggesting *RAI1* haploinsufficiency causes SMS. Bioinformatics analyses of the dosage sensitive *RAI1* gene, and comparative genomics between human and mouse orthologs, revealed a zinc finger like-PHD domain at the carboxyl terminus that is conserved in the trithorax group of chromatin-based transcriptional regulators, suggesting that RAI1 might be involved in chromatin remodeling *(21)*. These findings suggest *RAI1* is involved in transcriptional control through a multi-protein complex, and its function may be altered in individuals with SMS.

Interestingly, despite a common deletion size, the only constant objectively defined features among patients with SMS are sleep disturbances, low adaptive functioning, and mental retardation. There is no pathognomonic clinical feature, no characteristic cardiovascular defect, renal anomaly, otolaryngological, nor ophthalmic abnormality in SMS *(22)*.

The Emerging Clinical Phenotype of the dup(17)(p11.2p11.2) Syndrome: The Homologous Recombination Reciprocal of the Common SMS Deletion

The common SMS deletion region is duplicated in patients with a milder, predominantly neurobehavioral phenotype and the reciprocal chromosome duplication—dup(17)(p11.2p11.2)

(5,23). Similar to SMS patients with common deletion, subjects with common duplication dup(17)(p11.2p11.2) also manifest marked variability in the physical features and behavioral profile. Clinical findings include dysmorphic craniofacial features, hypotonia and failure to thrive, oropharyngeal dysphasia, neurocognitive impairment, and behavioral problems including autistic, aggressive, and self-injurious behavior. Structural cardiac anomalies including aortic root enlargement, have been identified. However, the frequency of organ system developmental abnormalities appears to be less than that observed for patients deleted for this genomic interval (i.e., SMS). Sleep disturbances are seen in all patients yet the findings are distinct from those of deletion 17p11.2. It is predicted that the incidence of dup(17)(p11.2p11.2) may be equal to that of SMS given the reciprocal nature of the common rearrangements responsible for the conditions. However, as this duplication is difficult to detect by routine cytogenetic analysis, many of these patients are currently probably not ascertained. Systematic clinical evaluation of a cohort of patients with dup(17)(p11.2p11.2) will be necessary to determine the features most characteristic of this microduplication syndrome.

The relatively high frequency of constitutional genomic disorders in proximal chromosome 17p is further substantiated by the identification of an individual with two distinct megabase-sized DNA rearrangements of this genomic interval. These included both a *de novo* dup(17)(p11.2p11.2) and an inherited HNPP deletion on the other homolog. These rearrangements were associated with mild delay and a family history of autosomal dominant carpal tunnel syndrome *(24)*.

SMS-REPS, LCR LOCATED AT THE BREAKPOINTS OF THE COMMON DELETION

Physical mapping studies have demonstrated that the SMS common deletion interval is flanked by large (approx 200 kb), highly identical (>98%), LCR gene clusters termed proximal and distal SMS-REPs *(1,3,7)* that during either maternal or paternal gametogenesis act as substrates for NAHR *(8,25)*. To delineate the genomic structure (size, orientation, sequence identity, gene content) and evolution of the SMS-REPs, we constructed and sequenced a complete approx 5-Mb bacterial and P1-derived artificial chromosome (BAC/PAC) contig in 17p11.2-p12. Our analysis revealed that both the proximal SMS-REP (approx 256 kb) and the distal copy (approx 176 kb) are located in the same orientation and derived from a progenitor copy, whereas the middle SMS-REP (approx 241 kb) is inverted and appears to have been derived from the proximal copy. This architecture likely explains why the common SMS deletions occur between proximal and distal SMS-REPs.

There are four regions of significant stretches of identity between the proximal and the distal SMS-REPs (A, B, C, and D regions in Fig. 1A). The sum of these high sequence similarity regions is approx 170 kb (169,905 bp), and the identity is greater than 98% with the exception of the D region (>95%) (Table 1). The largest conserved segment (region A in Fig. 1A) is 126 kb in size. Two large sequence blocks (between A and B, and between C and D) in the proximal SMS-REP are absent in the distal SMS-REP. Two smaller blocks, flanking areas of the B region in the distal SMS-REP are absent in the proximal SMS-REP (Fig. 1A).

FISH analysis using SMS-REP-specific BAC clones as probes revealed strong hybridization signals on metaphase chromosomes 17p11.2 and three strong signals on the interphase chromosomes. However, SMS-REP-specific BACs also showed weaker hybridization signals in interphase analysis and metaphase spreads; these map to chromosome 17p13.1, 17p12,

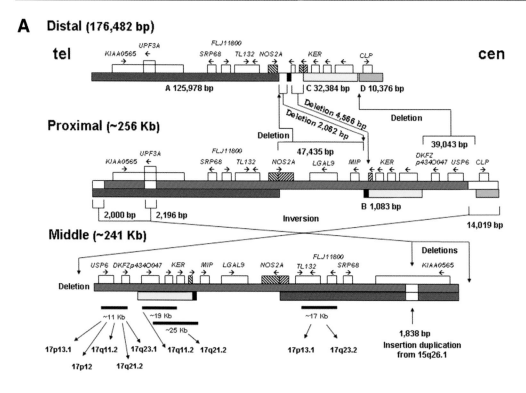

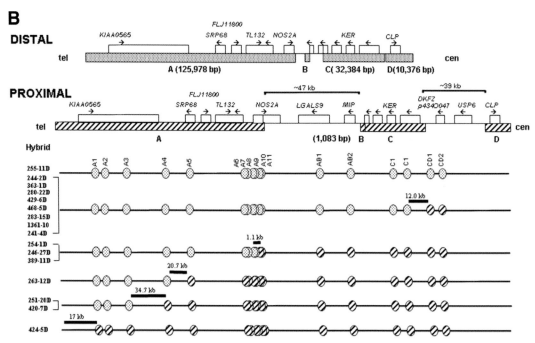

Fig. 1. Sequence-based genomic structure of the Smith-Magenis syndrome (SMS)-REPs. (A) There are four regions of sequence identity more than 95% between the proximal and the distal SMS-REPs (A, B, C, and D). The A, B, and C sequence blocks have more than 98% identity between distal and proximal REPs, whereas the D regions (green) show more than 95% identity. The thick blue lines represent the

17q11.2, 17q12, 17q21.2, and 17q23.2. In concordance with FISH results, BLAST analysis revealed that other approx 11–30 kb "SMS-REP-like" paralogous sequences, fragments of SMS-REPs, are localized on 17p13.1 (approx 28 kb), 17p12 (approx 11 kb), 17q11.2 (approx 30 kb), 17q12 (approx 11 kb), 17q21.2 (approx 25 kb), and 17q23.2 (approx 28 kb) (7).

Sequence analyses show that all three SMS-REPs within the SMS common deletion are not present in the mouse syntenic region (16). Apparently, except for a chromosome inversion of the region between the middle and proximal SMS-REP syntenic region in mouse, the gene order between SMS-REPs is conserved (16,26). Interestingly, transposition occurred for the TAC1 and KCNJ12 genes adjacent to the SMS-REPs. This rearrangement of gene order might have occurred during the evolution of the SMS-REPs, indicating that segmental duplications might transpose surrounding genes (16).

Reciprocal Crossovers and a Positional Preference for Strand Exchange in Recombination Events Resulting in Deletion or Duplication of Chromosome 17p11.2

Using restriction enzyme cis-morphisms and direct sequencing analyses in SMS patients with a common deletion, the regions of strand exchange were mapped in 16 somatic-cell hybrids that retain the deletion chromosome which effectively isolates the recombinant SMS-REP from the copies on the non-deleted homolog. The crossovers were distributed throughout the region of homology between the proximal and distal SMS-REPs. However, despite approx 170 kb of more than 98% identity, 50% of the recombinant junctions occurred in a 12.0-kb region within the KER gene clusters in the C region (Fig. 1B). DNA sequencing of this recombination hotspot (27), or positional preference for strand exchange, in seven recombinant SMS-REPs narrowed the crossovers to an approx 8-kb interval. Four of them occurred in a 1655-bp region rich in polymorphic nucleotides that could potentially reflect frequent gene

---

regions of homology between proximal and middle SMS-REPs. The proximal copy is the largest and is localized in the same orientations as the distal copy. The middle SMS-REP shows almost the same sequence and structure as the proximal copy except for two terminal deletions, an UPF3A gene interstitial deletion and a small (approx 2 kb) insertional duplication. However, it is inverted with respect to proximal and distal SMS-REPs. SMS-REP-specific CLP, TRE, and SRP cis-morphisms were confirmed by DNA sequencing. Fourteen genes/pseudogenes were found. The two additional KER copies in distal SMS-REP represent repeated fragments of the KER pseudogenes. Cross-hatched areas (NOS2A in the proximal and KER in the distal) denote two genes spanning the high homology and non-homology area between the distal and proximal SMS-REP copies, which suggest a three-step event for the hypothetical model of the evolution of the SMS-REPs. At the bottom, the chromosome 17 distribution of SMS-REP fragments, which constitute chromosome 17 LCR17s, is shown. The above data were obtained through BLAST analysis of sequence database. (B) Refining the regions of unequal crossover in somatic-cell hybrids. Top, the genomic structures of SMS-REPs, with the distal and proximal copies in direct orientation, telomere (tel) (left) and centromere (cen) (right). Bottom, regions of strand exchange within the recombinant SMS-REP of the deletion chromosome isolated in hybrids. Restriction cis-morphism markers enabling distinction between the distal and proximal SMS-REP copies are indicated (circles), with their positions corresponding to the proximal SMS-REP at the top of the figure. Some sites in the recombinant SMS-REP were derived from the distal SMS-REP (dotted circles), and others were derived from the proximal copy (hatched circles). For each somatic-cell hybrid, the region of strand exchange within the recombinant SMS-REP and its size are indicated (blackened horizontal bar). The recombination event in hybrid 255-11D is centromeric to the CLP region (D) in the distal SMS-REP.

Table 1
DNA Sequence Homology Comparison Among Different LCR17p Copies

	LCR17pB	LCR17pC	LCR17pD	Proximal CMT1A-REP	Middle SMS-REP	Distal SMS-REP
LCR17pA	98.70%	88.45%	98.57%	—	—	—
LCR17pC	—	—	88.03%	—	—	—
Distal CMT1A-REP	—	—	—	98.15%	—	—
Proximal SMS-REP	—	—	—	—	98.20%	98.13%
Middle SMS-REP	—	—	—	—	—	98.29%

SMS, Smith-Magenis syndrome; CMT1A, Charcot-Marie-Tooth disease type 1A.

conversion. For further evaluation of the strand exchange frequency in patients with SMS, novel junction fragments from the recombinant SMS-REPs were identified (8).

As predicted by the reciprocal-recombination model, junction fragments were also identified from this hotspot region in patients with dup(17)(p11.2p11.2), documenting reciprocity of the positional preference for strand exchange. Several potential cis-acting recombination-promoting sequences were identified within the hotspot. Of note, a 2.1-kb AT-rich inverted repeat was found flanking the proximal and middle KER gene clusters but not the distal one (8).

LCR17p Repeats

Recently, we provided evidence for the existence of additional LCRs in 17p11.2-p12 termed LCR17pA, LCR17pB, LCR17pC, LCR17pD, LCR17pE, LCR17pF, and LCR17pG (19,28) (Fig. 2). Segmental duplications constitute more than 23% of approx 7.5 Mb of genome sequence in proximal 17p, approx fourfold higher than predictions based on virtual analysis of the entire human genome. Based on the genomic sequence information spanning these LCRs, we determined the size, structure, orientation, and extent of homology for and between each copy. BLAST comparisons of LCR17p repeats revealed that LCR17pA is composed of three subunits, which we termed LCR17pA/B (approx 232 kb, homologous and in an inverted orientation with respect to LCR17pB) and adjacent to it on the centromeric side two overlapping sequences LCR17pA/C (approx 79 kb), and LCR17pA/D (approx 115 kb) (both homologous and directly oriented with respect to LCR17pC [approx 91 kb] and LCR17pD [approx 118 kb], respectively). Interestingly, the LCR17pC and LCR17pD copies directly flank the proximal SMS-REP (Fig. 2).

It is remarkable that despite different sizes, locations, orientations, and, most importantly, times of origin, proximal and distal CMT1A-REPs, proximal, middle, and distal SMS-REPs, LCR17pA/B and LCR17pB, and LCR17pA/D and LCR17pD, have retained very similar (approx 98.1–98.7%) nucleotide identity. Our studies show that in contrast to LCR17pA/D- and LCR17pD-mediated NAHR, resulting in recurrent SMS chromosome deletions (29), no deletions with breakpoint within similarly sized LCR17pA/C and LCR17pC have been found (19,30). We propose that during primate evolution, the DNA sequence homology between LCR17pA/C and LCR17pC copies must have dropped below a minimal misalignment/recombination stimulating threshold (<95%?) that in turn resulted in a lack of LCR/NAHR gene conversion events and DNA homogenization and a subsequent steady decrease of nucleotide identity to the current approx 88% value (Table 1).

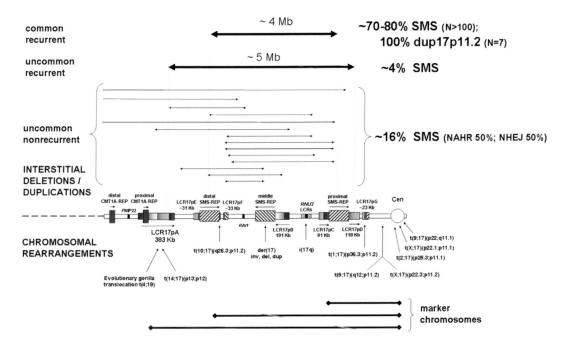

Fig. 2. Schematic diagram of breakpoints for DNA rearrangements in proximal chromosome 17p. (Top) Interstitial deletions and duplications are shown as horizontal arrows. Recurrent, common (approx 4 Mb) and unusual sized (approx 5 Mb) deletions are responsible for 70–80% and 4% of SMS cases, respectively. They both utilize low-copy repeats (LCRs) as substrates for nonallelic homologous recombination (NAHR). In approx 16% of SMS cases, uncommon nonrecurrent deletions have been found. Approximately half of them arise owing to NAHR mechanism between repetitive sequences and half through nonhomologous end-joining. (Bottom) LCR-associated chromosome translocations, isochromosome 17q, and marker chromosomes are depicted. The LCR17p structures are depicted in colors to better represent their positional orientation with respect to each other; the shaded rectangles and horizontal arrowheads represent the orientation of the LCRs (3,5–7,9,19,25,28–31,41–43).

Uncommon Deletions of the SMS Region Can Be Recurrent When Alternate LCRs Act as Homologous Recombination Substrates

LCR17ps predominate at breakpoints of uncommon nonrecurrent, or unusual sized chromosome deletions in proximal 17p. In fact, 64% of unusual sized SMS deletion breakpoints occur in LCRs (19,29,30). In some cases, the breakpoints of uncommon nonrecurrent deletions map to two different nonhomologous LCRs (e.g., SMS-REP and LCR17pA), indicating that they do not mediate the rearrangement by acting as homologous recombination substrates. However, genome architecture may stimulate rearrangements with nonrecurrent breakpoints, supporting the notion that chromosomal rearrangements are not random events but rather reflect structural features of the human genome.

A class of uncommon deletions were recurrent with breakpoints mapping to homologous LCRs. We identified a recombination hotspot within LCR17pA and LCR17pD, which serve as alternative substrates for NAHR that results in this recurrent large (approx 5 Mb) SMS deletion in 17p11.2 (29). Using polymerase chain reaction mapping of somatic cell hybrid lines, the breakpoints of six deletions within these LCRs were determined. Sequence analysis of the recombinant junctions revealed that all six strand exchanges occurred within a 524-bp interval, and four of them occurred within an *Alu*Sq/x element. This interval represents only 0.5% of the 124-kb stretch of 98.6% sequence identity between LCR17pA and LCR17pD. These findings indicate that alternative LCRs can mediate rearrangements, resulting in haploinsufficiency of the SMS critical region, and reimplicate homologous recombination as a major mechanism for genomic disorders *(29)*.

Uncommon, Nonrecurrent 17p11.2 Rearrangements Occur Via Both Homologous and Nonhomologous Mechanisms

To examine recombination mechanisms involved in uncommon, nonrecurrent rearrangements, we sequenced the products of strand exchange in hybrids retaining such rare deletion chromosomes from patients with SMS. Two of the four deletions are a product of *Alu–Alu* recombination, while the remaining two deletions result from a nonhomologous end-joining mechanism *(31)*. Of the breakpoints studied, 3/8 are located in LCRs, and 5/8 are within repetitive elements, including *Alu* and MER5B sequences. These findings suggest that higher-order genomic architecture, such as LCRs, and smaller repetitive sequences such as *Alu* elements, can mediate chromosomal deletions via homologous and nonhomologous mechanisms. These data further implicate homologous recombination as the predominant mechanism of deletion formation in this genomic interval *(31)*.

The Breakpoint Region of i(17q) in Human Neoplasia Is Characterized by a Complex Genomic Architecture With Large Palindromic LCRs

i(17q) is one of the most common recurrent structural abnormalities observed in human neoplasms including chronic myeloid leukemia and in solid tumors such as childhood primitive neuroectodermal tumors *(32,33)*. The i(17q) breakpoints were mapped in 11 cases with different hematological malignancies and the genomic structure of the involved region was determined. Our results revealed a complex genomic architecture in the i(17q) breakpoint cluster region characterized by large (approx 38–49 kb), palindromic, LCRs *(9)*, strongly suggesting that somatic rearrangements are not random events but rather reflect susceptibilities owing to the genomic structure *(34)*.

Molecular Genetic Basis and Animal Models of SMS and dup(17)(p11.2p11.2)

By examining the deleted regions in SMS patients with unusual-sized deletions, we refined the minimal SMS critical region (SMCR) to an approx 1.1-Mb genomic interval that contains 20 genes *(16,26)*. The number, order, and orientation of genes within the SMCR are highly conserved in mouse chromosome 11, 32–34 cM *(16)*. To identify the causative gene(s) in SMS, using chromosome engineering *(35)*, we generated chromosomes carrying either the deletion/ deficiency *(Df(11)17)* or duplication *(Dp(11)17)* of an approx 2-Mb genomic interval containing the mouse region syntenic to the SMCR *(36)*. These models partially reproduce the craniofacial and behavioral phenotype in humans *(36,37)*. The *Df(11)17/+* mice exhibit craniofacial abnormalities, seizures, marked obesity, abnormal circadian rhythm, and are hypoactive. The *Dp(11)17/+* animals are underweight, hyperactive, and have impaired contextual fear conditioning. Most of the phenotypes in the *Df(11)17/+* mice including craniofacial abnormalities, seizures, obesity, and some behavioral abnormities are rescued in *Df(11)17/Dp(11)17* mice, suggesting the existence of a dosage-sensitive gene(s) in this approx 2-Mb genomic interval *(37)*.

To refine regions responsible for different SMS phenotypic features, three lines of mice (*Df[11]17-1*, *Df[11]17-2*, and *Df[11]17-3*) with approx 590-kb deletions were generated *(38)* using retrovirus mediated chromosome engineering for constructing nested deletions *(39)*. Heterozygous mice with these smaller deletions manifest craniofacial anomalies and obesity *(38)*. The identification of *RAI1* point mutations in SMS patients suggest that haploinsufficiency of RAI1 causes the neurobehavioral, craniofacial, and otolaryngological phenotypes in SMS *(20,21)*. *Rai1*, the mouse homolog of *RAI1*, is located in the smaller deletion. The heterozygous mice with disruption of *Rai1* gene also exhibit a similar craniofacial phenotype and obesity *(40)*, suggesting that *Rai1* haploinsufficiency results in the craniofacial abnormalities and obesity in the smaller deletion mice.

Importantly, the severity and penetrance of the craniofacial phenotype were significantly reduced in the smaller deletion mice and *Rai1*[+/-] heterozygous mice in comparison to *Df(11)17/ + mice (38,40)*, indicating that genes or regulatory regions in the larger deletion that are not within the smaller deletion influence both the penetrance and expressivity of the phenotype. We observed phenotypic variation in these mouse models in both the same and different genetic backgrounds *(38)*, perhaps reflecting the variations in SMS patients. Our studies on mouse models suggest that in SMS even a single clinical endophenotype such as craniofacial features is affected by multiple genes, in which *RAI1* is the major causative gene, whereas other genes or regulatory regions within the SMCR, or located elsewhere, modify the phenotype. The molecular basis of dup(17)(p11.2p11.2) syndrome is still unknown. Examining whether the *Rai1* mutant allele can rescue the phenotype in *Dp(11)17/+* mice will help understand the role of *RAI1* in this disorder.

Serial Segmental Duplications During Primate Evolution Result in Complex Human Genome Architecture

Using multifaceted approaches, consisting of FISH studies in fibroblast and lymphoblast cell lines from several primate species and computational analyses of human genome sequence (molecular clock analysis), we investigated the complex structure and evolution of the genome architecture in an approx 7.5-Mb region of proximal 17p. Cumulative data from studies of different segmental duplications in proximal 17p suggest a potential model that most parsimoniously explains how the complex genomic architecture evolved (Fig. 3).

The complex genome architecture in proximal 17p results from a series of consecutive segmental duplications during primate evolution *(28)*. Both repetitive sequences and transposable elements were identified at the breakpoints of genome rearrangements, suggesting a potential role in their generation. Segmental duplications appear to influence genome evolution by a number of different mechanisms including the creation of novel fusion/fission genes at the LCR insertion site, as well as potentially enabling an increased mutation rate owing to LCR-mediated genomic inversion associated with reduced recombination. In essence, such genome architecture enables shuffling of the genome and generating new gene functions, both at segmental duplication breakpoints and by divergence of duplicated copies, providing ample diversity for selection to act upon during evolution.

SUMMARY

The proximal region of human chromosome 17p contains multiple LCRs, many of which have been identified at the breakpoints of DNA rearrangements associated with genomic

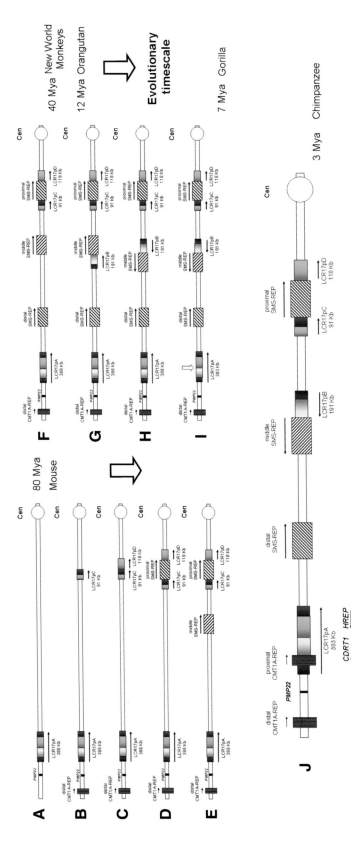

Fig. 3. Rearrangements of proximal 17p low-copy repeat (LCR) during primate evolution. Proximal chromosome 17p is depicted by two thin horizontal lines with the centromere (*white circle*) shown to the right. LCRs are shown as horizontal rectangles with the same color or black-and-white graphic, representing highly homologous sequence. (A) In the mouse genome only LCR17pA is present. (B,C) The proximal portion of LCR17pA was duplicated more than 25 million years ago (Mya). Note that LCR17pC and LCR17pD represent two overlapping portions of LCR17pA. (D) The proximal SMS-REP split the LCR17pC and LCR17pD copies resulting in three directly adjacent large LCRs. Two tandem duplication resulted in directly oriented middle (E) and distal (F) Smith-Magenis syndrome (SMS)-REPs (7). (G) After the divergence of orangutan and gorilla 7–12 Mya, the distal portion of LCR17p was tandemly duplicated creating a directly oriented LCR17pB copy. (H) Both middle SMS-REP and LCR17pB, adjacent to it, were inverted. (I) Following that, at the junction between LCR17pA/B and LCR17pD copies, the evolutionary translocation t(4:19) occurred in a pre-gorilla individual. 7–12 Mya (vertical open arrow). (J) Finally, between gorilla and chimpanzee, 3–7 Mya the proximal CMT1A-REP, present only in human and chimpanzee, resulted from the insertional duplication of the distal copy (44–46). To the right is shown a time line of mammalian, mainly primate evolution with Mya, as indicated.

disorders. The predominant mechanism for deletion and reciprocal duplication is NAHR utilizing homologous LCR as recombination substrates. Genome rearrangements can occur either during meiosis or mitosis, accompany genome evolution, and can cause genomic disorders. Chromosome rearrangements are not random events but instead reflect underlying genome architecture.

REFERENCES

1. Pentao L, Wise CA, Chinault AC, Patel PI, Lupski JR. Charcot-Marie-Tooth type 1A duplication appears to arise from recombination at repeat sequences flanking the 1.5 Mb monomer unit. Nat Genet 1992;2:292–300.
2. Chance PF, Abbas N, Lensch MW, et al. Two autosomal dominant neuropathies result from reciprocal DNA duplication/deletion of a region on chromosome 17. Hum Mol Genet 1994;3:223–228.
3. Chen K-S, Manian P, Koeuth T, et al. Homologous recombination of a flanking repeat gene cluster is a mechanism for a common contiguous gene deletion syndrome. Nat Genet 1997;17:154–163.
4. Reiter LT, Hastings PJ, Nelis E, De Jonghe P, Van Broeckhoven C, Lupski JR. Human meiotic recombination products revealed by sequencing a hotspot for homologous strand exchange in multiple HNPP deletion patients. Am J Hum Genet 1998;62:1023–1033.
5. Potocki L, Chen K-S, Park S-S, et al. Molecular mechanism for duplication 17p11.2- the homologous recombination reciprocal of the Smith-Magenis microdeletion. Nat Genet 2000;24:84–87.
6. Stankiewicz P, Park S-S, Inoue K, Lupski JR. The evolutionary chromosome translocation 4;19 in *Gorilla gorilla* is associated with microduplication of the chromosome fragment syntenic to sequences surrounding the human proximal CMT1A-REP. Genome Res 2001;11:1205–1210.
7. Park S-S, Stankiewicz P, Bi W, et al. Structure and evolution of the Smith-Magenis syndrome repeat gene clusters, SMS-REPs. Genome Res 2002;12:729–738.
8. Bi W, Park S-S, Shaw CJ, Withers MA, Patel PI, Lupski JR. Reciprocal crossovers and a positional preference for strand exchange in recombination events resulting in deletion or duplication of chromosome 17p11.2. Am J Hum Genet 2003;73:1302–1315.
9. Barbouti A, Stankiewicz P, Nusbaum C, et al. The breakpoint region of the most common isochromosome, i(17q), in human neoplasia is characterized by a complex genomic architecture with large, palindromic, low-copy repeats. Am J Hum Genet 2004;74:1–10.
10. Smith AC, McGavran L, Robinson J, et al. Interstitial deletion of (17)(p11.2p11.2) in nine patients. Am J Med Genet 1986;24:393–414.
11. Stratton RF, Dobyns WB, Greenberg F, et al. Interstitial deletion of (17)(p11.2p11.2): report of six additional patients with a new chromosome deletion syndrome. Am J Med Genet 1986;24:421–432.
12. Greenberg F, Guzzetta V, Montes de Oca-Luna R, et al. Molecular analysis of the Smith-Magenis syndrome: a possible contiguous-gene syndrome associated with del(17)(p11.2). Am J Hum Genet 1991;49:1207–1218.
13. Chen K-S, Potocki L, Lupski JR. The Smith-Magenis syndrome [del(17)p11.2]: clinical review and molecular advances. Ment Retard Dev Disabil Res Rev 1996;2:122–129.
14. Greenberg F, Lewis RA, Potocki L, et al. Multi-disciplinary clinical study of Smith-Magenis syndrome (deletion 17p11.2). Am J Med Genet 1996;62:247–254.
15. Juyal RC, Figuera LE, Hauge X, et al. Molecular analyses of 17p11.2 deletions in 62 Smith-Magenis syndrome patients. Am J Hum Genet 1996;58:998–1007.
16. Bi W, Yan J, Stankiewicz P, et al. Genes in the Smith-Magenis syndrome critical deletion interval on chromosome 17p11.2 and the syntenic region of the mouse. Genome Res 2002;12:713–728 .
17. Trask BJ, Mefford H, van den Engh G, et al. Quantification by flow cytometry of chromosome-17 deletions in Smith-Magenis syndrome patients. Hum Genet 1996;98:710–718.
18. Vlangos CN, Yim DKC, Elsea SH. Refinement of the Smith-Magenis syndrome critical region to ~950 kb and assessment of 17p11.2 deletions. Are all deletions created equally? Mol Genet Metab 2003;79:134–141.
19. Stankiewicz P, Shaw CJ, Dapper JD, et al. Genome architecture catalyzes nonrecurrent chromosomal rearrangements. Am J Hum Genet 2003;72:1101–1116.
20. Slager RE, Newton TL, Vlangos CN, Finucane B, Elsea SH. Mutations in *RAI1* associated with Smith-Magenis syndrome. Nat Genet 2003;33:466–468.
21. Bi W, Saifi GM, Shaw CJ, et al. Mutations of RAI1, a PHD-containing protein, in nondeletion patients with Smith-Magenis syndrome. Hum Genet 2004;115:515–524.

22. Potocki L, Shaw CJ, Stankiewicz P, Lupski JR. Variability in clinical phenotype despite common chromosomal deletion in Smith-Magenis syndrome [del(17)(p11.2p11.2)]. Genet Med 2003;5:430–434.

23. Potocki L, Treadwell-Deering D, Krull K, et al. The emerging clinical phenotype of the dup(17)(p11.2p11.2) syndrome: the homologous recombination reciprocal of the Smith-Magenis microdeletion. Polish Society of Human Genetics, Gdansk, Poland.

24. Potocki L, Chen K-S, Koeuth T, et al. DNA rearrangements on both homologs of chromosome 17 in a mildly delayed individual with a family history of autosomal dominant carpal tunnel syndrome. Am J Hum Genet 1999;64:471–478.

25. Shaw CJ, Bi W, Lupski JR. Genetic proof of unequal meiotic crossovers in reciprocal deletion and duplication of 17p11.2. Am J Hum Genet 2002;71:1072–1081.

26. Probst FJ, Chen K-S, Zhao Q, et al. A physical map of the mouse shaker-2 region contains many of the genes commonly deleted in Smith-Magenis syndrome (del17p11.2p11.2). Genomics 1999;55–348–352.

27. Lupski JR. Hotspots of homologous recombination in the human genome: not all homologous sequences are equal. Genome Biol 2004;5:242.

28. Stankiewicz P, Shaw CJ, Withers M, Inoue K, Lupski JR. Serial segmental duplications during primate evolution result in complex human genome architecture. Genome Res 2004;14:2209–2220.

29. Shaw CJ, Withers MA, Lupski JR. Uncommon Smith-Magenis syndrome deletions can be recurrent by utilizing alternate LCRs as homologous recombination substrates. Am J Hum Genet 2004;75:75–81.

30. Shaw CJ, Shaw CA, Yu W, et al. Comparative genomic hybridisation using a proximal 17p BAC/PAC array detects rearrangements responsible for four genomic disorders. J Med Genet 2004;41:113–119.

31. Shaw CJ, Lupski JR. Non-recurrent 17p11.2 deletions are generated by homologous and non-homologous mechanisms. Hum Genet 2004;116:1–7.

32. Fioretos T, Strömbeck B, Sandberg T, et al. Isochromosome 17q in blast crisis of chronic myeloid leukemia and in other hematologic malignancies is the result of clustered breakpoints in 17p11 and is not associated with coding TP53 mutations. Blood 1999;4:225–232.

33. Scheurlen WG, Schwabe GC, Seranski P, et al. Mapping of the breakpoints on the short arm of chromosome 17 in neoplasms with an i(17q). Genes Chromosomes Cancer 1999;25:230–240.

34. Stankiewicz P, Inoue K, Bi W, et al. Genomic disorders - genome architecture results in susceptibility to DNA rearrangements causing common human traits. Cold Spring Harb Symp Quant Biol 2003;LXVIII:445–454

35. Ramirez-Solis R, Liu P, Bradley A. Chromosome engineering in mice. Nature 1995;378:720–724.

36. Walz K, Caratini-Rivera S, Bi W, et al. Modeling del(17)(p11.2p11.2) and dup(17)(p11.2p11.2) contiguous gene syndromes by chromosome engineering in mice: phenotypic consequences of gene dosage imbalance. Mol Cell Biol 2003;23:3646–3655.

37. Walz K, Spencer C, Kaasik K, Lee CC, Lupski JR, Paylor R. Behavioral characterization of mouse models for Smith-Magenis syndrome and dup(17)(p11.2p11.2). Hum Mol Genet 2004;13:367–378.

38. Yan J, Keener VW, Bi W, et al. Reduced penetrance of craniofacial anomalies as a function of deletion size and genetic background in a chromosome engineered partial mouse model for Smith-Magenis syndrome. Hum Mol Genet 2004;13:2613–2624.

39. Su H, Wang X, Bradley A. Nested chromosomal deletions induced with retroviral vectors in mice. Nat Genet 2000;24:92–95.

40. Bi W, Ohyama T, Nakamura H, et al. Inactivation of Rai1 in mice recapitulates phenotypes observed in chromosome engineered mouse models for Smith-Magenis syndrome. Hum. Mol. Genet 2005;14:983–995.

41. Stankiewicz P, Park S-S, Holder SE, et al. Trisomy 17p10-p12 resulting from a supernumerary marker chromosome derived from chromosome 17: Molecular analysis and delineation of the phenotype. Clin Genet 2001;60:336–344

42. Shaw CJ, Stankiewicz P, Bien-Willner G, et al. Small marker chromosomes in two patients with segmental aneusomy for proximal 17p. Hum Genet 2004;115:1–7.

43. Yatsenko SA, Treadwell-Deering D, Krull K, et al. Trisomy 17p10-p12 due to mosaic supernumerary marker chromosome: delineation of molecular breakpoints and clinical phenotype and comparison to other proximal 17p segmental duplications. Am J Med Genet 2005;138A:175–180.

44. Kiyosawa H, Chance PF. Primate origin of the CMT1A-REP repeat and analysis of a putative transposon-associated recombinational hotspot. Hum Mol Genet 1996;5:745–753.

45. Reiter LT, Murakami T, Koeuth T, Gibbs RA, Lupski JR. The human COX10 gene is disrupted during homologous recombination between the 24 kb proximal and distal CMT1A-REPs. Hum Mol Genet 1997;6:1595–1603.
46. Inoue K, Dewar K, Katsanis N, et al. The 1.4-Mb CMT1A duplication/HNPP deletion genomic region reveals unique genome architectural features and provides insights into the recent evolution of new genes. Genome Res 2001;11:1018–1033.

13 Chromosome 22q11.2 Rearrangement Disorders

Bernice E. Morrow, PhD

INTRODUCTION

Meiotic unequal crossover events between blocks of low-copy repeats (LCRs) may lead to gene dosage imbalance resulting in genomic disorders. Genomic disorders are frequently associated with mental retardation or learning disabilities and mild to severe congenital anomalies. Chromosome 22q11.2 is particularly susceptible to chromosome rearrangements leading to several genomic disorders including velocardiofacial syndrome/DiGeorge syndrome (VCFS/DGS), der(22) syndrome, and cat-eye syndrome (CES), associated with a monosomy, trisomy, and tetrasomy of 22q11.2, respectively. Most VCFS/DGS patients have a similar hemizygous 3-Mb deletion mediated by meiotic interchromosomal homologous recombination events between LCRs termed LCR22s. The reciprocal duplication of the same interval, predicted on expected products of unequal crossover events, results in a more mild condition termed dup(22)(q11.2; q11.2) syndrome. In contrast to VCFS/DGS, dup(22)(q11.2; q11.2) and CES, der(22) syndrome is caused by a different molecular mechanism. Der(22) disorder

From: *Genomic Disorders: The Genomic Basis of Disease*
Edited by: J. R. Lupski and P. Stankiewicz © Humana Press, Totowa, NJ

arises in offspring of normal carriers of the constitutional t(11;22) (q23.3; q11.2) translocation by recombination between AT-rich (high AT sequence composition) palindromic sequences on 11q23.3 and 22q11.2. The palindromic sequence on 22q11.2 is within one of the LCR22s. Interestingly, both recurrent and novel breakpoints occur most often in LCR22s, making them an important architectural feature associated with susceptibility to genome rearrangements. To gain further insight into the mechanisms of how the LCR22s are involved in chromosome rearrangements, efforts are underway to determine the molecular evolution, structure, size, orientation, and their level of variability in humans.

MEIOTIC 22q11.2 REARRANGEMENTS

Diseases resulting from rearrangements of the human genome are referred to as genomic disorders and most are mediated by region-specific LCRs *(1–5)*. The 22q11.2 region is particularly susceptible to meiotic chromosome rearrangements associated with genomic disorders including VCFS/DGS (OMIM192430/OMIM188400) *(6–8)*; the reciprocal duplication syndrome, dup(22)(q11.2; q11.2) *(9–12)*, CES(MIM 115470); 13, and der(22) syndrome *(14,15)*. All of these are congenital anomaly disorders with varying levels of learning disabilities and mental retardation. An illustration of the chromosomal breakpoints for these disorders is shown in Fig. 1.

22q11.2 Deletion Syndrome

In 1965, a disorder in a group of infants with thymus gland aplasia and neonatal hypocalcemia was described and termed DiGeorge syndrome *(6)*. In the 1970s other sets of patients were ascertained with related, but more mild sets of clinical findings and were termed VCFS (Shprintzen et al. *[7]*) and separately, conotruncal anomaly face syndrome *(16)*. In early 1990s, when molecular cytogenetic technologies became available, it was realized that all these clinically similar disorders shared a hemizygous deletion on chromosome 22q11.2 *(17–19)*. These disorders occur quite frequently in different populations, in approx 1/4000 live births *(20)*. The main clinical findings are learning and behavioral abnormalities, craniofacial anomalies, thymus gland hypoplasia, and cardiovascular malformations. Many other clinical findings occur in association with the disorders but with variable expressivity. The great majority of the cases are sporadic owing to *de novo* deletions. When inherited, it is in an autosomal dominant manner and the penetrance is complete. Integrated physical and genetic maps were constructed and it was found that most VCFS/DGS patients have a similar 3-Mb deletion, whereas some have nested distal deletion breakpoints, the most common of which is a 1.5-Mb deletion (Fig. 1) *(21–25)*. The severity of the phenotype did not depend on the size of the deletion, suggesting that gene(s) within the smaller 1.5-Mb interval are responsible for its etiology. To understand the mechanism responsible for the recurrent deletion, the chromosome breakpoints for common features were analyzed. Three blocks of LCRs termed LCR22 were found to be associated with the breakpoints *(9,26,27)*.

Cat-Eye Syndrome and Der(22) Syndrome

CES is a more rare disorder that the 22q11.2 deletion syndrome and it is associated with ocular colobomata, anal atresia, congenital heart defects, renal malformations, craniofacial anomalies, male genital anomalies, skeletal defects, and mild mental retardation *(15,28)*. CES patients carry a supernumerary bisatellited chromosome 22, resulting in a tetrasomy of 22pter-

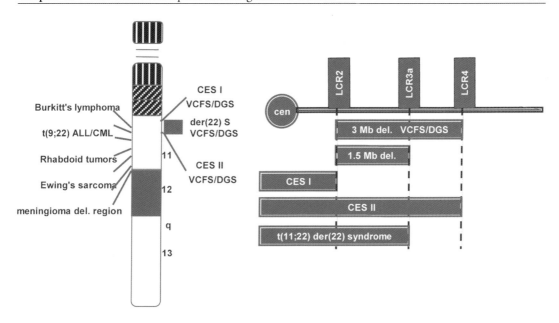

Fig. 1. Chromosome rearrangements on 22q11.2. To the left of the ideogram of chromosome 22, the list of human cancers breakpoint mapping in the 22q11q12 interval. On the right side, the list of the recurrent congenital anomaly disorders (dup(22)(q11.2; q11.2) disorder maps to the same interval as the 3 Mb VCFS/DGS deletion). Other duplication breakpoints occur more telomerically (not shown). The blue box represents the 3-Mb region associated with all three disorders. On the right, the horizontal line represents chromosome 22q11.2, with the centromere to the left. The recurrent chromosome rearrangement breakpoints are shown.

q11.2 (29–31). There are two common breakpoints in CES, type I and type II, and they occur in the same regions as for the common 3-Mb VCFS/DGS deletion breakpoints (26,31).

Der(22) syndrome is also a rare congenital anomaly disorder associated with similar features to CES, although there are some minor differences such as the absence of ocular colobomata and more severe mental retardation than in CES patients (32,33). Der(22) syndrome arises in offspring of normal carriers of the constitutional t(11;22) translocation, the most common recurrent non-Robertsonian constitutional translocation in humans (14). Patients with this disorder have a partial trisomy of the 11q23.3qter and 22pter-q11.2 regions (34,35). The recurrent t(11;22) translocation breakpoint occurs in the same region as for the 1.5 Mb distal deletion breakpoint in VCFS/DGS patients (Fig. 1), suggesting that this region is particularly labile (34).

Somatic Rearrangements Associated With Malignant Disorders on 22q11.2

The most common recurrent rearrangement on 22q11.2 associated with malignant tumors is the balanced t(9;22) translocation in patients with acute lymphocytic leukemia and chronic myeloid leukemia (Fig. 1). A characteristic Philadelphia chromosome der(22)t(9;22)(q34;q11) is present in tumor cells. A balanced t(8;22) translocation is associated with Burkitt's lymphoma and it disrupts the immunoglobulin light chain locus on 22q11.2 (36). Other rearrangements in malignant tumors include the t(11;22) translocation in Ewing sarcoma and the deletions or translocations in malignant rhabdoid tumors and meningiomas (Fig. 1). Thus, it is likely that sequences in the 22q11.2 region are prone to breakage also during mitosis. Detailed molecular characterization of the breakpoints remains to be performed.

SEGMENTAL DUPLICATIONS
AND 22q11.2 REARRANGEMENT DISORDERS

The establishment of physical maps of chromosome 22 made it possible to determine the position of the common recurrent breakpoints associated with chromosome 22q11.2 rearrangement disorders (Fig. 1). Probes used to screen filters containing large genomic insert bacterial artificial chromosome (BAC) clones identified clones mapping to several locations on 22q11.2 including clones in the vicinity of the breakpoints. LCRs have been noted already on 22q11.2 over 16 years ago (Heisterkamp and Groffen [78]) and in the general vicinity of VCFS/DGS locus over 10 years ago (37), but the connection between them was not made until integrated physical maps were generated (9,26).

Interchromosomal recombination events lead to the 22q11.2 deletion and a reciprocal duplication, both associated with congenital anomalies. Using microsatellite genetic markers and screening more than 150 VCFS/DGS patients and their unaffected family members, it was possible to narrow the region containing the common recurrent 1.5- and 3-Mb deletions (23). Further analysis of the breakpoints occurring in VCFS/DGS and CES patients suggested that they occurred in the same regions (38). More recently, the constitutional t(11;22) breakpoint on 22q11.2 was placed in the vicinity of the distal deletion breakpoint in VCFS/DGS patients with the nested 1.5 Mb deletion (34).

Blocks of region-specific segmental duplications or LCR22-2, LCR22-3a and LCR22-4; also known as LCR22-A, -B, and -D, respectively were found to map to the three regions of breakage, associated with VCFS/DGS, CES, and der(22) syndrome, all 1.5 Mb apart, implicating them in their etiology (Fig. 1) (9,24,25–27,34). The LCR22-2 and LCR22-4 are more than 240 kb in size and more than 99% identical in sequence. This suggested that misalignment of nonallelic copies of the homologs could occur during meiosis and through the mechanism of nonallelic homologous recombination (NAHR) resulting in a deletion.

Both intrachromosomal and interchromosomal unequal crossover events were found to be responsible for the 3-Mb deletion (Fig. 2) (26,38,39). This was determined by performing haplotype analysis with microsatellite markers, of three generations, the patient, parents, and grandparents. For interchromosomal events, which are more predominant (Baumer et al. [38]; Siatta et al. [39]), there should be individuals with the reciprocal duplication, dup(22)(q11.2q11.2). An analogous mechanism has been described for chromosome 17p11.2 for Smith-Magenis syndrome (SMS) (40). Indeed, interchromosomal unequal recombination events between two misaligned chromosomes 22 during meiosis resulted in a reciprocal duplication, dup(22)(q11.2)(11.2), (Fig. 2) (11,12,26). Unrelated dup(22)(q11.211.2) patients had been ascertained based on suspicion that they had VCFS/DGS. Dup(22)(q11.2q11.2) disorder is associated with some clinical findings occurring in VCFS/DGS, but also with other features which are distinct including characteristic facial features with mild craniofacial anomalies, hearing loss, and urogenital malformations (9,11,12).

Thus, based on mechanisms proposed, a newly recognized genetic syndrome was identified. Interestingly, unlike for VCFS/DGS which are characterized by deletions between LCR22-2 and LCR22 (LCR22-A–D), the size of the duplications vary in size, extending to more distal LCR22s (11) suggesting that larger duplications are more tolerated than larger deletions or that the mechanism for deletion and duplication may involve other sequences within LCR22s.

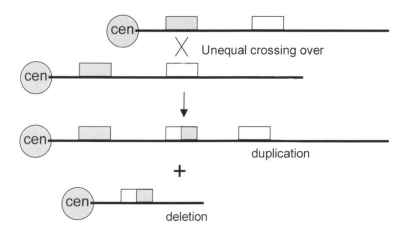

Fig. 2. Molecular mechanism for 22q11.2 rearrangements. Unequal crossover between two homologs can generate a duplication or a deletion *(26)*. The filled box represents LCR22-2 and the open box represents LCR22-4. Both LCR22s are more than 225 kb in size and are 3 Mb apart.

MOLECULAR MECHANISM MEDIATING
THE CONSTITUTIONAL t(11;22) TRANSLOCATION

In contrast to VCFS/DGS, CES and dup(22)(q11.2q11.2), mediated by NAHR events between LCR22s (Fig. 2), a different mechanism is responsible for the balanced recurrent t(11;22) translocation leading to the der(22) syndrome. The site of breakage for the constitutional t(11;22) translocation is within the center of AT-rich palindromes on chromosomes 11q23 and 22q11.2 (Figs. 3 and 4) *(35,41–45)*. The AT-rich palindrome on 22q11.2 is in LCR22-3a, which is equidistant between LCR22-2 and LCR22-4 that mediate the 3 Mb VCFS/DGS deletion (Fig. 1). Two cases of t(17;22)(q11.2;q11.2) with AT-rich palindromes on chromosome 17 at the breakpoints were reported *(9,43,46,47)*. Because the same sequences are present at the translocation breakpoints, a similar molecular mechanism is likely responsible for the t(11;22) and t(17;22) translocations based on one shown in experimental systems *(48,49)*.

The model (Fig. 4) proposes that palindromic sequences can form unstable cruciform structures (Fig. 3) susceptible to double-stranded breaks and repair by nonhomologous end-joining (NHEJ) mechanisms. As part of the repair, a translocation may ensue, thereby stabilizing the DNA. Therefore, both homologous and nonhomologous (NAHR and NHEJ) mechanisms are responsible for recurrent genomic disorders caused by LCR22s.

Seven LCR22s map to the 22q11.2 region *(24,26,42,44)*, suggesting that there might be individuals with breakpoints or chromosome rearrangements within LCR22s in addition to the ones harboring the more common rearrangement endpoints. Rare individuals with deletion breakpoints in these LCR22s have been identified *(50–53)*. Based on the analysis of chromosome breakpoints, the LCR22s are sequences that result in susceptibility to recurrent rearrangement mutations and understanding the molecular mechanisms should shed light on this process.

NOVEL 22Q11.2 TRANSLOCATIONS

Chromosome regions harboring breakpoints in cell lines from individuals carrying novel translocations within the 22q11.2 region were mapped to ascertain whether there could share

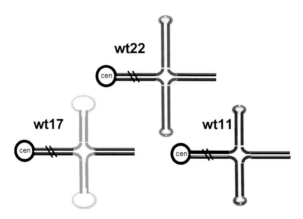

Fig. 3. AT-rich palindromes mediate the t(11;22) and the t(17;22) translocation. AT-rich palindromes on chromosomes 11q23.3, 17q11.2, and 22q11.7 can form cruciform structures as shown. The regions on chromosomes 11 and 22 form perfect palindromes, whereas the region on chromosome 17 contains non-palindromic sequences in the center of the cruciform structure, depicted as a look. Although the sequences in all three chromosomes are AT-rich, they are not homologous to each other.

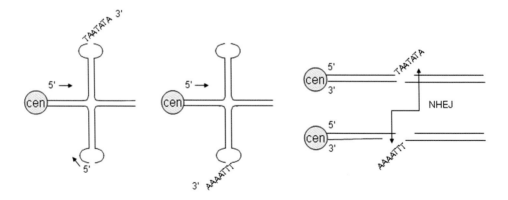

Fig. 4. Model of mechanism for translocations mediated by AT-rich palindromes. Palindromes are prone to double strand breaks which lead to translocations repaired by non-homologous end-joining (NHEJ). Although the sequences in all three chromosomes are AT-rich, they are not homologous to each other. When a breakpoint occurs in the labile loop created at the tips of the cruciform structure, a translocation may occur, resulting in a more stable non-palindromic sequence *(43)*. The arrows depict the orientation of DNA sequence with respect to the centromere. (Modified from refs. *48,49*.)

common features. Most breakpoints occurred in the proximal half of chromosome 22q11.2. Of these, half map to the LCR22s. Among the LCR22s, most were in LCR22-3a, the LCR22 associated with the t(11;22) translocation *(54)*. In two reports of translocations disrupting LCR22-3a (LCR22-B), one showed the breakpoint occurred between AT-rich palindromes in LCR22-3a and on the partner chromosome 4q35 *(55)* but the other did not (chromosome X) *(56)*, implicating different mechanisms. In our study, half of the translocations disrupting 22q11.2 occurred distal to the most telomeric unique sequence probe *(54)*. The breakpoints on the partner chromosomes occurred more frequently in telomeric bands, supporting the epidemiological data that breakpoints in telomeric bands are more common events than other regions within chromosomes. Previous reports have noted a higher rate of telomeric rearrangements than other chromosomal bands *(57)*. Telomeric regions are very dynamic and have shuffled during evolution between nonhomologous chromosomes *(58,59)*. An ascertainment bias toward imbalance of smaller segments as opposed to larger segments could explain the occurrence of 22q11.2 and telomeric rearrangements, but it is also possible that two susceptible regions misalign and pair following chromosome breakage.

INVERSION POLYMORPHISMS CAN OCCUR IN REGIONS HARBORING LCRS

In chromosome 7q11.23, associated with Williams-Beuren syndrome *(60,61)* and chromosome 15q11-q13 associated with Prader-Willi and Angelman syndromes (PWS/AS) *(62)*, polymorphic inversions between flanking inverted LCRs have been described. Two reports have shown that such an inversion polymorphism do not occur on 22q11.2 *(39,63)*. This is not surprising as 80% of the LCR22-2 and LCR22-4 sequences are in the direct, not indirect, orientation.

EVOLUTION OF LCR22S

To determine the evolutionary origin of LCR22s, high- resolution fluorescence *in situ* hybridization (FISH) mapping was performed. Utilizing human chromosomal paints, orthologs to human chromosome 22 were identified were not rearranged in Great Apes, Old and New World monkeys *(64,65)*. Using LCR22-specific probes derived from large insert genomic clones, multiple signals were detected in interphase nuclei from the different primate species including apes *Pan troglodytes* (common chimpanzee), *Pan paniscus*, (pygmy chimpanzee or bonobo), *Gorilla gorilla* (gorilla), and Old World monkeys (rhesus monkey [*Macaca mulatta*]) *(24)*. These data are similar to what was ascertained for other genomic disorders mediated by LCRs, such as PWS/AS, and SMS, showing that multiple copies of LCRs predate the divergence of Great Apes from Old World monkeys, at least 20–25 million years ago *(66)*. The LCRs that are associated with human genomic disorders are not present in the mouse. This suggests that they have evolved after the divergence of the common ancestor between mouse and primates.

MODULAR STRUCTURE OF LCR22S

To better understand mechanisms involved in the evolutionary origin of LCR22s, their sequence composition and architectural features were analyzed. The LCR22s comprise 12% of the 22q11.2 interval and are composed of blocks or modules harboring known genes, pseudogenes, and predicted genes *(26,67)*. They are 10–250 kb in size, contain a variety of blocks in direct and inverted orientations (Fig. 5). The genes within (*USP18, GGT, BCR, GGTLA*) have become duplicated during evolution, thereby shaping the architecture of LCR22s (Fig. 5). The full-length functional genes each lie in different LCR22s, whereas duplicated copies are present in many of them *(68)*. Because the genes comprise a significant part of the LCR22s, they can be used to understand their evolution. Although important for the evolution of LCR22s, they are not likely candidates for the malformations in VCFS/DGS patients as the copies in the deleted region are non-functional pseudogenes.

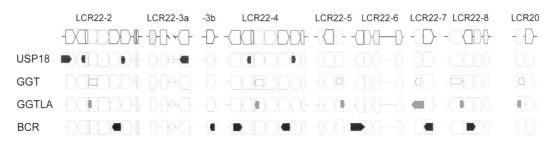

Fig. 5. Block structure of the LCR22s and genes within. The known genes, *USP18 (68a)*, *GGT (77)*, *GGTLA (78)*, and *BCR (79)* and their pseudogene copies, comprise part of the LCR22s. We performed a comparative computational analysis of all the clones spanning the 22q11.2 region to identify similarities. We also took into account a recent annotation of the LCRs in chromosome 22 *(67)*. The different regions of similarity are depicted by different colors. The genes and predicted genes, in their normal genomic organization with respect to the centromeres are shown. LCR22-3a has an uncloned region. The LCR22s are drawn to scale.

The three proximal LCR22s mediate the recurrent chromosome 22q11.2 rearrangement disorders (Fig. 1). Low stringency FISH mapping with LCR22 probes, revealed multiple signals on 22q11.2 and a few other chromosomes suggesting that they have been unstable during evolution (Fig. 6; *[67–68]*). As previously stated, the genes are present in a single copy in the mouse, on different chromosomes, and have therefore evolved more recently in primates. The sequences of the LCR22 genes and copies therein were compared by examining the 22q11.2 region to determine if there was a specific mechanism responsible for gene duplication *(68)*.

ALU-MEDIATED RECOMBINATION EVENTS ARE RESPONSIBLE FOR GENE DUPLICATION

The results of a genome-wide effort to identify sequence elements at the junctions between LCRs and unique sequences were reported *(69)*. A total of 9464 junctions and 2366 duplication alignments were examined throughout the genome and a significant enrichment of *Alu* elements in the vicinity of the junctions was found (27% of all LCRs had an *Alu* at least one end). This suggested that the duplication process forming the LCRs coincided with a primate-specific burst of *Alu* retroposition activity. Because the *Alu* sequences were identical in sequence, it was possible that they could undergo *Alu–Alu* based unequal recombination events forming mosaic *Alu* products. In the case of 22q11.2, the breakpoints in some of the *Alu* elements involved in the rearrangements occurred by unequal crossover mechanisms, whereas others occurred by different mechanisms, resulting in breakpoints at the end of *Alu* elements as opposed to the middle of *Alu* for unequal crossover events *(68)*.

The *IGSF3* gene maps to chromosome 1p13.1. Part of this gene became copied onto 22q11.2, to LCR22-2 and LCR22-4. It is adjacent to the *GGT* locus in these LCR22s. The rearrangement responsible for this "*trans*" rearrangement involving non-homologous chromosomes appeared to have been created in meiosis by a replication-dependent mechanism similar to the model proposed by Richardson et al. *(70)*. In this model, recombination occurs by *Alu*-mediated misalignment of two different chromosomes. A gene conversion then takes place, thereby avoiding crossovers, which would lead to aberrant translocations. These results suggest that mammalian genomes have a mechanism scanning the entire genome to find stretches of homology *(70,71)*.

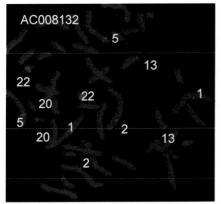 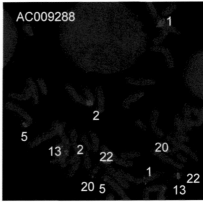

Fig. 6. Low-stringency FISH mapping. Probes from LCR22-2 (GenBank AC008132) and LCR22-4 (GenBank AC009288) were used for low-stringency FISH mapping. Hybridization signals were detected on chromosomes 1p13, 2p11, 5p13, 13p11, and 20p12. The strongest signals were detected on chromosome 22q11 owing to the presence of multiple copies of sequences contained within the LCR22s *(68)*.

ARCHITECTURAL FEATURES IN LCR22S

Besides genes and pseudogenes, there are other architectural features in the LCR22s that are noteworthy. As mentioned, LCR22-3a harbors an AT-rich palindrome that mediates the recurrent t(11;22) translocation and perhaps the 1.5-Mb deletion in VCFS/DGS patients (Fig. 1). The AT-rich sequence and surrounding sequences have remained uncloned and are missing from the human genome libraries. It is likely that they are absent because of the palindromic nature of the AT-rich stretch of sequence in humans. Interestingly, a similar pattern of AT-rich sequences, although non-palindromic, is present in LCR22-2 and LCR22-4. It is possible that in some humans, they could be palindromic in nature but have rearranged in bacteria during library formation, thereby deleting sequences. The presence of potential palindromic sequences in LCR22-2 and LCR22-4 is particularly interesting as recently palindromic sequences have been found near the hotspot for the common 17p11.2 deletion associated with SMS and its reciprocal duplication dup(17)(p11.2 p11.2) syndrome *(72)*.

GENE CONVERSION BETWEEN THE LCR22S

The LCR22s are more than 98% identical in sequence. Of all LCR22s, LCR22-2 and LCR22-4 are the most similar, and they are more than 99% identical over large regions. The high level of identity between the two may be the reason why unequal homologous recombination events cause 22q11.2 rearrangements. Another type of recombination that is possible in regions of high sequence similarity is gene conversion, where one sequence invades and replaces another.

Paralogs are defined as sequence elements, which are present more than once per genome, arising by duplication processes during evolution. The different LCR22s are examples of paralogs. A nucleotide variation in one vs another LCR is termed a paralogous sequence variant (PSV; such as an A in LCR22-2 and a T in LCR22-4). A series of contiguous PSVs would represent a signature for a particular LCR22. A single nucleotide alteration in LCR22-2 (A/T) and in LCR22-4 (A/T), suggests that gene conversion could have been taking place. This is especially significant if there is a consecutive series of such nucleotide variants in *cis*. DNA

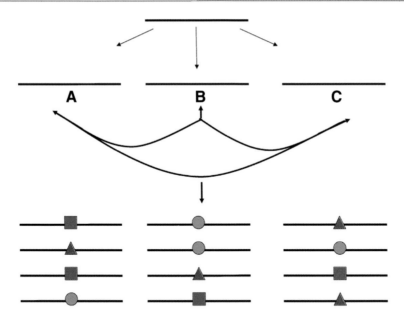

Fig. 7. Model of gene conversion. An original locus duplicated to copies 1, 2, and 3 during primate evolution. The colored shapes represent individual SNPs, which developed over time. The gene conversion events between copies 1, 2, and 3 result in a homogenization process whereby variation occurs in different individuals. (Modified from ref. *59.*)

sequence analyses support the occurrence of gene conversion events in LCR22-2 and LCR22-4 based on our analysis of overlapping BAC clones from different genomic libraries spanning the interval (Morrow et al., unpublished data). The evidence is quite similar to that for the large olfactory receptor gene family segmental duplication and for telomere associated repeats *(58,73)*. A model has been proposed to explain how segmental duplications can become homogenized during evolution (Fig. 7) *(59,73,74)*. This process was hypothesized from data generated in studies of the HERV sequences involved in the *AZFa* microdeletion on chromosome Y and the CMT1A rearrangement on chromosome 17p12 *(75,76)*. Recently, it has been suggested that regions harboring higher rates of gene conversion might be hotspots for common rearrangements in LCRs *(72)*.

A gene conversion event, detected as a simultaneous loss and gain of a single nucleotide variation, would confirm that the LCR22-2 and LCR22-4 are more dynamic than originally believed. Gene conversion could cause stretches of homology to become larger in length and could more strongly stimulate unequal crossover events, thus leading to a deletion or duplication. It is therefore important to define the rate of gene conversion and identify subregions within LCR22s that have altered rates of gene conversion. Long stretches of sequence identity, perhaps created by gene conversion events, between the two LCR22s might serve as a point for unequal crossover. Based on recent studies of the SMS deletion and reciprocal duplication, there is a potential association between the positions of the unequal crossover and an increased rate of gene conversion *(72)*.

SUMMARY

The majority of recurrent chromosome 22q11.2 rearrangements are mediated by recombination events between LCR22s. In contrast to the deletion and duplication disorders, recurrent translocations result from nonhomologous recombination between AT-rich palindromic sequences or other mechanisms, but not homologous recombination events. LCR22s have evolved during primate speciation and this has been mediated, in part, by misalignment between highly repetitive *Alu* SINE elements. Because *Alu* elements have diverged in sequence over time, one may wonder whether such elements could stimulate recombination events in meiosis in humans. One possibility would be that gene conversion events could serve to erase divergences between *Alu* elements or other sequences in the vicinity of labile motifs or elements. Besides *Alu* SINEs, there may be other sequences or sequence elements involved with the complex evolutionary pathway for LCR22 evolution and they will likely be uncovered by mapping the genomes of primate species.

There is supporting evidence that chromosome breakage associated with recurrent genomic disorders may occur in specific regions or hotspots in LCRs *(61,62,72)*. The same may be true for VCFS/DGS, dup(22)(q11.2; q11.2), and CES. How can one find these hotspots? It may be possible that hotspots for chromosome rearrangements have higher gene conversion rates. In this way, premeiotic germ cells from some individuals will be more or less susceptible to rearrangements than others. To determine this, it would be necessary to compare sequences of parental DNAs in a large number of trios, with the child harboring a *de novo* deletion.

In addition to the seven LCR22s, there are other LCR blocks, mostly smaller in size as compared to the ones described here, containing different genes or pseudogenes, in the same interval of 22q11.2 *(67)* but they have not been associated yet with any particular human disorder. It would also be of interest to determine their evolutionary origin in primates to compare this with the larger, disease associated LCR22s.

REFERENCES

1. Lupski JR. Genomic disorders, structural features of the genome can lead to DNA rearrangements and human disease traits. Trends Genet 1998;14:417–422.
2. Stankiewicz P, Lupski JR. Molecular-evolutionary mechanisms for genomic disorders. Curr Opin Genet Dev 2002;12:312–319.
3. Stankiewicz P, Lupski JR. Genome architecture, rearrangements and genomic disorders. Trends Genet 2002;18:74–82.
4. Lupski JR. 2002 Curt Stern Award Address. Genomic disorders recombination-based disease resulting from genomic architecture. Am J Hum Genet 2003;72:246–252.
5. Shaw CJ, Lupski JR. Implications of human genome architecture for rearrangement-based disorders: the genomic basis of disease. Hum Mol Genet 2004;13:57–64.
6. DiGeorge A. A new concept of the cellular basis of immunity. J Pediatr 1965;67:907.
7. Shprintzen RJ, Goldberg RB, Lewin ML, et al. A new syndrome involving cleft palate, cardiac anomalies, typical facies, and learning disabilities, velo-cardio-facial syndrome. Cleft Palate J 1978;15:56–62.
8. Emanuel BS, McDonald-McGinn D, Saitta SC, Zackai EH. The 22q11.2 deletion syndrome. Adv Pediatr 2001;48:39–73.
9. Edelmann L, Pandita RK, Spiteri E, et al. A common molecular basis for rearrangement disorders on chromosome 22q11.2. Hum Mol Genet 1999;8:1157–1167.
10. Bergman A, Blennow E. Inv dup(22), del(22)(q11) and r(22) in the father of a child with DiGeorge syndrome. Eur J Hum Genet 2000;8:801–804.
11. Ensenauer RE, Adeyinka A, Flynn HC, et al. Microduplication 22q11.2, an emerging syndrome, clinical, cytogenetic, and molecular analysis of thirteen patients. Am J Hum Genet 2003;73:1027–1040.
12. Hassed SJ, Hopcus-Niccum D, Zhang L, Li S, Mulvihill JJ. A new genomic duplication syndrome complementary to the velocardiofacial (22q11 deletion) syndrome. Clin Genet 2004;65:400–404.
13. Guanti G. The aetiology of the cat eye syndrome reconsidered. J Med Genet 1981;18:108–118.
14. Zackai EH, Emanuel BS. Site-specific reciprocal translocation t(11;22)(q23;q11), in several unrelated families with 3, 1 meiotic disjunction. Am J Med Genet 1980;7:507–521.

15. Schinzel A, Schmid W, Auf der Maur P, et al. Incomplete trisomy 22. I. Familial 11/22 translocation with 3, 1 meiotic disjunction. Delineation of a common clinical picture and report of nine new cases from six families. Hum Genet 1981;56:249–262.

16. Burn J, Takao A, Wilson D, et al. Conotruncal anomaly face syndrome is associated with a deletion within chromosome 22q11. J Med Genet 1993;30:822–824.

17. Scambler PJ, Kelly D, Lindsay E, et al. Velo-cardio-facial syndrome associated with chromosome 22 deletions encompassing the DiGeorge locus. Lancet 1992;339:1138–1139.

18. Driscoll DA, Spinner NB, Budarf ML, et al. Deletions and microdeletions of 22q11.2 in velo-cardio-facial syndrome. Am J Med Genet 1992;44:261–268.

19. Matsuoka, R., Takao, A., Kimura, M., et al. Confirmation that the conotruncal anomaly face syndrome is associated with a deletion within 22q11.2. Am J Med Genet 1994;53:285–259.

20. Burn J, Goodship J. Congenital heart disease. In: *Principles and Practice of Medical Genetics, 3rd edition, Vol. 1* (Rimoin DL, Connor JM, Pyeritz RE, eds.) Edinburgh: Churchill Livingston, 1996; pp. 767–828.

21. Lindsay EA, Goldberg R, Jurecic V, et al. Velo-cardio-facial syndrome, frequency and extent of 22q11 deletions. Am J Med Genet 1995;57:514–522.

22. Morrow B, Goldberg R, Carlson C, et al. Molecular definition of the 22q11.2 deletions in velo-cardio-facial syndrome. Am J Hum Genet 1995;56:1391–1403.

23. Carlson C, Sirotkin H, Pandita R, et al. Molecular definition of 22q11.2 deletions in 151 velo-cardio-facial syndrome patients. Am J Hum Genet 1997;61:620–629.

24. Shaikh TH, Kurahashi H, Saitta SC, et al. Chromosome 22-specific low copy repeats and the 22q11.2.2 deletion syndrome, genomic organization and deletion endpoint analysis. Hum Mol Genet 2000;9:489–501.

25. Emanuel BS, Shaikh TH. Segmental duplications, an 'expanding' role in genomic instability and disease. Nat Rev Genet 2001;2:791–800.

26. Edelmann L, Pandita RK, Morrow BE. Low-copy repeats mediate the ommon 3-Mb deletion in patients with velo-cardio-facial syndrome. Am J Hum Genet 1999;64:1076–1086.

27. Shaikh TH, Kurahashi H, Emanuel BS. Evolutionarily conserved low copy repeats (LCRs) in 22q11 mediate deletions, duplications, translocations, and genomic instability, an update and literature review. Genet Med 2001;3:6–13.

28. Berends MJ, Tan-Sindhunata G, Leegte B, van Essen AJ. Phenotypic variability of Cat-Eye syndrome. Genet Couns 2001;12: 23–34.

29. Reiss JA, Weleber RG, Brown MG, Bangs CD, Lovrien EW, Magenis RE. Tandem duplication of proximal 22q, a cause of cat-eye syndrome. Am J Med Genet 1985;20:165–171.

30. Mears AJ, Duncan AM, Budarf ML, et al. Molecular characterization of the marker chromosome associated with cat eye syndrome. Am J Hum Genet 1994;55:134–142.

31. McTaggart KE, Budarf ML, Driscoll DA, Emanuel BS, Ferreira P, McDermid HE. Cat eye syndrome chromosome breakpoint clustering, identification of two intervals also associated with 22q11.2 deletion syndrome breakpoints. Cytogenet Cell Genet 1998;81:222–228.

32. Fraccaro M, Lindsten J, Ford CE, Iselius L. The 11q;22q translocation, a European collaborative analysis of 43 cases. Hum Genet 1980;56:21–51.

33. Van Hove JL, McConkie-Rosell A, Chen YT, et al. Unbalanced translocation 46,XY, 15,+der(22)t(15;22) (q13;q11)pat, case report and review of the literature. Am J Med Genet 1992;44:24–30.

34. Funke B, Edelmann L, McCain N, et al. Der(22) syndrome and velo-cardio-facial syndrome/DiGeorge syndrome share a 1.5 Mb region of overlap on chromosome 22q11.2. Am J Hum Genet 1999;64:747–758.

35. Shaikh TH, Budarf ML, Celle L, Zackai EH, Emanuel BS. Clustered 11q23 and 22q11 breakpoints and 3, 1 meiotic malsegregation in multiple unrelated t(11;22) families. Am J Hum Genet 1999;65:1595–1607.

36. Emanuel BS, Selden JR, Wang E, Nowell PC, Croce CM. In situ hybridization and translocation breakpoint mapping. I. Nonidentical 22q11.2 breakpoints for the t(9;22) of CML and the t(8;22) of Burkitt lymphoma. Cytogenet Cell Genet 1984;38:127–131.

37. Halford S, Lindsay E, Nayudu M, Carey AH, Baldini A, Scambler PJ. Low-copy-number repeat sequences flank the DiGeorge/velo-cardio-facial syndrome loci at 22q11. Hum Mol Genet 1993;2:191–196.

38. Baumer A, Dutly F, Balmer D, et al. High level of unequal meiotic crossovers at the origin of the 22q11.2. 2 and 7q11.23 deletions. Hum Mol Genet 1998;7: 887–894.

39. Saitta SC, Harris SE, Gaeth AP, et al. Aberrant interchromosomal exchanges are the predominant cause of the 22q11.2 deletion. Hum Mol Genet 2004;13:417–428.

40. Potocki L, Chen KS, Park SS, et al. Molecular mechanism for duplication 17p11.2- the homologous recombination reciprocal of the Smith-Magenis microdeletion. Nat Genet 2000;24:84–87.

41. Edelmann L, Spiteri E, McCain N, et al. A common breakpoint on 11q23 in carriers of the constitutional t(11;22) translocation. Am J Hum Genet 1999;65:1608–1616.

42. Kurahashi H, Shaikh TH, Hu P, Roe BA, Emanuel BS, Budarf ML. Regions of genomic instability on 22q11.2 and 11q23 as the etiology for the recurrent constitutional t(11;22). Hum Mol Genet 2000;9:1665–1670.

43. Edelmann L, Spiteri E, Koren K, et al. AT-rich palindromes mediate the constitutional t(11;22) translocation. Am J Hum Genet 2001;68:1–13.

44. Kurahashi H, manuel BS. Long AT-rich palindromes and the constitutional t(11;22) breakpoint. Hum Mol Genet 2001;10:2605–2617.

45. Gotter AL, Shaikh TH, Budarf ML, Rhodes CH, Emanuel BS. A palindrome-mediated mechanism distinguishes translocations involving LCR-B of chromosome 22q11.2. Hum Mol Genet 2004;13:103–115.

46. Kehrer-Sawatzki H, Haussler J, Krone W, et al. The second case of a t(17;22) in a family with neurofibromatosis type 1, sequence analysis of the breakpoint regions. Hum Genet 1997;99:237–247.

47. Kurahashi H, Shaikh T, Takata M, Toda T, Emanuel BS. The constitutional t(17;22), another translocation mediated by palindromic AT-rich repeats. Am J Hum Genet 2003;72:733–738.

48. Akgun E, Zahn J, Baumes S, et al. Palindrome resolution and recombination in the mammalian germ line. Mol Cell Biol 1997;17:5559–5570.

49. Richardson C, Jasin M. Frequent chromosomal translocations induced by DNA double-strand breaks. Nature 2000;405:697–700.

50. Kurahashi H, Nakayama T, Osugi Y, et al. Deletion mapping of 22q11.2 in CATCH22 syndrome, identification of a second critical region. Am J Hum Genet 1996;58:1377–1381.

51. Kurahashi H, Tsuda E, Kohama R, et al. Another critical region for deletion of 22q11, a study of 100 patients. Am J Med Genet 1997;72:180–185.

52. O'Donnell H, McKeown C, Gould C, Morrow B, Scambler P. Detection of an atypical 22q11 deletion that has no overlap with the DiGeorge syndrome critical region. Am J Hum Genet 1997;60:1544–1548.

53. Rauch A, Pfeiffer RA, Leipold G, Singer H, Tigges M, Hofbeck M. A novel 22q11.2.2 microdeletion in DiGeorge syndrome. Am J Hum Genet 1999;64:659–666.

54. Spiteri E, Babcock M, Kashork CD, et al. Frequent translocations occur between low copy repeats on chromosome 22q11.2 (LCR22s) and telomeric bands of partner chromosomes. Hum Mol Genet 2003;12:1823–1837.

55. Nimmakayalu MA, Gotter AL, Shaikh TH, Emanuel BS. A novel sequence-based approach to localize translocation breakpoints identifies the molecular basis of a t(4;22). Hum Mol Genet 2003;12:2817–2825.

56. Debeer P, Mols R, Huysmans C, Devriendt K, Van de Ven WJ, Fryns JP. Involvement of a palindromic chromosome 22-specific low-copy repeat in a constitutional t(X; 22)(q27;q11). Clin Genet 2002;62:410–414.

57. Aurias A, Prieur M, Dutrillaux B, Lejeune J. Systematic analysis of 95 reciprocal translocations of autosomes. Hum Genet 1978;45:259–282.

58. Mefford HC, Linardopoulou E, Coil D, van den Engh G, Trask BJ. Comparative sequencing of a multicopy subtelomeric region containing olfactory receptor genes reveals multiple interactions between non-homologous chromosomes. Hum Mol Genet 2001;10:2363–2372.

59. Mefford HC, Trask BJ. The complex structure and dynamic evolution of human subtelomeres. Nat Rev Genet 2002;3:91–102.

60. Osborne LR, Li M, Pober B, et al. A 1.5 million-basepair inversion polymorphism in families with Williams-Beuren syndrome. Nat Genet 2001;29:321–325.

61. Bayes M, Magano LF, Rivera N, Flores R, Perez Jurado LA. Mutational mechanisms of Williams-Beuren syndrome deletions. Am J Hum Genet 2003;73:131–151.

62. Chai JH, Locke DP, Greally JM, et al. Identification of four highly conserved genes between breakpoint hotspots BP1 and BP2 of the Prader-Willi/Angelman syndromes deletion region that have undergone evolutionary transposition mediated by flanking duplicons. Am J Hum Genet 2003;73:898–925.

63. Gebhardt GS, Devriendt K, Thoelen R, et al. No evidence for a parental inversion polymorphism predisposing to rearrangements at 22q11.2 in the DiGeorge/Velocardiofacial syndrome. Eur J Hum Genet 2003;11:109–111.

64. Tarazami ST, Kringstein AM, Conte RA, Verma RS. Comparative mapping of the cri du chat and DiGeorge syndrome regions in the great apes. Genes Genet Syst 1998;73:135–136.

65. Stanyon R, Consigliere S, Muller S, Morescalchi A, Neusser M, Wienberg J. Fluorescence in situ hybridization (FISH) maps chromosomal homologies between the dusky titi and squirrel monkey. Am J Primatol 2000;50:95–107.

66. Park SS, Stankiewicz P, Bi W, et al. Structure and evolution of the Smith-Magenis syndrome repeat gene clusters, SMS-REPs. Genome Res 2002;12:729–738.
67. Bailey JA, Yavor AM, Viggiano L, et al. Human-specific duplication and mosaic transcripts: the recent paralogous structure of chromosome 22. Am J Hum Genet 2002;70:83–100.
68. Babcock M, Pavlicek A, Spiteri E,et al. Genome shuffling of genes in low copy repeats on 22q11.2 (LCR22) by Alu-mediated recombination events during evolution. Genome Res 2003;13:2519–2532.
68a.Schwer H, Liu LO, Zhou L, et al. Cloning and characterization of a novel human ubiquiitin-specific protease, a homologue of murine UBP43 (USP 18). Genomics 2000;65:44–52.
69. Bailey JA, Liu G, Eichler EE. An Alu transposition model for the origin and expansion of human segmental duplications. Am J Hum Genet 2003;73:823–834.
70. Baker MD, Read LR, Beatty BG, Ng P. Requirements for ectopic homologous recombination in mammalian somatic cells. Mol Cell Biol 1996;16: 7122–7132.
71. Richardson C, Moynahan ME, Jasin M. Double-strand break repair by interchromosomal recombination, suppression of chromosomal translocations. Genes Dev 1998;12:3831–3842.
72. Bi W, Park SS, Shaw CJ, Withers MA, Patel PI, Lupski JR. Reciprocal crossovers and a positional preference for strand exchange in recombination events resulting in deletion or duplication of chromosome 17p11.2. Am J Hum Genet 2003;73:1302–1315.
73. Newman T, Trask BJ. Complex Evolution of 7E Olfactory Receptor Genes in Segmental Duplications. Genome Res 2003;13:781–793.
74. Samonte RV, Eichler EE. Segmental duplications and the evolution of the primate genome. Nat Rev Genet 2002;3:65–72.
75. Blanco P, Shlumukova M, Sargent CA, Jobling MA, Affara N, Hurles ME. Divergent outcomes of intrachromosomal recombination on the human Y chromosome: male infertility and recurrent polymorphism. J Med Genet 2000;37:752–758.
76. Hurles ME. Gene conversion homogenizes the CMT1A paralogous repeats. BMC Genomics 2001;2:11.
77. Courtay C, Heisterkamp N, Siest, G, Groffen J. Expression of multiple gamma-glutamyltransferase genes in man. Biochem J 1994;297:503–508.
78. Heisterkamp N, Groffen J. Duplication of the bcr and gamma-glutamyl transpeptidase genes. Nucl Acids Res 1998;16:8045–8056.
79. Croce CM, Huebner K, Isobe M, et al. Mapping of four distinct BCR-related loci to chromosome region 22q11: order of BCR loci relative to chronic myelogenous leukemia and acute lymphoblastic leukemia breakpoints. Proc Natl Acad Sci USA 1987;84:7174–7178.
80. Parsons JD. Miropeats: graphical DNA sequence comparisons. Comput Appl Biosci 1995;11: 615–619.

14 Neurofibromatosis 1

Karen Stephens, PhD

CONTENTS

INTRODUCTION

Among genomic disorders, submicroscopic deletions underlying neurofibromatosis 1 (NF1) are unusual because they involve the deletion of a tumor suppressor gene (*NF1*), they show a different preference for low-copy repeats (LCR) as substrates for meiotic vs mitotic recombination events, and they account for only a small fraction of mutations that cause the disorder. The *NF1* gene at chromosome 17q11.2 is flanked by two sets of LCRs in direct orientation that undergo paralogous recombination. A pair of NF1-REPs mediate the recurrent constitutional 1.4-Mb microdeletion that occurs preferentially during maternal meiosis, whereas a pair of *JJAZ1* pseudogene and functional gene mediate the recurrent 1.2-Mb microdeletion that occurs preferentially during postzygotic mitosis in females. Breakpoints have been mapped at the nucleotide level for both deletions and sequence features that may contribute to the choice of discrete sites for strand exchange have been identified. NF1-REP-mediated *NF1* microdeletions involve 13 additional genes, whereas *JJAZ1*-mediated microdeletions involve the same genes but one. *NF1* microdeletions are of great interest because they predispose to a heavy tumor burden, malignancy, and possibly other severe manifestations.

In 1992, the first report of a NF1 patient with a submicroscopic contiguous gene deletion spanning the *NF1* tumor suppressor gene provided direct evidence that this common autosomal dominant disorder was caused by haploinsufficiency of the *NF1* protein product, neurofibromin *(1)*. Here, subsequent molecular, genetic, and clinical studies of *NF1* microdeletions are reviewed, which have made significant contributions to our understanding of the mutational mechanisms and pathogenesis of this common multisystemic, progressive, tumor predisposition disorder, and to genomic disorders in general.

From: *Genomic Disorders: The Genomic Basis of Disease*
Edited by: J. R. Lupski and P. Stankiewicz © Humana Press, Totowa, NJ

MOLECULAR BASIS OF NEUROFIBROMATOSIS 1

Virtually all subjects affected with NF1 develop multiple benign neurofibromas, which are tumors of superficial and deep peripheral nerves that increase in number with age, along with pigmentation changes of café au lait macules, axillary/inguinal freckling, and hamartomas of the iris of the eye *(2)*. Neurofibromas are unpredictable with regards to number, location, rate of growth, and potential for malignant transformation. Additional complications unrelated to neurofibroma development are legion, and include learning disabilities, scoliosis and other bone abnormalities, optic glioma, and malignancies of various organ systems, such as malignant peripheral nerve sheath tumors (MPNST), rhabdomyosarcoma, and myeloid leukemias *(3)*. Although a deletion or other constitutional inactivating mutation of one *NF1* allele predisposes to benign or malignant tumorigenesis, a somatic inactivating mutation of the remaining *NF1* allele in a tumor progenitor cell is an early, if not initiating, event in most, if not all, NF1-associated tumors. The tumor progenitor cell of the cellularly heterogeneous neurofibroma and the MPNST is the Schwann cell *(4)*. A second requirement for neurofibroma development in a mouse model is the presence of heterozygous $Nf1^{+/-}$ murine cells in the micro-tumor environment *(4)*. The requirement of different neurofibromin levels in target cells vs supportive cells results in modulation of the RAS signaling pathway, as neurofibromin is a guanosine-5'-triphosphatase (GTPase)-activating protein that catalyzes the conversion of active RAS-GTP to inactive RAS-GDP *(5)*. The requirement for *Nf1* heterozygosity in the mouse brain for the development of optic nerve glioma by *Nf1* ablated astrocytes *(6)* extends the emerging paradigm that neurofibromin haploinsufficiency in cells of the micro-tumor environment is critical.

The NF1 Mutational Profile

The mutational profile of the *NF1* gene at chromosome 17q11.2 is complex, as both constitutional and somatic mutations occur that result in generalized or segmental (localized) NF1 disease and tumor development (Table 1). NF1 is inherited as an autosomal dominant trait, but also occurs sporadically in approx 30–50% of cases. In 80–90% of cases owing to intragenic *NF1* inactivating mutations, no correlation has been detected between mutation type and/or location and the development of specific manifestations *(7–9)*. Approximately 5% of NF1 cases are because of submicroscopic, contiguous gene deletions *(10–12)*. Most *NF1* microdeletions are *de novo* and are predominantly of maternal origin, although familial cases do occur *(13–17)*. Subjects with *NF1* microdeletions tend to have a high tumor burden and may have facial anomalies, early age at onset of dermal neurofibromas, vascular anomalies, learning disabilities, astrocytomas, and malignancy *(12–14,18,19)*. Formal studies regarding *NF1* microdeletion genotype/phenotype correlations await a comprehensive clinical and molecular evaluation of a cohort of *NF1* microdeletion subjects ascertained in an unbiased manner. One such study has shown that *NF1* microdeletion doubles the lifetime risk of MPNST relative to nondeletional genotypes *(20)*. One confounding factor in such studies is that approx 25% of *NF1* microdeletions occur as postzygotic mutations and different levels of mosaicism in patient tissues can result in generalized or localized NF1 (*see* LCR-Mediated Somatic *NF1* Microdeletions) *(21)*. A major area of research is focused on identifying genes in the deleted region that modify NF1-related tumorigenesis or other manifestations of the disorder. As summarized in Table 1, somatic second hit inactivating mutations of *NF1* are typically owing to loss of heterozygosity by recombination, chromosomal deletion that is not known to be LCR-mediated or intragenic inactivating mutations (Table 1).

Table 1
Mutational Profile of the *NF1* Gene

NF1 mutation category	Patient phenotype/ tissue	Mode of inheritance	NF1 *mutation type*	Selected references
Constitutional	NF1	familial or *de novo*	LCR-mediated contiguous gene deletion (approx 5%)	*10*
			Nonsense, splicing defects, missense (85–90%)	*39–41*
Somatic mosaicism	NF1	*de novo*	LCR-mediated contiguous gene deletion	*21,38,42–44*
	Localized NF1	*de novo*	LCR-mediated contiguous gene deletion, multi-exonic deletion	*21,38,45*
Germline mosaicism	Unaffected	*de novo*	Intragenic deletion	*46*
Somatic 2nd hits in tumor tissue[a]	Neurofibroma	*de novo*	Splicing defects, LOH[b]	*47–49*
	MPNST	*de novo*	LOH[b], deletion	*48–52*
	Myeloid leukemia	*de novo*	Nonsense, others that predict premature truncation	*7*

[a]Reviewed in ref. *52*.
[b]Loss of heterozygosity via recombination or deletion.

RECURRENT NF-REP-MEDIATED *NF1* MICRODELETIONS

An estimated (50–60%) of constitutional *NF1* microdeletions have a common recurrent 1.4-Mb deletion that includes *NF1* and at least 13 other genes (Fig. 1; Table 2) (11). Both centromeric and telomeric deletion breakpoints cluster within two LCR sequences, or paralogs, termed NF1-REP-P1 and NF1-REP-M (Fig. 1). The direct orientation of these two NF1-REPs suggested a mechanism consistent with the existing paradigm whereby deletions occur by nonallelic homologous recombination, or paralogous recombination, between misaligned paralogs on the interchromosomal, intrachromosomal, or intrachromatidal level *(22)*. For *NF1*, this mechanism was confirmed by mapping NF1-REP-mediated deletion breakpoints at the nucleotide level *(17,23)* and by haplotype analyses *(16)*.

NF1-REPs are complex assemblies of paralogs from different sequence families consisting of expressed genes, pseudogenes, gene fragments, and non-coding sequence (Fig. 2) *(24)*. NF1-REP-P1 and NF1-REP-M share a 51-kb segment of 97.5% sequence identity, termed NF1-REP-51, which serves as the substrate for paralogous recombination events. Two other components of the NF1-REP family include NF1-REP-P2, which is centromeric to *NF1*, and NF1-REP-E19 located on chromosome 19p13.13 (Fig. 2) *(24,25)*. *NF1* microdeletions owing to apparent paralogous recombination between NF1-REP-P2 and -M have been reported, but their breakpoints have not been mapped at the nucleotide level *(26)*. Large kilobase-sized polymorphisms have not been observed in the NF1-REPs, although certain structural features, such as the inverted repeats in *KIAA0563rel*-ψ of NF1-REP-P1 that could mediate an inversion event, may generate such polymorphisms in the general population. There is no evidence of constitutional or somatic chromosomal translocations that could be attributable to recombina-

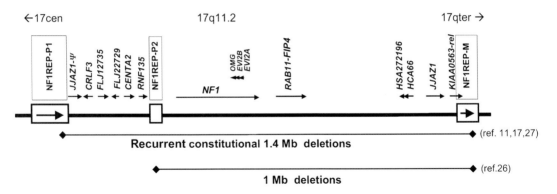

Fig. 1. Genomic structure of the *NF1* microdeletion region in chromosome 17q11.2 and the recurrent constitutional 1.4-Mb deletion. The 350-kb *NF1* gene, and other regional genes, are indicated by arrows showing their direction of transcription. *OMG*, *EVI2A*, and *EVI2B* are within an *NF1* intron and are transcribed on the alternate strand. Table 2 details the genes in this region. Boxes designate the 3 NF1-REPs, with arrows indicating direct repeat orientation of NF1-REP-P1 and -M. Genomic length from NF1-REP-P1 through NF1-REP-M is 1.5 Mb and the most frequent constitutional deletions are 1.4 Mb. Two approx 1-Mb deletions have been reported apparently because of recombination between NF1-REP-P2 and -M (*see* Recurrent NF-REP-Mediated *NF1* Microdeletions; *26*). NF1-REP-P1, -P2, -M are 131, 43, and 75 kb in length, respectively (*see* Fig. 2 for details). Gene names are from May 2004 assembly of the human genome (http://genome.ucsc.edu/) and may differ from names on previously published maps of the region (*23,25,26*).

Table 2

Functional Genes Within the Recurrent 1.4-Mb *NF1* Microdeletion Region

Gene/marker[a]	Description	REFSEQ mRNA accession number
CRLF3	Cytokine receptor-like factor 3	NM_015986.2
FLJ12735	Putative ATP(GTP)-binding protein[b]	NM_024857.3
FLJ2279	Hypothetical protein, unknown function	NM_024683.1
CENTA2	Centaurin alpha 2, binds phosphatidylinositol 3,4,5-triphosphate and inositol 1,3,4,5,-tetrakisphophate	NM_018404.1
RFN135	Ring finger protein 135	NM_032322.3 NM_197939.1
NF1	Ras GTPase stimulating protein	NM_000267.1
OMG	Oligodendrocyte myelin glycoprotein; cell adhesion molecule contributing to myelination in the central nervous system	NM_002544.2
EVI2B	Ecotropic viral integration site 2B, membrane protein	NM_006495.2
EVI2A	Ecotropic viral integration site 2A, membrane protein	NM_014210.1
RAB11-FIP4	Putative Rab11 family interacting protein 3	NM_032932.2
HSA272196	Hypothetical protein, unknown function	NM_018405.2
HCA66	Hepatocellular carcinoma-associated antigen 66	NM_018428.2
JJAZ1	Protein with zinc finger domain and homology to Drosophia Polycomb protein SUZ12	NM_015355.1
KIAA0563-rel	KIAA0563-related, unknown function	NM_014834.2

[a]From the May 2004 genome assembly (http://genome.ucsc.edu/).

[b]ATP, adenosine-5'-triphosphate; GTP, guanosine-5'-triphosphate.

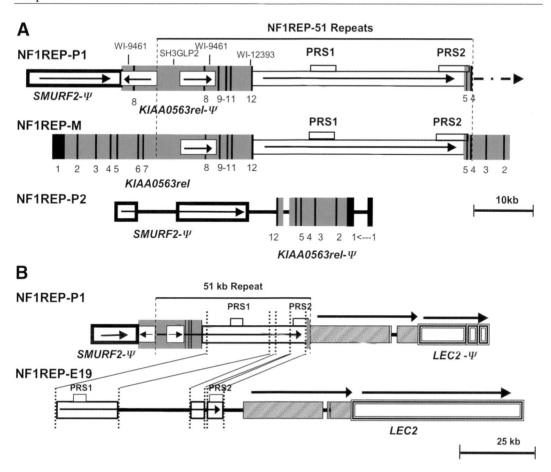

Fig. 2. The structure of the NF1-REP paralogs. (A) The structure of NF1-REP-P1 (131 kb) and a partial structure of NF1-REP-M (*see* B for complete structure) are shown. These serve as paralogous recombination substrates for the common 1.4-Mb *NF1* microdeletion. The 51-kb high sequence identity region, designated NF1-REP-51 harbors the recombination hotpots PRS1 and PRS2. Gray blocks indicate the *KIAA0563rel* functional gene and related pseudogene (ψ) fragments with numbered black bars designating exons or exon-derived sequences. White boxes with arrows inside *KIAA0563rel* sequences designate the orientation of a 5.9-kb inverted repeats with two copies in NF1-REP-P1 and one in NF1-REP-M. STS in KIAA0563rel are shown as landmarks. Open blocks with bold margins are *SMURF2*-derived pseudogene (ψ) fragments. The arrow at the telomeric end of NF1-REP-P1 indicates that it is truncated; see panel B for full-length structure. NF1-REP-P2 is a partial NF1-REP with fragments derived from *SMURF2* and *KIAA0563* pseudogenes. Figures are oriented from centromere (left) to telomere. BAC identities and accession numbers for each NF1-REP are given in Forbes et al. *(24)*. (B) Comparison of NF1-REP-P1 and NF1-REP-E19, at chromosome 19p13.13. Boxes are labeled as in (A), in addition to *LEC2* and its pseudogene (open blocks with borders of multiple lines) and non-coding sequences between PRS2 and *LEC2* (blocks filled with diagonal lines); sequence orientations are shown with arrows. The *SMURF2*, non-coding, and *LEC2* sequences flanking the 51-kb repeat are considered part of NF1-REP-P1 based on paralogy with NF1-REP-P2 and NF1-REP–E19. BAC identities and accession numbers for each NF1-REP are given in Forbes et al. *(24)*. Note difference in scales between panels A and B. (Adapted with permission from ref. *24*.)

tion between chromosome 17 NF1-REPs and NF1-REP-E19, although NF1-REP-P1-51 and NF1-REP-E19 share 94–95% sequence identity that includes the recombination hotspots PRS1 and PRS2 (*see* next section) (Fig. 2) *(24)*. Additional NF1-REP-like elements with KIAA0563 fragments are at chromosome 17q12 and 17q24, but they do not share any other sequences with NF1-REP-P1, -P2, or –M *(11,24,25)*. Whether these LCRs mediate chromosomal rearrangements is unknown. Similar to those of other LCRs that mediate genomic disorders on chromosome 17, the segmental duplications giving rise to NF1-REPs originated in recent hominoid evolution about 25 million years ago before the separation of orangutan from the human lineage *(25)*. Fluorescent *in situ* hybridization (FISH) studies showed the presence of NF1-REP-P1 and NF1-REP-M orthologs flanking the *NF1* gene in the Great Apes *(27)*.

Discrete Paralogous Recombination Sites

Despite 51 kb of 97.5% sequence identity between NF1-REP-P1-51 and NF1-REP-M-51, paralogous recombination occurred preferentially at two discrete sites. *NF1* microdeletion breakpoints were mapped at the nucleotide level to intervals defined by paralogous sequence variants (PSV; also known as NF1-REP-specific variants). The product of paralogous recombination is a chimeric NF1-REP-P1/NF1-REP-M and shows a pattern of PSVs with transition from NF1-REP-P1 PSVs to NF1-REP-M PSVs at the breakpoint interval. Breakpoint mapping was facilitated by use of human/rodent somatic hybrid cell lines that carried only the deleted homolog 17 of the patient *(17,23)*. Sixty-nine percent ($N = 78$) of *NF1* microdeletion cases had breakpoints that clustered at paralogous recombination sites 1 and 2 (PRS1 and PRS2) (Fig. 3) *(17,23,24) (23)*. PRS2 harbored 51% of breakpoints, whereas PRS1 harbored 18%. A single case UWA160-1 had a distinct breakpoint centromeric to PRS sites (Fig. 3). The PRS1 and PRS2 regions are 4.1 and 6.3 kb in length, respectively, and are 14.5 kb apart. Each PRS has a hotspot where the majority of breakpoints mapped; PRS2 has a 2.3-kb hotspot that accounts for 93% of breakpoints, whereas PRS1 has a 0.5-kb hotspot accounting for 60% of breakpoints. During sequence analysis of recombinant PRS in several cases, instead of a perfect transition of PSVs from NF1-REP-P1 to -M, the PSVs were in "patches" with a complex transition from NF1-REP-P1 to -M to -P1 to -M *(17,23)*, indicating apparent gene conversion events. These regions were relatively short (<627 bp) and, like similar events of REP-mediated rearrangements in CMT1A and *AZFa* and *IDS (28–31)*, are considered consistent with a mechanism of double-strand break repair.

There was no significant difference between PRS1- and PRS2-mediated microdeletions for the parent of origin or for *de novo* vs familial cases *(17,23)*. In a series of 59 *NF1* microdeletion cases for which clinical evaluation of the parents was available, 10% inherited the disease, and presumably the microdeletion, from an affected parent. Among 45 *de novo* cases where parental origin could be determined, 80% were of maternal origin. The recent development of deletion-specific amplification assays that detect the recurrent *NF1* microdeletions at PRS1 and PRS2 will facilitate the assembly of patient cohorts of the same genotype for clinical evaluation and will quickly identify those patients with variant deletions, which will be important to narrow the critical region of the deletion responsible for the increased tumor load and malignancy risk of microdeletion patients *(17,23)*.

Genomic Context and Sequence Analysis of Paralogous Recombination Sites

Detailed analysis of the PRS and the NF1-REP-51 paralogs at the nucleotide level identified interesting features, but lacked compelling evidence for why breakpoints preferentially occur at these sites *(24)*. There were no obligate local sequence features shared by PRS1 and PRS2.

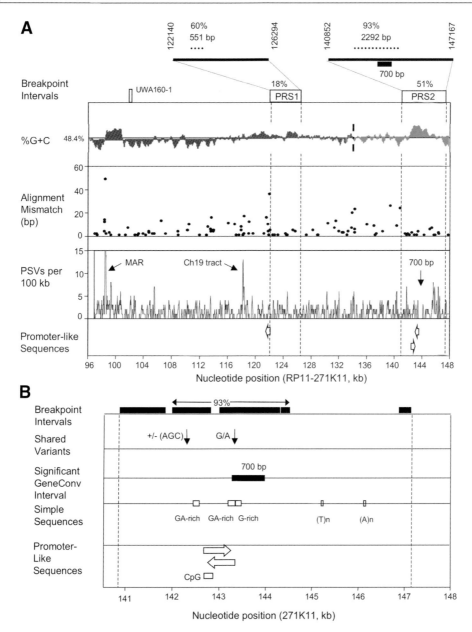

Fig. 3. Genomic context of the paralogous recombination hotspots for *NF1* microdeletion. (A) Alignment, identity, and sequence features of the 51-kb high identity NF1-REP-P1-51 and NF1-REP-M-51 paralogs. Alignment mismatch panel shows gap alignments ranging from 1 to 50 bp between NF1-REP-P1-51 and NF1-REP-M-51 in BACs RP11-271K11 and RP11-640N20, respectively. PSVs for each REP, indels excluded, with a sliding 100-bp window are shown, including a matrix attachment site (MAR), an apparent gene conversion tract with variants matching NF1-REP-E19, and a 700-bp segment of perfect match with statistical evidence of gene conversion. The positions of promoter like sequences not associated with known genes are indicated in the lower panel. (B) Detailed structure of the PRS2 region. Breakpoint intervals are shown along with the 2.3-kb hotspot, which harbors 93% of breakpoint intervals in PRS2 region. Finer localization of the 700-bp gene conversion tract and the promoter like sequences from (A) are shown. Nucleotide positions for both panels refer to the NF1-REP-P1-51 in BAC RP11-271K11. (Adapted from ref. *24* with permission.)

Basic Local Alignment Search Tool (BLAST; www.ncbi.nlm.nib.gov/blast) comparison of PRS1 and PRS showed no significant sequence identity with the exception of *Alu* elements, LINES and other high-copy repeats, which typically shared less than 80% identity in short segments *(24)*. PRS1 and 2 regions have quite different patterns of G+C content; the PRS2 hotspot is very G+C rich, while the PRS1 hotspot is not (Fig. 3). Both PRS hotspots are 1–2 kb distal to relative large alignment gaps (Fig. 3A), yet these did not suppress pairing as recombination in at least a few cases occurred within less than 1 kb from the gaps. The PRS regions are not of greater or lesser paralogous sequence identity as shown by the spatial distribution of PSVs, which are relatively evenly distributed across the NF1-REP-51 segment (Fig. 3) *(24)*. Numerous tests for the presence of motifs with demonstrated or suspected roles in recombination, transcription, or translation were performed. A *Chi* element within PRS2 was identified *(17)*, but this association is not preferential, as it is one of four evenly spaced *Chi* elements in NF1-REP-51 *(24)*. Figure 3B shows the location of a CpG island and two promoter-like sequences, which although not associated with any known gene, may function to provide chromatin accessibility. Statistical tests for gene conversion identified the 700-bp perfect match between NF1-REP-P1-51 and NF1-REP-M-51 that coincided with PRS2 (Fig. 3B). Although perfect sequence match may contribute to breakpoint localization, these results suggest that perfect tracts at paralogous recombination hotspots may be a result of gene conversion at sites at which preferential pairing occurs for other unknown reasons *(24)*. A search for palindromes, which are associated with other genomic rearrangements *(32–35)*, found no palindromes larger than 18 bp and separated by 63 bp. The palindromes within the KIAA0563-ψ of NF1-REP-P1 are considered too distant to influence recombination at the PRS regions (Fig. 2A).

UNIQUE, NON-LCR-MEDIATED *NF1* MICRODELETIONS

A subset of submicroscopic *NF1* microdeletions have breakpoints outside of the NF1-REP paralogs (Fig. 4) and appear to arise by a mechanism other than paralogous recombination. Among the five larger deletions, all except the BUD case (patient B in Fig. 4) have a telomeric breakpoint within the *ACCN1* gene. BUD has a telomeric breakpoint in the *SLFN* gene cluster. At least four of these deletions also have different centromeric breakpoint intervals. Only breakpoints in case six have been mapped at the nucleotide level with the centromeric breakpoint between *BLMH* and *CPD* and the telomeric breakpoint in *ACCN1* intron 1. The breakpoints were not located within LCR elements. However, there were stretches of 20–21 bp of *Alu*-like elements at the two breakpoints and LINE and short interspersed nuclear element (SINE) elements within several hundred bp from the breakpoints. Together, these data provide support for a mechanism of nonhomologous end-joining (NHEJ) *(36)*. Because LCRs are not known to be located in/near the breakpoints of the other *NF1* microdeletions shown in Fig. 4, they may well arise by NHEJ also. As more such deletions are identified, it will be of interest to determine if there is a preferential parent of origin effect. In these examples, UWA106-3, BUD, and 96-2 have paternally derived deletions, whereas 372A was maternally derived. In general, larger deletions tend to occur in NF1 patients with severe or additional complications, but phenotypic information is limited and the extent of an *NF1* deletion has no predictive value to date.

The smaller deletions depicted on Fig. 4 are of interest because precise breakpoint mapping and full clinical evaluation of such patients may serve to narrow the critical region between NF1-REP-P1 and NF1-REP-M that confers the phenotype of heavy tumor load and increased

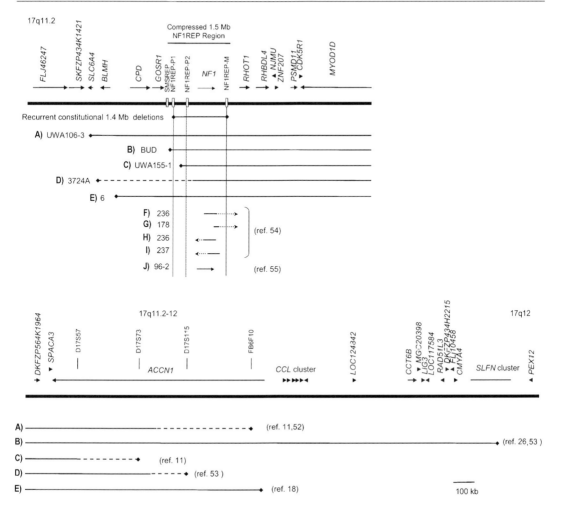

Fig. 4. Nonrecurrent *NF1* microdeletions. A schematic of the 5.6-Mb region from *FLJ46247* to *PEX12* is diagrammed in two panels. Figures are drawn to scale with the exception of the 1.5-Mb NF1-REP region, which is compressed for space considerations. Gene names and gene clusters are written above arrows indicating their direction of transcription. The three NF1-REP (open boxes) and an adjacent SMS REP (gray box) are indicated. Four markers within *ACCN1* are shown that serve to differentiate the extent of deletions with breakpoints within this large gene. Below the map, the recurrent 1.4-Mb deletion is shown compared to that of 10 cases (A–J) with unique breakpoints. Solid lines indicated deleted region and dashed lines indicate uncertainty in the precise endpoint (*see* text for details). Gene names in this figure are from a May, 2004 assembly of the human genome (http://genome.ucsc.edu/) and may differ from names on previously published maps of the region *(23,25,26,36).*

malignancy risk to deletion patients. Patients 236, 178, 236, and 237 have at least one breakpoint within the *NF1* gene, but the extent of the deletion and position of the other breakpoints are not known. Patient 96-2 is deleted for much of the *NF1* gene, but whether other genes are involved in this deletion is not known.

LCR-MEDIATED SOMATIC *NF1* MICRODELETIONS

An estimated 25% of *NF1* microdeletions occur as postzygotic mutations during mitosis resulting in tissue mosaicism *(21)* and a phenotype that can vary from the classical generalized

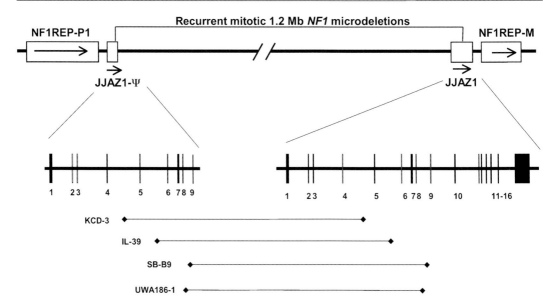

Fig. 5. Recurrent mitotic *NF1* microdeletions. The schematic shows the pair of *JJAZ1* low-copy repeats (LCRs) that mediate recurrent mitotic microdeletions of the *NF1* region (refer to Fig. 1 for genomic context of the region). These LCRs share 46 kb of homology with 97% sequence identity and are located just "internal" to the NF1-REP-P1 and –M *(26)*. Breakpoints are drawn for four cases of 1.2-Mb deletions mediated by paralogous recombination between the *JJAZ1*-ψ pseudogene and the *JAZZ1* functional gene. (Three from ref. *21* and UWA186-1 as an additional unpublished case from my laboratory.)

NF1 to localized or segmental NF1 *(37,38)*. Like the common recurrent meiotic *NF1* microdeletions, somatic rearrangements occur by paralogous recombination; however, the site of preferential exchange was different. Seven of eight mitotic *NF1* microdeletions had breakpoints that clustered at the *JJAZ1*-ψ pseudogene and the *JJAZ1* functional gene, which are direct repeats located adjacent and NF1-REP-P1 and NF1-REP-M (Fig. 1) *(21)*. The *JJAZ1*-ψ has 9 exons that share 46-kb homology at 97% identity with the functional *JJAZ1* gene (Fig.5) *(26)*. In three cases, breakpoint intervals were mapped at the nucleotide level by use of PSVs and the microdeletions occurred at different sites (Fig. 5). Consistent with this observation is the breakpoint of a somatic mosaic female patient in my laboratory, UWA186-1, whose breakpoint in intron 8 is approx 2 kb proximal to that of SB-B9 (Stephens, unpublished observations). The *JJAZ1*-ψ/*JJAZ1* fusion product of the recombination is expressed in human-rodent somatic cell lines, but unlikely to be translated owing to stop codons in the pseudogene *(21)*.

The level of somatic mosaicism for *JJAZ1*-mediated *NF1* microdeletions varied significantly in different patient tissues. The percentage of deleted cells as determined by FISH was quite high in peripheral blood (91–100%) and significantly lower in buccal cells or skin fibroblasts (51–59%) *(21)*. These data suggest that a selective growth advantage of hematopoetic stem cells carrying *NF1* microdeletions. Different levels of mosaicism significantly compound both the diagnosis and counseling of patients with *JJAZ1*-mediated mosaic *NF1* microdeletions.

JJAZ1- and NF1-REP-mediated *NF1* microdeletions have striking differences and parallels. First, paralogous recombination at *JJAZ1* LCRs is preferentially mitotic, whereas that at NF1-REP LCRs is meiotic. Second, *JJAZ1* paralogous recombination is intrachromosomal in two cases examined *(21)*, whereas NF1-REP paralogous recombination is primarily interchromosomal *(16)*. Third, small inverted repeats of 75–127 bp flank the intronic *JJAZ1* breakpoints in two cases and may cause double strand breaks by forming hairpins *(21)*. Parallels between the two types of microdeletions include paralogous recombination, and deletion of the same set of contiguous genes, except for the functional *KIAA0563-rel* gene near NF1-REP-M, which is not deleted in *JJAZ1*-mediated rearrangements (Fig. 1). Furthermore, both paralogous recombination events occur preferentially in females for reasons that are not known *(15,17,21)*.

FUTURE DIRECTIONS

It will be important to determine the molecular basis for the different preferences for LCR substrates during meiotic vs mitotic recombination. Furthermore, does *JJAZ1*-mediated recombination contribute to somatic *NF1* second hit mutations at NF1-associated tumors? Does this site represent a mitotic recombination hotspot in the genome, perhaps in the female genome? And why is maternal recombination more prevalent for both LCR-mediated microdeletions? Clinical studies to identify the putative modifying gene that confers the increased risk for tumorigenesis and malignancy remain a priority. These studies will be facilitated by new assays and approaches to identify patient cohorts of the same deletion genotype and exclude mosaic cases that would confound the analyses.

SUMMARY

Submicroscopic deletions at chromosome 17q11.2 underlying the common genetic disorder NF1 are of great interest because they predispose to a heavy neurofibroma burden, malignancy, and possibly other severe manifestations. The NF1 microdeletion phenotype, which remains to be defined in detail, is thought to be owing to the deletion of the *NF1* tumor suppressor gene and an additional unidentified flanking gene(s). Surprisingly, there is a different preference for LCR recombination substrates for recurrent meiotic versus recurrent mitotic *NF1* microdeletion events. Paralogous recombination between a pair of 51-kb NF1-REPs mediate the recurrent common constitutional 1.4-Mb microdeletion that occurs preferentially during maternal meiosis. Recombination between the *JJAZ1* pseudogene and functional gene mediate the recurrent 1.2-Mb microdeletion, which occurs preferentially during postzygotic mitosis in females. NF1-REP-mediated *NF1* microdeletions involve 13 additional genes, whereas *JJAZ1*-mediated microdeletions involve the same genes but one. Breakpoints of both deletions mapped at the nucleotide level identify several potential sequence features that may contribute to the choice of discrete sites for strand exchange.

REFERENCES

1. Kayes LM, Riccardi VM, Burke W, Bennett RL, Stephens K. Large de novo DNA deletion in a patient with sporadic neurofibromatosis 1, mental retardation, and dysmorphism. J Med Genet 1992;29:686–690.
2. Friedman JM. Neurofibromatosis 1: clinical manifestations and diagnostic criteria. J Child Neurol 2002;17: 548–554.
3. Friedman JM, Gutmann DH, MacCollin M, Riccardi VM, (eds.) *Neurofibromatosis. Phenotype, Natural History, and Pathogenesis, 3rd edition.* Baltimore: The Johns Hopkins University Press, 1999.
4. Zhu Y, Ghosh P, Charnay P, Burns DK, and Parada LF. Neurofibromas in NF1: Schwann cell origin and role of tumor environment. Science 2002;296:920–922.
5. Dasgupta B, Gutmann DH. Neurofibromatosis 1: closing the GAP between mice and men. Curr Opin Genet Dev 2003;13:20–27.

6. Bajenaru ML, Hernandez MR, Perry A, et al. Optic nerve glioma in mice requires astrocyte Nf1 gene inactivation and Nf1 brain heterozygosity. Cancer Res 2003;63:8573–8577.
7. Side L, Taylor B, Cayouette M, et al. Homozygous inactivation of the NF1 gene in bone marrow cells from children with neurofibromatosis type 1 and malignant myeloid disorders. N Engl J Med 1997;336:1713–1720.
8. Kluwe L, Friedrich RE, Mautner VF. Allelic loss of the NF1 gene in NF1-associated plexiform neurofibromas. Cancer Genet Cytogenet 1999;113:65–69.
9. Messiaen L, Riccardi, V, Peltonen, J, et al. Independent NF1 mutations in two large families with spinal neurofibromatosis. J Med Genet 2003;40:122–126.
10. Kluwe L, Siebert R, Gesk S,et al. Screening 500 unselected neurofibromatosis 1 patients for deletions of the NF1 gene. Hum Mutat 2004;23:111–116.
11. Dorschner MO, Sybert VP, Weaver M, Pletcher BA, Stephens K. NF1 microdeletion breakpoints are clustered at flanking repetitive sequences. Hum Mol Genet 2000;9:35–46.
12. Kayes LM, Burke W, Riccardi VM, et al. Deletions spanning the neurofibromatosis 1 gene: identification and phenotype of five patients. Am J Hum Genet 1994;54:424–436.
13. Leppig K, Kaplan P, Viskochil D, Weaver M, Orterberg J, Stephens K. Familial neurofibromatosis 1 gene deletions: cosegregation with distinctive facial features and early onset of cutaneous neurofibromas. Am J Med Genet 1997;73:197–204.
14. Wu BL, Schneider GH, Korf BR. Deletion of the entire NF1 gene causing distinct manifestations in a family. Am J Med Genet 1997;69:98–101.
15. Upadhyaya M, Ruggieri M, Maynard J, et al. Gross deletions of the neurofibromatosis type 1 (NF1) gene are predominantly of maternal origin and commonly associated with a learning disability, dysmorphic features and developmental delay. Hum Genet 1998;102:591–597.
16. Lopez-Correa C, Brems H, Lazaro C, Marynen P, Legius E. Unequal Meiotic Crossover: A Frequent Cause of NF1 Microdeletions. Am J Hum Genet 2000;66:1969–1974.
17. Lopez-Correa C, Dorschner M, Brems H, et al. Recombination hotspot in NF1 microdeletion patients. Hum Mol Genet 2001;10:1387–1392.
18. Venturin M, Guarnieri P, Natacci F, et al. Mental retardation and cardiovascular malformations in NF1 microdeleted patients point to candidate genes in 17q11.2. J Med Genet 2004;41:35–41.
19. Gutmann DH, James CD, Poyhonen M, et al. Molecular analysis of astrocytomas presenting after age 10 in individuals with NF1. Neurology 2003;61:1397–1400.
20. De Raedt T, Brems H, Wolkenstein P, et al. Elevated risk for MPNST in NF1 microdeletion patients. Am J Hum Genet 2003;72:1288–1292.
21. Kehrer-Sawatzki H, Kluwe L, Sandig C, et al. High frequency of mosaicism among patients with neurofibromatosis type 1 (NF1) with microdeletions caused by somatic recombination of the JJAZ1 gene. Am J Hum Genet 2004;75:410–423.
22. Stankiewicz P, Lupski JR. Genome architecture, rearrangements and genomic disorders. Trends Genet 2002;18:74–82.
23. Dorschner MO, Brems H, Le R, et al. Tightly clustered breakpoints permit detection of the recurrent 1.4 Mb NF1 microdeletion by deletion-specific amplification. 2005; submitted.
24. Forbes SH, Dorschner MO, Le R Stephens K. Genomic context of paralogous recombination hotspots mediating recurrent NF1 region microdeletion. Genes Chromosomes Cancer 2004;41:12–25.
25. De Raedt T, Brems H, Lopez-Correa C, Vermeesch JR, Marynen P, Legius, E. Genomic organization and evolution of the NF1 microdeletion region. Genomics 2004;84:346–360.
26. Jenne DE, Tinschert S, Dorschner MO, et al. Complete physical map and gene content of the human NF1 tumor suppressor region in human and mouse. Genes Chromosomes Cancer 2003;37:111–120.
27. Jenne DE, Tinschert S, Reimann H, et al. Molecular Characterization and Gene Content of Breakpoint Boundaries in Patients with Neurofibromatosis Type 1 with 17q11.2 Microdeletions. Am J Hum Genet 2001;69:3.
28. Lagerstedt K, Karsten SL, Carlberg BM, et al. Double-strand breaks may initiate the inversion mutation causing the Hunter syndrome. Hum Mol Genet 1997;6:627–633.
29. Lopes J, Ravise N, Vandenberghe A, et al. Fine mapping of de novo CMT1A and HNPP rearrangements within CMT1A-REPs evidences two distinct sex-dependent mechanisms and candidate sequences involved in recombination. Hum Mol Genet 1998;7:141–148.
30. Reiter LT, Hastings PJ, Nelis E, De Jonghe P, Van Broeckhoven C, Lupski JR. Human meiotic recombination products revealed by sequencing a hotspot for homologous strand exchange in multiple HNPP deletion patients. Am J Hum Genet 1998;62:1023–1033.

31. Sun C, Skaletsky H, Rozen S, et al. Deletion of azoospermia factor a (AZFa) region of human Y chromosome caused by recombination between HERV15 proviruses. Hum Mol Genet 2000;9:2291–2296.
32. Repping S, Skaletsky H, Lange J, et al. Recombination between palindromes P5 and P1 on the human Y chromosome causes massive deletions and spermatogenic failure. Am J Hum Genet 2002;71:906–922.
33. Kurahashi H, Emanuel BS. Long AT-rich palindromes and the constitutional t(11;22) breakpoint. Hum Mol Genet 2001;10:2605–2617.
34. Kurahashi H, Inagaki H, Yamada K, et al. Cruciform DNA structure underlies the etiology for palindrome-mediated human chromosomal translocations. J Biol Chem 2004;279:35,377–35,383.
35. Nag DK, Kurst A. A 140-bp-long palindromic sequence induces double-strand breaks during meiosis in the yeast Saccharomyces cerevisiae. Genetics 1997;146:835–847.
36. Venturin M, Gervasini C, Orzan F, et al. Evidence for non-homologous end joining and non-allelic homologous recombination in atypical NF1 microdeletions. Hum Genet 2004;115:69–80.
37. Ruggieri M, Huson SM. The clinical and diagnostic implications of mosaicism in the neurofibromatoses. Neurology 2001;56:1433–1443.
38. Petek E, Jenne DE, Smolle J, et al. Mitotic recombination mediated by the JJAZF1 (KIAA0160) gene causing somatic mosaicism and a new type of constitutional NF1 microdeletion in two children of a mosaic female with only few manifestations. J Med Genet 2003;40:520–525.
39. Mattocks C, Baralle D, Tarpey P, French-Constant C, Bobrow M, Whittaker J. Automated comparative sequence analysis identifies mutations in 89% of NF1 patients and confirms a mutation cluster in exons 11-17 distinct from the GAP related domain. J Med Genet 2004;41:e48.
40. Messiaen LM, Callens T, Mortier G, et al. Exhaustive mutation analysis of the NF1 gene allows identification of 95% of mutations and reveals a high frequency of unusual splicing defects. Hum Mutat 2000;15:541–555.
41. Ars E, Kruyer H, Morell M, et al. Recurrent mutations in the NF1 gene are common among neurofibromatosis type 1 patients. J Med Genet 2003;40:e82.
42. Streubel B, Latta E, Kehrer-Sawatzki H, Hoffmann GF, Fonatsch C, Rehder H. Somatic mosaicism of a greater than 1.7-Mb deletion of genomic DNA involving the entire NF1 gene as verified by FISH: further evidence for a contiguous gene syndrome in 17q11.2. Am J Med Genet 1999;87:12–16.
43. Tinschert S, Naumann I, Stegmann E, et al. Segmental neurofibromatosis is caused by somatic mutation of the neurofibromatosis type 1 (NF1) gene. Eur J Hum Genet 2000;8:455–459.
44. Colman SD, Rasmussen SA, Ho VT, Abernathy CR, Wallace MR. Somatic mosaicism in a patient with neurofibromatosis type 1. Am J Hum Genet 1996;58:484–490.
45. van den Brink HJ, van Zeijl CM, Brons JF, van den Hondel CA, van Gorcom RF. Cloning and characterization of the NADPH cytochrome P450 oxidoreductase gene from the filamentous fungus Aspergillus niger. DNA Cell Biol 1995;14:719–729.
46. Lazaro C, Gaona A, Lynch M, Kruyer H, Ravella A, Estivill X. Molecular characterization of the breakpoints of a 12-kb deletion in the NF1 gene in a family showing germ-line mosaicism. Am J Hum Genet 1995;57:1044–1049.
47. Serra E, Ars E, Ravella A, et al. Somatic NF1 mutational spectrum in benign neurofibromas: mRNA splice defects are common among point mutations. Hum Genet 2001;108:416–429.
48. Rasmussen SA, Overman J, Thomson SA, et al. Chromosome 17 loss-of-heterozygosity studies in benign and malignant tumors in neurofibromatosis type 1. Genes Chromosomes Cancer 2000;28:425–431.
49. Serra E, Rosenbaum T, Nadal M, et al. Mitotic recombination effects homozygosity for NF1 germline mutations in neurofibromas. Nat Genet 2001;28:294–296.
50. Legius E, Marchuk DA, Collins FS, Glover TW. Somatic deletion of the neurofibromatosis type 1 gene in a neurofibrosarcoma supports a tumour suppressor gene hypothesis. Nature Genet 1993;3:122–126.
51. Frahm S, Mautner VF, Brems H, et al. Genetic and phenotypic characterization of tumor cells derived from malignant peripheral nerve sheath tumors of neurofibromatosis type 1 patients. Neurobiol Dis 2004;16:85–91.
52. Stephens K. Genetics of neurofibromatosis 1- associated peripheral nerve sheath tumors. Cancer Invest 2003;21:901–918.
53. Kehrer-Sawatzki H, Tinschert S, Jenne DE. Heterogeneity of breakpoints in non-LCR-mediated large constitutional deletions of the 17q11.2 NF1 tumor suppressor region. J Med Genet 2003;10:e116.
54. Fang LJ, Vidaud D, Vidaud M, Thirion JP. Identification and characterization of four novel large deletions in the human neurofibromatosis type 1 (NF1) gene. Hum Mutat 2001;18:549–550.
55. Lopez Correa C, Brems H, Lazaro C, et al. Molecular studies in 20 submicroscopic neurofibromatosis type 2 gene deletions. Hum Mutat 1999;14:387–393.

15

Williams-Beuren Syndrome

Stephen W. Scherer, PhD and Lucy R. Osborne, PhD

CONTENTS

INTRODUCTION

Williams-Beuren syndrome (WBS; also called Williams syndrome) is a multisystem developmental disorder that is almost always associated with an approx 1.5-Mb deletion of chromosome 7q11.23 (OMIM no. 194050). The deletion was identified in 1993 based on the observation of phenotypic overlap with supravalvular aortic stenosis (SVAS), a distinct autosomal dominant disorder affecting the cardiovascular system *(1)*. It has since been shown that SVAS arises because of the disruption of one copy of the elastin gene, through either deletion, translocation or point mutation *(2–4)*, but the genes contributing to the remaining aspects of WBS have not yet been definitively determined.

The 7q11.23 chromosomal region that is commonly deleted in WBS contains more than 25 genes and, as might be expected, is flanked by chromosome-specific low-copy repeats (LCRs) *(5,6)*. The nature of these repeats are such that in addition to deletions (and presumably the reciprocal duplications), inversions of the region are also mediated, one of which exists as a polymorphism that seems to predispose to the deletion *(7,8)*. The increasing number of genomic rearrangements being discovered to be associated with this region are, therefore, not only expanding the repertoire of molecular diagnostic tests for WBS and its associated phenotypes, but also impacting on genetic counseling for this disorder. To facilitate future molecular genetic studies involving the WBS locus, we are actively cataloging chromosome rearrangements involving the WBS-LCRs and associated phenotypes. The clinical and molecular data can be found at http://www.chr7.org/.

From: *Genomic Disorders: The Genomic Basis of Disease*
Edited by: J. R. Lupski and P. Stankiewicz © Humana Press, Totowa, NJ

CLINICAL OVERVIEW

The WBS phenotype is quite variable, as would be expected for a developmental disorder, but there are a number of core clinical features that are present in the vast majority of affected individuals. These include both physical and neurological elements that combine to produce a unique and therefore characteristic clinical picture. The frequency of WBS has been estimated at between 1 in 20,000 and 1 in 7500, with the second statistic likely a more accurate reflection of the population frequency because it was generated from a larger data set (9,10).

Physical manifestations of WBS usually include involvement of the cardiovascular system, most often as a narrowing of the ascending aorta (SVAS) although a generalized arteriopathy can lead to vascular stenoses in other vessels, and hypertension is common in later life. Stellate irides, flat nasal bridge, short, up-turned nose with anteverted nostrils, long philtrum, full lips and lower cheeks, and a small chin are the recognizable facial features. Other symptoms include hernias, visual impairment, hypersensitivity to sound, chronic otitis media, malocclusion, small or missing teeth, renal anomalies, constipation, vomiting, growth deficiency, infantile hypercalcemia, musculoskeletal abnormalities, and a hoarse voice (11,12). As WBS individuals grow older they may also present with premature graying of the hair, diabetes and impaired glucose tolerance, decreased bone mineral density, sensorineural hearing loss, and a high frequency of psychiatric symptoms (13).

Individuals with WBS usually have mild mental retardation, with an average intelligence quotient (IQ) of between 55 and 60, although there is a wide range of recorded values. The most striking aspect of the WBS phenotype is the distinct behavioral profile, which encompasses a unique combination of both friendliness and anxiety (11,14). It is characterized by impaired cognition, hyperreactivity, sensory integration dysfunction, delayed expressive and receptive language skills, and multiple developmental motor disabilities affecting balance, strength, coordination, and motor planning (12). In addition, approx 70% of WBS individuals suffer from attention deficit and hyperactivity disorder and there is a high incidence of anxiety and simple phobias (12,15,16).

WBS was linked to chromosome 7q11.23 through the occurrence of a part of the phenotypic spectrum, SVAS, as an independent autosomal dominant disorder. SVAS was mapped to 7q11.23 through linkage analysis (17) and the elastin gene (ELN) was then found to be disrupted in an individual with a t(6;7) chromosome translocation (2). The vast majority of individuals presenting with the classic symptoms of WBS harbor a deletion of 7q11.23 (18–21). Individuals without rearrangements of 7q11.23, or with rearrangements of other regions of the genome have been reported, but these are likely misdiagnoses or perhaps phenocopies of WBS (22–28).

GENOMIC STRUCTURE OF THE WBS REGION

Human Chromosome 7q11.23

The WBS deletion region is comprised of around 1.2 Mb of unique DNA sequence, including at least 24 protein-coding genes, flanked by large LCRs; one on the centromeric side and two on the telomeric side (Fig. 1). These LCRs, which predispose the region to non-allelic homologous recombination (NAHR), are between 300 and 400 kb in size and are comprised of both transcribed and non-transcribed genes and pseudogenes. The structure of each LCR is complex, but has been subdivided into segments of homologous sequence termed blocks A, B, and C (29–31). The centromeric, medial, and telomeric copies of each block can be distin-

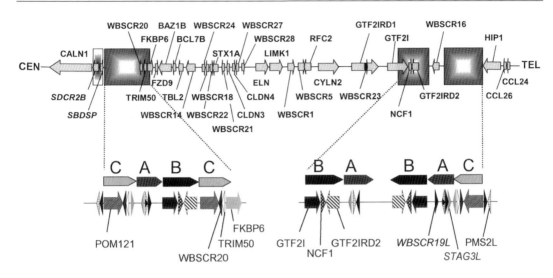

Fig. 1. The Williams-Beuren syndrome (WBS) deletion region at 7q11.23. The gene organization of the WBS region is shown, with genes represented as arrows that indicate the orientation of their transcription. A segment containing pseudogenes (*SBDSP*; *SDCRBP*) that has been duplicated from 7q11.22 lies adjacent to the centromeric low-copy repeats (LCR). The centromeric, medial and telomeric WBS LCRs are depicted as shaded boxes and expanded below to reveal the genomic structure of each. The locations of the three repeat blocks, designated A, B, and C are shown with their orientation indicated by the direction of the arrow. The individual gene components of the LCRs are shown with different shaded arrows. The actual genes are those that are labeled, while the unlabeled segments represent pseudogenes. The exceptions to this are *STAG3L* and *WBSCR19L*, whose actual genes lie outside the region.

guished from each other by single nucleotide differences, or paralagous sequence variants, although the sequence identity can be as high as 99.6% over large stretches of DNA.

The individual blocks are made up of genes and sequences that are present in duplicated copies, both within the WBS region and at other sites on chromosome 7. These genes include general transcription factor 2I (*GTF2I*), GTF2I repeat domain-containing protein 2 (*GTF2IRD2*), neutrophil cytosolic factor 1 (*NCF1*), stromal antigen 3 (*STAG3*), POM121 membrane glycoprotein (*POM121*), FK506-binding protein 6 (*FKBP6*), Williams-Beuren syndrome chromosome region 20 (*WBSCR20*), tripartite motif-containing 50 (*TRIM50*), and a number of highly related postmeiotic segregation increased 2-like (*PMS2L*) genes. Of these, functional copies of *WBSCR20*, *TRIM50*, and *FKBP6* are disrupted or deleted near the centromeric breakpoint. *GTF2I* is always disrupted or deleted at the telomeric breakpoint, with *NCF1* and *GTF2IRD2* variably deleted depending on the location of the distal deletion breakpoint.

Three *STAG3* pseudogenes are present within the LCRs, but the functional copy lies distal to the WBS region at 7q22, along with two other pseudogenes *(32)*. Several POM121 transcription units are also present within the LCRs, but it is unknown which of these corresponds to the functional gene. Further complexity is added by the presence of fusion transcripts between POM121 and Zona pellucida sperm-binding protein 3 (ZP3) *(33)*, which maps close, but distal, to the WBS region *(34*; http://www.chr7.org/), and numerous other POM121-like sequences scattered throughout the genome. Intriguingly, POM121-like sequences are also found within the LCRs that flank the 22q11.2 deletion region *(35)*.

Gene clusters of highly similar transcription units, the PMS2L genes are also contained within the LCRs. Because of the large number and high homology of these genes, it is still unknown exactly how many exist and which are actively transcribed, but many different transcripts have been demonstrated *(36,37)*. *PMS2L* gene clusters are also present in two other locations on human chromosome 7; 7q11.22 and 7q22 *(5)*.

Syntenic Region in Nonhuman Species

The gene content and order of the WBS deletion region is conserved within the syntenic region of mouse chromosome 5, band G1. As with other chromosome regions involved in genomic disorders, the LCRs seen on human chromosome 7q11.23 are absent in the mouse, but interestingly their positions correspond to evolutionary inversion breakpoints *(30)* (Fig. 2). This coincidence of LCRs and evolutionary chromosome breakpoints has also been reported in the Smith-Magenis syndrome region on human chromosome 17p11.2 and mouse chromosome 11 *(38,39)*, and in the Prader-Willi/Angelman syndrome region on human chromosome 15q11-q13 and mouse chromosome 7 *(40)*.

Because the LCRs are absent in the mouse, so are the multiple psuedogenes. Any genes or pseudogenes contained within the human LCRs are single copy in the mouse and located either within the WBS syntenic region (in the case of *Gtf2i*, *Gtf2ird2*, *Ncf1*, *Wbscr20*, *Trim50*, *Pom121*, and *Fkbp6*) or within the region of synteny with their functional human gene copy (*Pms2* and *Stag3*). Of the commonly deleted genes, only one is not present in the mouse— *WBSCR23*. There is evidence from sequence homology for the presence of this gene in apes but not in Old World monkeys, suggesting that it arose within the last 25 million years *(41)*. The presence of an ape-specific gene within the common deletion raises the intriguing thought that it may contribute to some of the more "human" features seen in WBS, such as gregarious personality or descriptive language, but the expression of *WBSCR23* appears to be restricted to the skin and some internal organs, making it unlikely to be involved in the alteration of brain function *(42)*.

The high DNA sequence similarity between the LCRs at 7q11.23 suggests that they appeared only recently, leaving little time for divergence. Although these LCRs are not present in the mouse, there is evidence for their existence in closer relatives of modern humans, most notably the nonhuman primates. Comparative analysis in a variety of species has revealed that the LCRs evolved in the hominoid lineage sometime after the divergence of Old World monkeys, which happened approx 25 million years ago. Macaques (Old World monkeys), like mice, do not have these duplicated segments of DNA present at the syntenic regions of 7q11.23, however, apes such as orangutans and gorillas do show multiple copies of sequences from this region *(43)*. Further expansion of the LCR copy number is estimated to have occurred between 5 and 10 million years ago, because fluorescence *in situ* hybridization (FISH) analysis of nonhuman primate chromosomes show that the gorilla and chimpanzee have more signals than orangutan and gibbon *(43)*. A more detailed analysis of the LCR sequences using FISH and sequence-specific polymerase chain reaction suggests that the evolution of the LCRs has been complex *(43a)*. In the orangutan and gorilla, two copies of the C-block and two copies of the A-block are present, although not always at the same locus. Even in our closest ancestor, the chimpanzee, there are two C-blocks and two A-blocks, but only one B-block. This indicates that the duplication of the B-block, which contains the highest level of sequence identity within the human LCRs and is the site for the majority of the non-allelic homologous recombinations, was duplicated less than 5 million years ago.

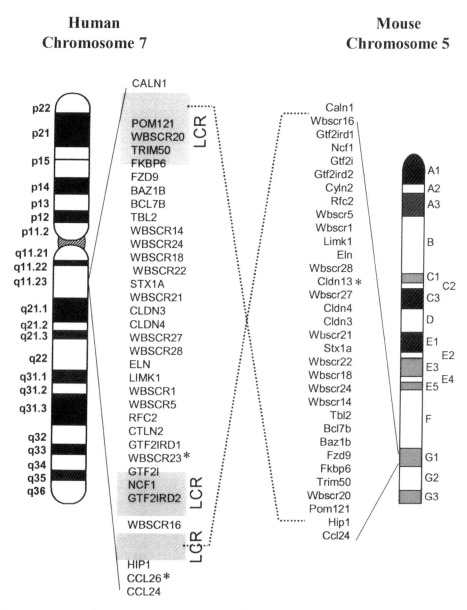

Fig. 2. Synteny between human chromosome 7q11.23 and mouse chromosome 5G. The gene order of both regions is shown and the low-copy repeats present at human 7q11.23 are shaded. The region has undergone an evolutionary inversion between mouse and human as indicated by the dashed lines. Asterisks indicate genes that are present in one species but not the other.

DELETIONS

Deletions of the WBS region occur because of unequal meiotic recombination in grandparental chromosomes *(44–46)*. Approximately two-thirds of these recombinations are interchromosomal rearrangements between chromosome 7 homologs, whereas the remainder are intrachromosomal and involve sister chromatids of the same chromosome 7. A survey of all reported cases where inheritance was determined reveals no bias in inheritance of the

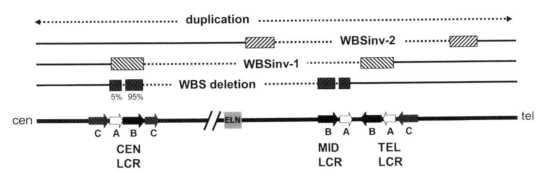

Fig. 3. Genomic rearrangements of the Williams-Beuren syndrome (WBS) region. All documented, recurrent rearrangements of the WBS region are shown. The block components of the flanking low-copy repeats (LCRs) are shown, along with the relative position of *ELN*, which lies at the center of the commonly deleted region. The regions to which the breakpoints have been localized are indicated by boxes. The WBSinv-2 inversion does not appear to be an LCR-mediated event. The duplication extends beyond the WBS region in both directions.

deletion, as it apparently occurs with equal frequency on maternally or paternally inherited chromosomes *(47–49)*.

Common Deletions

The polymorphic marker *D7S1870*, which lies within the proximal part of *GTF2I*, was initially shown to be deleted in every patient with a diagnosis of classic WBS. *D7S489B*, however, which lies near Frizzled 9 (*FZD9*), was shown to be present in all such patients *(6,47,48,50,51)*. Subsequently, it has been shown that in approx 95% of WBS patients, the deletion occurs between highly homologous sequences within the centromeric and medial B-blocks, whereas in the remainder it occurs between sequences in the adjacent A-blocks (Fig. 3) *(31)*. These two block pairs are the only ones that are directly oriented with respect to each other (Fig. 1). The predominance of recombination between the B-blocks, rather than the A-blocks is postulated to occur because of the higher sequence identity (99.6 vs 98.2%), more contiguous homology (there are two interstitial deletions of the medial A-block), and the shorter distance between the blocks (1.55 vs 1.84 Mb). In addition, the active transcription of all three of the GTF2I genes within the testes and in blastocysts suggests that they are transcribed in germ cells, which could induce an open chromatic formation that is conducive to recombination *(6,52)*.

The exceptionally high identity between repeat-block sequences copies has made it extremely difficult to identify the exact deletion breakpoints in patients. Site-specific nucleotide differences (SSNs) between the repeats, also referred to as paralagous sequence variants or *cis*-morphisms, have been utilized to study the relative copy number of different segments of the B-block, allowing the sites of recombination to be mapped *(31)*. These elegant studies have revealed a 1.4-kb recombination hotspot within *GTF2I*, which accounts for one-third of all deletions arising on a noninverted chromosome *(53)*. Other breakpoints exist throughout the remainder of *GTF2I*, *NCF1*, and *GTF2IRD2*, with additional hot spots associated with both paternally inherited and maternally inherited deletions *(53)*. This translates into a variable number of genes within the deletion; 26 if the recombination occurs in *GTF2I*, up to 28 if it

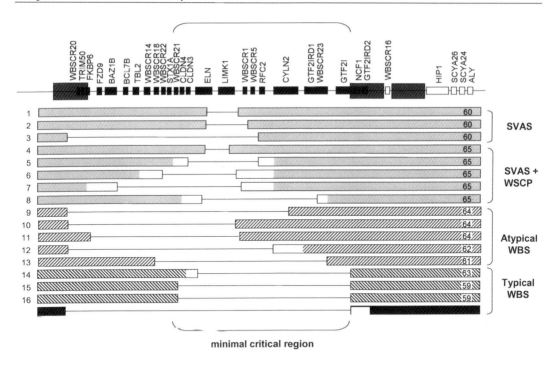

Fig. 4. Genotype–phenotype correlation in Williams-Beuren syndrome (WBS). The WBS region is shown including all the known genes and the flanking repeats depicted as shaded boxes. Seventeen patients with smaller deletions of the region are listed beneath (with references) and the extent of their deletions are represented as lines between non-deleted blocks (unknown breakpoints lie within the white areas). They are shown in groups of increasing phenotypic complexity, with patients showing the classic WBS phenotype at the bottom of the page. The proposed WBS minimal critical region is indicated with brackets.

occurs within *GTF2IRD2* or the A-block. The inclusion of *NCF1* within the deletion is supported by two reports of patients with WBS and chronic granulomatous disease (OMIM no. 233700), presumably owing to a mutation of the intact *NCF1* gene *(54,55)*. A recent correlation has been made between the deletion of *NCF1* and reduced incidence of hypertension in WBS *(56)*. It has also been suggested that hypertension is linked to parent-of-origin *(57)*, however, this may reflect the predominance of paternally inherited deletions that have recombination breakpoints within the *GTF2I* hotspot, thereby leaving *NCF1* intact *(53)*.

Smaller Deletions

Although the vast majority of WBS individuals have the common deletion, there are some who carry partial deletions of the region, most being associated with a subset of the WBS phenotype *(58–65)*. The extent of the smaller deletions in these individuals are summarized in Fig. 4. With relatively few patients, none of whom are deleted for exactly the same interval, it is hard to make precise correlations between the genotype and the phenotype. Even very distinctive characteristics such as the WBS cognitive profile, with its verbal strengths and weakness in spatial abilities, do not appear to correlate with deletion size. Initial reports of two families with small deletions and the WBS cognitive profile suggested that hemizygosity for the LIM Kinase 1 gene *(LIMK1)* was responsible for deficits in visuospatial processing *(58)*.

A subsequent study, however, identified three families with deletions spanning *LIMK1* that showed no evidence of visuospatial deficits *(60)*. Yet a third study identified another three families with deletions of *LIMK1* who did exhibit the WBS cognitive profile *(65)*. This typifies the difficulties in making accurate genotype–phenotype correlations where patients are seen by different physicians in different countries and where often there is only one affected family member being analyzed. Moreover, for any such genomic examination it will be imperative to scan the entire region for potential chromosomal micro-rearrangements (including noncontiguous ones), mutations, or complex alterations, before any firm conclusions are drawn.

Some general conclusions can be drawn from the patients with smaller deletions. It appears that a minimal deletion region of approx 10–12 genes is necessary for the full phenotypic spectrum of WBS to be expressed (Fig. 4). In addition, it is likely that the more telomeric end of the deletion makes a significant contribution to the developmental delay seen in these patients, because individuals with this region intact do not have significant cognitive impairment.

Larger Deletions

A small number of larger deletions of 7q11.23, which include the WBS commonly deleted region have been reported, but the boundaries of most are not yet well delineated. From the published reports, however, it would seem that patients with deletions that extend either proximally or distally from the WBS region have a more severe phenotype, often with significant developmental delay and seizures (*[66–69]*; personal observation). It is likely that the characteristic WBS phenotypes are still present, although many of the behavioral and cognitive features are masked by severe mental retardation.

INVERSIONS

WBSinv-1 Inversion of the WBS Region

The highly related blocks flanking the WBS region are arranged not only in direct orientation (centromeric and medial copies) but also in inverted orientation (centromeric and telomeric copies) with respect to each other. The presence of these blocks in an inverted orientation can mediate unequal meiotic recombination events that result in the balanced inversion of the intervening region (without the loss of any part of the chromosome) *(7)* (Fig. 3). This inversion, named WBSinv-1, is found in approx 25–30% of parents who transmit a deleted chromosome to their WBS child, and can be readily detected by three-color interphase FISH analysis or by pulsed-field gel electrophoresis (PFGE) followed by Southern blot analysis *(7,31)*. In carriers of WBSinv-1, the inversion can be visualized directly using three differentially labeled probes using FISH analysis of interphase spreads of cells. Two of the probes lie within the commonly deleted region, while the third lies outside, either proximally or distally, and acts as an anchor with which to orient the other two signals. Using PFGE, a junction fragment can be detected on digestion of genomic DNA with *Not*I restriction enzyme and hybridization with a probe for the *GTF2I* gene.

WBSinv-1 can also be inferred in a parental chromosome, based on analysis of the deleted chromosome in their WBS offspring. For this, analysis of the same SSNs used for mapping the deletion breakpoints is used. If the deletion occurred through interchromosomal recombination between a normal and WBSinv-1 chromosome, the pattern of SSNs is different than if it occurred through either interchromosomal recombination between two normal chromosomes 7, or through intrachromosomal recombination *(31)*.

A model has been developed that predicts the possible regions undergoing NAHR based on SSN analysis in WBS families where the inversion status of the transmitting parent has been established by FISH *(31)* (Fig. 5). The WBSinv-1 inversion is predicted to occur as an intrachromosomal rearrangement during meiosis, or perhaps during mitosis (Fig. 5A), while the subsequent deletion is thought to be restricted to interchromosomal rearrangements (Fig. 5B). Analysis of SSNs has narrowed the region of inversion recombination to the B-block or A-block in some individuals, but it is unknown whether NAHR is restricted to these blocks or if it also occurs in the C-block. This implies that size of the inverted region could be anywhere between 1.8 and 2.5 Mb. Based on this analysis of deletions, it is predicted that the most likely region to undergo unequal exchange during the generation of the WBSinv-1 chromosome would be the B-block, because it shows the highest nucleotide identity. Alternatively, there may be specific hot spots of recombination associated with this rearrangement, as there are for the deletions *(53)*.

All WBSinv-1 chromosomes that subsequently undergo deletion show recombination within the terminal 38 kb of B-block, which is not present in the centromeric copy *(31)*. This requires the recombination event leading to WBS to take place between homologous sequences in the medial and telomeric B-block (Fig. 5B).

WBSinv-1 has also been identified in three individuals with clinical features that show some similarity to WBS *(7)*. In one such patient, the junction fragment detected by PFGE was smaller (approx 500 kb) than that seen in three WBSinv-1 carriers (approx 600 kb), suggesting that the inversion breakpoints may differ in this patient or that the rearrangement may be more complex (with the simplest definition being that a deletion is also present). Alternatively, the WBSinv-1 breakpoints could be quite variable and the clinical features of these patients may, therefore, be unrelated to the inversion.

WBSinv-1 As a Risk Factor for Having a Child With WBS

The finding that one-fourth to one-third of transmitting WBS parents are carriers for the WBSinv-1 polymorphism suggests that it predisposes to unequal meiotic recombination. A thorough evaluation of the population frequency is needed in order to accurately assign a numerical risk factor to carrier status for WBSinv-1, but preliminary data do support a significant increase in risk associated with the inverted chromosome. The population frequency has been estimated at 5% based on the analysis of 200 families with a classic WBS deletion member, where both transmitting and nontransmitting parents had their WBSinv-1 carrier status determined *(70)*. The same study took the frequency of WBS to be 1 in 7500 (based on data from ref. *10*) and generated a risk factor of 4.5-fold for an inversion carrier. This gives an overall chance of having an affected child of 1 in 2000 for WBSinv-1 carriers and 1 in 9200 for noncarriers.

A second study looked at the WBSinv-1 status of the transmitting parent in two families with multiple affected children *(71)*. In one family, there were no inversion carriers, but in the second family, both affected siblings had inherited a deleted WBSinv-1 chromosome from their father, who was a carrier for WBSinv-1.

Together, these data indicate that the WBSinv-1 polymorphism seems to be a significant risk factor for WBS. Although the increase in risk associated with the inversion is substantial, the absolute risk of having a child with WBS is still well below the risk of fetal loss associated with prenatal diagnosis procedures, making widespread carrier testing unfeasible at this time. However, as prenatal diagnostic techniques improve and their associated risks decrease, carrier testing for WBSinv-1 may become part of a standard screening panel for those planning families *(72)*.

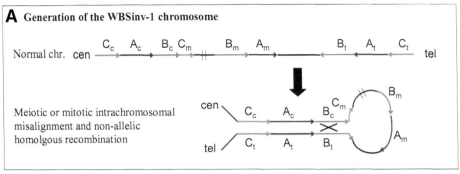

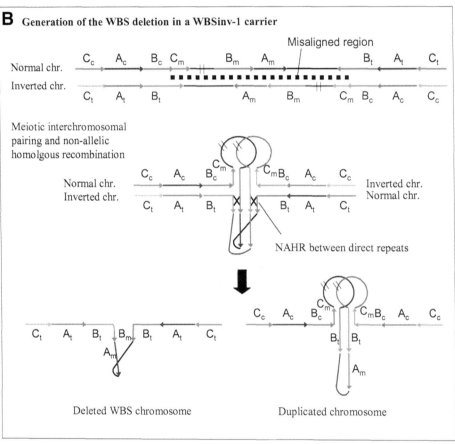

Fig. 5. A model for the generation of WBSinv-1 and the subsequent Williams-Beuren syndrome (WBS) deletion. (A) Generation of the WBSinv-1 chromosome. The region predicted to undergo nonallelic homologous recombination (NAHR) is indicated by X. Unique DNA within the WBS region is represented by a black line and the 1.5-Mb commonly deleted region between the centromeric and medial low-copy repeats (LCRs) and is represented by a blue line. The LCRs are indicated by green (for block A), red (for block B), and yellow (for block C) lines. They are labeled with the respective block letter where the suffix indicates whether the block is centromeric (c), medial (m), or telomeric (t). (B) Generation of the WBS deletion in a WBSinv-1 carrier. The predicted alignment of the WBSinv-1 and normal chromosomes is shown. The two regions that are predicted to correctly align and enable recombination to occur, are indicated with X. The products of such a recombination event are shown. The NAHR event depicted should result in the generation of both a deleted and a duplicated chromosome.

Pathogenic WBSinv-2

A second micro-inversion of the WBS region, named WBSinv-2, has been identified in several patients with clinical features of WBS, but not in any unaffected individual *(8)* (Fig. 3). One of the patients with WBSinv-2 also carried a deletion of 7q31.2-q32 making the comparison of her phenotype to that seen in WBS difficult. A second patient, however, showed no other genomic rearrangement and presented with a history of developmental delay, short stature, coarse facial features, stellate irides, and a very friendly affect. She also exhibited hypersensitivity to sound, mild joint laxity, a love of music, and had an IQ of approx 50 (phenotype and breakpoints are found at http://chr7.org).

WBSinv-2 has breakpoints that lie within apparently unique sequences, one between *LIMK1* and *GTF2IRD1* within the commonly deleted interval, and the other between *HIP1* and *POR*, distal to the telomeric LCR. The location of the breakpoints does not immediately suggest an LCR-mediated mechanism for inversion (as is the case for WBSinv-1). Indeed, because the breakpoints are still only roughly mapped in these patients, it may be that their coincidence is owing to phenotypic selection. A WBSinv-2 breakpoint could directly interrupt at least one gene within the commonly deleted interval. There may also be wider reaching effects on nearby genes, and this could explain the similarity in clinical features.

DUPLICATIONS

Based on the repeat-mediated mechanism of deletion at the WBS locus, the reciprocal duplication event of 7q11.23 is expected to occur at an equal frequency (which is reflected in the 1 in 7500 to 1 in 20,000 occurrence of WBS). However, analysis of numerous patients with WBS-like features without deletion has not yielded evidence of duplication of the region. The fact that duplications have not been observed suggests either that there is no associated phenotype, that they are incompatible with life, or that they result in a phenotype that is quite different from WBS. Reciprocal duplications of both del(17)(p11.2) and del(22)(q11.2) have been identified, and in both cases the phenotypic features are less severe, particularly in dup(17)(p11.2), which can manifests with any one of a range of neurological or psychological disorders alongside variable physical features *(73,74)*.

Recently a large duplication of approx 16 Mb spanning 7q11.22 to 7q21.11 was identified in a boy with clinical features quite unlike WBS *(75)*. This patient presented at the age of 7 months with hypotonia and dysmorphic features. At 18 months old he has developmental delay, with greatest deficits in gross and oral motor skills, including expressive language. His facial features are not typical of WBS, with low set ears and a very small mouth, and he has no vocalization pattern and has not been weaned from the bottle. Because this duplication extends much further than the WBS region, it remains to be seen whether a smaller duplication of just the WBS interval would lead to similar or less complex features. The characterization of this patient does tell us that such a duplication is unlikely to result in any of the hallmark features of WBS, and that as such the search for dup(7)(q11.23) should be expanded to other phenotypic groups. Somerville et al. describes a reciprocal WBS duplication *(75a)*.

FUTURE DIRECTIONS

The repeat laden genomic structure of the WBS region predisposes to susceptibility for deletions, inversions, and, quite possibly, other more complex rearrangements. In order to develop the most accurate diagnostic tests and fully understand statistical relevance, it will be important to resolve all of the possible normal and disease-associated chromosomal variants associated with this region. Unpublished data from our group and collaborators (LA Pérez-Jurado, personal communication) indicate that in addition to the anomalies described in this chapter, there can also be variation in the number of LCRs, smaller rearrangements between the two adjacent LCRs, and duplications at this locus. In addition, there appears to be a background of gene conversion within these blocks, which makes identification of LCR-specific sequences impossible in some individuals *(31)*.

Subregions of the WBS segmental duplications also exist at other locations on chromosome 7, suggesting that additional rearrangements of this chromosome may occur through NAHR. These rearrangements could occur either as *de novo* or inherited germline events, or as somatic changes that may be involved in cancer initiation or progression. Indeed, more than 30 rearrangement breakpoints associated with malignancies have already been mapped to the 7q22.1 segmental duplication that includes WBS-like LCRs *(8)*.

Linking additional genes to WBS-subphenotypes will be an arduous task, and will likely necessitate the study of both patient samples and animal models. Several single gene mouse mutants have been generated already, but although some show aspects of WBS, no combination fully recapitulates the full phenotypic spectrum of this disorder *(76–79)*. It is likely that a multiple gene deletion knockout will provide a better model for WBS. Ultimately, however, the screening of patients with atypical WBS for smaller deletions or point mutations at specific sites, will provide the most definitive evidence of the genes contributing to the underlying molecular basis of this fascinating genomic and clinical condition.

SUMMARY

The WBS region on chromosome 7q11.23 is subject to numerous genomic rearrangements, including deletions, inversions, and duplications. A commonly deleted interval is present in the vast majority of individuals with the classic features of the disorder and encompasses between 26 and 28 genes, although the minimal critical region is thought to span only around 10–12 genes. Smaller deletions and inversions can give rise to subsets of the phenotype, but there is no clear-cut genotype–phenotype correlation, and the only gene definitely implicated in any aspect of the clinical features is *ELN*. There is a polymorphic inversion (WBSinv-1) present in between one-fourth to one-third of WBS parents, which predisposes the region to subsequent deletion and may have implications for genetic counseling. Deletion breakpoint mapping has shown that the nonallelic homologous recombination that leads to the common deletion often occurs within defined hotspots, some of which are gender-specific and one of which occurs only on the WBSinv-1 chromosome.

REFERENCES

1. Ewart AK, Morris CA, Atkinson D, et al. Hemizygosity at the elastin locus in a developmental disorder, Williams syndrome. Nat Genet 1993;5:11–16.
2. Curran ME, Atkinson DL, Ewart AK, Morris CA, Leppert MF, Keating MT. The elastin gene is disrupted by a translocation associated with supravalvular aortic stenosis. Cell 1993;73:159–168.
3. Li DY, Toland AE, Boak BB, et al. Elastin point mutations cause an obstructive vascular disease, supravalvular aortic stenosis. Hum Mol Genet 1997;6:1021–1028.
4. Tassabehji M, Metcalfe K, Donnai D, et al. Elastin: genomic structure and point mutations in patients with supravalvular aortic stenosis. Hum Mol Genet 1997;6:1029–1036.

5. Osborne LR, Herbrick JA, Greavette T, Heng HH, Tsui LC, Scherer SW. PMS2-related genes flank the rearrangement breakpoints associated with Williams syndrome and other diseases on human chromosome 7. Genomics 1997;45:402–406.

6. Pérez Jurado LA, Wang YK, Peoples R, Coloma A, Cruces J, Francke U. A duplicated gene in the breakpoint regions of the 7q11.23 Williams-Beuren syndrome deletion encodes the initiator binding protein TFII-I and BAP-135, a phosphorylation target of BTK. Hum Mol Genet 1998;7:325–334.

7. Osborne LR, Li M, Pober B, et al. A 1.5 million-base pair inversion polymorphism in families with Williams-Beuren syndrome. Nat Genet 2001;29:321–325.

8. Scherer SW, Cheung J, MacDonald JR, et al. Human chromosome 7: DNA sequence and biology. Science 2003;300:767–772.

9. Greenberg F. Williams syndrome professional symposium. Am J Med Genet Suppl 1990;6:85–88.

10. Stromme P, Bjornstad PG, Ramstad K. Prevalence estimation of Williams syndrome. J Child Neurol 2002;17:269–271.

11. Morris CA, Demsey SA, Leonard CO, Dilts C, Blackburn BL. Natural history of Williams syndrome: physical characteristics. J Pediatr 1988;113:318–326.

12. Pober BR, Dykens EM. Williams syndrome: an overview of medical, cognitive, and behavioral features. Child Adolesc Psych Clinics N Am 1996;5:929–943.

13. Cherniske E, Carpenter TO, Klaiman C, et al. Multisystem study of 20 older adults with Williams Syndrome. Am J Med Genet 2004;131A:255–264.

14. Mervis CB, Robinson BF, Bertrand J, Morris CA, Klein-Tasman BP, Armstrong SC. The Williams syndrome cognitive profile. Brain Cogn 2000;44:604–628.

15. Dilts CV, Morris CA, Leonard CO. Hypothesis for development of a behavioural phenotype in Williams syndrome. Am J Med Genet Suppl 1990;6:126–131.

16. Bellugi U, Bihrle A, Jernigan T, Trauner D, Doherty S. Neuropsychological, neurological and neuroanatomical profile of Williams syndrome. Am J Med Genet 1990;6:115–125.

17. Olson TM, Michels VV, Lindor NM, et al. Autosomal dominant supravalvular aortic stenosis: localization to chromosome 7. Hum Mol Genet 1993;2:869–873.

18. Kotzot D, Bernasconi F, Brecevic L, et al. Phenotype of the Williams-Beuren syndrome associated with hemizygosity at the elastin locus. Eur J Pediatr 1995;154:477–482.

19. Lowery MC, Morris CA, Ewart A, et al. Strong correlation of elastin deletions, detected by FISH, with Williams syndrome: evaluation of 235 patients. Am J Hum Genet 1995;57:49–53.

20. Mari A, Amati F, Mingarelli R, et al. Analysis of the elastin gene in 60 patients with clinical diagnosis of Williams syndrome. Hum Genet 1995;96:444–448.

21. Nickerson E, Greenberg F, Keating MT, McCaskill C, Shaffer LG. Deletions of the elastin gene at 7q11.23 occur in ~90% of patients with Williams syndrome. Am J Hum Genet 1995;56:1156–1161.

22. Jefferson RD, Burn J, Gaunt KL, Hunter S, Davison EV. A terminal deletion of the long arm of chromosome 4 [46,XX,del(4)(q33)] in an infant with phenotypic features of Williams syndrome. J Med Genet 1976;23:474–480.

23. Miles JH, Michalski KA. Familial 15q12 duplication associated with Williams phenotype. Am J Hum Genet 1983;35:144A.

24. Kaplan LC, Wharton R, Elias E, Mandell F, Donlon T, Latt SA. Clinical heterogeneity associated with deletions in the long arm of chromosome 15: Report of 3 new cases and their possible genetic significance. Am J Med Genet 1987;28:45–53.

25. Bzduch V, Lukacova M. Interstitial deletion of the long arm of chromosome 6(q22.2q23) in a boy with phenotypic features of Williams syndrome. Clin Genet 1989;35:230–231.

26. Colley A, Thakker Y, Ward H, Donnai D. Unbalanced 13;18 translocation and Williams syndrome. J Med Genet 1992;29:63–65.

27. Tupler R, Maraschio P, Gerardo A, Mainieri R, Lanzi G, Tiepolo L. A complex chromosome rearrangement with 10 breakpoints: tentative assignment of the locus for Williams syndrome to 4q33-q35.1. J Med Genet 1992;29:253–255.

28. Joyce CA, Zorich B, Pike SJ, Barber JC, Dennis NR. Williams-Beuren syndrome: phenotypic variability and deletions of chromosomes 7, 11, and 22 in a series of 52 patients. J Med Genet 1996;33:986–992.

29. Peoples R, Franke Y, Wang YK, et al. A physical map, including a BAC/PAC clone contig, of the Williams-Beuren syndrome—deletion region at 7q11.23. Am J Hum Genet 2000;66:47–68.

30. Valero MC, de Luis O, Cruces J, Pérez-Jurado LA. Fine-scale comparative mapping of the human 7q11.23 region and the orthologous region on mouse chromosome 5G: the low-copy repeats that flank the Williams-Beuren syndrome deletion arose at breakpoint sites of an evolutionary inversion(s). Genomics 2000;69:1–13.

31. Bayés M, Magano LF, Rivera N, Flores R, Pérez-Jurado LA. Mutational mechanisms of Williams-Beuren syndrome deletions. Am J Hum Genet 2003;73:131–151.

32. Pezzi N, Prieto I, Kremer L, et al. STAG3, a novel gene encoding a protein involved in meiotic chromosome pairing and location of STAG3-related genes flanking the Williams-Beuren syndrome deletion. FASEB J 2000;14:581–592.

33. Kipersztok S, Osawa GA, Liang LF, Modi WS, Dean J. POM-ZP3, a bipartite transcript derived from human ZP3 and a POM121 homologue. Genomics 1995;25:354–359.

34. DeSilva U, Elnitski L, Idol JR, et al. Generation and comparative analysis of approximately 3.3 Mb of mouse genomic sequence orthologous to the region of human chromosome 7q11.23 implicated in Williams syndrome. Genome Res 2002;12:3–15.

35. Edelmann L, Pandita RK, Morrow BE. Low-copy repeats mediate the common 3-Mb deletion in patients with velo-cardio-facial syndrome. Am J Hum Genet 1999;64:1076–1086.

36. Horii A, Han HJ, Sasaki S, Shimada M, Nakamura Y. Cloning, characterization and chromosomal assignment of the human genes homologous to yeast PMS1, a member of mismatch repair genes. Biochem Biophys Res Commun 1994;204:1257–1264.

37. Nicolaides NC, Carter KC, Shell BK, Papadopoulos N, Vogelstein B, Kinzler KW. Genomic organization of the human PMS2 gene family. Genomics 1995;30:195–206.

38. Probst FJ, Chen KS, Zhao Q, et al. A physical map of the mouse shaker-2 region contains many of the genes commonly deleted in Smith-Magenis syndrome (del17p11.2p11.2). Genomics 1999;55:348–352.

39. Bi W, Yan J, Stankiewicz P, et al. Genes in a refined Smith-Magenis syndrome critical deletion interval on chromosome 17p11.2 and the syntenic region of the mouse. Genome Res 2002;12:713–728.

40. Gimelli G, Pujana MA, Patricelli MG, et al. Genomic inversions of human chromosome 15q11-q13 in mothers of Angelman syndrome patients with class II (BP2/3) deletions. Hum Mol Genet 2003;12:849–858.

41. Goodman M. The genomic record of Humankind's evolutionary roots. Am J Hum Genet 1999;64:31–39.

42. Merla G, Ucla C, Guipponi M, Reymond A. Identification of additional transcripts in the Williams-Beuren syndrome critical region. Hum Genet 2002;110:429–438

43. DeSilva U, Massa H, Trask BJ, Green ED. Comparative mapping of the region of human chromosome 7 deleted in Williams syndrome. Genome Res 1999;9:428–436.

43a. Antonell A, de Luis O, Domingo-Roura X, Pérez-Jurado LA. Evolutionary mechanisms shaping the genomic structure of the Williams-Beuren syndrome chromosomal region at human 7q11.23. Genom Res 2005;15:1179–1188.

44. Dutly F, Schinzel A. Unequal interchromosomal rearrangements may result in elastin gene deletions causing the Williams-Beuren syndrome. Hum Mol Genet 1996;5:1893–1898.

45. Urban Z, Helms C, Fekete G, et al. 7q11.23 deletions in Williams syndrome arise as a consequence of unequal meiotic crossover. Am J Hum Genet 1996;59:958–962.

46. Baumer A, Dutly F, Balmer D, et al. High level of unequal meiotic crossovers at the origin of the 22q11.2 and 7q11.23 deletions. Hum Mol Genet 1998;7:887–894.

47. Pérez Jurado LA, Peoples R, Kaplan P, Hamel BC, Francke U. Molecular definition of the chromosome 7 deletion in Williams syndrome and parent-of-origin effects on growth. Am J Hum Genet 1996;59:781–792.

48. Wu YQ, Sutton VR, Nickerson E, et al. Delineation of the common critical region in Williams syndrome and clinical correlation of growth, heart defects, ethnicity, and parental origin. Am J Med Genet 1998;78:82–89.

49. Wang MS, Schinzel A, Kotzot D, et al. Molecular and clinical correlation study of Williams-Beuren syndrome: No evidence of molecular factors in the deletion region or imprinting affecting clinical outcome. Am J Med Genet 1999;86:34–43.

50. Robinson WP, Waslynka J, Bernasconi F, et al. Delineation of 7q11.2 deletions associated with Williams-Beuren syndrome and mapping of a repetitive sequence to within and to either side of the common deletion. Genomics 1996;34:17–23.

51. Gilbert-Dussardier B, Bonneau D, Gigarel N, et al. A novel microsatellite DNA marker at locus D7S1870 detects hemizygosity in 75% of patients with Williams syndrome. Am J Hum Genet 1995;56:542–544.

52. Wang YK, Pérez-Jurado LA, Francke U. A mouse single-copy gene, Gtf2i, the homolog of human GTF2I, that is duplicated in the Williams-Beuren syndrome deletion region. Genomics 1998;48:163–170.

53. Rivera N, Lucena J, Bayés M, Pérez-Jurado LA. Sex-preferential hotspots for non-allelic homologous recombination within segmental duplications in Williams-Beuren syndrome deletions. Am Soc Hum Genet 2004;A:849.
54. Kabuki T, Kawai T, Kin Y, et al. [A case of Williams syndrome with p47-phox-deficient chronic granulomatous disease] Nihon Rinsho Meneki Gakkai Kaishi 2003;26:299–303.
55. Gilbert-Barness E, Fox T, Morrow G, Luquette M, Pomerance H. Williams syndrome associated with crohn disease, multiple infections, and chronic granulomatous disease. Pediatr Pathol Mol Med 2004;23:29–37.
56. Antonell A, Del Campo M, Magano LF, et al. Hemizygosity at the NCF1 gene in Williams-Beuren syndrome patients decreases their risk of hypertension. Am Soc Hum Genet 2004;A:622.
57. Antoine HJ, Wijesuriya H, Appelbaum M, et al. Hypertension: risk in Williams syndrome is determined by gender and parent of origin. Am Soc Hum Genet 2004;A:221.
58. Frangiskakis JM, Ewart AK, Morris CA, et al. LIM-kinase1 hemizygosity implicated in impaired visuospatial constructive cognition. Cell 1996;86:59–69.
59. Botta A, Novelli G, Mari A, et al. Detection of an atypical 7q11.23 deletion in Williams syndrome patients which does not include the STX1A and FZD3 genes. Am J Med Genet 1999;36:478–480.
60. Tassabehji M, Metcalfe K, Karmiloff-Smith A, et al. Williams syndrome: use of chromosomal microdeletions as a tool to dissect cognitive and physical phenotypes. Am J Hum Genet 1999;64:118–125.
61. Del Campo M, Magano LF, Martinez Iglesias J, Pérez-Jurado LA. Partial features of Williams-Beuren syndrome in a family with a novel 700 kb 7q11.23 deletion. Eur J Hum Genet 2001;9:C055.
62. Gagliardi C, Bonaglia MC, Selicorni A, Borgatti R, Giorda R. Unusual cognitive and behavioural profile in a Williams syndrome patient with atypical 7q11.23 deletion. J Med Genet 2003;40:526–530.
63. Heller R, Rauch A, Luttgen S, Schroder B, Winterpacht A. Partial deletion of the critical 1.5 Mb interval in Williams-Beuren syndrome. J Med Genet 2003;40:E99.
64. Hirota H, Matsuoka R, Chen XN, et al. Williams syndrome deficits in visual spatial processing linked to GTF2IRD1 and GTF2I on chromosome 7q11.23. Genet Med 2003;5:311–321.
65. Morris CA, Mervis CB, Hobart HH, et al. GTF2I hemizygosity implicated in mental retardation in Williams syndrome: genotype-phenotype analysis of five families with deletions in the Williams syndrome region. Am J Med Genet 2003;123A:45–59.
66. Mizugishi K, Yamanaka K, Kuwajima K, Kondo I. Interstitial deletion of chromosome 7q in a patient with Williams syndrome and infantile spasms. J Hum Genet 1998;43:178–181.
67. Wu YQ, Nickerson E, Shaffer LG, Keppler-Noreuil K, Muilenburg A. A case of Williams syndrome with a large, visible cytogenetic deletion. J Med Genet 1999;36:928–932.
68. Morimoto M, An B, Ogami A, et al. Infantile spasms in a patient with Williams syndrome and craniosynostosis. Epilepsia 2003;44:1459–1462.
69. Stock AD, Spallone PA, Dennis TR, et al. Heat shock protein 27 gene: chromosomal and molecular location and relationship to Williams syndrome. Am J Med Genet 2003;120A:320–325.
70. Hobart HH, Gregg RG, Mervis CB, et al. Heterozygotes for the microinversion of the Williams-Beuren syndrome region have an increased risk for affected offspring. Am Soc Hum Genet 2004;A:891.
71. Scherer SW, Gripp KW, Lucena J, et al. Observation of a parental inversion variant in a rare Williams-Beuren syndrome family with two affected children. Hum Genet 2005;117:383–388.
72. Osborne LR, Joseph-George AM, Scherer SW. Williams-Beuren syndrome. In: *Congenital Heart Disease: Molecular Diagnostics* (Kearns-Jonker, M, ed.) Totowa, NJ: Humana, in press.
73. Potocki L, Chen KS, Park SS, et al. Molecular mechanism for duplication 17p11.2- the homologous recombination reciprocal of the Smith-Magenis microdeletion. Nat Genet 2000;24:84–87.
74. Ensenauer RE, Adeyinka A, Flynn HC, et al. Microduplication 22q11.2, an emerging syndrome: clinical, cytogenetic, and molecular analysis of thirteen patients. Am J Hum Genet 2003;73:1027–1040.
75. Seo EJ, Lanphear NE, Scherer SW, Osborne LR. Tandem duplication of chromosome 7q11.22-q21.11 in a patient with developmental delay. Am Soc Hum Genet 2004;A:731.
75a. Somerville MJ, Mervis CB, Young EJ, et al. Duplication of the Williams-Beuren locus related to severe expressive language delay. N Engl J Med, in press.
76. Li DY, Brooke B, Davis EC, et al. Elastin is an essential determinant of arterial morphogenesis. Nature 1998;393:276–280.

77. Hoogenraad CC, Koekkoek B, Akhmanova A, et al. Targeted mutation of Cyln2 in the Williams syndrome critical region links CLIP-115 haplo-insufficiency to neurodevelopmental abnormalities in mice. Nat Genet 2002;32:116–127.

78. Meng Y, Zhang Y, Tregoubov V, et al. Abnormal spine morphology and enhanced LTP in LIMK-1 knockout mice. Neuron 2002;35:121–133.

79. Onay T, Young E, Lipina T,et al. Mice heterozygous for the GTF2I transcription factors exhibit behaviours seen in Williams-Beuren syndrome. Am Soc Hum Genet 2004;A:67.

16 Sotos Syndrome

Naohiro Kurotaki, MD, PhD and
Naomichi Matsumoto, MD, PhD

INTRODUCTION

Sotos syndrome (SoS) is a well-known overgrowth syndrome with mental retardation, specific craniofacial features, and advanced bone age. Since *NSD1* haploinsufficiency was proven to be the major cause of SoS in 2002, many intragenic mutations and chromosomal microdeletions (MDs) involving the entire *NSD1* gene have been described. The sizes of most SoS MDs are identical and a specific genomic architecture around these MDs was found. Recently, precise analyses of the low-copy repeats (LCRs) flanking the SoS common deletion showed that the deletion arises through nonhomologous recombination (NAHR) utilizing the LCRs, and proved that SoS is a genomic disorder.

SoS (OMIM no. 117550), also known as cerebral gigantism, was originally reported by Sotos et al. *(1)* in 1964. SoS is characterized by overgrowth, characteristic craniofacial features, developmental delay, and advanced bone age *(2)*. In 2002, *NSD1* disruption was found in a patient with SoS and haploinsufficiency of *NSD1* has been shown to be a major cause of SoS *(3)*. In the Japanese population, about half cases have chromosomal MDs involving the entire *NSD1* gene *(3,4)*. The majority of MDs are identical *(4)* and the NAHR was shown to be a causative mechanism *(5,6)*. In this chapter, we focus on recent progress in clinical and genetic aspects of SoS. The genomic architecture around the common MD will be presented.

From: *Genomic Disorders: The Genomic Basis of Disease*
Edited by: J. R. Lupski and P. Stankiewicz © Humana Press, Totowa, NJ

CLINICAL FEATURES

SoS typically presents with overgrowth, characteristic craniofacial features, developmental delay, and advanced bone age *(2)*.

Overgrowth: overgrowth usually starts prenatally and can be observed especially in early infancy *(2)*. However, overgrowth seems to normalize during childhood and may not be found in adulthood *(7–9)*.

Craniofacial features: macrocephaly, a high hairline with coarse hair growth, high arched palate, and prominent jaw are common findings. The occipitofrontal circumference is more than 97th percentile in childhood *(2)*.

Developmental delay: developmental delay is a cardinal symptom and can be attributed to central nervous system abnormalities *(2)*. Speech delay and abnormal motor development are commonly observed. Dilatation of cerebral ventricles is sometimes noted. In neuroimaging studies of 40 SoS patients, prominence of the trigone and the occipital horns was found in 90 and 75%, respectively *(10)*.

Advanced bone age: advanced bone age was observed in 31 of 37 (84%) SoS patients *(2)* and does not appear to be associated with abnormalities of collagen metabolism *(11)*.

Others: cardiac, urogenital, musculoskeletal, and ophthalmologic anomalies have been observed also *(2,12–15)*. Neoplasms in SoS have been found with a frequency of 2.2–3.9% *(16)*.

DIAGNOSIS OF SOS

SoS has been diagnosed based on clinical manifestations, however, the diagnosis is difficult when craniofacial features are less remarkable or are similar to those of other overgrowth syndromes with overlapping phenotypes. Weaver and Beckwith-Wiedemann syndromes associated with *NSD1* abnormalities showed similar facial features to those of SoS *(17,18)*. Overgrowth tends to normalize in adulthood *(9)*, thus, the diagnosis is easier in early life *(19)*. Objective diagnosis of SoS has been substantially improved, since the discovery of *NSD1* mutations in SoS *(3)*. The major diagnostic criteria proposed by Cole and Hughes *(2)* include pre- and postnatal characteristic overgrowth with advanced bone age, and developmental delay. However, a recent report by Rio et al. *(20)* indicated that typical facial appearance and macrocephaly were consistently recognized but overgrowth or advanced bone age was not always observed in patients with *NSD1* mutations. Therefore, the diagnostic criteria for SoS likely need to be carefully revised after collecting more data on the phenotypic spectrum in SoS patients with known *NSD1* abnormalities. "Sotos-like syndrome" usually has been referred to a large spectrum of patients that do not fulfill the major criteria for SoS *(2,17,20,21)*.

MOLECULAR GENETICS

NSD1 Structure and Functions

Mouse *Nsd1* was originally isolated in 1998 as one of the nuclear proteins interacting with retinoic acid receptors and thyearsoid hormone receptors *(22)*. The human *NSD1* was identified at the 5q35 breakpoint of a SoS patient with an apparently balanced translocation t(5;8)(q35;q24.1) *(23,24)*. *NSD1* has an 8088-bp open reading frame consisting of 23 exons and is translated into a 2696 amino-acid protein. NSD1 protein has at least six functional domains, a su[var]3-9,enhancer-of-zest,trithorax (SET) domain, two proline-tryptophan-tryptophan-proline (PWWP) domains, and three plant homeodomain protein-finger (PHD) domains with nuclear localization signals. The SET domain of NSD1 showed methyl transferase activity for Lys36 of histone H3 (H3-K36) and Lys20 of histone H4 (H4-K20), whose methylation may result in transcriptional silencing of developmentally regulated genes *(25)*. PHD finger domains are found in a large number of chromatin regulatory factors like CBP/ p300, and chromatin remodeling protein ACF *(26)*. The PWWP domain was initially identified in the protein encoded by the Wolf-Hirschhorn syndrome candidate gene 1 *(WHSC1) (27)*. The essential function is still unknown, however, the PWWP domain is often associated with SET domains and is thought to be an essential for development *(28)*. Thus, these six protein domains are suggested to regulate chromatin formations and gene transcriptions *(23)*. Homozygous knockout of *Nsd1* in mice led to embryonic death at 10.5 days and gastrulation failure, suggesting that Nsd1 may be a protein regulating development especially in an early post-implantation period *(25)*.

The NSD1 is a portion of a fusion protein in a recurrent translocation t(5;11)(q35;p15.5) found in childhood acute myeloid leukemia *(29–31)*. Six non-SoS cases of acute myeloid leukemia had fusion transcripts of *NSD1* and *NUP98* (nucleoporin 98 gene) *(29–31)*. SoS has been suggested to be associated with neoplasms *(32)*. It is also important to address whether *NSD1* abnormality in itself can cause tumorigenesis in the near future.

NSD1 Mutations

NSD1 mutations in SoS have been reported by several groups *(3,4,17,20,33–36)*. To date, among a total of 91 point mutations (PM) have been identified in 241 patients suspected of SoS. Seventy-one protein truncation mutations and 20 missense mutations have been reported with 62 being *de novo* (Fig. 1). Five protein truncation mutations were found in 23 Sotos-like patients *(17,20)*. Protein truncation mutations are spread throughout the entire *NSD1* coding regions; however, missense mutations cluster at the 3' part of *NSD1* where most of the known functional domains are located. In SoS, six missense mutations have been identified in the SET domain, three in the PHD domains and three in the PWWP domains.

Thus, among different world populations, *NSD1* mutations have been consistently shown to be the major cause of SoS. Interestingly, the frequency of MDs involving *NSD1* is quite different. In the Japanese population, about half of the cases (49/95) had MDs, whereas microdeletions are observed in only 11% of cases (13/118) analyzed in European populations *(3,4,17,20,33–36)*. The reason for this observed difference remains to be elucidated.

Genotype/Phenotype Correlation

Interestingly, some clinical differences between SoS patients with PMs and MDs have been reported *(14,17,20)*. Nagai et al. *(14)* compared clinical phenotypes between 5 PM and 21 MD SoS patients. Both PM and MD cases showed typical craniofacial features. Remarkably, the peak height at younger than 6 years of age and the intelligence quotient/developmental quotient (IQ/ DQ) in patients older than 6 years were significantly different between PM and MD patients. The values of the standard deviation (SD) scores were 3.3 (PM) and 2.2 (MD), and IQ/DQ (mean) were 78 ± 12 (PM) and 57 ± 12 (MD), respectively. In addition, MD patients predominantly showed cardiovascular and urogenital abnormalities, and recurrent convulsions.

Rio et al. *(20)* compared 16 PM and 6 MD patients. Two MD patients showed typical SoS, but the other four patients were diagnosed as Sotos-like syndrome because they did not have overgrowth (height less than +2 SDs), or advanced bone age. Four out of six MD patients had severe mental retardation with no speech at all. Cardiovascular anomalies were found in three

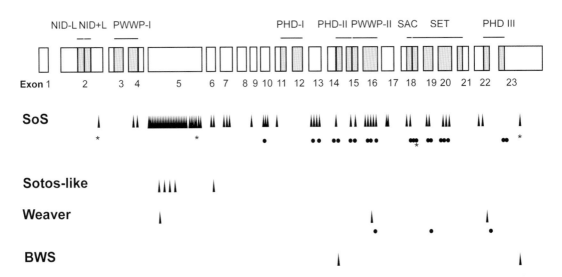

Fig. 1. The structure of *NSD1* with mutations in Sotos syndrome, Sotos-like syndrome, and other syndromes. Each box indicates exon, gray regions show functional domains (SET, PWWP, and PHD) and nuclear receptor interacting domains, NID^{-L} and NID^{+L}. Start and stop codons are located at exon 2 and 23, respectively. Arrowheads and filled circles indicate protein truncation mutations and missense mutations. Asterisks below arrowhead or circle show familial mutations. The same mutation in different individuals was shown as different arrowheads.

out of six MD cases. Among 16 PM cases, 14 were diagnosed as typical SoS and 2 as Sotos-like syndrome owing to the absence of advanced bone age. The degree of mental retardation was variable and 2 out of 16 patients had cardiac septal defect. Both reports suggested that mental retardation in SoS patients with MD is more severe than in patients with PM and cardiovascular complications in SoS patients with MD are more frequent than in those with PM.

NSD1 Mutations in Other Overgrowth Syndromes

Notably, in six cases of Weaver syndrome, whose phenotype overlaps significantly with SoS *(17,18,37)* and in two cases of another overgrowth syndrome, Beckwith-Wiedemann syndrome (BWS), *NSD1* mutations were identified *(18)*. In Weaver syndrome, 6 cases out of 13 had *NSD1* intragenic PM *(17,20)*, suggesting that SoS and Weaver syndrome are allelic. The majority of BWS is caused by either genetic alterations (11p15 paternal uniparental disomy or *CDKN1C* mutations) or epigenetic defects (demethylation of the *KvDMR1* region of *KCNQ1OT* and hypermethylation of *H19) (38–40)*. Interestingly, in addition to two BWS cases with *NSD1* mutations, two SoS cases without *NSD1* abnormality showed abnormal status of the 11p15 region (demethylation of *KCNQ1OT* and a paternal isodisomy of 11p15) *(18)*. These data indicate challenges for proper clinical diagnosis of even well-established overgrowth syndromes. Another possibility is an unknown common pathway among the three syndromes. It is very important to evaluate *NSD1* status in other overgrowth syndromes to elucidate whether *NSD1* mutations are specific not only for SoS.

IS SOS A GENOMIC DISORDER?

Fifty MDs have been analyzed using fluorescence *in situ* hybridization and microarray comparative genomic hybridization *(4)*. Three different types of microdeletions were delineated, among which, the approx 2-Mb MD I (Fig. 2A) was the most common (found in 46 out of 50 patients). In the other four cases two smaller MDs were recognized. Highly homologous regions at each deletion breakpoints of the MD I were identified *(4–6)*. These LCRs were termed Sotos syndrome distal-repeat (SoS-DREP, approx 429 kb) and proximal-repeat (SoS-PREP, approx 390 kb) (Fig. 2). Sequence comparisons of SoS-DREP and SoS-PREP revealed that six sequence homology subunits (A–F) of PREP showed more than 96% identity to DREP (Fig. 2B). Their sizes of SoS-PREP subunits were 123.6 kb (A), 20.1 kb (B), 62.8 kb (C), 7.8 kb (D), 8.2 kb (E), and 93.9 kb (F) and those of SoS-DREP subunits were 119.1 kb (A), 19.7 kb (B), 68.7 kb (C), 7.8 kb (D), 8.3 kb (E), 82.8 kb (F), and 50.1 kb (C'). Each of the homologous subunits, with the exception of one, is located in an inverted orientation and the order of subunits is different between the two SoS-REPs. Only the subunit C' in SoS-DREP is oriented directly with respect to the subunit C in SoS-PREP. These subunits are more than 99% identical. Two recent reports showed that the subunit C' in SoS-DREP and the subunit C in SoS-PREP, were utilized as a substrate of NAHR of the SoS common deletion *(5,6)*. In addition, the reports indicated that the crossover events occurred in those subunits and that an approx 80% of crossover hotspots were within an approx 3-kb genomic sequence in those subunits *(5,6)* (Fig. 2).

These data established that SoS is a new genomic disorder and an NAHR mechanism is a consistent mechanism for generation of the SoS common deletion as in other genomic disorder reported *(41–43)*.

IS SOS A CONTIGUOUS GENE SYNDROME?

There are at least 22 genes that map within the common deleted region (UCSC Genome Browser, May 2004 Assembly, http://genome.ucsc.edu/cgi-bin/hgGateway) (Fig. 2). Both SoS-REPs contain two genes, *THOC3* and *NY-REN-7* (Fig. 2). *THOC3* and *NY-REN-7* have open reading frames that are completely conserved in SoS-PREP and SoS-DREP. The *PROP1* gene maps only to SoS-DREP between subunit E and C' (Fig. 2A). Among those 22 genes deleted, *NSD1*, the plasma coagulation factor 12 gene (*F12*, OMIM +234000), the prophet of the *PIT-1* gene (*PROP1*, OMIM +601538), and the xylosylprotein β 1,4-galactosyltransferase, polypeptide 7 gene (*B4GALT7*, also known as xylosylprotein 4-β-galactosyltransferase I gene, *XGTP1*, OMIM *604327) may be directly related to human phenotypes.

F12 encodes the coagulation factor XII, also known as Hageman factor. Heterozygous deletion of *F12* may result in partial F12 deficiency, which could present with a slight to moderate bleeding tendency *(44,45)*. Low levels of factor XII activity may also be a risk factor for repeated spontaneous abortions or skin ulcers *(46,47)*. A common polymorphism in the 5'-untranslated region of *F12*, the c.46C > T substitution, was found to be associated with low F12 level *(48)*. In cases of c.46T/T, the value of F12 was remarkably decreased. Soria et al. *(49)* reported that the 5q33-qter region is a quantitative risk factor for thrombosis using genome wide linkage analysis. A novel homozygous p.W484C mutation was shown to induce low F12 levels *(50)*. It is important to evaluate F12 in SoS patients with MDs, although such a risk has not been known in SoS.

Homozygous or compound-heterozygous defects of *PROP1* result in combined pituitary hormone deficiency including GH, PRL, TSH, LH and FSH (OMIM +601538) *(51)*. So far,

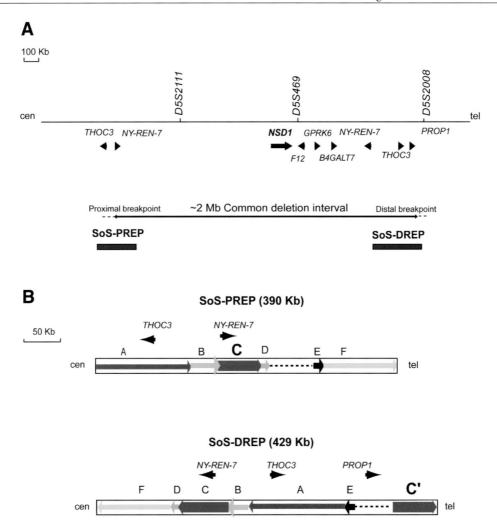

Fig. 2. (A) Physical map depicting microdeletions found in Sotos syndrome (SoS) and two low-copy repeat sequences, termed proximal-repeat (SoS-PREP) and distal-repeat (SoS-DREP) at 5q35. The Sos-REPs, indicated as black boxes, are proximal and distal to *NSD1*. Among 22 genes that map within the deletion interval, *NSD1*, the SoS-REP-specific predicted genes (*THO3*, *NY-REN-7*, and *PROP1*), and possible human phenotype-related genes (*F12*, *GPRK6*, *B4GAL4T7*) are presented. *THOC3* and *NY-REN-7* map to both SoS-PREP and SoS-DREP. Bold bi-directional arrow represents a deleted region. An approx 2-Mb microdeletion is the most commonly observed in SoS. (B) There are six subunits of more than 96% sequence identity between the proximal and the distal SoS-REPs (A–F); their orientation is depicted as arrow. All subunits except C' are inverted with respect to each other. Dotted lines indicate unique sequence in low-copy repeats. Three relevant genes are shown.

three SoS cases associated with hypothyearsoidism have been reported *(52,53)*. Unmasking of the recessive allele is possible when one allele harbors a PM and the other is deleted. It may be worth investigating *PROP1* if hypothyearsoidism is observed.

   B4GALT7 regulates the synthesis of various glycosaminoglycans (GAGs). GAGs are basic components of heparin/heparan sulfate or those of chondroitin sulfate/dermatan sulfate and have an important role in the formation of various tissues and organs *(54)*. Defects of GAGs may be possibly responsible for the various forms of so-called mucopoly-saccharidoses. In the progeroid type of Ehlers-Danlos syndrome, compound heterozygosity for p.A186D and p.L206P mutations of *B4GALT7* was confirmed. The father was heterozy-gous for the p.L206P allele and mother heterozygous for the p.A186D allele *(55,56)*. Although only one case with such mutations has been reported, carrier status for such PMs in contributions with hemizygous deletion of *B4GALT7* in SoS patients with MDs could contribute to phenotypic variability.

GPRK6 encodes G protein-coupled receptor kinase 6 protein (GPRK6) (OMIM *600869), which can regulate G protein-coupled receptors. Using immunohistochemistry, GPRK6 expression was confirmed in striatal neurons receiving dopaminergic input and postsynaptic D2/D3 dopamine receptors were targets of GPRK6 *(57)*. Investigation of *GPRK6* by gene targeting to create a knockout animal shows higher sensitivity to psychostimulants including cocaine and amphetamine especially in homozygous mice rather than heterozygous, suggest-ing that such high sensitivity may be related to some potential psychiatric diseases in human *(58)*. It would be interesting to evaluate for different psychiatric and behavioral aspects between SoS cases with MD versus PM.

The influence of the deletion of 21 genes other than *NSD1* needs to be carefully evaluated, as some genes may affect the severity of phenotypes in MD patients.

FUTURE DIRECTION

Rearrangement-prone regions of the human genome including LCRs have been challenging to sequence *(59,60)*. Validation and mapping of MD breakpoints at the nucleotide level should provide further insights into the mechanisms of DNA rearrangement. Functional studies of *NSD1* are required for elucidating pathophysiological aspects of SoS. Intensive molecular analyses of 282 patients with SoS, Sotos-like syndrome, and Weaver syndrome revealed the *NSD1* abnormalities in 168 cases; *NSD1* was intact in the other remaining 114 cases. Improved methods to detect other types of *NSD1* abnormalities, including partial deletion and nucleotide changes of introns and promoter regions, and more data of clinical phenotypes observed in patients with MDs and PMs should reveal further genotype/phenotype correlations and pro-vide insights into SoS pathophysiological mechanisms.

ACKNOWLEDGMENT

We would like to express our gratitude to Dr. Remco Visser, MD (Department of Human Genetics, Nagasaki University Graduate School of Biomedical Sciences) for critical reviewing of this manuscript. Naohiro Kurotaki is a recipient of the grant for Medical Research of Alumni Association of Nagasaki University School of Medicine and a Nagasaki Medical Association Research Subsidy.

REFERENCES

1. Sotos JF, Dodge PR, Muirhead D, Crawford JD, Talbot NB. Cerebral gigantism in childhood: a syndrome of excessively rapid growth with acromegalic features and a nonprogressive neurologic disorder. N Eng J Med 1964;271:109–116.
2. Cole TRP, Hughes HE. Sotos syndrome: a study of the diagnostic criteria and natural history. J Med Genet 1994;31:20–32.

3. Kurotaki N, Imaizumi K, Harada N, et al. Haploinsufficiency of NSD1 causes Sotos syndrome. Nat Genet 2002;30:365–366.

4. Kurotaki N, Harada N, Shimokawa O, et al. Fifty microdeletions among 112 cases of Sotos syndrome: low copy repeats possibly mediate the common deletion. Hum Mutat 2003;22:378–387.

5. Visser R, Shimokawa O, Harada N, et al. Identification of a 3.0-kb major recombination hotspot in patients with Sotos Syndrome who carry a common 1.9-Mb microdeletion. Am J Hum Genet 2005;76:52–67.

6. Kurotaki N, Stankiewicz P, Wakui K, Niikawa N, Lupski JR. Sotos syndrome common deletion is mediated by directly oriented subunits within inverted Sos-REP low-copy repeat. Hum Mol Genet 2005;14:532–542.

7. Chen C-P, Lin S-P, Chang T-Y, et al. Perinatal imaging findings of inherited Sotos syndrome. Prenat Diagn 2002;22:887–892.

8. Cole TRP, Hughes HE. Sotos syndrome. J Med Genet 1990;27:571–576.

9. Agwu JC, Shaw NJ, Kirk J, Chapman S, Ravine D, Cole TRP. Growth in Sotos syndrome. Arch Dis Child 1999;80:339–342.

10. Schaefer GB, Bodensteiner JB, Buehler BA, Lin A, Cole TRP. The neuroimaging findings in Sotos syndrome. Am J Med Genet 1997;68:462–465.

11. Rao VH, Buehler BA, Schaefer GB. Accelerated linear growth and advanced bone age in Sotos syndrome is not associated with abnormalities of collagen metabolism. Clin Biochem 1998;31:241–249.

12. Noreau DR, Al-Ata J, Jutras L, Teebi AS. Congenital heart defects in Sotos syndrome. Am J Med Genet 1998;79:327–328.

13. Tsukahara M, Murakami K, Iino H, Tateishi H, Fujita K, Uchida M. Congenital heart defects in Sotos syndrome. Am J Med Genet 1999;84:172.

14. Nagai T, Matsumoto N, Kurotaki N, et al. Sotos syndrome and haploinsufficiency of NSD1: clinical features of intragenic mutations and submicroscopic deletions. J Med Genet 2003;40:285–289.

15. Maino DM, Kofman J, Flynn MF, Lai L. Ocular manifestations of Sotos syndrome. J Am Optom Assoc 1994;65:339–346.

16. Visser R, Matsumoto N. Genetics of Sotos syndrome. Curr Opin Pediatr 2003;15:598–606.

17. Douglas J, Hanks S, Temple IK, et al. NSD1 mutations are the major cause of Sotos syndrome and occur in some cases of Weaver syndrome but are rare in other overgrowth phenotypes. Am J Hum Genet 2003;72:132–143.

18. Baujat G, Rio M, Rossignol S, et al. Paradoxical NSD1 mutations in Beckwith-Wiedemann syndrome and 11p15 anomalies in Sotos syndrome. Am J Hum Genet 2004;74:715–720.

19. Tatton-Brown K, Rahman N. Clinical features of NSD1-positive Sotos syndrome. Clin Dysmorphol 2004;13:199–204.

20. Rio M, Clech L, Amiel J, et al. Spectrum of NSD1 mutations in Sotos and Weaver syndromes. J Med Genet 200340:436–440.

21. Amiel J, Faivre L, Wilson L, et al. Dysmorphism, variable overgrowth, normal bone age, and severe developmental delay: a "Sotos-like" syndrome? J Med Genet 2002;39:148–152.

22. Huang N, vom Baur E, Garnier J-M, et al. Two distinct nuclear receptor interaction domains in NSD1, a novel SET protein that exhibits characteristics of both corepressors and coactivators. Embo J 1998;17:3398–3412.

23. Kurotaki N, Harada N, Yoshiura K-I, Sugano S, Niikawa N, Matsumoto N. Molecular characterization of NSD1, a human homolog of the mouse Nsd1 gene. Gene 2001;279:197–204.

24. Imaizumi K, Kimura J, Matsuo M, et al. Sotos syndrome associated with a de novo balanced reciprocal translocation t(5;8)(q35;q24.1). Am J Med Genet2002;107:58–60.

25. Rayasam GV, Wendling O, Angrand P-O, et al. NSD1 is essential for early post-implantation development and has a catalytically active SET domain. Embo J 2003;22:3153–3163.

26. Gozani O, Karuman P, Jones DR, et al. The PHD finger of the chromatin-associated protein ING2 functions as a nuclear phosphoinositide receptor. Cell 2003;114:99–111.

27. Stec I, Wright TJ, van Ommen G-JB, et al. WHSC1, a 90 kb SET domain-containing gene, expressed in early development and homologous to a Drosophila dysmorphy gene maps in the Wolf-Hirschhorn syndrome critical region and is fused to IgH in t(4;14) multiple myeloma. Hum Mol Genet 1998;7:1071–1082.

28. Ge Y-Z, Pu M-T, Gowher H, Wu H-P, Ding J-P, Jeltsch A, and Xu G-L (2004) Chromatin targeting of de novo DNA methyltransferases by the PWWP domain. J Biol Chem, 279, 25447-25454.

29. Jaju RJ, Fidler C, Haas OA, et al. A novel gene, NSD1, is fused to NUP98 in the t(5;11)(q35;p15.5) in de novo childhood acute myeloid leukemia. Blood 2001;98:1264–1267.

30. Brown J, Jawad M, Twigg SRF, et al. A cryptic t(5;11)(q35;p15.5) in 2 children with acute myeloid leukemia with apparently normal karyotypes, identified by a multiplex fluorescence in situ hybridization telomere assay. Blood 2002;99:2526–2531.

31. Panarello C, Rosanda C, Morerio C. Cryptic translocation t(5;11)(q35;p15.5) with involvement of the NSD1 and NUP98 genes without 5q deletion in childhood acute myeloid leukemia. Genes Chromosomes Cancer 200235:277–281.

32. Cohen MM, Jr. Tumor and nontumors in Sotos syndrome. Am J Med Genet 1998;84:173–175.

33. Höglund P, Kurotaki N, Kytölä S, Miyake N, Somer M, Matsumoto N. Familial Sotos syndrome is caused by a novel 1 bp deletion of the NSD1 gene. J Med Genet 2003;40:51–54.

34. Kamimura J, Endo Y, Kurotaki N, et al. Identification of eight novel NSD1 mutations in Sotos syndrome. J Med Genet 2003;40:e126.

35. Türkmen S, Gillessen-Kaesbach G, Meinecke P, et al. Mutations in NSD1 are responsible for Sotos syndrome, but are not a frequent finding in other overgrowth phenotypes. Eur J Hum Genet 2003;11:858–865.

36. de Boer L, Kant SG, Karperien M, et al. Genotype-phenotype correlation in patients suspected of having Sotos syndrome. Horm Res 2004;62:197–207.

37. Opitz JM, Weaver DW, Reynolds JFJr. The syndromes of Sotos and Weaver: reports and review. Am J Med Genet 1998;79:294–304.

38. Li M, Squire JA, Weksberg R. Molecular genetics of Wiedemann-Beckwith syndrome. Am J Med Genet 1998;79:253–259.

39. Weksberg R, Smith AC, Squire J, Sadowski P. Beckwith-Wiedemann syndrome demonstrates a role for epigenetic control of normal development. Hum Mol Genet 2003;12:R61–R68.

40. Jiang Y-H, Bressler J, Beaudet AL. Epigenetics and human disease. Annu Rev Genomics Hum Genet 2004;5:479–510.

41. Inoue K, Lupski JR. Molecular mechanisms for genomic disorders. Annu Rev Genomics Hum Genet 2002;3:199–242.

42. Stankiewicz P, Lupski JR. Genome architecture, rearrangements and genomic disorders. Trends Genet 2002;18:74–82

43. Shaw CJ, Lupski JR. Implications of human genome architecture for rearrangement-based disorders: the genomic basis of disease. Hum Mol Genet 2004;13:R57–R64.

44. Miwa S, Asai I, Tsukada T, Shimizu M, Teramura K, Sunaga Y. Hageman factor deficiency. Report of a case found in a Japanese girl. Acta Haematol 1968;39:36–41.

45. Egeberg O. Factor XII defect and hemorrhage. Evidence for a new type of hereditary hemostatic disorder. Thromb Diath Haemorrh 1970;23:432–440.

46. Pauer H-U, Burfeind P, Köstering H, Emons G, Hinney B. Factor XII deficiency is strongly associated with primary recurrent abortions. Fertil Steril 2003;80:590–594.

47. Sato-Matsumura KC, Matsumura T, Hayashi H, Atsumi T, Kobayashi H. Factor XII deficiency: a possible cause of livedo with ulceration? Br J Dermatol 2000;143:897–899.

48. Kanaji T, Okamura T, Osaki K, et al. A common genetic polymorphism (46 C to T substitution) in the 5'-untranslated region of the coagulation factor XII gene is associated with low translation efficiency and decrease in plasma factor XII level. Blood 1998;91:2010–2014.

49. Soria JM, Almasy L, Souto JC, et al. A quantitative-trait locus in the human factor XII gene influences both plasma factor XII levels and susceptibility to thrombotic disease. Am J Hum Genet 2002;70:567–574.

50. Wada H, Nishioka J, Kasai Y, et al. Molecular characterization of coagulation factor XII deficiency in a Japanese family. Thromb Haemost 2003;90:59–63.

51. Rodriguez R, Andersen B. Cellular determination in the anterior pituitary gland: PIT-1 and PROP-1 mutations as causes of human combined pituitary hormone deficiency. Minerva Endocrinol 2003;28:123–133.

52. Sotos JF, Romshe CA, Cutler EA. Cerebral gigantism and primary hypothyearsoidism: pleiotropy or incidental concurrence. Am J Med Genet 1978;2:201–205.

53. Hulse JA. Two children with cerebral gigantism and congenital primary hypothyearsoidism. Dev Med Child Neurol 1981;23:242–246.

54. Amado M, Almeida R, Schwientek T, Clausen H. Identification and characterization of large galacto-syltransferase gene families: galactosyltransferases for all functions. Biochim Biophys Acta 1999;1473:35–53.

55. Okajima T, Fukumoto S, Furukawa K, Urano T. Molecular basis for the progeroid variant of Ehlers-Danlos syndrome. Identification and characterization of two mutations in galactosyltransferase I gene. J Biol Chem 1999;274:28,841–28,844.

56. Almeida R, Levery SB, Mandel U, et al. Cloning and expression of a proteoglycan UDP-galactose:beta-xylose beta1,4-galactosyltransferase I. A seventh member of the human beta4-galactosyltransferase gene family. J Biol Chem 1999;274:26,165–26,171.
57. Haribabu B, Snyderman R. Identification of additional members of human G protein-coupled receptor kinase multigene family. Proc Natl Acad Sci USA 1993;90:9398–9402.
58. Gainetdinov RR, Bohn LM, Sotnikova TD, et al. Dopaminergic supersensitivity in G protein-coupled receptor kinase 6-deficient mice. Neuron 2003;38:291–303.
59. Cheung J, Estivill X, Khaja R, et al. Genome-wide detection of segmental duplications and potential assembly errors in the human genome sequence. Genome Biol 2003;4:R25
60. Eicher EE, Clark RA, She X. Assessment of the sequence gaps: unfinished business in a finished human genome. Nat Rev Genet 2004;5:345–354.

17 X Chromosome Rearrangements

Pauline H. Yen, PhD

CONTENTS

BACKGROUND

X chromosome rearrangements usually convey clinical manifestations in the hemizygous males and are, thus, readily ascertained. They are found in all parts of the X chromosome and are associated with more than 20 disorders. Some of the rearrangements are the results of homologous recombination between low-copy repeats (LCRs) on the X chromosome or between large homologous regions on the X and Y chromosome, whereas others are caused by nonhomologous end-joining (NHEJ). For most large deletions associated with contiguous gene syndromes, the deletion breakpoints remain uncharacterized. The deletions, as well as inversions and duplications on the X chromosome, occur mainly in male germ cells, indicating intrachromatid or sister chromatid exchange as the underlying mechanism.

INTRODUCTION

Among all human chromosomes, the X chromosome seems to have more than its share of genomic disorders identified so far *(1)*. There are two main reasons for the apparent prevalence of genomic disorders on the X chromosome. The hemizygous status of the X chromosome in males allows phenotypic manifestation of rare recessive genomic disorders that would have escaped detection if they were present on an autosome. In addition, high homology shared between the X and the Y chromosome makes the X chromosome specifically prone to X/Y translocation, resulting in the deletion of the terminal sequences *(2)*. To date, more than 20 genomic disorders have been identified on the X chromosome. Deletions associated with the genomic disorders can be easily detected in the males by polymerase chain reaction or Southern

From: *Genomic Disorders: The Genomic Basis of Disease*
Edited by: J. R. Lupski and P. Stankiewicz © Humana Press, Totowa, NJ

blotting, whereas the carrier status of a female is usually determined by fluorescence *in situ* hybridization (FISH) analysis *(3–6)*. In this chapter, X-linked genomic disorders are grouped according to the underlying mechanisms such as nonallelic homologous recombination (NAHR) between direct LCRs, NAHR between inverted LCRs, and NHEJ. For most of the *Short Stature Homeobox* (*SHOX*) deletions and contiguous gene syndromes, the breakpoints have not been characterized and, thus, the mechanisms remain unclear.

DELETIONS/DUPLICATIONS CAUSED BY NAHR BETWEEN DIRECT LCRS

Most cases of X-linked ichthyosis (XLI), color blindness, and incontinential pigmenti (IP) are caused by recurrent deletions resulting from NAHR between direct LCRs *(7–9)*. In XLI the LCRs flank the steroid sulfatase (*STS*) gene, in color blindness the color pigment genes reside within the LCRs, and in IP the LCRs are one within and one outside the nuclear factor *(NF)*-κB *essential modulator* (*NEMO*) gene. When NAHR occurs between two direct repeats on the same chromatid, it generates only deletion (Fig. 1A). If the recombination involves two X chromosome homologs or sister chromatids, it generates both duplication and deletion (Fig. 1A). Reciprocal duplications have been identified at the color pigment gene cluster and the *NEMO* locus *(8,10)*. Although duplications at the *STS* locus have also been reported, whether they involve the same LCRs as the recurrent deletion remains to be determined *(11)*. Studies on *de novo NEMO* deletions in IP patients show that most cases occur in the paternal germ cells, indicating unequal crossover between sister chromatids or intrachromatid recombination as the underlying mechanism *(9)*.

X-Linked Ichthyosis and the STS Gene at Xp22.3

XLI (MIM 308100) affects approx 1 in 5000 males worldwide *(12)*. It is caused by a deficiency of the microsomal enzyme steroid sulfatase (STS) that hydrolyzes a variety of 3β-hydroxysteroid sulfates. The *STS* gene at Xp22.3 consists of 10 exons and spans approx 135 kb of genomic DNA *(13)*. There is a truncated *STS* pseudogene at Yq11 that contains sequences homologous to five of the exons.

XLI is one of the first genomic disorders found to have recurrent deletions flanked by LCR elements *(7)*. Up to 90% of XLI patients have the entire *STS* gene deleted *(14)*. The deletions are heterogeneous in size and the breakpoints spread over several megabases. A majority of the deletions have common breakpoints within two direct LCRs, S232A and S232B, that are 1.6 Mb apart (Fig. 1B). The common recurrent 1.6-Mb deletion is present in approx 87% of *STS* deletion patients in the Unites States and Japan, and 30% of the patient population in Mexico *(15–18)*. One-third of the Mexican patients appear to have a smaller recurrent deletion with the distal breakpoint at S232A and the proximal breakpoint somewhere between S232B and another LCR G1.3 (DXF22S1) *(18)*. The 1.6-Mb segment between S232A and S232B contains four genes, HDHD1A*(GS1)*, PNPLA4*(GS2)*, VCX-8r/VCX-A, and LOC392425 in addition to *STS (19–21)*. Interestingly, patients with the 1.6-Mb deletion have the same phenotype as those with mutations within the *STS* gene, indicating that removal of the additional genes around *STS* has no apparent phenotypic consequences.

There are six copies of S232 repeats within the human genome, four at Xp22.3 flanking *STS* and two at Yq11. The X-linked S232 repeats are highly polymorphic in length. They span more than 2 Mb and are oriented in different directions (Fig. 1B). The 1.6-Mb deletion breakpoints

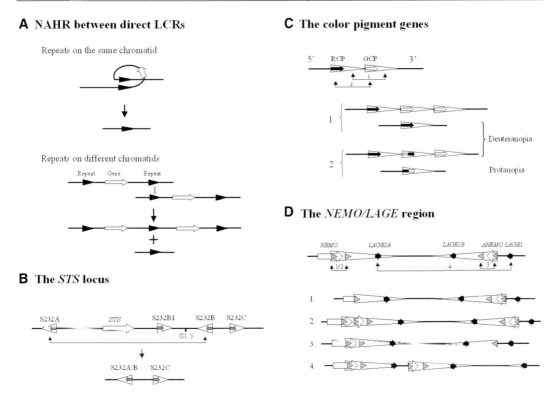

Fig. 1. Nonallelic homologous recombination (NAHR) between direct low-copy repeats. Horizontal arrows depict genes in the 5' to 3' direction and arrowheads depict repeats. (A) Models of NAHR. Recombination between repeats on different chromatids produces both deletion and duplication, whereas recombination between repeats on the same chromatid produces only deletion. (B) The steroid sulfatase (*STS*) gene and its flanking S232 repeats. The solid arrows within the arrowheads represent the *Variable Charge X* genes within the S232 repeats. Vertical arrows connect the repeats that are involved in the NAHR to generate the *STS* deletion. (C) Tandem array of the color pigment genes. Only one green color pigment (GCP) gene in addition to the red color pigment gene is shown. Recombination between the intergenic regions (rearrangement 1) changes the copy number of the GCP gene in the recombinant chromosomes. Recombination between the genes (rearrangement 2) results in hybrid genes in addition to changed gene copy number. (D) Complex structure of the *NEMO/LAGE* region. Gray unlabeled arrowheads depict the *int3h* repeats that are present in introns 3 and the 3' flanking regions of *NEMO* (depicted as open arrow) as well as the truncated Δ*NEMO* pseudogene. Open arrowheads depict the large inverted repeats that contain the 3' portion of *NEMO* and the *LAGE2* (solid arrow) genes. The recombination products involving the various pairs of repeats are shown. The drawings are not to scale.

fall within S232A and S232B, which are in the same direction and share more than 11 kb of 95% identity. The structure of the S232 repeats is quite complex. Each S232 repeat contains 5 kb of unique sequence in addition to two elements, RU1 and RU2, that are composed of variable number of tandem repeats *(22)*. The repeating unit of RU2 is of highly asymmetric sequence and in itself contains a variable number of a GGGA repeat. The size of RU2 varies from 0.6 kb to more than 23 kb among different individuals, accounting entirely for the observed polymorphism at the S232 loci. RU1 consists of a 30-bp repeat unit and is a part of a testis-specific gene, *Variable Charge X (VCX)* or *Variable Charge Y (VCY)*, that is complete embedded in the S232 repeat *(21)*. The *VCX/Y* family encodes basic proteins that appear to play a role in the regulation of ribosome assembly during spermatogenesis *(23)*. The RU2 VNTR sequences as well as the open chromatin structure associated with active transcription of the *VCX* genes may facilitate homologous recombination between S232A and S232B, though the exact locations of the deletion breakpoints within the S232 repeats have not been determined *(22,24)*.

Color Blindness and the Red and Green Pigment Genes at Xq28

Color blindness affects approx 5% of the male population worldwide, and a vast majority of the cases are caused by defects in the color pigment genes on the X chromosome *(8)*. Of the genes encoding the three color pigments in humans, the blue pigment gene is located on chromosome 7, and the red pigment (*Opsin 1 Long-wave-sensitive, OPN1LW*) and green pigment (*Opsin 1 Middle-wave-sensitive, OPN1MW*) genes are embedded in head-to-tail tandem-arrayed repeating units at Xq28. Such tandem arrangement predisposes the red and green pigment genes to NAHR and genomic rearrangement. The pigment genes consist of six exons spanning 14 kb. They are derived from a duplication event 30 million years ago and share 98% similarity throughout the entire gene. The repeating unit in the tandem array includes a single pigment gene at the 5' end and 25 kb of intergenic sequences. The red pigment gene is located at the 5' end of the array, followed by one or more copies of the green pigment gene (Fig. 1C). Unequal crossover within the 25-kb intergenic regions would generate X chromosomes with increased or decreased copies of the green pigment gene (Fig. 1C1). This accounts for the variable copy number of the green pigment gene in the human population. Of the X chromosomes in the normal population with trichromatic vision, the percentages carrying one, two, three, four, and more copies of the green pigment gene are 25, 50, 20, and 5%, respectively. Regardless of the number of the green pigment gene, only the one next to the red pigment gene is expressed. This limited expression is attributed to the presence of a locus control region 5' of the red and green pigment gene array. Men with only one red pigment gene but no green pigment gene are dichromatic with deuteranopia (green vision defects). This occurs in 2–3% of the male population. Intragenic crossovers between the color pigment genes occur mainly within introns, resulting in distinct hybrid gene types (Fig. 1C1). Because exon 5 plays the largest role in spectral tuning, men would have deuteranopia when the hybrid genes contain exon 5 of the red pigment gene, and protanopia (red vision defects) when the hybrid genes contain exon 5 of the green pigment gene.

Incontinential Pigmenti and the NEMO Gene at Xq28

Familial IP (MIM 308310) is a rare X-linked dominant disorder affecting approx 1 in 50,000 newborns. It is characterized by abnormalities of the skin, hair, nails, teeth, eyes, and central nervous system, with a distinctive pattern of hyperpigmentation and dermal scarring *(25)*. Affected males die *in utero,* whereas affected females have extremely skewed X-inactivation owing to the death of cells carrying the mutation on the active X chromosome. The disorder is caused by defects in the *NEMO* gene that encodes a regulator of the NF-κB signal pathway *(9,26)*. The gene spans 23 kb and consists of 10 exons. A recurrent 10-kb deletion that removes exons 4–10 accounts for 70–80% of the mutations identified in IP patients *(9,26)*. This deletion is flanked at the ends by two identical 878-bp MER67B repeats (termed *int3h* repeats), one located within intron 3 of the gene and the other in the 3' flanking region (Fig. 1D1). In most of the *de novo* cases, the deletion occurred in the paternal germline, indicating intra-chromosomal recombination between the repeats.

In addition to the recurrent deletion previously described, there are other arrangements around the *NEMO* gene that are promoted by the complex structure in the region *(10)*. The 3' portion of *NEMO* is in fact included in a 35.5-kb segmental duplication that occurred 10–15 million years ago after divergence of the great ape lineage (Fig. 1D). The duplicated regions are present in opposite orientation and include exons 3–10 of *NEMO* (designated Δ*NEMO*) and the *LAGE2* gene. The inverted repeats share more than 99% sequence identity that is believed to be maintained through frequent gene conversion. Immediately distal to the repeats is the *LAGE1* gene that is related to *LAGE2*. Molecular analyses of normal controls and IP patients had identified rare rearrangements in the region, including *int3h* duplication in *NEMO* (Fig. 1D2), *int3h* deletion in Δ*NEMO* (Fig. 1D3), and *LAGE1-LAGE2A* inversion (Fig. 1D4). Both the *int3h* duplication and *LAGE1-LAGE2A* inversion are nonpathogenic because they were found in normal individuals. It is unclear whether *int3h* deletion in Δ*NEMO* is also nonpathogenic because the rare mutation has only been identified in IP patients with a mutated *NEMO* gene. However, Δ*NEMO* appears to be a nonfunctional pseudogene by several criteria.

INVERSIONS CAUSED BY NAHR BETWEEN INVERTED LCRS

NAHR between indirect repeats on the same chromatid results in inversion of the intervening sequence (Fig. 2A). When one or both of the repeats are within a gene, the inversion would disrupt the gene structure and result in a phenotype, such as seen in the X-linked hemophilia A and Hunter syndrome. When both repeats are situated outside a gene, the inversion would generate a polymorphism, such as the one associated with the emerin (*EMD*) gene. The inversions usually create altered restriction fragments that are easily detected by Southern blotting. It is interesting that all three genes associated with recurrent inversions are located at Xq28, close to the end of the X chromosome long arm. Studies on *de novo* mutations of hemophilia A showed that the inversions occur almost exclusively in male germ cells *(27)*. It is suggested that pairing of the X chromosomes in female germ cells inhibits mispairing of the inverted repeats. The proximity of the locus to the free end of the chromosome could also facilitate chromosome looping required for the alignment of the inverted repeats.

Hemophilia A and the F8 Gene at Xq28

Hemophilia A (HEMA, MIM 306700) is a common X-liked coagulation disorder affecting 1 in 5000 males *(28)*. It is caused by defects in the factor VIII (*F8*) gene, located approx 1 Mb from the Xq telomere. The *F8* gene consists of 26 exons and spans more than 141 kb *(29)*. Within its intron 22 reside two genes, *factor VIII-associated gene A* (*F8A*) and *factor VIII-associated gene B* (*F8B*), that are transcribed in the opposite and the same direction, respectively, as *F8*. *F8A* is a small 1.8-kb intronless gene that is ubiquitously expressed. There are two additional copies of *F8A* situated approx 300 and 400 kb, respectively, 5' and telomeric to *F8* (Fig. 2B). These genes are transcribed in the same direction as *F8*. The homology between *F8* intron 22 (*int22h-1*) and the 5' regions (*int22h-2* and *int22h-3*) extends beyond the *F8A* genes, and the inverted repeats share 9.5 kb of 99.9% sequence similarity *(30)*. About 45% of severe hemophilia A cases (25% of all cases of hemophilia A) have an inversion of the *F8* gene caused by NAHR between *int22h-1* and *int22h-2* or *int22h-3 (31)*. The inversions are detected by Southern blotting that gives different fragments for inversions involving *int22h-2* or *int22h-3*. No DNA is lost or gained during the inversion process. Interestingly, inversions involving the more distal *int22h-3* are four times more common than those involving the more

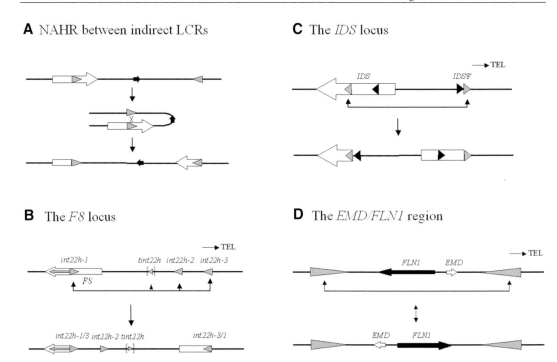

Fig. 2. Nonallelic homologous recombination (NAHR) between inverted low-copy repeats. (A) A model of NAHR. Recombination between inverted repeats on the same chromatid results in the inversion of the intervening sequence. When one or both repeats are within a gene (the open arrow), the inversion disrupts the gene structure and may produce a phenotype. When both repeats are outside a gene (the solid arrow) the inversion creates a polymorphism without disrupting the gene. (B) The *F8* gene and its flanking repeats. The open arrow depicts the *F8* gene with the included gray arrow depicting the *F8B* gene. The gray arrowheads represent the *int22h* repeats, and the *F8A* genes inside the repeats. The truncated *int22h* (*tint22h*) that has been identified in a single family is bracketed. Recombination occurs mainly between *int22h1* and *int22h3*, and its product is depicted. (C) The *IDS* gene and its pseudogene *IDS*ψ. *IDS*ψ contains sequences homologous to exon2-intron3 (black arrowhead) and intron7 (gray arrowhead) of *IDS*. All *IDS* inversions characterized so far result from recombination between the intron7 homologous sequences. (D) The *EMD/FLN1* region and its flanking repeats. Recombination between the repeats generates an inversion polymorphism of the region.

proximal *int22h-2*. It is possible that the longer distance between *int22h-1* and *int22h-3* favors the looping of the DNA strand that brings the LCRs together. In addition to inversions involving *int22h-2* and *int22h-3*, a hemophilia A patient was found to have a third kind of inversion disrupting *F8 (32)*. This inversion involves an extra-truncated copy of *int22h* (*tint22h*) located between *int22h-2* and *F8* (Fig. 2B). The *tint22h* repeat contains only 1.9 kb of the 9.5 kb *int22h* sequence. It is detected only in the patient's family and does not appear to be a common polymorphism in the UK population studied.

Hunter Syndrome and the IDS Gene at Xq28

Hunter syndrome (or mucopolysaccharidosis type II, MPS II, MIM 309900) is a rare X-linked lysosomal storage disorder that affects about 1 in 132,000 male live births *(33)*. It is caused by iduronate-2-sulfatase (IDS) deficiency, which results in the deposits of mucopolysaccharides in the lysosomes and the excretion of large amounts of chondroitin sulfate B and heparitin sulfate in the urine. The *IDS* gene consists of 9 exons spanning 23 kb *(34)*. About 20 kb 5' and telomeric to the *IDS* gene is an *IDS* pseudogene (*IDS*ψ) arranged in the opposite direction (Fig. 2C) *(35)*. *IDS*ψ is homologous to two discontinuous segments of *IDS*; a 1.3-kb segment with 98.4% homology to the 3' portion of exon 2 through the first half of intron 3, and a 1.6 kb segment with 96% homology to intron 7. About 13% of Hunter syndrome patients have a recurrent inversion caused by NAHR between *IDS* and *IDS*ψ *(35–37)*. Of the *IDS/IDS*ψ inversions characterized to date, all have the breakpoints mapped within the intron 7 homologous regions. Therefore, similar to the recurrent inversion at *F8*, recombination at *IDS* also prefers the homologous regions more distant from each other. Because of the rarity of the disorder, it has not been studied whether the *IDS* inversion also occurs exclusively in male germ cells.

Emery-Dreifuss Muscular Dystrophy and the EMD Gene at Xq28

Emery-Dreifuss muscular dystrophy (EMD, MIM310300) is an X-linked degenerative myopathy, characterized by progressive weakening and atrophy of muscle and cardiomyopathy *(38)*. It is caused by defects in the emerin (*EMD*) gene, which encodes a nuclear lamina-associated protein involved in the anchorage of nuclear membrane to the cytoskeleton *(39)*. The *EMD* gene consists of six exons and spans 2 kb. *EMD*, together with its neighboring filamin (*FLN1*) gene, are flanked by two 11.3-kb inverted repeats that share more than 99% sequence similarity (Fig. 2D) *(40)*. A polymorphism consisting of inversion of the 48-kb *FLN1/EMD* region, likely caused by NAHR between the two long inverted repeats, was discovered during characterization of the molecular defects in EMD patients. The inversion is present in 18% of the X chromosomes in the Caucasian population and does not seem to increase the risk of DNA rearrangement in the region *(41)*. However, it could dramatically reduce recombination in females heterozygous for the inversion and is thought to account for the discrepancy between the physical map and the genetic map of the region.

DELETIONS/DUPLICATIONS CAUSED BY NHEJ

Duchenne/Becker muscular dystrophy and Pelizaeus-Merzbacher disease are two additional X-linked disorders with deletions/duplications as the major molecular defects *(42,43)*. However, deletions/duplications in these disorders lack repetitive sequences at the breakpoints, suggesting that they result from nonhomologous end joining. This chapter focuses on Duchenne/Becker muscular dystrophy and the dystrophin gene at Xp22. Pelizaeus-Merzbacher disease is covered elsewhere in Chapter 18.

Duchenne muscular dystrophy (DMD; MIM 310200) is the most common form of muscular dystrophy, affecting approx 1 in 3500 newborn males *(42)*. About one-third of the cases represent *de novo* new mutations. The disorder is characterized by a progressive muscle weakening, and patients rarely survive beyond the age of 20 years. Becker muscular dystrophy is a milder allelic form of DMD with a later age of onset and slower progression of the disease. The gene underlying both disorders, *DMD*, is the largest gene in the human genome *(44)*. It consists of 79 exons spanning more than 2.2 Mb. Its protein product, dystrophin, is associated with integral membrane glycoproteins on the inner surface of muscle fibers and links the inner cytoskeleton to the extracellular matrix.

Deletion of one or more exons of the *DMD* gene accounts for 60% of mutations in DMD/BMD patients in the European and North American populations and much less in other populations *(45,46)*. The deletions are heterogeneous in size and they cluster at two hotspots. About

30% of the deletions are located in the 5' region centered around exon 7, and the remaining 70% are mapped to the middle of the gene centered around exons 40–50 *(45–47)*. However, the deletion breakpoints scatter throughout the "hotspots" and no extensive homology is present at the ends of the majority of the deletions *(48,49)*. The *DMD* deletions, thus, appear to occur mainly by NHEJ. The unusual high incidence of deletion at *DMD* is thought to be promoted by the high recombination rate within the gene. *DMD* has a recombination rate about four times the rate that would be expected for a gene of its size, and the major meiotic recombination hotspots coincide with the deletion hotspots *(50)*. Partial duplication of the *DMD* gene accounts for approx 6% of the mutations *(51)*. Similar to the deletions, no extensive homology is present at the ends of the duplicated segments in most cases. In all cases studied, the duplications were found to occur in the paternal germline, indicating unequal sister-chromatid exchange as the underlying mechanism.

THE *SHOX* GENE DELETIONS

The *SHOX* gene, also known as the *pseudoautosomal homeobox-containing osteogenic gene (PHOG)*, is another gene with a high deletion frequency, yet the underlying mechanisms remain unclear *(52,53)*. The gene is located within the pseudoautosomal region of the X chromosome short arm (PAR1), approx 500 kb proximal from the telomere. It consists of seven exons spanning approx 40 kb, and encodes a member of the paired-like homeodomain protein family that acts as a transcriptional activator in osteogenic cells and plays an important role in limb development *(54)*.

SHOX mutations have been found in three disorders: idiopathic short stature (SS; MIM 604271), Leri-Weill dyschondrosteosis (LWD; MIM127300), and Langer mesomelic dysplasia (MIM 249700) *(55)*. In addition, *SHOX* haploinsufficiency is responsible for the skeletal anomaly in Turner syndrome patients. Approximately 2–7% of individuals with idiopathic SS and 60–100% of LWD patients have *SHOX* mutations *(56–59)*. The rare and more severe Langer mesomelic dysplasia has homozygous or compound heterozygous mutations of the *SHOX* gene *(56)*. A striking feature of *SHOX* mutations is that there is considerable phenotypic heterogeneity among the patients, and no correlation exists between the type and position of a mutation within the gene and the resulting phenotype. Complete gene deletion or the same point mutations could result in SS or LWD, and there is a significant inter- and intrafamilial variation in the severity of the phenotype, indicating the involvement of modifiers *(58)*.

Deletions involving the entire *SHOX* gene account for a vast majority (>70%) of *SHOX* mutations regardless of the clinical manifestation. Most of the deletions were detected by FISH, however, and the extents of the deletions have not been determined. For those that have been characterized, they were both terminal and interstitial deletions, and their sizes ranged from 150 kb to more than 9 Mb *(52,56,58)*. Deletions that extend beyond the PAR1 boundary are associated with contiguous gene syndromes, to be described in the next section. The high frequency of *SHOX* deletion has been attributed to the prevalence of repetitive sequences within the PAR1 region, although none of the deletion breakpoints have been isolated and sequenced *(60)*.

CONTIGUOUS GENE SYNDROMES

A large fraction of contiguous gene syndromes (CGSs) identified to date are located on the X chromosome. The CGSs map to all regions of the X chromosome (Table 1). Their clinical

Table 1
Contiguous Gene Syndromes on the X Chromosome

Location	Genes deleted	Clinical features	Refs.
Xp22.3	SHOX, ARSE, VCX-A, STS, KAL1, GPR143, MID1, HCCS	Short stature/Leri-Weill dyschondrosteosis, condrodysplasia punctata, mental retardation, ichthyosis, hypogonadism/anosmia, ocular albinism, microphthalmia/linear skin defects	61–64
Xp21	IL1RAPL1, NR0B1, GK, DMD, XK, CYBB, OTC	Mental retardation, adrenal hypoplasia, glycerol kinase deficiency, muscular dystrophy, McLeod phenotype (acanthocytosis, compensated hemolytic anemia), chronic granulomatous disease, ornithine transcarbamylase deficiency	81–84
Xp11.3	NDP, MAOA, MAOB	Norrie disease (congenital blindness, hearing loss, mental retardation), disruptive behavior, abnormal sexual maturation, seizures, hypotonia	88–90
Xq12	AR, OPHN1	Androgen insensitivity, mental retardation	91,92
Xq21.1	REP1, POU3F4, RPS6KA6	Deafness, mental retardation, choroideremia	93–96
Xq21.3	BTK, DDP	Agammaglobulinemia, sensorineural deafness	97
Xq22.3	COL4A6, COL4A5	Alport syndrome (hematuria, hearing loss), leiomyomatosis	98
Xq22.3	COL4A5, FACL4, AMMECR1, KCNE1L	AMME: Alport syndrome, mental retardation, midface hypoplasia, elliptocytosis	99–102
Xq28	ABCD1, BCAP31 (DXS1357E)	Adrenoleukodystrophy, onset before 3 years of age	103
Xq28	MTM1, F18	Myotubular myopathy, intersexual genitalia	104,105

manifestations depend largely on the gene contents of the deletions, though some genes can be deleted with little consequences. With some exceptions, most CGS patients are males, and female carriers for the same deletions are phenotypically normal. Some of the CGSs are quite rare and only a few cases have been reported. The more common ones at Xp22.3 and Xp21 are described in some detail next.

Contiguous Gene Syndromes at Xp22.3

More than 40 patients with contiguous gene syndromes at Xp22.3 have been reported (61–64). These patients have clinical manifestations associated with two or more disorders mapped to Xp22.3, including SS, LWD, X-linked chondrodysplasia punctata (CDPX, MIM 302950), mental retardation (MR), XLI, X-linked Kallmann syndrome (KAL1, MIM 308700), ocular albinism type 1 (OA1, MIM 300500), and microphthalmia with linear skin defects (MLS, MIM 309801). CDPX, KAL1, OA1, and MLS are caused by defects in the *arylsulfatase E* (*ARSE*), *KAL1*, *G protein-coupled receptor 143* (*GPR143*), and *holocytochrome c-type synthetase* (*HCCS*) gene, respectively (65–69). A mental retardation locus (*MRX*) was mapped to a 15-kb critical region between *ARSE* and *STS* based on phenotype-genotype correlation *(70)*. However, the only gene identified within the critical region is *VCX-A*, a member of a gene family with testis-specific expression *(21)*. It is possible that an unidentified nonprotein-coding or microRNA gene within the region is responsible for the mental retardation phenotype *(71)*. With the exceptions of *SHOX, STS,* and *HCCS* mutations, complete gene deletion accounts for only small fractions of the mutations identified in patients with isolated disorders within the region.

Patients with CGSs at Xp22.3 have large deletions that span several megabases, and their phenotypes correlate with the genes that are eliminated by the deletions (Fig. 3A). Most of the patients are males. However, MLS is found almost exclusively in females because of embryonic lethality for the hemizygous males (72). All of the affected MLS individuals are monosomy from Xpter to Xp22 owing to unbalanced translocations or terminal deletions of the X chromosome that remove more than 10 Mb of Xp terminal sequences. In addition to MLS, these females have SS because of haploinsufficiency of the *SHOX* gene.

A large fraction of the deletions associated with Xp22.3 CGSs is terminal, resulting from X/Y or X/autosomal translocation. X/Y translocations occur rarely in the human population, and the majority have breakpoints at Xp22 and Yq11 *(73)*. These regions share 89–94% sequence similarity over an extended area *(2,74)*. *ARSD, ARSE, VCX-A, STS,* and *KAL1* at Xp22 all have homologous sequences at Yq11 *(13,21,75,76)*. Mapping and characterization of the breakpoints indicate that some of these X/Y translocations result from recombination between homologous sequences at these regions *(73)*. No breakpoints of the interstitial deletions associated with Xp22.3 CGSs have been isolated and sequenced, and it is not known whether these deletions are formed through NAHR or NHEJ. Two families of LCR are known to be present at Xp22; the S232 family that are involved in the recurrent deletion of *STS,* and the G1.3 family *(77–80)*. There are four clusters of G1.3 related sequences at Xp22, one between *STS* and *KAL1*, two between *KAL1* and *GPR143*, and one proximal to *Midline 1* (*MID1*). Similar to the S232 repeats, the G1.3 repeats also contain a gene family, *family with sequence similarity 9* (*FAM9*), that is expressed exclusively in the testis *(80)*. There may be additional LCRs in the region waiting to be discovered.

Contiguous Gene Syndromes at Xp21

Close to 100 patients with Xp21 contiguous deletion syndromes have been reported *(81–84)*. About two-thirds of the patients have DMD, glycerol kinase deficiency (GKD; MIM 307030), and adrenal hypoplasia congenital (AHC; MIM 300200), 25% have AHC and GKD, and the rest have GKD and DMD, or the more proximally located disorders such as the McLeod phenotype (MIM 314850), chronic granulomatous disease (CGD; MIM 306400), and ornithine transcarbamylase (OTC) deficiency (MIM 311250). AHC is caused by defects in the *nuclear receptor subfamily 0 group B, member 1* (*NROB1*) gene, also known as *DAX1*, which when present in double dosage causes XY sex reversal *(85,86)*. CGD is caused by defects in the *cytochrome b β subunit* (*CYBB*) gene *(87)*. The sizes of the deletions range from less than 1 Mb to more than 14 Mb, and the deletion breakpoints spread over a wide range (Fig. 3B) *(81)*. A boy with AHC and mental retardation was reported to have a 2-Mb deletion extending from the *NROB1* gene to the distal *interleukin-1 receptor accessory protein-like* (*IL1RAPL*) gene, which is 1.4 Mb in size *(84)*, implicating *IL1RAPL* in nonspecific mental retardation. None of the deletion breakpoints have been isolated and the mechanism(s) underlying the deletions remains unclear.

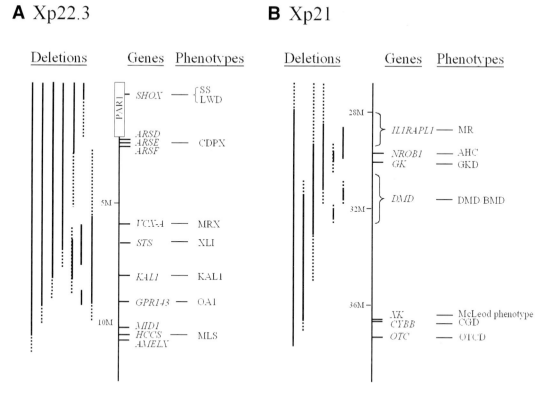

Fig. 3. Contiguous gene syndromes at two regions of the X chromosome. The maps show the distances (in megabases) of the genes from Xp telomere, taken from the NCBI map viewer. Not all genes in the areas are shown. Lines at the left side of the maps depict regions deleted in the patients. A line in most cases represents deletions in a collection of patients who have the same phenotype but different deletion breakpoints. The dashed ends of the line cover the regions where the breakpoints may be located since most breakpoints of the deletions have not been well mapped. PAR1, pseudoautosomal region 1; SS, short stature; LWD, Leri-Weill dyschondrosteosis; CDPX, X-linked chondrodysplasia punctata; MR, mental retardation; XLI, X-linked ichthyosis, KAL1, X-linked Kallmann syndrome; OA1, Ocular albinism type 1; MLS, microphthalmia with linear skin defects; AHC, adrenal hypoplasia congenital; GKD, glycerol kinase deficiency; DMD, Duchenne muscular dystrophy; BMD, Becker muscular dystrophy; CGD, chronic granulomatous disease; OTCD, ornithine transcarbamylase deficiency.

SUMMARY

Through the combined efforts of many researchers worldwide over the last two decades, we are beginning to understand the molecular mechanisms underlying several X-linked genomic disorders. Both NAHR and NHEJ play significant roles in the genesis of these genomic rearrangements. However, for a majority of deletions associated with contiguous gene syndromes, the breakpoints are undefined and the mechanisms remain unclear. With the sequence of the entire X chromosome determined, it is now much easier to map and characterize deletion breakpoints. Future work on delineating sequences at the breakpoints should provide us with a better understanding of the structures and etiology of X chromosome rearrangements.

REFERENCES

1. Stankiewicz P, Lupski JR. Genome architecture, rearrangements and genomic disorders. Trends Genet 2002;18:74–82.
2. Skaletsky H, Kuroda-Kawaguchi T, Minx PJ, et al. The male-specific region of the human Y chromosome is a mosaic of discrete sequence classes. Nature 2003;423:825–837.
3. Hentemann M, Reiss J, Wagner M, Cooper DN. Rapid detection of deletions in the Duchenne muscular dystrophy gene by PCR amplification of deletion-prone exon sequences. Hum Genet 1990;84:228–232.
4. Voskova-Goldman A, Peier A, Caskey CT, Richards CS, Shaffer LG. DMD-specific FISH probes are diagnostically useful in the detection of female carriers of DMD gene deletions. Neurology 1997;48:1633–1638.
5. Nomura K, Nakano H, Umeki K, et al. A study of the steroid sulfatase gene in families with X-linked ichthyosis using polymerase chain reaction. Acta Derm Venereol 1995;75:340–342.
6. Valdes-Flores M, Kofman-Alfaro SH, Jimenez-Vaca AL, Cuevas-Covarrubias SA (2001) Carrier identification by FISH analysis in isolated cases of X-linked ichthyosis. Am J Med Genet 2001;102:146–148.
7. Yen PH, Li XM, Tsai SP, Johnson C, Mohandas T, Shapiro LJ. Frequent deletions of the human X chromosome distal short arm result from recombination between low copy repetitive elements. Cell 1990;61: 603–610.
8. Nathans J. The evolution and physiology of human color vision: insights from molecular genetic studies of visual pigments. Neuron 1999;24:299–312.
9. Smahi A, Courtois G, Vabres P, et al. Genomic rearrangement in NEMO impairs NF-kappaB activation and is a cause of incontinentia pigmenti. The International Incontinentia Pigmenti (IP) Consortium. Nature 2000;405:466–472.
10. Aradhya S, Bardaro T, Galgoczy P, et al. Multiple pathogenic and benign genomic rearrangements occur at a 35 kb duplication involving the NEMO and LAGE2 genes. Hum Mol Genet 2001;10:2557–2567.
11. Shaw-Smith C, Redon R, Rickman L, et al. Microarray based comparative genomic hybridization (array-CGH) detects submicroscopic chromosomal deletions and duplications in patients with learning disability/mental retardation and dysmorphic features. J Med Genet 2004;41:241–248.
12. Shapiro LJ. Steroid sulfatase deficiency and the genetics of the short arm of the human X chromosome. Adv Hum Genet 1985;14:331–381.
13. Yen PH, Marsh B, Allen E, et al. The human X-linked steroid sulfatase gene and a Y-encoded pseudogene: evidence for an inversion of the Y chromosome during primate evolution. Cell 1988;55:1123–1135.
14. Hernandez-Martin A, Gonzalez-Sarmiento R, de Unamuno P. X-linked ichthyosis: an update. Brit J Dermat 1999;141:617–627.
15. Shapiro LJ, Yen P, Pomerantz D, Martin E, Rolewic L, Mohandas T. Molecular studies of deletions at the human steroid sulfatase locus. Proc Natl Acad Sci USA 1989;86:8477–8481.
16. Ballabio A, Carrozzo R, Parenti G, et al. Molecular heterogeneity of steroid sulfatase deficiency: a multicenter study on 57 unrelated patients, at DNA and protein levels. Genomics 1989;4:36–40.
17. Saeki H, Kuwata S, Nakagawa H, Shimada S, Tamaki K, Ishibashi Y. Deletion pattern of the steroid sulphatase gene in Japanese patients with X-linked ichthyosis. Br J Dermatol 1998;139:96–98.
18. Jimenez Vaca AL, Valdes-Flores Mdel R, Rivera-Vega MR, Gonzalez-Huerta LM, Kofman-Alfaro SH, Cuevas-Covarrubias SA. Deletion pattern of the STS gene in X-linked ichthyosis in a Mexican population. Mol Med 2001;7:845–849.
19. Yen PH, Ellison J, Salido EC., Mohandas T, Shapiro L. Isolation of a new gene from the distal short arm of the human X chromosome that escapes X-inactivation. Hum Mol Genet 1992;1:47–52.
20. Lee W-C, Salido E, and Yen PH (1994) Isolation of a new gene GS2 (DXS1283E) from a CpG island between STS and KAL1 on Xp22.3. Genomics 22, 372—376.
21. Lahn BT, Page DC. A human sex-chromosomal gene family expressed in male germ cells and encoding variably charged proteins. Hum Mol Genet 2000;9:311–319.
22. Li XM, Yen PH, Shapiro LJ. Characterization of a low copy repetitive element S232 involved in the generation of frequent deletions of the distal short arm of the human X chromosome. Nucl Acids Res 1992;20: 1117–1122.

23. Zou SW, Zhang JC, Zhang XD, et al. Expression and localization of VCX/Y proteins and their possible involvement in regulation of ribosome assembly during spermatogenesis. Cell Res 2003;13:171–177.
24. Wu TC, Lichten M. Meiosis-induced double-strand break sites determined by yeast chromatin structure. Science 1994;263:515–518.
25. Berlin AL, Paller AS, Chan LS. Incontinentia pigmenti: a review and update on the molecular basis of pathophysiology. J Am Acad Dermatol 2002;47:169–187.
26. Aradhya S, Woffendin H, Jakins T, et al. A recurrent deletion in the ubiquitously expressed NEMO (IKK-gamma) gene accounts for the vast majority of incontinentia pigmenti mutations. Hum Mol Genet 2001;10:2171–2179.
27. Rossiter JP, Young M, Kimberland ML, et al. Factor VIII gene inversions causing severe hemophilia A originate almost exclusively in male germ cells. Hum Mol Genet 1994;3:1035–1039.
28. Hoyer LW. Hemophilia A. New Engl J Med 1994;330:38–47.
29. Antonarakis SE, Kazazian HH, Tuddenham EG. Molecular etiology of factor VIII deficiency in hemophilia A. Hum Mutat 1995;5:1–22.
30. Naylor JA, Buck D, Green P, Williamson H, Bentley D, Giannelli F. Investigation of the factor VIII intron 22 repeated region (int22h) and the associated inversion junctions. Hum Mol Genet 1995;4:1217–1224.
31. Lakich D, Kazazian HH Jr, Antonarakis SE, Gitschier J. Inversions disrupting the factor VIII gene are a common cause of severe haemophilia A. Nat Genet 1993;5:236–241.
32. Naylor JA, Nicholson P, Goodeve A, Hassock S, Peake I, Giannelli F. A novel DNA inversion causing severe hemophilia A. Blood 1996;87:3255–3261.
33. Young ID, Harper PS. Incidence of Hunter's syndrome. Hum Genet 1982;60:391–392.
34. Flomen RH, Green EP, Green PM, Bentley DR, Giannelli F. Determination of the organisation of coding sequences within the iduronate sulphate sulphatase (IDS) gene. Hum Mol Genet 1993;2:5–10.
35. Bondeson ML, Dahl N, Malmgren H, et al. Inversion of the IDS gene resulting from recombination with IDS-related sequences is a common cause of the Hunter syndrome. Hum Mol Genet 1995;4:615–621.
36. Timms KM, Bondeson ML, Ansari-Lari MA, et al. Molecular and phenotypic variation in patients with severe Hunter syndrome. Hum Mol Genet 1997;6:479–486.
37. Bunge S, Rathmann M, Steglich C, et al. Homologous nonallelic recombinations between the iduronate-sulfatase gene and pseudogene cause various intragenic deletions and inversions in patients with mucopolysaccharidosis type II. Eur J Hum Genet 1998;6:492–00.
38. Emery AEH. Emery-Dreifuss syndrome. J Med Genet 1989;26:637–641.
39. Bione S, Maestrini E, Rivella S, et al. Identification of a novel X-linked gene responsible for Emery-Dreifuss muscular dystrophy. Nat Genet 1994;8:323–327.
40. Small K, Iber J, Warren ST. Emerin deletion reveals a common X-chromosome inversion mediated by inverted repeats. Nat Genet 1997;16:96–99.
41. Small K, Warren ST. Emerin deletions occurring on both Xq28 inversion backgrounds. Hum Mol Genet 1998;7:135–139.
42. O'Brien KF, Kunkel LM. Dystrophin and muscular dystrophy: past, present, and future. Mol Genet Metab 2001;74:75–88.
43. Inoue K, Osaka H, Thurston VC, et al. Genomic rearrangements resulting in PLP1 deletion occur by nonhomologous end joining and cause different dysmyelinating phenotypes in males and females. Am J Hum Genet 2002;71:838–853.
44. Tennyson CN, Klamut HJ, Worton RG. The human dystrophin gene requires 16 hours to be transcribed and is cotranscriptionally spliced. Nat Genet 1995;9:184–190.
45. Den Dunnen JT, Grootscholten PM, Bakker E, et al. Topography of the Duchenne muscular dystrophy (DMD) gene: FIGE and cDNA analysis of 194 cases reveals 115 deletions and 13 duplications. Am J Hum Genet 1989;45:835–847.
46. Shomrat R, Gluck E, Legum C, Shiloh Y. Relatively low proportion of dystrophin gene deletions in Israeli Duchenne and Becker muscular dystrophy patients. Am J Med Genet 1994;49:369–373.
47. Baumbach LL, Chamberlain JS, Ward PA, Farwell NJ, Caskey CT. Molecular and clinical correlations of deletions leading to Duchenne and Becker muscular dystrophies. Neurology 1989;39:465–474.
48. Sironi M, Pozzoli U, Cagliani R, et al. Relevance of sequence and structure elements for deletion events in the dystrophin gene major hot-spot. Hum Genet 2002;112:272–288.
49. Toffolatti L, Cardazzo B, Nobile C, et al. Investigating the mechanism of chromosomal deletion: characterization of 39 deletion breakpoints in introns 47 and 48 of the human dystrophin gene. Genomics 2002;80:523–530.

50. Oudet C, Hanauer A, Clemens P, Caskey T, Mandel JL. Two hot spots of recombination in the DMD gene correlate with the deletion prone regions. Hum Mol Genet 1992;1:599–603.

51. Hu X, Ray PN, Murphy EG, Thompson MW, Worton RG. Duplicational mutation at the Duchenne muscular dystrophy locus: its frequency, distribution, origin, and phenotype genotype correlation. Am J Hum Genet 1990;46:682–695.

52. Rao E, Weiss B, Fukami M, et al. Pseudoautosomal deletions encompassing a novel homeobox gene cause growth failure in idiopathic short stature and Turner syndrome. Nat Genet 1997;16:54–63.

53. Ellison JW, Wardak Z, Young MF, Gehron Robey P, Laig-Webster M, Chiong W. PHOG, a candidate gene for involvement in the short stature of Turner syndrome. Hum Mol Genet 1997;6:1341–1347.

54. Rao E, Blaschke RJ, Marchini A, Niesler B, Burnett M, Rappold GA. The Leri-Weill and Turner syndrome homeobox gene SHOX encodes a cell-type-specific transcriptional activator. Hum Mol Genet 2001;10: 3083–3091.

55. Blaschke RJ, Rappold GA. SHOX: Growth, Leri-Weill and Turner syndromes. Trends Endocrinol Metab 2000;11:227–230.

56. Belin V, Cusin V, Viot G, et al. SHOX mutations in dyschondrosteosis (Leri-Weill syndrome). Nat Genet 1998;19:67–69.

57. Shears DJ, Vassal HJ, Goodman FR, et al. Mutation and deletion of the pseudoautosomal gene SHOX cause Leri-Weill dyschondrosteosis. Nat Genet 1998;19:70–73.

58. Schiller S, Spranger S, Schechinger B, et al. Phenotypic variation and genetic heterogeneity in Leri-Weill syndrome. Eur J Hum Genet 2000;8:54–62.

59. Flanagan SF, Munns CFJ, Hayes M, et al. Prevalence of mutations in the short stature homeobox containing gene (SHOX) in Madulung deformity of childhood. J Med Genet 2002;39:758–763.

60. Rappold GA, Fukami M, Niesler B, et al. Deletions of the homeobox gene SHOX (Short Stature Homeobox) are an important cause of growth failure in children with short stature. J Clin Encocrinol Metab 2002;87: 1402–1406.

61. Ballabio A. Contiguous deletion syndromes. Curr Opin Genet Dev 1991;1:25–29.

62. Schaefer L, Ferrero GB, Grillo A, et al. A high resolution deletion map of human chromosome Xp22. Nat Genet 1993;4:272–279.

63. Seidel J, Schiller S, Kelbova C, et al. Brachytelephalangic dwarfism due to the loss of ARSE and SHOX genes resulting from an X;Y translocation. Clin Genet 2001;59:115–121.

64. Frints SG, Fryns J, Lagae L, Syearsrou M, Marynen P, Devriendt K. Xp22.3; Yq11.2 chromosome translocation and its clinical manifestations. Ann Genet 2001;44:71–76.

65. Franco B, Meroni G, Parenti G, et al. A cluster of sulfatase genes on Xp22.3: Mutations in chondrodysplasia punctata (CDPX) and implications for warfarin embryopathy. Cell 1995;81:5–25.

66. Legouis R, Hardelin J-P, Levilliers J, et al. The candidate gene for the X-linked Kallmann syndrome encodes a protein related to adhesion molecules. Cell 1991;67:423–435.

67. Franco B, Guioli S, Pragliola A, et al. A gene deleted in Kallmann's syndrome shares homology with neural cell adhesion and axonal path-finding molecules. Nature 1991;353:529–536.

68. Bassi MT, Schiaffino MV, Renieri A, et al. Cloning of the gene for ocular albinism type 1 from the distal short arm of the X chromosome. Nat Genet 1995;10:13–19.

69. Prakash SK, Cormier TA, McCall AE, et al. Loss of holocytochrome c-type synthetase causes the male lethality of X-linked dominant microphthalmia with linear skin defects (MLS) syndrome. Hum Mol Genet 2002;11:3237–3248.

70. Fukami M, Kirsch S, Schiller S, et al. A member of a gene family on Xp22.3, VCX-A, is deleted in patients with X-linked nonspecific mental retardation. Am J Hum Genet 2000;67:563–573.

71. Bartel DP. MicroRNAs: genomics, biogenesis, mechanism, and function. Cell 2004;116:281–297.

72. Lindsay EA, Grillo A, Ferrero GB, et al. Microphthalmia with linear skin defects (MLS) syndrome: clinical, cytogenetic, and molecular characterization. Am J Med Genet 1994;49:229–234.

73. Yen PH, Tsai SP, Wenger SL, Steele MW, Mohandas TK, Shapiro LJ. X/Y translocations resulting from recombination between homologous sequences on Xp and Yq. Proc Natl Acad Sci USA 1991;88:8944–8948.

74. Lahn BT, Page DC. Four evolutionary strata on the human X chromosome. Science 1999;286:964–967.

75. Meroni G, Franco B, Archidiacono N, et al. Characterization of a cluster of sulfatase genes on Xp22.3 suggests gene duplications in an ancestral pseudoautosomal region. Hum Mol Genet 1996;5:423–431.

76. Incerti B, Guioli S, Pragliola A, et al. Kallmann syndrome gene on the X and Y chromosomes: implications for evolutionary divergence of human sex chromosomes. Nat Genet 1992;2:311–314.

77. Knowlton RG, Nelson CA, Brown VA, Page DC, Donis-Keller H. An extremely polymorphic locus on the short arm of the human X chromosome with homology to the long arm of the Y chromosome. Nucl Acids Res 1989;17:423–437.

78. Bardoni B, Guioli S, Raimondi E, et al. Isolation and characterization of a family of sequences dispersed on the human X chromosome. Genomics 1988;3:32–38.

79. Ballabio A, Bardoni B, Guioli S, Basler E, Camerino G. Two families of low-copy-number repeats are interspersed on Xp22.3:implications for the high frequency of deletions in this region. Genomics 1990;8: 263–270.

80. Martinez-Garay I, Jablonka S, Sutajova M, Steuernagel P, Gal A, Kutsche K. A new gene family (FAM9) of low-copy repeats in Xp22.3 expressed exclusively in testis: implications for recombinations in this region. Genomics 2002;80:259–267.

81. McCabe ER, Towbin JA, van den Engh G, Trask BJ. Xp21 contiguous gene syndromes: deletion quantitation with bivariate flow karyotyping allows mapping of patient breakpoints. Am J Hum Genet 1992;51: 1277–1285.

82. Sjarif DR, Ploos van Amstel JK, Duran M, Beemer FA, Poll-The BT. Isolated and contiguous glycerol kinase gene disorders: a review. J Inherit Metab Dis 2000;23:529–547.

83. Hellerud C, Adamowicz M, Jurkiewicz D, et al. Clinical heterogeneity and molecular findings in five Polish patients with glycerol kinase deficiency: investigation of two splice site mutations with computerized splice junction analysis and Xp21 gene-specific mRNA analysis. Mol Genet Metab 2003;79:149–159.

84. Sasaki R, Inamo Y, Saitoh K, Hasegawa T, Kinoshita E, Ogata T. Mental retardation in a boy with congenital adrenal hypoplasia: a clue to contiguous gene syndrome involving DAX1 and IL1RAPL. Endocr J 2003;50:303–307.

85. Zanaria E, Muscatelli F, Bardoni B, et al. An unusual member of the nuclear hormone receptor superfamily responsible for X-linked adrenal hypoplasia congenita. Nature 1994;372:635–641.

86. Bardoni B, Zanaria E, Guioli S, et al. A dosage sensitive locus at chromosome Xp21 is involved in male to female sex reversal. Nat Genet 1994;7:497–501.

87. Royer-Pokora B, Kunkel LM, Monaco AP, et al. Cloning the gene for an inherited human disorder—chronic granulomatous disease—on the basis of its chromosomal location. Nature 1986;322:32–38.

88. Collins FA, Murphy DL, Reiss AL, et al. Clinical, biochemical, and neuropsychiatric evaluation of a patient with a contiguous gene syndrome due to a microdeletion Xp11.3 including the Norrie disease locus and monoamine oxidase (MAOA and MAOB) genes. Am J Med Genet 1992;42:127–134.

89. Chen ZY, Denney RM, Breakefield XO. Norrie disease and MAO genes: nearest neighbors. Hum Mol Genet 1995;4:1729–1737.

90. Suarez-Merino B, Bye J, McDowall J, Ross M, Craig IW. Sequence analysis and transcript identification within 1.5 MB of DNA deleted together with the NDP and MAO genes in atypical Norrie disease patients presenting with a profound phenotype. Hum Mutat 2001;17:523.

91. Davies HR, Hughes IA, Savage MO, et al. Androgen insensitivity with mental retardation: a contiguous gene syndrome? J Med Genet 1997;34:158–160.

92. Schueler MG, Higgins AW, Nagaraja R, et al. Large-insert clone/STS contigs in Xq11-q12, spanning deletions in patients with androgen insensitivity and mental retardation. Genomics 2000;66:104–109.

93. Merry DE, Lesko JG, Sosnoski DM, et al. Choroideremia and deafness with stapes fixation: a contiguous gene deletion syndrome in Xq21. Am J Hum Genet 1989;45:530–540.

94. Kandpal G, Jacob AN, Kandpal RP. Transcribed sequences encoded in the region involved in contiguous deletion syndrome that comprises X-linked stapes fixation and deafness. Somat Cell Mol Genet 1996;22: 511–517.

95. de Kok YJ, Vossenaar ER, Cremers CW, et al. Identification of a hot spot for microdeletions in patients with X-linked deafness type 3 (DFN3) 900 kb proximal to the DFN3 gene POU3F4. Hum Mol Genet 1996;5: 1229–1235.

96. Yntema HG, van den Helm B, Kissing J, et al. A novel ribosomal S6-kinase (RSK4; RPS6KA6) is commonly deleted in patients with complex X-linked mental retardation. Genomics 1999;62:332–343.

97. Richter D, Conley ME, Rohrer J, et al. A contiguous deletion syndrome of X-linked agammaglobulinemia and sensorineural deafness. Pediatr Allergy Immunol 2001;12:107–111.

98. Garcia-Torres R, Cruz D, Orozco L, Heidet L, Gubler MC. Alport syndrome and diffuse leiomyomatosis. Clinical aspects, pathology, molecular biology and extracellular matrix studies. A synthesis. Nephrologie 2000;21:9–12.

 99. Jonsson JJ, Renieri A, Gallagher PG, et al. Alport syndrome, mental retardation, midface hypoplasia, and elliptocytosis: a new X linked contiguous gene deletion syndrome? J Med Genet 1998;35:273–278.
100. Piccini M, Vitelli F, Bruttini M, et al. FACL4, a new gene encoding long-chain acyl-CoA synthetase 4, is deleted in a family with Alport syndrome, elliptocytosis, and mental retardation. Genomics 1998;47: 350–358.
101. Vitelli F, Piccini M, Caroli F, et al. Identification and characterization of a highly conserved protein absent in the Alport syndrome (A), mental retardation (M), midface hypoplasia (M), and elliptocytosis (E) contiguous gene deletion syndrome (AMME). Genomics 1999;55:335–340.
102. Piccini M, Vitelli F, Seri M, et al. KCNE1-like gene is deleted in AMME contiguous gene syndrome: identification and characterization of the human and mouse homologs. Genomics 1999;60:251–257.
103. Corzo D, Gibson W, Johnson K, et al. Contiguous deletion of the X-linked adrenoleukodystrophy gene (ABCD1) and DXS1357E: a novel neonatal phenotype similar to peroxisomal biogenesis disorders. Am J Hum Genet 2002;70:1520–1531.
104. Hu LJ, Laporte J, Kress W, et al. Deletions in Xq28 in two boys with myotubular myopathy and abnormal genital development define a new contiguous gene syndrome in a 430 kb region. Hum Mol Genet 1996;5: 139–143.
105. Bartsch O, Kress W, Wagner A, Seemanova E. The novel contiguous gene syndrome of myotubular myopathy (MTM1), male hypogenitalism and deletion in Xq28:report of the first familial case. Cytogenet Cell Genet 1999;85:310–314.

18

Pelizaeus-Merzbacher Disease and Spastic Paraplegia Type 2

Ken Inoue, MD, PhD

CONTENTS

BACKGROUND

Pelizaeus-Merzbacher disease (PMD) is a genomic disorder that is caused by altered dosage of a single gene, proteolipid protein 1 *(PLP1)*. Either duplication or deletion of *PLP1*-containing genomic regions on chromosome Xq22.2 results in a severe leukodystrophy characterized by deficits of myelination in the central nervous system (CNS). In this chapter, the molecular and genomic mechanisms for rearrangements causing PMD are reviewed, emphasizing differences in comparison to Charcot-Marie-Tooth disease type 1A (CMT1A) and hereditary neuropathy with liability to pressure palsies (HNPP).

INTRODUCTION

Gene dosage is a unique mechanism underlying some genetic disorders of myelin in the CNS and peripheral nervous systems (PNS). Alterations in gene dosage often are a consequence of genomic rearrangements such as duplication and deletion, which respectively result in an increased or decreased production of proteins encoded by the genes within the altered genomic interval *(1)*. At least, two myelin genes are known to be dosage sensitive and the changes in their copy number can cause dramatic disturbance of myelin development and maintenance. The first and best characterized gene is the peripheral myelin protein 22 gene *(PMP22)*; duplication of *PMP22* causes CMT1A, whereas the reciprocal deletion leads to HNPP *(2)*.

From: *Genomic Disorders: The Genomic Basis of Disease*
Edited by: J. R. Lupski and P. Stankiewicz © Humana Press, Totowa, NJ

The *PLP1* is the second example of a dosage-sensitive myelin gene. Altered dosage of *PLP1*, which can arise from gene duplication or gene deletion, causes PMD (MIM 312080) *(3–9)*. PMD is characterized by arrest of oligodendrocyte differentiation and failure to produce myelin in the CNS, resulting in developmental delay usually beginning in the first year of life (reviewed in refs. *10,11*). PMD patients also develop additional neurological features including nystagmus, pyramidalm and extrapyramidal signs and cerebellar symptoms. Sequence alterations in the *PLP1* coding regions and splice junctions can also cause PMD (reviewed in refs. *12,13*) or spastic paraplegia type 2 (SPG2; MIM 312920), a clinically distinct and milder disorder that has some similarities to PMD *(14,15)*. In this chapter, genomic mechanisms underlying *PLP1* duplication and deletion are compared to those of *PMP22* duplication and deletion.

PLP1 AND *PMP22*

Both *PLP1* and *PMP22* encode major myelin proteins. Each appears to play an important role in the development and maintenance of myelin, although the exact functions of these proteins remain elusive (Table 1). PLP1 is primarily expressed in oligodendrocytes that form myelin in the CNS, whereas PMP22 is predominantly expressed in the Schwann cells that produce myelin in the PNS. *PLP1* spans an approx 17-kb genomic interval on chromosome Xq22.2 and is composed of seven coding exons. PLP1 contains 276 amino acids, of which 35 residues encoded in the latter half of exon 3 are alternatively spliced out in DM20 *(16)*. DM20 is predominantly expressed in oligodendrocyte precursors before the initiation of myelin production, whereas major PLP1 expression occurs after birth in conjunction with myelin maturation.

PMP22 is located on chromosome 17p12 and is composed of four coding exons. There are two alternatively spliced non-coding first exons that are transcribed from independent promoters *(17,18)*. Both transcript variants encode the same protein sequence that is 116 residues shorter than PLP1.

Expression levels of both *PLP1* and *PMP22* are tightly regulated during development. Modest expression of both genes is observed in nonmyelin lineage cells, but the major expression occurs at the stage of terminal differentiation and myelin formation in the CNS or PNS (reviewed in refs. *11,19*).

PLP1/DM20 and PMP22 are tetra-span membrane proteins with both the amino and carboxyl termini located in the cytoplasm. During the process of protein synthesis in the endoplasmic reticulum (ER), both proteins are properly folded before being transported through Golgi apparatus to the myelin membrane. PMP22 undergoes post-translational glycosylation, whereas PLP/DM20 does not. Disease-causing amino acid substitutions in both PLP1/DM20 and PMP22 result in protein misfolding and accumulation in the ER *(20–22)*. Despite the different glycosylation status of each protein, calnexin, a molecular chaperone in the ER, appears to play a role in quality control of both proteins *(23,24)*. Interestingly, abnormal accumulation of mutant PLP/DM20, but not PMP22, evokes the unfolded protein response, subsequently leading to apoptotic cell death *(23,25)*. Nevertheless, accumulation of misfolded proteins in ER leads to toxic gain-of-function effects in both proteins, which is consistent with the observation that patients with point mutations in either *PLP1* or *PMP22* generally have more severe disease.

PMD/SPG2 AND CMT1A/HNPP

PMD/SPG2 and CMT1A/HNPP result from a variety of disease-causing mutations in either *PLP1* or *PMP22* that occur through distinct mechanisms (Table 1). Genomic duplication is the

Table 1
Similarities and Differences Between PMD/SPG2 and CMT1A/HNPP[a]

		PMD/SPG2	CMT1A/HNPP
Prevalence		<1/100,000[a]	~1/2500
Gene (locus)		PLP1 (Xq22.2)	PMP22 (17p12)
Expression		Oligodendrocyte in CNS myelin	Schwann cells in PNS myelin
Protein		Tetra-span membrane protein	Tetra-span membrane protein
Mutations, frequency and mechanism			
Duplication	Frequency	60–70% of PMD	>70% of CMT1
	Gene dosage	Twice (in males)	1.5 times
	Severity	Moderate	Moderate
	Cellular pathology	Accumulation in late endosomes	Accumulation in late endosomes
Deletion	Frequency	Rare	>90% of HNPP
	Gene dosage	Null	Half
	Severity	Mild	Mild
	Cellular pathology	Protein deficit	Haploinsufficiency
Point mutation	Frequency	~20%	Rare
	Severity	Mostly severe	Mostly severe
	Cellular pathology	Protein misfolding and ER accumulation	Protein misfolding and ER accumulation
Genomic mechanisms for recombination		NHEJ	NAHR
Clustered breakpoints		Proximal end: no Distal end: yes	Yes
Order of duplication		Tandem/inverted	Tandem
Origin of recombinant products		Sister chromatid exchange	Crossover between two homologous chromosomes
Involvement of LCRs in the recombination		Probably yes	Yes
Presence of flanking LCRs		No	Yes

[a]Estimated from ref. 58.

most frequent mutation in both PMD and CMT1A. *PLP1* duplications account for approx 60–70% of PMD patients. Similarly, more than 70% of CMT1 patients have a *PMP22* duplication. *PLP1* genomic deletion has only been reported in three families, whereas *PMP22* deletion causes the common trait HNPP.

Duplication of *PLP1* doubles gene dosage in males owing to X-chromosome hemizygosity (Table 1). This contrasts with the autosomal *PMP22* duplication that increases the gene dosage by half. As shown by increased severity in rare patients with either a triplication of *PLP1* or a homozygous duplication of *PMP22* (3,9,26,27), disease severity is proportionate to gene copy number. Consistent with these observations, mice with homozygous *Plp1* transgenes have a prominent dysmyelinating phenotype and shortened lifespan (28,29), whereas heterozygotes develop a late-onset demyelinating disease (30,31). Similarly, *Pmp22* transgenic murine models have shown that the expression level of *Pmp22* correlated with the degree of demyelination *(32)*.

In contrast to the severe phenotype observed with duplications, deletions of either gene results in a milder phenotype (Table 1). This is especially surprising in *PLP1* deletion, because it results in a *PLP1* null genotype in males. Male patients with *PLP1* deletion show mild PMD or SPG2 *(6,7)*. Similarly, mice lacking *Plp1* revealed minimal dysmyelinating changes *(33)*, accompanied by slowly progressive axonal degradation *(34)*. Heterozygous deletion of *PMP22* results in HNPP, a milder disease than duplication-causing CMT1A *(35)*. Mice heterozygous or homozygous for Pmp22 null alleles also recapitulate HNPP with a different degree of severity *(36,37)*.

In summary, a gene dosage defines the severity for diseases involving both *PLP1* and *PMP22*. It is worth noting that having an extra copy of *PLP1* or *PMP22* conveys a more toxic effect than not having enough of them, which appears to be a unique feature of these two genes. However, the molecular and cellular bases for the pathophysiology of the gene dosage effect remain largely unknown. Interestingly, recent studies on overexpression of both genes revealed aggregation of proteins within late endosomes coupled with sequestration of myelin membrane components *(38–42)*. This common cellular phenotype suggests a similar cellular pathology probably underlies both *PLP1* and *PMP22* duplications.

MOLECULAR TOOLS TO VISUALIZE DUPLICATIONS AND DELETIONS

Unlike structural chromosomal abnormalities caused by constitutional chromosomal rearrangement, genomic duplications and deletions associated with PMD/SPG2 and CMT1A/HNPP are "submicroscopic" and not resolved by routine chromosome banding analyses. On the other hand, DNA sequencing cannot detect the gene dosage differences, because the rearrangement does not create a sequence-based abnormality. Therefore, detection of duplication and deletion require other specific molecular technologies.

Interphase fluorescent *in situ* hybridization (FISH) with specific probes that contain the *PLP1* genomic locus with an intrachromosomal control has been applied widely for molecular diagnostics of PMD *(4,9,43,44)*. Interphase FISH can clearly visualize difference in copy number both in male patients and in female carriers. Alternatively, quantitative polymerase chain reaction can be utilized as an indirect measurement of gene dosage *(5,45,46)*. Recent advances in real-time polymerase chain reaction quantification technologies have dramatically improved sensitivity, accuracy, and efficiency of such quantitative dosage determinations. Finally, microarray-based comparative genomic hybridization analysis has emerged as a novel technology that enables detection and determination of the size of the duplicated or deleted genomic intervals in one experiment *(47–49)*. Such technologies can provide an enormous amount of information for genomic rearrangements and promote elucidation of the underlying genomic mechanisms.

MECHANISMS FOR DUPLICATIONS AND DELETIONS

PMD/SPG2 and CMT1A/HNPP are similar in the types of mutations causing disease, in the relationship between gene dosage and phenotypes, and in the cellular pathology. In contrast, recombination mechanisms for disease-associated genomic rearrangement appear to be significantly different between these diseases.

In the majority of genomic disorders, a precise genomic rearrangement commonly results in a uniform recombinant product with clustered breakpoints *(1,50)*. The CMT1A duplication and the HNPP deletion represent a prototype for this model of genomic rearrangement. A 1.4-Mb genomic interval, which encompasses *PMP22* and 20 other genes, is flanked by highly homologous 24-kb low-copy repeat (LCR) units, called proximal and distal CMT1A-REPs *(51,52)*. Homologous recombination between nonallelic (or paralogous) copies of CMT1A-REPs (i.e., nonallelic homologous recombination [NAHR]) and resolution of its intermediates (i.e., Holliday junctions) results in unequal crossover that causes the CMT1A-associated duplication and the reciprocal HNPP-associated deletion. Because the CMT1A-REP repeat-specific genomic feature conveys the susceptibility to NAHR at this locus, the CMT1A duplication and the HNPP deletion recur with high frequency. The same mechanism appears to underlie many other genomic disorders *(53)*.

The molecular mechanisms for the genomic rearrangements that cause *PLP1* duplication and deletion remain largely elusive, but current knowledge suggests that the involvement of NAHR is unlikely. FISH mapping of the duplicated genomic intervals in individuals with PMD revealed no common recombinant duplicated genomic segments (Fig. 1) *(4,9)*. It has been thought that the duplications are mainly tandem in nature, but our recent findings also suggest that some are inverted duplications (Lee, Inove, and Lupski, unpublished data). In contrast to CMT1A, duplicated genomic segments often originate from a single chromosome rather than two homologous chromosomes, as shown by identical haplotypes within the duplicated genomic intervals *(4,9)*. In addition, the origin of the *de novo* duplication events can often be traced to male spermatogenesis *(46)*. Each of these findings suggests that *PLP1* duplications are commonly generated by sister-chromatid exchange in male meiosis *(4,9,46)*. Unlike observations in CMT1A and HNPP, extensive genome sequence analysis of this interval identified no flanking pair of tandem LCRs that could serve as substrates for NAHR *(4,6,54)*. Instead, an inverted pair of LCRs was found approx 180-kb distal to *PLP1*; these have been named LCR-PMDA and LCR-PMDB (Fig. 1) *(6)*.

An analysis of recombination breakpoints associated with the rare *PLP1* deletions has provided a potential model for the genomic rearrangements causing the more common *PLP1* duplications *(6)*. The precise mapping and sequencing of recombination junction fragments in three *PLP1* deletion families revealed the involvement of the following complex and distinct processes, including (1) inheritance of an unbalanced insertional translocation, (2) sister-chromatid exchange in male meiosis, and (3) complex rearrangement. Nevertheless, the products of recombination in each family, when the strand exchange products were analyzed at the nucleotide sequence level, revealed that the recombination process appeared to occur by nonhomologous end-joining (NHEJ) *(6)*.

Unlike homologous recombination, NHEJ, a major pathway for repairing double-strand DNA breaks, does not require a stretch of homologous sequences for initiating recombination. Thus, recombination can occur anywhere on a chromosome arm. Based on the observation that the recombination breakpoints for *PLP1* duplication are not confined to specific positions but spread across the *PLP1* region and that pairs of tandem LCRs do not flank the duplicated genomic interval, it is likely that NHEJ mediates the genomic rearrangements that lead to *PLP1* duplications *(6)*. Supporting this hypothesis, DNA sequence analyses of several duplication junction fragments appeared to show absence of homology at the recombination breakpoints, evidence for NHEJ and not NAHR *(55,56)*.

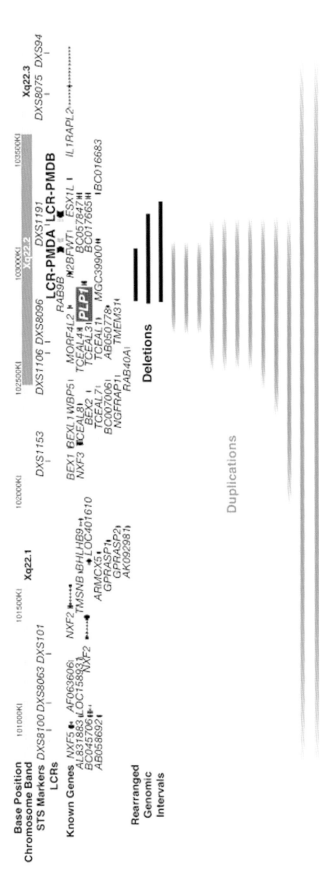

Fig. 1. Structure of proteolipid protein 1 (*PLP1*) genomic region. The top rectangles represent chromosomal bands and the numbers above show the physical distance from the telomeric end of the short arm (left). Representative steroid sequence-tagged site are shown. A pair of low-copy repeats (LCRs), LCR-PMDA and LCR-PCMB, are present distal to *PLP1*. Arrows indicate orientation of each unit and different tones show the level of homology. Genes are listed with vertical lines showing each exon. Horizontal bars (bottom) represent genomic intervals that are rearranged in each PMD patient with either deletion (black horizontal bar with sharp ends) or duplication (dark gray horizontal bar with shaded ends). Recombination breakpoints are defined by DNA sequence for deletions and by fluorescent *in situ* hybridization mapping for duplications. Note that the distal ends of recombinant genomic intervals are accumulated at LCR-PMDs, whereas the proximal breakpoint ends are more diffuse. (Information for the physical map was obtained from University of California, Santa Cruz, Genome Browser of Human Genome May 2004 at http://genome.ucsc.edu.)

THE ROLE OF HUMAN GENOMIC ARCHITECTURE

One of the characteristic features of the human genome is its structural complexity with a large number of LCRs. This higher order genomic architecture has been implicated in the pathomechanisms of genomic disorders *(53)*. It has been demonstrated repeatedly in different genomic disorders that locus-specific LCRs serve as substrates for NAHR, thus, genomic architecture plays a direct and significant role in common and recurrent genomic rearrangements. Meanwhile, it is less understood as to whether such genomic architecture can also convey susceptibility to *PLP1* duplication and, if so, what is the mechanism underlying the susceptibility to NHEJ. The distal recombination breakpoints for *PLP1* duplications and deletions appear to accumulate around LCR-PMDs by FISH mapping (Fig. 1) *(4,6)*. Moreover, the distal breakpoints for two out of three *PLP1* deletions examined were mapped within the LCR-PMDs at the DNA sequence level *(6)*. In addition, our preliminary genomic analysis of *PLP1* duplications using pulsed-field gel electrophoresis suggests that LCR-PMDs are involved in duplication event as well *(54)*. Furthermore, the extensive genomic analysis uncovered a number of scattered, small (approx 5 kb) LCRs in an approx 1-Mb genomic interval proximal to *PLP1*, most of which are not homologous to any sequence composing either LCR-PMDA or LCR-PMDB *(54)*. Further studies are required to determine whether these proximal small LCRs are involved in the genomic recombination events. Nevertheless, current findings are in support of our working hypothesis that human genomic architecture may also convey susceptibility to NHEJ-mediated genomic disorders by stimulating disease-causing genomic rearrangements *(6,54,57)*.

SUMMARY

In contrast to the major advances in elucidating the mechanisms for NAHR-mediated genomic disorders, there is a paucity of information regarding molecular mechanisms underlying the NHEJ-based genomic disorders. However, similar to what has been revealed in NAHR-mediated genomic disorders, it has become evident that human genomic architecture also is involved in the mechanism for NHEJ-based genomic disorders. Using the available human genome sequence together with advanced molecular technologies, further studies on PMD will clarify the disease mechanisms for the NHEJ-based genomic disorders.

ACKNOWLEDGMENTS

I appreciate all the patients and families for their contribution to our research projects on PMD. I also thank Dr. Neal Boerkoel for his critical review and Drs. Hitoshi Osaka, Kimiko Deguchi, and Lisa Shaffer for their long-term collaboration and advice.

REFERENCES

1. Lupski JR. Genomic disorders: structural features of the genome can lead to DNA rearrangements and human disease traits. Trends Genet 1998;14:417–422.
2. Chance PF, Abbas N, Lensch MW, et al. Two autosomal dominant neuropathies result from reciprocal DNA duplication/deletion of a region on chromosome 17. Hum Mol Genet 1994;3:223–228.
3. Ellis D, Malcolm S. Proteolipid protein gene dosage effect in Pelizaeus-Merzbacher disease. Nat Genet 1994;6:333–334.
4. Inoue K, Osaka H, Imaizumi K, et al. Proteolipid protein gene duplications causing Pelizaeus-Merzbacher disease: molecular mechanism and phenotypic manifestations. Ann Neurol 1999;45:624–632.

5. Inoue K, Osaka H, Sugiyama N, et al. A duplicated *PLP* gene causing Pelizaeus-Merzbacher disease detected by comparative multiplex PCR. Am J Hum Genet 1996;59:32–39.

6. Inoue K, Osaka H, Thurston VC, et al. Genomic rearrangements resulting in *PLP1* deletion occur by non-homologous end-joining and cause different dysmyelinating phenotypes in males and females. Am J Hum Genet 2002;71:838–853.

7. Raskind WH, Williams CA, Hudson LD, Bird TD. Complete deletion of the proteolipid protein gene (PLP) in a family with X-linked Pelizaeus-Merzbacher disease. Am J Hum Genet 1991;49:1355–1360.

8. Cremers FPM, Pfeiffer RA, van de Pol TJR, et al. An interstitial duplication of the X chromosome in a male allows physical fine mapping of probes from the Xq13-q22 region. Human Genetics 1987;77:23–27.

9. Woodward K, Kendall E, Vetrie D, Malcolm S. Pelizaeus-Merzbacher disease: identification of Xq22 proteolipid-protein duplications and characterization of breakpoints by interphase FISH. Am J Hum Genet 1998;63:207–217.

10. Hudson LD. Pelizaeus-Merzbacher disease and the allelic disorder X-linked spastic paraplegia type 2. In: *The Metabolic and Molecular Bases of Inherited Diseases. 8th ed.* (Scriver CR, Beaudet AL, Sly WS, Valle D, eds.), New York: McGraw-Hill, 2001; pp 5789–5798.

11. Inoue K. *PLP1*-related inherited dysmyelinating disorders: Pelizaeus-Merzbacher disease and spastic paraplegia type 2. Neurogenetics 2005;6:1–16.

12. Hodes ME, Pratt VM, Dlouhy SR. Genetics of Pelizaeus-Merzbacher disease. Dev Neurosci 1993;15:383–394.

13. Garbern J, Cambi F, Shy M, Kamholz J. The molecular pathogenesis of Pelizaeus-Merzbacher disease. Arch Neurol 1999;56:1210–1214.

14. Saugier-Veber P, Munnich A, Bonneau D, et al. X-linked spastic paraplegia and Pelizaeus-Merzbacher disease are allelic disorders at the proteolipid protein locus. Nat Genet 1994;6:257–262.

15. Osaka H, Kawanishi C, Inoue K, et al. Novel nonsense proteolipid protein gene mutation as a cause of X-linked spastic paraplegia in twin males. Biochem Biophys Res Commun 1995;215:835–841.

16. Nave KA, Lai C, Bloom FE, Milner RJ. Splice site selection in the proteolipid protein (PLP) gene transcript and primary structure of the DM-20 protein of central nervous system myelin. Proc Natl Acad Sci USA 1987;84:5665–5669.

17. Maier M, Berger P, Nave KA, Suter U. Identification of the regulatory region of the peripheral myelin protein 22 (PMP22) gene that directs temporal and spatial expression in development and regeneration of peripheral nerves. Mol Cell Neurosci 2002;20:93–109.

18. Suter U, Snipes GJ, Schoener-Scott R, et al. Regulation of tissue-specific expression of alternative peripheral myelin protein-22 (PMP22) gene transcripts by two promoters. J Biol Chem 1994;269:25,795–25,808.

19. Lupski JR, Garcia CA. Charcot-Marie-Tooth peripheral neuropathies and related disorders. In: *The Metabolic and Molecular Bases of Inherited Diseases. 8th ed.* (Scriver CR, Beaudet AL, Sly WS, Valle D, eds.), New York: McGraw-Hill, 2001; pp 5759–5788.

20. Gow A, Lazzarini RA. A cellular mechanism governing the severity of Pelizaeus-Merzbacher disease. Nat Genet 1996;13:422–428.

21. Gow A, Southwood CM, Lazzarini RA. Disrupted proteolipid protein trafficking results in oligodendrocyte apoptosis in an animal model of Pelizaeus-Merzbacher disease. J Cell Biol 1998;140:925–934.

22. D'Urso D, Prior R, Greiner-Petter R, Gabreëls-Festen AA, Müller HW. Overloaded endoplasmic reticulum-Golgi compartments, a possible pathomechanism of peripheral neuropathies caused by mutations of the peripheral myelin protein PMP22. J Neurosci 1998;18:731–740.

23. Dickson KM, Bergeron JJ, Shames I, et al. Association of calnexin with mutant peripheral myelin protein-22 ex vivo: a basis for "gain-of-function" ER diseases. Proc Natl Acad Sci USA 2002;99:9852–9857.

24. Swanton E, High S, Woodman P. Role of calnexin in the glycan-independent quality control of proteolipid protein. EMBO J 2003;22:2948–2958.

25. Southwood CM, Garbern J, Jiang W, Gow A. The unfolded protein response modulates disease severity in Pelizaeus-Merzbacher disease. Neuron 2002;36:585–596.

26. Lupski JR, Montes de Oca-Luna R, Slaugenhaupt S, et al. DNA duplication associated with Charcot-Marie-Tooth disease type 1A. Cell 1991;66:219–232.

27. LeGuern E, Gouider R, Mabin D, et al. Patients homozygous for the 17p11.2 duplication in Charcot-Marie-Tooth type 1A disease. Ann Neurol 1997;41:104–108.

28. Readhead C, Schneider A, Griffiths I, Nave KA. Premature arrest of myelin formation in transgenic mice with increased proteolipid protein gene dosage. Neuron 1994;12:583–595.

29. Kagawa T, Ikenaka K, Inoue Y, et al. Glial cell degeneration and hypomyelination caused by overexpression of myelin proteolipid protein gene. Neuron 1994;13:427–442.

30. Inoue Y, Kagawa T, Matsumura Y, Ikenaka K, Mikoshiba K. Cell death of oligodendrocytes or demyelination induced by overexpression of proteolipid protein depending on expressed gene dosage. Neurosci Res 1996;25:161–172.

31. Anderson TJ, Schneider A, Barrie JA, et al. Late-onset neurodegeneration in mice with increased dosage of the proteolipid protein gene. J Comp Neurol 1998;394:506–519.

32. Huxley C, Passage E, Robertson AM, et al. Correlation between varying levels of PMP22 expression and the degree of demyelination and reduction in nerve conduction velocity in transgenic mice. Hum Mol Genet 1998;7:449–458.

33. Klugmann M, Schwab MH, Puhlhofer A, et al. Assembly of CNS myelin in the absence of proteolipid protein. Neuron 1997;18:59–70.

34. Griffiths I, Klugmann M, Anderson T, et al. Axonal swellings and degeneration in mice lacking the major proteolipid of myelin. Science 1998;280:1610–1613.

35. Chance PF, Alderson MK, Leppig KA, et al. DNA deletion associated with hereditary neuropathy with liability to pressure palsies. Cell 1993;72:143–151.

36. Adlkofer K, Frei R, Neuberg DH, Zielasek J, Toyka KV, Suter U. Heterozygous peripheral myelin protein 22-deficient mice are affected by a progressive demyelinating tomaculous neuropathy. J Neurosci 1997;17: 4662–4671.

37. Adlkofer K, Martini R, Aguzzi A, Zielasek J, Toyka KV, and Suter U. Hypermyelination and demyelinating peripheral neuropathy in Pmp22-deficient mice. Nat Genet 1995;11:274–280.

38. Niemann S, Sereda MW, Suter U, Griffiths IR, Nave KA. Uncoupling of myelin assembly and schwann cell differentiation by transgenic overexpression of peripheral myelin protein 22. J Neurosci 2000;20:4120–4128.

39. Chies R, Nobbio L, Edomi P, Schenone A, Schneider C, Brancolini C. Alterations in the Arf6-regulated plasma membrane endosomal recycling pathway in cells overexpressing the tetraspan protein Gas3/PMP22. J Cell Sci 2003;116:987–999.

40. Ryan MC, Shooter EM, Notterpek L. Aggresome formation in neuropathy models based on peripheral myelin protein 22 mutations. Neurobiol Dis 2002;10:109–118.

41. Simons M, Kramer EM, Macchi P, et al. Overexpression of the myelin proteolipid protein leads to accumulation of cholesterol and proteolipid protein in endosomes/lysosomes: implications for Pelizaeus-Merzbacher disease. J Cell Biol 2002;157:327–336.

42. Simons M, Kramer EM, Thiele C, Stoffel W, Trotter J. Assembly of myelin by association of proteolipid protein with cholesterol- and galactosylceramide-rich membrane domains. J Cell Biol 2000;151:143–154.

43. Inoue K, Kanai M, Tanabe Y, et al. Prenatal interphase FISH diagnosis of *PLP1* duplication associated with Pelizaeus-Merzbacher disease. Prenat Diagn 200121:1133–1136.

44. Hodes ME, Woodward K, Spinner NB, et al. Additional copies of the proteolipid protein gene causing Pelizaeus-Merzbacher disease arise by separate integration into the X chromosome. Am J Hum Genet 2000;67:14–22.

45. Regis S, Filocamo M, Mazzotti R, et al. Prenatal diagnosis of Pelizaeus-Merzbacher disease: detection of proteolipid protein gene duplication by quantitative fluorescent multiplex PCR. Prenat Diagn 2001;21: 668–671.

46. Mimault C, Giraud G, Courtois V, et al. and The Clinical European Network on Brain Dysmyelinating Disease. Proteolipoprotein gene analysis in 82 patients with sporadic Pelizaeus-Merzbacher disease: duplications, the major cause of the disease, originate more frequently in male germ cells, but point mutations do not. Am J Hum Genet 1999;65:360–369.

47. Shaw CJ, Shaw CA, Yu W, et al. Comparative genomic hybridisation using a proximal 17p BAC/PAC array detects rearrangements responsible for four genomic disorders. J Med Genet 2004;41:113–119.

48. Albertson DG, Pinkel D. Genomic microarrays in human genetic disease and cancer. Hum Mol Genet 2003;12:R145–R152.

49. Mantripragada KK, Buckley PG, de Stahl TD, Dumanski JP. Genomic microarrays in the spotlight. Trends Genet 2004;20:87–94.

50. Inoue K, Lupski JR. Molecular mechanisms for genomic disorders. Annu Rev Genomics Hum Genet 2002;3:199–242.

51. Pentao L, Wise CA, Chinault AC, Patel PI, Lupski JR. Charcot-Marie-Tooth type 1A duplication appears to arise from recombination at repeat sequences flanking the 1.5 Mb monomer unit. Nat Genet 1992;2:292–300.

52. Inoue K, Dewar K, Katsanis N, et al. The 1.4-Mb CMT1A duplication/HNPP deletion genomic region reveals unique genome architectural features and provides insights into the recent evolution of new genes. Genome Res 2001;11:1018–1033.
53. Stankiewicz P, Lupski JR. Genome architecture, rearrangements and genomic disorders. Trends Genet 2002;18:74–82.
54. Lee J, Dean M, Gold B, Inoue K, Lupski JR. Role of genomic architecture in *PLP1* duplication causing Pelizaeus-Merzbacher disease. American Society of Human Genetics, 54th Annual Meeting. Toronto, 2004; pp A103.
55. Hobson G, Cundall M, Sperle K, et al. Fine mapping of duplication endpoints in Pelizaeus-Merzbacher disease. American Society of Human Genetics, 53rd Annual Meeting. Los Angels, 2003; pp A1009.
56. Iwaki A, Kondo J, Ototsuji M, Kurosawa K, Fukumaki Y. Characterization of the breakpoints of PLP1 duplication in three cases of Pelizaeus-Merzbacher disease. American Society of Human Genetics, 53rd Annual Meeting. Los Angels, 2003; pp A2229.
57. Shaw CJ, Lupski JR. Implications of human genome architecture for rearrangement-based disorders: the genomic basis of disease. Hum Mol Genet 2004;13:R57–R64.
58. Heim P, Claussen M, Hoffmann B, et al. Leukodystrophy incidence in Germany. Am J Med Genet 1997;71: 475–478.

19 Y-Chromosomal Rearrangements and Azoospermia

Matthew E. Hurles, PhD and Chris Tyler-Smith, PhD

CONTENTS

BACKGROUND

Approximately 0.03% of men carry a Y-chromosomal defect that leads to azoospermia, the absence of sperm cells from semen. Deletion mapping of the Y chromosomes of azoospermic or oligozoospermic men suggested that loss of three nonoverlapping regions, *AZFa*, *AZFb*, and *AZFc*, could be responsible. When the finished Y-chromosomal reference sequence became available, the recurrent deletion of each of these intervals could be explained largely by non-allelic homologous recombination between direct repeats. However, in contrast to the conclusion from deletion mapping, *AZFb* deletions were found to overlap with *AZFc* deletions. In addition, a background level of nonhomologous recombination was found to generate a minority of deletions of these intervals. *USP9Y* appears to be the critical gene underlying the *AZFa* phenotype, but the critical genes lost in the *AZFb* and *AZFc* deletions have not yet been identified. Inspection of the sequence allowed additional duplications, inversions, and partial deletions of the *AZF* intervals to be anticipated, and many of the predicted structures have subsequently been identified in the population. The phenotypic consequences of these additional rearrangements of the *AZFc* region are unclear. High levels of gene conversion homogenize duplicated sequences in both direct and inverted orientations on the Y, which could potentiate subsequent rearrangements. The Y chromosome provides an excellent model for understanding genomic disorders; however, more finished sequences and new methodologies are needed.

From: *Genomic Disorders: The Genomic Basis of Disease*
Edited by: J. R. Lupski and P. Stankiewicz © Humana Press, Totowa, NJ

INTRODUCTION

"Azoospermia" is the absence of sperm cells (spermatozoa) from the semen. It is found in as many as 1–2% of men and is a heterogeneous condition with diverse causes. It has been classified in a number of ways, for example, according to whether there is a failure of sperm cell production, or a failure of transport from the testes tubules to the semen fluid. Among the underlying causes are genetic factors, and this chapter focuses on one subset of these: microdeletions of Y-chromosomal DNA loci. After Klinefelter syndrome (approx 0.1% of births), such deletions are the second most frequent cause of spermatogenic failure and may be present in approx 0.03% of men.

The link between azoospermia and Y defects has been recognized for almost three decades. We outline some aspects of the historical development of the field in the next section, but because the finished DNA sequence of most of the euchromatic portion of the Y chromosome is now available *(1)*, in the remainder of the chapter we emphasize two themes: the way that known deletions can be explained by the DNA sequence, and, in a complementary fashion, the way that the sequence can suggest additional possible deletions or other rearrangements that can then be experimentally verified and investigated further. We end with a discussion of findings that are not so readily explained and outline some possible future directions for the field.

IDENTIFICATION OF *AZF* LOCI ON THE Y CHROMOSOME

The Azoospermia Phenotype

The complete absence of sperm cells from semen may seem like a simple phenotype, unambiguously ascertained by an examination of semen, but sperm count can be affected by many factors (such as time since the last ejaculation, substance abuse, frequency of hot baths, and even dental caries) and can, thus, vary considerably in a single individual *(2)*. A discussion of this variation lies outside the scope of the present chapter; here we note that sperm count can be regarded as a continuous trait (Fig. 1) with azoospermia grading into oligozoospermia (few sperm) and the normozoospermic state, and will not distinguish between the first two, so that the phenotype under consideration here would more accurately be described as "azoo- or oligozoospermia." Although azoospermia, in the strict sense, leads to infertility under natural conditions (this can sometimes be overcome by assisted reproduction), the relationship between oligozoospermia and fertility (producing offspring) is complex but can only be discussed briefly in this chapter.

Deletion Mapping of AZF *Loci on the Y Chromosome*

The idea that azoospermia was linked to the Y chromosome was initially established by the cytogenetic observations of Tiepolo and Zuffardi in 1976 *(3)*, who detected visible deletions of the distal euchromatic region of Yq in 5/1170 infertile males and an additional male of unknown fertility; four of the six were *de novo* events. The authors, therefore, presciently suggested that factors (in the plural, later designated *AZF*s for *AZoospermia Factors*) controlling spermatogenesis were contained within the deleted region. The availability of DNA hybridization probes and subsequently sequence-tagged sites (STSs) detecting Y-specific loci allowed the construction of deletion maps from rearranged chromosomes *(4)*. Deletion mapping provides a clear ordering of loci into deletion intervals when the underlying sequences are

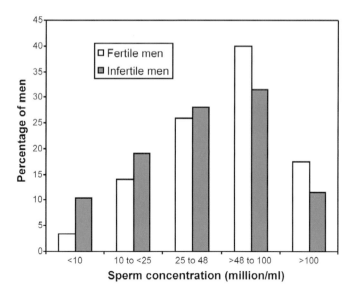

Fig. 1. Distribution of sperm counts in fertile and infertile men. Note the broad ranges and overlap between the two samples. (Modified from data in ref. *42*.)

unique, but the results can be misleading when the sequences are present in multiple copies. Some regions of the Y chromosome are entirely multicopy and difficulties in deletion map interpretation underlie some of the problems discussed below. Individuals with cytogenetically normal Ys and idiopathic infertility were characterized using this approach, and microdeletions were identified in a subset of them; however, these did not all overlap *(5)*. An extensive compilation of data from 370 men with azoospermia or oligozoospermia led to a widely held view that three nonoverlapping deletions, designated *AZFa*, *AZFb*, and *AZFc* in the order centromere to Yq telomere, could be defined *(6)*. It was expected that further work would refine the locations of the individual genes within these intervals that were responsible for the spermatogenic failure, using a combination of finer deletion mapping and the subsequent detection of point mutations. Although this expectation has been largely fulfilled for *AZFa* (*see* The *AZFa* Deletion), the *AZFb* and *AZFc* intervals have proved more refractory to analysis and the identity of the key genes within them remains unclear.

Early Clues to Yq Complexity

As attempts to identify *AZF* genes progressed, it became clear that several lines of evidence could not be incorporated into a simple picture of an intact "normal" Y chromosome with sporadic deletion mutations leading to azoospermia.

PHENOTYPIC VARIABILITY

The sperm count associated with any Y-chromosomal genotype is variable. The variation within a single individual has been previously mentioned, so it should not be surprising that considerable variation is also seen in the phenotypes of individuals with deletions that are indistinguishable at the molecular level. Nevertheless, it is striking that men with *AZFc* deletions, where independent events lead to a common structure (*see* The *AZFc* Deletion) and are usually associated with spermatogenic failure, can occasionally conceive children naturally

(6–9). In one family, an *AZFc*-deleted man fathered four sons, the last at the age of 38, although at the time of analysis when he was aged 63, he was azoospermic *(7)*; the three sons tested were all oligozoospermic. These observations underscore the complexity of the relationship between microdeletions and fertility. Moreover, fertility is a property of couples, not individual males, so there are many additional genetic and environmental factors that can complicate the relationship between low sperm count and fertility.

POLYMORPHIC DELETIONS AND DUPLICATIONS

Y-chromosomal deletions have also been found in the population as polymorphisms. For example, deletion of the locus 50f2/C within the *AZFc* region (now known to be part of the single-copy sequence "u3" that is also removed by *de novo* azoospermia-associated deletions; *see* Fig. 2) was initially reported in the normal father of a 46,XY female *(10)*, and further investigation showed that both deletion and duplication of this locus were common: 6.4 and 1.4%, respectively, in a worldwide sample *(11)*. Furthermore, different sequences were codeleted or coduplicated with 50f2/C in different individuals, and when the haplotypic background was taken into account, six independent deletion events and four duplications could be identified. Although the spermatogenic status of the men investigated was unknown, one deletion was present at approx 55% in the Finns, and thus was unlikely to be associated with spermatogenic failure.

Surveys of infertile patients and controls (either fertile or normozoospermic individuals) provided further examples of deletions that were not associated with azoospermia, either because they were found only in controls, or were transmitted by the fathers of infertile patients. In one large-scale evaluation using 48 STSs and 920 fertile individuals, 11 men (1.2%) were found to show deletions of single STSs that removed one of four different loci *(12)*. One of these was Amelogenin on Yp, but the other three (sY207, sY269, and sY272) are repeated sequences with copies lying within *AZFb* or *AZFc*, as defined at that time. These four deletions were assumed to represent polymorphisms, but in the same study, deletions of other single STSs (e.g., sY75, sY126) were found only in infertile patients. Are these related to the patient's infertility or not?

DELETION MAP COMPLEXITIES: *AZFd*

Interpretation of the meaning and order of the intervals defined by deletion mapping proved to be difficult, irrespective of the phenotype associated with any particular deletion. These complexities are illustrated by the proposed designation of a fourth deletion interval, *AZFd*. This was identified by Kent-First et al. in a study of 514 infertile males *(12)*. Six men who retained *DAZ* lacked only one STS, sY152, and eight lacked only the adjacent STS, sY153; one of the latter deletions was a *de novo* event. This was taken as evidence for a distinct deletion interval located between *AZFb* and *AZFc*. Yet on the finished sequence *(1)*, all copies of sY152 and sY153 are located within *AZFc* as defined by the common b2/b4 deletion (Fig. 2). Current European guidelines for molecular diagnosis of Y-chromosomal microdeletions consider that "a putative fourth *AZFd* region postulated by Kent-First et al. . . . does not exist" *(13)*. The deletion maps and yeast artificial chromosome contigs in many repeated parts of Yq that were available at the time have not been scrutinized in such detail, but may be equally unreliable.

The Importance of High-Quality Finished Sequence

Lessons to be drawn from the preceding section are that: (1) reliable sequence information is essential for interpreting the structures of deletions and other rearrangements involving

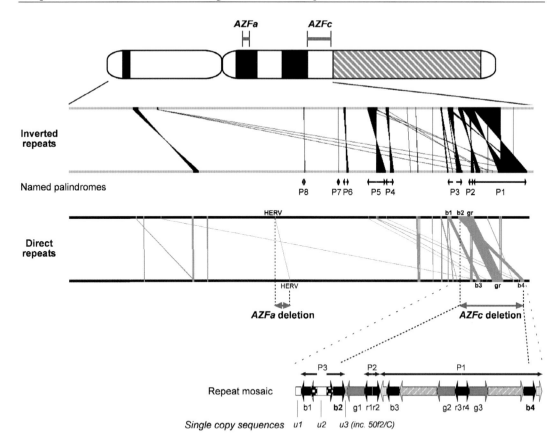

Fig. 2. Classical *AZF* deletions mapped onto the finished Y chromosome sequence. (Top) Approximate locations of the *AZFa* and *AZFc* deletion intervals on the Y chromosome. (Middle) Visualization of duplicated sequences with greater than 900 bp of identity in inverted (upper middle) and direct (lower middle) orientation on the Y chromosome-specific euchromatic reference sequence. This image was generated using the GenAlyzer software *(43)* and places diagonal lines between aligned chromosomes to show the location of inverted and direct repeats. Underneath the inverted repeats are shown the eight palindromes identified within the Y sequence. The visualization of direct repeats is annotated with the positions of the repeats promoting the *AZFa* and *AZFc* deletions, HERV-HERV and b2/b4 elements, respectively. (Bottom) Expanded view of the *AZFc* region and adjacent sequences, showing the mosaic of smaller repeats referred to in the text and including the nonrepeated segment u3 that contains 50f2/C.

repeated Y regions; (2) the sequence should be based on the Y chromosome of a single man in order to avoid confusion between polymorphisms and variants in different copies of repeated sequences within the same chromosome; but (3) sequence may be needed from more than one individual in order to understand the extent of normal polymorphic variation. The first two of these requirements have largely been met by the near-complete euchromatic sequence reported by Skaletsky et al. *(1)*, which the authors estimated had an error rate of less than 1 in 10,000 bases, and was mostly obtained from bacterial artificial chromosomes derived from a single individual, the RPCI-11 donor. Exceptions, however, included nine clones spanning the *AZFa* region. Relevant details of the *AZF* region sequences are discussed next. Here, we note that approx 25% of the euchromatic Y sequence is made up of eight palindromes (the largest spanning 2.9 Mb; Figs. 2 and 3) with arm-to-arm sequence identities of 99.94–99.997%.

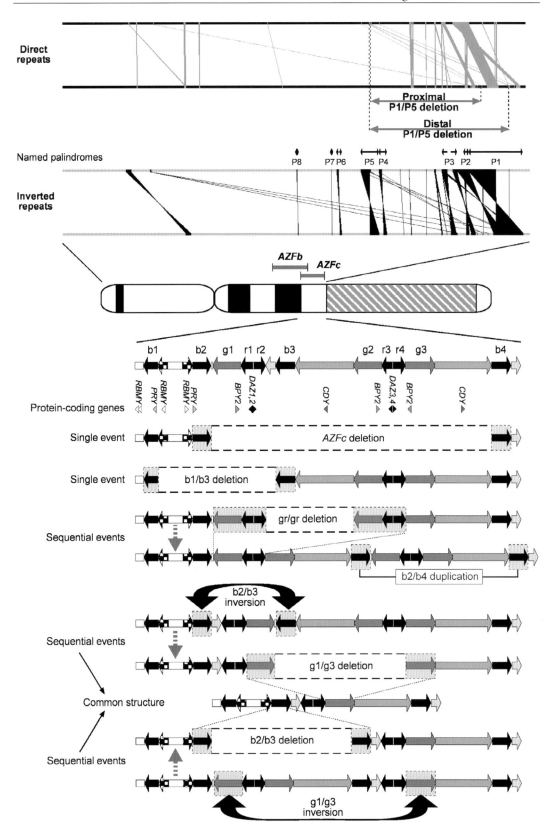

Although *AZFa* is made up of unique sequence, much of *AZFb* consists of palindromes and *AZFc* is made up almost entirely of such sequences. Only 27 proteins were identified as being encoded by the male-specific portion of the Y, but many of these have multicopy genes. In addition, the male-specific portion of the Y contains 28 non-coding transcripts, again many with multicopy genes. Genes coding for 14 different proteins lie in the *AZF* regions.

CONFIRMATION OF "CLASSICAL" *AZF* DELETIONS BY GENOMIC SEQUENCE DATA

The AZFa *Deletion*

The first *AZF* deletion characterized at the sequence level was *AZFa*. Iterative fine-mapping of the breakpoints of the most commonly deleted interval eventually led three groups to identify the same junction sequences in 2000 *(14–16)*. These fall within an approx 10-kb human endogenous retroviral (HERV) sequence that is duplicated on either side of the *AZFa* interval. The sequence similarity between these two HERVs varies dramatically along their length, with all the sequenced breakpoints clustering within two smaller "hotspots" that contain by far the longest lengths of absolute identity between the two HERVs. The HERVs provide the largest blocks of sequence identity in this part of the chromosome (Fig. 2). As with other genomic disorders, the clustering of rearrangement breakpoints within duplicated sequences and the association between sequence identity and junction sequences implicates nonallelic homologous recombination (NAHR) between these two HERVs as the mechanism underlying the deletion event.

The *AZFa* deletion removes two protein-coding genes, *USP9Y* and *DBY*, and one non-coding transcript, and results in a complete absence of germ cells known as the sertoli cell only phenotype. A single infertile male with a *de novo* null mutation (a 4-bp deletion) that produces a truncated *USP9Y* protein has the less severe, spermatid arrest, phenotype *(17)*, which implicates one or more additional sequences, most likely *DBY (18)*, in the more severe sertoli cell only phenotype.

The AZFc *Deletion*

Deletions of the *AZFc* interval are the most common Y-chromosomal lesion seen in infertile males. The highly duplicated nature of the *AZFc* interval—only 7% of which is single copy—hindered efforts to refine the position of the breakpoints of the common *AZFc* deletion using

---

Fig. 3. *(left)* Novel rearrangements mapped onto the finished Y chromosome sequence. (Top) Visualization of duplicated sequences with more than 900 bp of identity on the Y-specific euchromatic reference sequence. This image was generated using the GenAlyzer software *(43)* and places diagonal lines between aligned chromosomes to show the location of inverted and direct repeats. The visualization of direct repeats is annotated with the positions of the repeats promoting the two recurrent *AZFb*-encompassing deletions described in the text, P1 and P5. Above inverted repeats are shown the eight palindromes identified within the Y sequence. (Middle) Approximate locations of the *AZFb* and *AZFc* deletion intervals on the Y chromosome. (Bottom) Expanded view of the *AZFc* region and adjacent sequences showing some of the rearrangements described in the text. The *AZFc* (b2/b4), b1/b3, and gr/gr deletions can each arise from the reference sequence by a single event, and one example of a subsequent duplication (b2/b4 duplication following gr/gr deletion) is shown. Other deletions (g1/g3, b2/b3) appear to take place on substrates that differ from the reference sequence by inversion events. Alternative inversion-deletion routes leading to the same structure are shown.

STSs. Only when the entire region had been sequenced using clones derived from a single male could the position of these breakpoints be localized *(19)*. Although most of the duplicated sequence in distal Yq resides in near-identical palindromes, there are a number of long highly similar sequences in direct orientation, including some within the *AZFc* interval that could potentially promote NAHR-mediated deletions. The common *AZFc* deletion occurs between 229-kb direct repeats, which share 99% sequence identity and are denoted b2 and b4 in Figs. 2 and 3. Precise breakpoint junctions within these repeats have not been identified, but it is assumed that NAHR is the causal mechanism of this approx 3.5-Mb deletion *(19)*.

Unlike the *AZFa* deletion, the specific gene(s) responsible for variable phenotype associated with the *AZFc* deletion have not been identified. Nine protein-coding genes and 12 non-coding transcripts are removed by the *AZFc* deletion, and these include all the members of eight different gene families *(19,20)*. Unfortunately, expression patterns cannot be used to differentiate between these candidate genes as all are expressed in the testes. Furthermore, the partial *AZFc* deletions characterized thus far (and discussed in Partial *AZFc* Deletions Predicted From the Reference Sequence) do not remove all the members of any of these gene families; the high level of redundancy of gene copies in this region hinders the identification of the critical loci underlying the *AZFc* phenotype.

DISCOVERY OF ADDITIONAL COMPLEXITY

Rearrangements Related to Classical Deletions

AZFa DUPLICATION AND HERV HOMOGENIZATION

If NAHR is the causal mechanism of a recurrent deletion, it is commonly presumed that the reciprocal event, a duplication, will also be generated *(21)*. The finding of this duplication is often regarded as proof that NAHR is indeed the mutational mechanism underlying both rearrangements. Duplications are often harder to detect than their reciprocal deletions, as they are more rarely pathogenic and require a quantitative rather than a qualitative assay. Duplications of the *AZFa* interval that appear to be compatible with fertility have been identified during a population survey of simple tandem repeats (STRs) diversity on the Y chromosome *(22)*. In two unrelated individuals, STRs within the *AZFa* interval exhibited unusual electrophero-grams suggestive of their being duplicated relative to other YSTRs outside the *AZFa* interval. Junction sequences that could only derive from a hybrid HERV at the duplication breakpoint were also identified in the same individuals. As these duplications were identified in a survey of population diversity, there was no phenotypic information available. However, the duplicated STR haplotypes within the two *AZFa* intervals on the same chromosome were not identical, which suggests that sufficient time must have elapsed for these haplotypes to diverge, implying that, unlike their reciprocal deletions, these duplications are compatible with fertility. It is worth noting that on a constitutively haploid chromosome such as the Y, duplications must be caused by NAHR between sister chromatids.

In addition to the deletion and duplication events within the *AZFa* interval, NAHR has been involved in the homogenization of the HERV sequences that promote the rearrangements *(14,23)*. In two independent lineages of the Y chromosome phylogeny, the maximal length of absolute identity that is shared between the HERVs has been expanded fivefold as a result of homogenization of the approx 4.5 kb of sequence between the two NAHR hotspots *(14)*. This homogenization process most likely occurred because of an *AZFa* deletion on a chromosome that had previously undergone an *AZFa* duplication. This dramatic polymorphism for the absolute length of sequence identity between the HERVs, and the apparent relationship between the length of sequence identity and hotspots of NAHR activity, together suggest that some males may have higher rates of *AZFa* deletion/duplication than others.

PARTIAL *AZFC* DELETIONS PREDICTED FROM THE REFERENCE SEQUENCE:
b1/b3, gr/gr, AND THEIR PHENOTYPIC CONSEQUENCES

Although early studies *(11)* and several subsequent analyses had provided evidence for partial deletions and duplications within the *AZFc* region, their structures and phenotypic consequences were unclear. The availability of the sequence and an understanding of the mechanism of the *AZFc* (b2/b4) deletion led to the prediction that two partial deletions might arise by homologous recombination between other direct repeats: b1/b3, or the various green and red repeats, now collectively abbreviated as gr/gr *(24)* (Fig. 3). A search strategy based on the presence or absence of STSs spanning amplicon boundaries and thus providing some specificity in this highly repeated region was used to characterize 689 men *(25)*. STS patterns indicative of both of the predicted deletions were found: one b1/b3 deletion and 22 gr/gr deletions, and all those that could be tested (1/1 and 20/22, respectively) were confirmed to be deletions by fluorescent *in situ* hybridization. In addition, two of the gr/gr deletions showed duplications interpreted as b2/b4 events (Fig. 3). The spermatogenic phenotype of the man with the b1/b3 deletion was not reported, but gr/gr deletions were found in 9/246 men with total sperm counts less than 2×10^7 (or $<10^7$/mL) compared with 0/148 with total sperm counts more than 4×10^7, a difference that achieves statistical significance ($p < 0.014$, Fisher exact test). This finding led the authors to suggest that the gr/gr deletion, which removes some but not all members of three protein-coding and five non-coding gene families, exists within the population at a lower than expected frequency as a result of mutation/ selection balance. However, statistical significance would be lost if the 149th man with normal spermatogenesis were to carry the deletion (9/246 vs 1/149, $p > 0.05$), a conservative consideration often applied in the statistical interpretation of forensic evidence. This factor and the prevalence of the deletion in the general population mean that the association of the gr/gr deletion with spermatogenic failure must be considered uncertain until more data are available, particularly in the light of results from other deletions discussed next. Irrespective of the phenotype associated with the gr/gr deletions, their genomic properties are of considerable interest. The Y chromosome outside the pseudoautosomal regions evolves along stable lineages that are not disrupted by recombination and can be identified and organized into a phylogenetic tree using neutral polymorphisms. gr/gr deletions were found in 14 branches of a tree that resolved 43 lineages and had apparently arisen independently in each of these branches, although the locations of the recombination events within the gr repeats are unknown and could differ between lineages: for example, some could remove *DAZ1/DAZ2*, wereas others could remove *DAZ3/DAZ4*. The deleted chromosomes made up a small proportion of most lineages, but in one, D2b, all 12 chromosomes examined carried the deletion, and this lineage is known to be present in approx 30% of men in Japan *(26)*. Such a frequency can be achieved by a neutral marker by genetic drift, but is unlikely to be attained by a lineage that is selected against even to the extent of 1% *(27)*, the selective disadvantage estimated by the authors. Possible explanations are that: (1) some or all gr/gr deletions have no significant effect on spermatogenesis; (2) they reduce sperm numbers but have no significant effect on fertility; or (3) a compensatory mutation has arisen. Such a mutation would be most effective if it was located on the Y chromosome and was, thus, permanently linked to the deletion, and the b2/b4 duplication reported in 2/30 gr/gr deletions (*see* Fig. 3) provides a candidate for such a mutation since it restores gene copy numbers to their original levels or higher *(25)*. Unfortunately, it is not yet known whether or not D2b gr/gr deletions carry a b2/b4 duplication.

Ironically, although the gr/gr deletion may not be in mutation/selection balance, the *AZFc* deletion characterized by the same authors provides a clear example of such a balance. The incomplete penetrance of the *AZFc* deletion leads to its infrequent but recurrent transmission from father to son (*see* The *AZFa* Deletion) and results in the *AZFc* deletion reaching a population frequency higher than its *de novo* mutation rate, but being kept in check by the deletion's substantial fitness costs.

PARTIAL *AZFc* DELETIONS NOT PREDICTED FROM THE REFERENCE SEQUENCE: g1/g3 (=b2/b3)

The detection in the population of deletions predicted from the sequence provides a powerful illustration of the usefulness of sequence data. Further surveys, however, have discovered additional partial *AZFc* deletions that were not predicted. A major class lacks two apparently discontinuous regions, one including u3 (and thus 50f2/C) and the other the *DAZ3* and *DAZ4* genes, which lie in the distal *DAZ* cluster *(20,28)*. Neither deletion could arise by homologous recombination from the reference sequence, but a combination of two events, an inversion followed by a deletion, involving both the b2/b3 and g1/g3 repeats, could remove all the missing sequences by either of two pathways (*see* Fig. 3). This deletion product has been identified in four lineages, but most deleted chromosomes belong to one of them, N, where it appears to be fixed. The N lineage is even more widespread than D2b, predominating in northern Asia and making up 12% of Y chromosomes in one worldwide survey *(29)*. The proposed mechanism of deletion gains credence from the detection of both of the possible intermediate inverted structures in nondeleted chromosomes, with b2/b3 inversions showing at least two independent origins in a 44-branch tree and gr/gr inversions 5; additional duplications were found in 3 of the 14 deleted chromosomes *(20)*. Genes removed by the deletion (known either as g1/g3 or b2/b3) include some but not all members of three protein-coding and five non-coding gene families, but with the loss of more family members than the gr/gr deletion. The success of the N lineage is easily understood under the hypothesis that such partial deletions are neutral events—it is entirely owing to chance genetic drift—but requires more convoluted explanations involving compensating mutations other than the known duplications under the hypothesis that such partial deletions are associated with spermatogenic failure.

Deletions Encompassing the **AZFb** *Interval*

The relatively simple relationship observed for *AZFa* and *AZFc* between a deletion interval mapped using STSs and a single common deletion structure does not hold true for *AZFb*. There are at least two recurrent deletions that remove the *AZFb* interval defined by STS mapping, as well as additional nonrecurrent deletions *(30)*. All of these deletions also remove part of the *AZFc* region, suggesting that the *AZFb* interval is not a discrete block as was originally supposed *(6)*. NAHR is again the most likely mechanism underlying the recurrent deletions, although the lack of homology at the breakpoints of a nonrecurrent deletion indicates a low background level of nonhomologous recombination.

As with *AZFc*, the direct repeats responsible for both of the recurrent deletions lie within different palindromes in distal Yq. The 6.2-Mb recurrent deletion that removes only a small portion of the *AZFc* locus in addition to the *AZFb* region occurs between approx 100-kb direct repeats that reside in the proximal copies of palindromes P1 and P5 *(30)* (*see* Fig. 3). The 7.7-Mb recurrent deletion that removes a much greater proportion of the *AZFc* region occurs between the corresponding repeats in the distal copies of palindromes P1 and P5 (Fig. 3). There is evidence that within the approx 100-kb repeats lies a 933-bp hotspot in which the deletion breakpoints are preferentially located, although more *AZFb*-deleted chromosomes need to be characterized at the sequence level for unambiguous identification of hotspot activity.

Twenty-one protein-coding genes and 11 non-coding transcripts are removed by the proximal P1/P5 deletion, which represents all the family members of 15 different genes *(20,30)*. In the larger distal P1/P5 deletion, an additional four protein-coding genes and six non-coding transcripts are deleted, with the result that 19 gene families are lost in their entirety.

When overlapping deletions elsewhere in the genome result in similar phenotypes, it is usual to assume that the critical genes underlying the phenotype map to the region of overlap. This viewpoint has not been adopted for the overlapping *AZFb/AZFc* deletions causing male infertility on Yq, probably for historical reasons. The overlap of the deletions contains only members of gene families and not entire families. Is loss of these members primarily responsible for the phenotype, with modifications by flanking genes, or do similar phenotypes arise from the loss of genes in the nonoverlapping regions?

FURTHER *AZFB* COMPLEXITY: 50f2/E DUPLICATIONS

Perhaps unsurprisingly in view of the *AZFc* complexity, there are hints of a greater variety of *AZFb* rearrangements. One case of a duplication involving both 50f2/C (Fig. 2) and a second locus approx 1.4 Mb proximal, 50f2/E, was detected in a population screen of 595 normal individuals *(11)*, and may represent an example of one of the predicted P1/P5 duplications *(31)*. It seems likely that systematic searches would reveal a wealth of further inversions, duplications, and deletions.

CURRENT QUESTIONS AND FUTURE DIRECTIONS

AZF *Genes and Spermatogenic Failure*

IDENTIFICATION OF CRITICAL *AZF* GENES

The recurrent *AZF* deletions previously discussed account for most of those understood at a molecular level, but there are exceptions for all three regions. Partial deletions of *AZFa* have been described *(32)*; out of a sample of 11 deletions removing *AZFb*, 2 could not be explained by homologous recombination *(30)*; and 1 out of 48 *AZFc* deletions was smaller than the common size shared by the other 47 *(19)*. Although these findings require further investigation and interpretation in the light of the large variety of possible deletion substrates, they do suggest that there is a low level of more diverse and sometimes nonhomologous deletion. Although of less clinical significance because of their rarity, they may be highly informative in pinpointing the functionally important genes in the large regions identified by the recurrent mutations.

An alternative way of identifying the critical genes is offered by some of the variant structures. Despite searches, point mutations have not so far been found in *AZFb* or *AZFc*, and one possible explanation for this failure is that inactivation of a single copy of any of the genes present, which are all multicopy in the reference sequence, would be insufficient to lead to spermatogenic failure. In some lineages, however, such as N, the genes *BPY2* and *CDY1* are present in single copies, and *DAZ* is reduced to two copies (Fig. 3). Men belonging to lineage N might therefore experience spermatogenic failure as a result of inactivation of the last copy of one of these genes by a point mutation, so a screening program focusing on this lineage might prove fruitful.

UNDERSTANDING THE SIGNIFICANCE OF PARTIAL *AZF* DELETIONS

Independent replication of the association study between gr/gr deletions and spermatogenic failure is needed, and further work should identify the deletion breakpoints and thus the individual members of gene families that are lost. In addition, more thorough investigation of the effect of the common partial deletions within *AZFc* on spermatogenesis is desirable, taking into account both the phylogenetic background and any associated duplications. Lineages Db2 and N would be of particular interest. Population genetic approaches might also provide information: have these lineages experienced negative selection and expanded less rapidly than expected for a neutral lineage? Methods that compare the age of a lineage with its frequency and determine whether the observed pattern is compatible with neutrality *(33,34)* could be used to address this question. If some partial deletions are associated with fitness costs, these might indicate the underlying selective pressures that have operated to favor multicopy genes on the Y chromosome.

The Limitations of a Single Sequence

It should be apparent from the previous discussion that the mosaic pattern of direct and inverted repeats capable of promoting rearrangements generates substantial structural polymorphism on the long arm of the Y chromosome. The principle that it is possible to predict potential variants is well established *(24,31)* and we have not cataloged them further here. However, it is worth emphasizing that not every structure observed in the population can be explained by a single mutational step from the reference sequence, and that in many cases there are alternative recombinatorial routes to the same structure (*see* Fig. 3).

Because most rearrangements are expected to occur more frequently than one in 3 billion meioses, we can reasonably expect that most, if not all, of these structures could be found in the current global population of more than 3 billion males. However, we would like to know how prevalent these different events and structures are, the locations of the recombination events within the repeated regions, and what their effects are on both spermatogenesis and further Y-chromosomal rearrangements. Some of the rearrangements may predispose to further pathogenic rearrangements, but others are likely to protect against them: for example, the b1/b3 deletion removes the b2 repeat and presumably prevents the common *AZFc* deletion. In view of the likely complexity of rearrangement events, it will be important to understand them in their phylogenetic context.

It is worth considering the consequences of the choice of reference sequence: if this had been derived from lineage N, our view of the *AZFc* region would be simpler and we would have no sequence data from sections like u3. In the same way, the current reference sequence may lack regions present on other chromosomes. Additional sequences and/or structural maps of other Y-chromosomal lineages are therefore desirable. Selection of high-priority lineages could be directed by the phylogeny, perhaps choosing the most divergent—known as haplogroup A *(35)*—or by preliminary mapping experiments to identify the most distinct structures. Unfortunately, such duplicated structures cannot be sequenced efficiently using current high-throughput methods that rely on the assembly of short reads.

The Utility of a Haploid Chromosome

In many respects the constitutive haploidy of the Y chromosome renders it a useful model for understanding chromosomal dynamics. There is no need to generate somatic cell hybrids to separate a rearranged chromosome away from its unaltered homolog. This saves time and effort in the study of individual rearrangements. The unusual evolutionary history of the Y chromosome also facilitates studies of the origins of rearrangements. The lack of allelic recombination over the entire male-specific portion of the Y chromosome makes it possible to relate all extant chromosomes with a single phylogeny *(35)*. Structural polymorphisms can be shown to have multiple independent origins if they lie on different lineages of this well-characterized phylogeny *(14,22)*. In principle, the origin of a specific polymorphic rearrangement can be placed in both time and space, albeit with a substantial degree of imprecision *(22,29)*.

Having emphasized the positive qualities of the Y chromosome, it is necessary to add the caveat that it is presently unclear how good a model the Y chromosome will be for other regions of the genome enriched for segmental duplications. The generality of the Y-chromosome is called into question by its paucity of genes, its high repeat content and especially its absence of a meiotic pairing partner over most of its length. As a consequence of all of these factors, rearrangement is the dominant mode of pathogenic mutation on this chromosome, an observation that is unlikely to hold true for other chromosomes. Nevertheless, the lessons learned from studying distal Yq may well be informative for the interpretation of other complex mosaics of inverted and direct repeats, where rearrangements of different types and sizes are associated with different phenotypic outcomes, and the concept of a single wild-type structure breaks down.

The Chimpanzee Y Chromosome

Much can be learned about the nature of mutational processes from the comparative analyses of homologous sequences between species. Thus, the prospect of a finished Y-chromosomal sequence from the common chimpanzee represents an opportunity to infer the evolutionary history of the structure and sequence of the human Y chromosome, and to explore how mutational processes differ between duplicated and single-copy sequences. Already, limited sequencing of palindromes and their flanking sequences have revealed extensive gene conversion between the palindromes in distal Yq *(36)*. Similarly, comparative sequences from chimpanzees and gorillas have revealed localized concerted evolution in and around the rearrangement hotspots within the HERVs that promote the *AZFa* rearrangement *(37)*.

Y-Chromosomal Gene Conversion

As previously described, studies of both sequence variation within species and sequence divergence between species have revealed that much of the duplicated sequence on the Y chromosome undergoes sequence homogenization. In principle, two different mechanisms could account for this observation. The first is gene conversion, which represents one resolution of a homologous recombination intermediate in which no rearrangement results, but sequence information is transferred in a nonreciprocal fashion from one repeat to another. The second process is unequal crossover in which successive duplication and deletion events generate hybrid repeats that are more similar to one another than the ancestral repeats. Both of these processes have been observed at Y-chromosomal loci *(14,22,36)*, although only gene conversion is capable of homogenizing repeats in inverted orientation.

It has been suggested that the palindromic nature of distal Yq is functionally important because it allows gene conversion to maintain the integrity of critical genes *(36)*. However, this suggestion ignores the fact that gene conversion does not require a palindromic structure; it also occurs between direct repeats. In addition, gene conversion is blind to the ancestral state of a mutation, so would not be biased toward maintaining integrity. It is more likely that the Yq palindromes owe their predominance to either a mutational bias in the duplication mechanism toward inverted duplications, or to a selective bias toward repeats in inverted orientation because these are more stable structures.

It has been observed that gene conversion between duplicated sequences is capable of altering patterns of sequence divergence between orthologous sequences *(37,38)*. In the case of the Yq palindromes, gene conversion seems to reduce sequence divergence beneath that observed at single-copy Y-chromosomal sequences *(36)*. The reverse is true at the *AZFa*-HERVs, where gene conversion elevates sequence divergence between humans, chimpanzees, and gorillas *(37)*. More theoretical modeling and data from elsewhere in the genome are required to explain these opposing outcomes.

Sequence similarity between duplicated sequences potentially influences the rate of NAHR between them *(14,39)*. Gene conversion generates variation in the degree of sequence similarity between duplicated sequences. Consequently, it will be interesting to see whether past gene conversion events are capable of potentiating future rearrangement events. Such studies will require rates of NAHR-promoted rearrangement to be accurately ascertained in individuals with varying levels of duplicate sequence similarity.

The Need for New Technologies

As befits the emergence of a new discipline, there are many questions that remain unanswered. Why do some pairs of repeats promote NAHR much more readily than others? What underlies the existence of rearrangement hotspots? What phenotypic consequences result from the altered copy number of which genes? Some of these questions can be answered using existing methods, for example the functional characterization of candidate genes in model organisms. However, many of the questions relating to duplicated sequences in the human genome require the development of a whole new set of techniques. Among these desired methods are those that will allow us to rapidly characterize megabase-sized chromosomal structures, to efficiently capture long paralog-specific sequences, to type inversions without resorting to fluorescent *in situ* hybridization and to quantify rates of NAHR in different individuals. The haplotyping of single molecules of DNA derived from sperm and other tissues are likely to be central to the development of many of these methods *(40,41)*.

SUMMARY

The abundance and chromosome-wide distribution of segmental duplications on the Y allows an enormous variety of further duplications, deletions, and rearrangements to take place by NAHR. The nonessential nature of the chromosome (it is absent from females) and its low gene content mean that many of these rearrangements are compatible with life and may persist in the population as polymorphisms. A subset of rearrangements removes genes required for spermatogenesis and therefore leads to the recognizable genomic disorders of azoospermia. The finished sequence of the chromosome has allowed the molecular basis of several *AZF* deletions to be elucidated and led to the discovery of additional structural variation. It highlights the need for structural information from diverse Y chromosomes and further studies of both the mechanisms that generate rearrangements and the phenotypes associated with each structure.

ACKNOWLEDGMENTS

We thank Jim Cummins, Rune Eliasson, and members of an e-mail discussion group for helpful insights, and Peter Vogt for useful comments on the manuscript.

REFERENCES

1. Skaletsky H, Kuroda-Kawaguchi T, Minx PJ, et al. The male-specific region of the human Y chromosome is a mosaic of discrete sequence classes. Nature 2003;423:825–837.
2. Eliasson R. Basic semen analysis. In: *Current Topics in Andrology* (Matson P, ed.), Perth, Australia: Ladybrook Publishing, 2003; pp. 35–89.
3. Tiepolo L, Zuffardi O. Localization of factors controlling spermatogenesis in the nonfluorescent portion of the human Y chromosome long arm. Hum Genet 1976;34:119–124.
4. Vergnaud G, Page DC, Simmler MC, et al. A deletion map of the human Y chromosome based on DNA hybridization. Am J Hum Genet 1986;38:109–124.
5. Vogt P, Chandley AC, Hargreave TB, Keil R, Ma K, Sharkey A. Microdeletions in interval 6 of the Y chromosome of males with idiopathic sterility point to disruption of AZF, a human spermatogenesis gene. Hum Genet 1992;89:491–496.
6. Vogt PH, Edelmann A, Kirsch S, et al. Human Y chromosome azoospermia factors (AZF) mapped to different subregions in Yq11. Hum Mol Genet 1996;5:933–943.
7. Chang PL, Sauer MV, Brown S. Y chromosome microdeletion in a father and his four infertile sons. Hum Reprod 1999;14:2689–2694.
8. Saut N, Terriou P, Navarro A, Levy N, Mitchell MJ. The human Y chromosome genes BPY2, CDY1 and DAZ are not essential for sustained fertility. Mol Hum Reprod 2000;6:789–793.
9. Gatta V, Stuppia L, Calabrese G, Morizio E, Guanciali-Franchi P, Palka G. A new case of Yq microdeletion transmitted from a normal father to two infertile sons. J Med Genet 2002;39:E27.
10. Disteche CM, Casanova M, Saal H, et al. Small deletions of the short arm of the Y chromosome in 46,XY females. Proc Natl Acad Sci USA 1986;83.7841–7844.
11. Jobling MA, Samara V, Pandya A, et al. Recurrent duplication and deletion polymorphisms on the long arm of the Y chromosome in normal males. Hum Mol Genet 1996;5:1767–1775.
12. Kent-First M, Muallem A, Shultz J, et al. Defining regions of the Y-chromosome responsible for male infertility and identification of a fourth AZF region (AZFd) by Y-chromosome microdeletion detection. Mol Reprod Dev 1999;53:27–41.
13. Simoni M, Bakker E, Krausz C. EAA/EMQN best practice guidelines for molecular diagnosis of Y-chromosomal microdeletions. State of the art 2004. Int J Androl 2004;27:240–249.
14. Blanco P, Shlumukova M, Sargent CA, Jobling MA, Affara N, and Hurles ME. Divergent outcomes of intrachromosomal recombination on the human Y chromosome: male infertility and recurrent polymorphism. J Med Genet 2000;37:752–758.
15. Kamp C, Hirschmann P, Voss H, Huellen K, Vogt PH. Two long homologous retroviral sequence blocks in proximal Yq11 cause AZFa microdeletions as a result of intrachromosomal recombination events. Hum Mol Genet 2000;9:2563–2572.
16. Sun C, Skaletsky H, Rezen S, et al. Deletion of azoospermia factor a (AZFa) region of human Y chromosome caused by recombination between HERV15 proviruses. Hum Mol Genet 2000;9:2291–2296.
17. Sun C, Skaletsky H, Birren B, et al. An azoospermic man with a de novo point mutation in the Y-chromosomal gene USP9Y. Nat Genet 1999;23:429–432.
18. Ditton HJ, Zimmer J, Kamp C, Rajpert-De Meyts E, Vogt PH. The AZFa gene DBY (DDX3Y) is widely transcribed but the protein is limited to the male germ cells by translation control. Hum Mol Genet 2004;13:2333–2341.
19. Kuroda-Kawaguchi T, Skaletsky H, Brown LG, et al. The AZFc region of the Y chromosome features massive palindromes and uniform recurrent deletions in infertile men. Nat Genet 2001;29:279–286.
20. Repping S, van Daalen SK, Korver CM, et al. A family of human Y chromosomes has dispersed throughout northern Eurasia despite a 1.8-Mb deletion in the azoospermia factor c region. Genomics 2004;83:1046–1052.
21. Potocki L, Chen K-S, Park S-S, et al. Molecular mechanism for duplication 17p11.2 - the homologous recombination reciprocal of the Smith-Magenis microdeletion. Nat Genet 2000;24:84–87.
22. Bosch E, Jobling MA. Duplications of the AZFa region of the human Y chromosome are mediated by homologous recombination between HERVs and are compatible with male fertility. Hum Mol Genet 2003;12: 341–347.
23. Bosch E, Hurles ME, Navarro A, Jobling MA. Dynamics of a human inter-paralog gene conversion hotspot. Genome Res 2004;14:835–844.
24. Yen P. The fragility of fertility. Nat Genet 2001;29:243–244.

25. Repping S, Skaletsky H, Brown L, et al. Polymorphism for a 1.6-Mb deletion of the human Y chromosome persists through balance between recurrent mutation and haploid selection. Nat Genet 2003;35:247–251.
26. Underhill PA, Shen P, Lin AA, et al. Y chromosome sequence variation and the history of human populations. Nat Genet 2000;26:358–361.
27. Tyler-Smith C, McVean G. The comings and goings of a Y polymorphism. Nat Genet 2003;35:201–202.
28. Fernandes S, Paracchini S, Meyer LH, Floridia G, Tyler-Smith C, Vogt PH. A large AZFc deletion removes DAZ3/DAZ4 and nearby genes from men in Y haplogroup N. Am J Hum Genet 2004;74:180–187.
29. Zerjal T, Dashnyam B, Pandya A, et al. Genetic relationships of Asians and Northern Europeans, revealed by Y-chromosomal DNA analysis. Am J Hum Genet 1997;60:1174–1183.
30. Repping S, Skaletsky H, Lange J, et al. Recombination between palindromes P5 and P1 on the human Y chromosome causes massive deletions and spermatogenic failure. Am J Hum Genet 2002;71:906–922.
31. Hurles ME, Jobling MA. A singular chromosome. Nat Genet 2003;34:246–247.
32. Foresta C, Ferlin A, Moro E. Deletion and expression analysis of AZFa genes on the human Y chromosome revealed a major role for DBY in male infertility. Hum Mol Genet 2000;9:1161–1169.
33. Wilson IJ, Balding DJ. Genealogical inference from microsatellite data. Genetics 1998;150:499–510.
34. Sabeti PC, Reich DE, Higgins JM, et al. Detecting recent positive selection in the human genome from haplotype structure. Nature 2002;419:832–837.
35. Jobling MA, Tyler-Smith C. The human Y chromosome: an evolutionary marker comes of age. Nat Rev Genet 2003;4:598–612.
36. Rozen S, Skaletsky H, Marszalek JD, et al. Abundant gene conversion between arms of palindromes in human and ape Y chromosomes. Nature 2003;423:873–876.
37. Hurles ME, Willey D, Matthews L, Hussain SS. Origins of chromosomal rearrangement hotspots in the human genome: evidence from the AZFa deletion hotspots. Genome Biol 2004;5:R55.
38. Innan H. A method for estimating the mutation, gene conversion and recombination parameters in small multigene families. Genetics 2002;161:865–872.
39. Waldman AS, Liskay RM. Dependence of intrachromosomal recombination in mammalian cells on uninterrupted homology. Mol Cell Biol 1988;8:5350–5357.
40. Arnheim N, Calabrese P, Nordborg M. Hot and cold spots of recombination in the human genome: the reason we should find them and how this can be achieved. Am J Hum Genet 2003;73:5–16.
41. Mitra RD, Butty VL, Shendure J, Williams BR, Housman DE, Church GM. Digital genotyping and haplotyping with polymerase colonies. Proc Natl Acad Sci USA 2003;100:5926–5931.
42. Guzick DS, Overstreet JW, Factor-Litvak P, et al. Sperm morphology, motility, and concentration in fertile and infertile men. N Engl J Med 2001;345:1388–1393.
43. Choudhuri JV, Schleiermacher C, Kurtz S, Giegerich R. GenAlyzer: interactive visualization of sequence similarities between entire genomes. Bioinformatics 2004;20:1964–1965.

20 Inversion Chromosomes

Orsetta Zuffardi, PhD, Roberto Ciccone, PhD, Sabrina Giglio, MD, PhD, and Tiziano Pramparo, PhD

Contents

INTRODUCTION

A number of findings revealed that chromosome inversions are more frequent than deduced from classical cytogenetic studies. Indeed, some paracentric cryptic inversions have been found to be flanked by segmental duplications, either causing a Mendelian disease owing to the interruption of specific genes at inversion breakpoints or being present in the normal population as a polymorphism. In the latter case, in the heterozygous state they predispose to further unbalanced rearrangements such as inv dup rearrangements or simple deletions and duplications. The importance of this susceptibility factor has been well clarified with respect to some genomic disorders involving chromosome 8p and it is now emerging as a possible model that may explain the genetic basis of other recurrent chromosome rearrangements.

CLASSICAL CHROMOSOME INVERSIONS: EPIDEMIOLOGICAL DATA

Chromosome inversions are the most common rearrangement differentiating humans and the great ape species at the karyotypic level *(1–4)*. Inversions in which a breakpoint is in heterochromatic regions (1qh, 9qh, 16qh, and Yq) are relatively frequent and are regarded as variants. The most common inversion not involving centromeric heterochromatin is the

From: *Genomic Disorders: The Genomic Basis of Disease*
Edited by: J. R. Lupski and P. Stankiewicz © Humana Press, Totowa, NJ

inv(2)(p11q13) that is also considered a benign variant. Other polymorphic inversions are also frequent and include inv(5)(p13q13) and inv(10)(p11q21.2) *(5)*. Apart from these cases, inversions are approx 10 times more rare than the other balanced rearrangements (Robertsonian translocations: 1 in 1000; reciprocal translocations: 1 in 625; *[6]*) having a frequency ranging from approx 0.012 to 0.07% for the pericentric inversions and approx 0.01 to 0.05% for the paracentric inversions *(7)*. In contrast to translocations for which the most frequent cause of ascertainment is the presence of reproductive difficulties, the majority of inversions are ascertained at prenatal diagnosis or because of an abnormal phenotype *(5)*. The risk of unbalanced offspring from an inversion carrier, putting together the data of pericentric and the paracentric inversions, is approx 1%, much lower than that of reciprocal translocation carriers (2.7% in families ascertained through a balanced proband and 19.2% among the families ascertained through an unbalanced proband) *(5)*. Accordingly, the reproductive fitness of inversion carriers is 0.926 ± 0.085, higher than that of reciprocal translocation carriers (0.70 ± 0.048; *[8]*). Reproductive fitness in Robertsonian translocation carriers varies between 0.768 ± 0.056 for the D/D carriers and 0.921 ± 0.123 for the D/G carriers *(8)*.

RECOMBINANT CHROMOSOMES FROM CARRIERS OF CLASSICAL HETEROZYGOUS INVERSIONS

Studies on inversion heterozygotes in man and in other species have reported crossover suppression in the inverted region *(9)* and increased recombination elsewhere on the same chromosome *(10)*. When recombination occurs within the inverted region between the normal and the inverted chromosomes two complementary recombinant chromosomes arise. Each of them is duplicated for the distal region of one arm and deleted for the opposite one. In the case of paracentric inversions the two recombinants are dicentric and acentric. The size of the inversion seems to be the main factor influencing the type of synapsis between the inverted and the normal chromosome. For a more complete discussion on this topic, *see* ref. 7.

CRYPTIC INVERSIONS ASSOCIATED WITH SEGMENTAL DUPLICATIONS

In the last 15 years, a series of submicroscopic paracentric inversions have been discovered while studying specific genes at a genomic level. Some of these inversions lead to the breakage of a dosage sensitive gene and, therefore, cause a Mendelian disease, other inversions break within either an extragenic region or disrupt nondosage sensitive genes and are, thus, considered benign. Most of these cryptic inversions are mediated by large (usually >10 kb), highly homologous low-copy repeat (LCR) structures (also called segmental duplications or duplicons) that can act as recombination substrates in nonallelic homologous recombination (NAHR). There are clear evidences that some of the benign inversions are not mere neutral polymorphisms but may predispose to other rearrangements. The story began in 1993 when Lakich et al. *(11)* discovered that nearly half of the patients with severe haemophilia A had a breakage of the factor VIII gene caused by an inversion mediated essentially by intrachromatid recombination between DNA sequences in the A gene in intron 22 and one or other of two inverted copies of this sequence (*int22h-2, int22h-3*) located, respectively, 500 and 600 kb more telomeric. A few years later a similar mechanism was shown to be responsible for 13% of Hunter disease patients. In this case the inversion occurs because of abnormal recombination between the *IDS* gene and its pseudogene located 90 kb away, resulting in the disruption of the gene *(12).* Other recurrent cryptic inversions mediated by homologous LCRs have been reported in normal individuals and, at least some of them, are regarded as benign. The inversion at the Xq28 emerin/filamin region was found while trying to elucidate the discrepancies observed between the genetic and physical map distances *(13).* This inversion, present in the heterozygous state in 33% of females and in the hemizygous state in 19% of males, is mediated by two 99% sequence identical segmental duplications flanking the emerin and filamin genes. Although inversion carriers are completely normal, some of the emerin deletions associated with Emery-Dreifuss muscular dystrophy have been hypothesized to be the result of inversion-mediated rearrangements *(14).* Moreover, it is not impossible that some of the dicentric X chromosomes pter-qter::qter-pter *(15)* are formed as a consequence of unequal crossovers between the same LCRs that mediate the inversions.

Another recurrent benign cryptic inversion has been detected at the region surrounding the NPHP1 locus at 2q13. Saunier et al. *(16)* discovered that homozygous deletion of 290 kb responsible for nephronophthisis 1 is mediated by two copies of segmental duplications with the same orientation. These LCRs are surrounded and partially embedded into two homologous segmental duplications having opposite orientation and mediating an approx 500-kb inversion present in 1.3% of the population in the homozygous state. No negative effect has been demonstrated in association with this inversion. It is obvious that embryos with any dicentric chromosome 2pter-2q13::2q13-2ptcr would not be viable.

The paradigmatic situation is that of the Y chromosome. This chromosome has an abundance of LCR (amplicons), which render this chromosome susceptible to a multitude of rearrangements that, when involving the long arm, are often the cause of spermatogenic failure (*see* Chapter 19) *(17).* It has been assumed that the polymorphisms observed at loci on the Y chromosome and mtDNA are selectively neutral and, therefore, existing patterns of molecular variation could be used to deduce the histories of populations in terms of drift, population movements, and cultural practices. However, Jobling et al. *(18)* demonstrated that the 3-Mb Yp inversion present in the male population is the preferential background for the *PRKX/PRKY* translocation underlying most XX males and some XY females (Fig. 1). This is a clear demonstration that this Y inversion "polymorphism" is not neutral. It seems likely that other cryptic inversions are responsible for the complex series of deletions and duplications mediated by several types of LCRs associated with the AZFc locus *(19,20).*

CRYPTIC INVERSION AT 8p23

The finding that a Y chromosome inversion was the basis for a recurrent translocation *(18)* was at first considered peculiar to the sex chromosomes. Further relevance of these data emerged following our studies *(21)* reporting that some recurrent chromosome rearrangements at 8p occur as a consequence of an 8p submicroscopic paracentric inversion present in the parent transmitting the abnormal chromosome. At that time, we already knew that the recurrent inv dup(8p) rearrangement, an inverted duplication of the chromosome 8 short arm associated with deletion of the very distal 8p (8p23.2-pter), was not the primary product of an abnormal recombination but instead was produced by the breakage of a dicentric chromosome 8qter-8p23.1::8p23.1-8qter *(22)* leading to the formation of an inv dup(8p) and, though formally not demonstrated, to a chromosome 8 deleted for part of its short arm (8p-) (Fig. 2). In the dicentric chromosome the two duplicated regions are separated by a small single copy region (Fig. 3). The fact that the original inv dup (8p) was a dicentric chromosome led us to hypothesize that

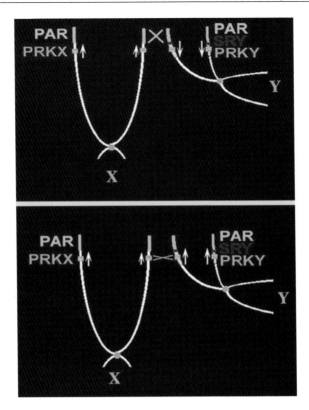

Fig. 1. Mechanism of the Xp/Yp translocation at the basis of XX males and XY females. (Top) Recombination between the Xp and Yp chromosome normally occurs at the pseudo-autosomal region 1 (PAR). *PRKX* gene lies on the X chromosome approx 1 Mb centromeric to PAR. On the Y chromosome the *SRY* gene is just centromeric to PAR. PRKY, homologous to PRKX, lies about 4.5 Mb centromeric to PAR and is included within a polymorphic inversion region (yellow region) of 3 Mb. In noninverted subjects *PRKX* and *PRKY* have opposite orientation, thus preventing any possible recombination event. In subjects with inverted PRKX and PRKY acquire the same orientation (Bottom), thus, allowing an ectopic recombination. The result is the transposition of *SRY* on the Xp chromosome and the absence of *SRY* on the Y chromosome.

the reciprocal analphoid chromosome might be present in some subjects who acquired of a neocentromere. From a literature review we were able to identify two of such cases where the analphoid chromosome was a supernumerary marker that was mosaic with a normal cell line. Molecular definition of this marker (+der[8p]) demonstrated that it was exactly the reciprocal of the dicentric chromosome 8 and that both rearrangements were mediated by a pair of olfactory receptor (OR)-gene clusters mapping to 8p23.1 *(21)* (Figs. 3 and 4). The refined distance between the two clusters (the single-copy region) is approx 3.5 Mb. We reasoned that, according to the classical cytogenetics, the production of two reciprocal rearrangements, one dicentric and the other acentric, could only result following a crossover within a paracentric inversion. We, thus, studied by fluorescent *in situ* hybridization the apparently normal chromosomes 8 in the parent-of-origin of several inv dup(8p)s (thus far 16 cases) and of one case of +der(8p) and discovered that a heterozygous paracentric inversion with the same breakpoints of the dicentric and the acentric chromosomes was present in all of them. The presence of the

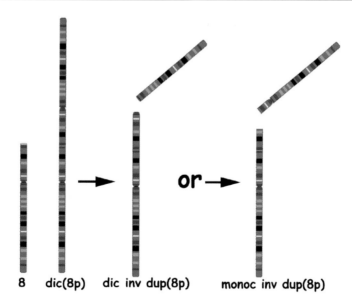

8   dic(8p)   dic inv dup(8p)   monoc inv dup(8p)

Fig. 2. The dicentric chromosome resulting from nonallelic homologous recombination can undergo a breakage at the level of the second centromere or a more proximal breakage, leading to an inv dup(8p)s and a del(8p). Note that the inv dup(8p)s may differ according to the duplication size

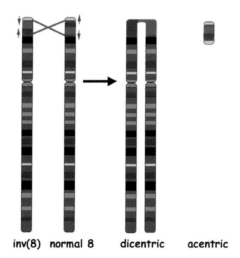

inv(8) normal 8   dicentric   acentric

Fig. 3. Cryptic paracentric inversion between the two pairs of olfactory receptor (OR) gene clusters mapping to 8p23.1. Non-allelic homologous recombination results in a dicentric and an acentric recombinant chromosome. The single copy region is delimited by the two OR gene clusters (red arrows).

inversion also explained a highly unlikely crossover pattern at 8p23 observed in members of some Centre d'Etude du Polymorphisme Humain families *(23)* that showed apparent triple recombination events in a very short region. Studies on normal populations revealed that the 8p23 inversion is present in the heterozygous state in 26% of the European population *(21)* and in 39% of the Japanese population *(24)*. Thus, the inversion represents a genomic polymorphism that,

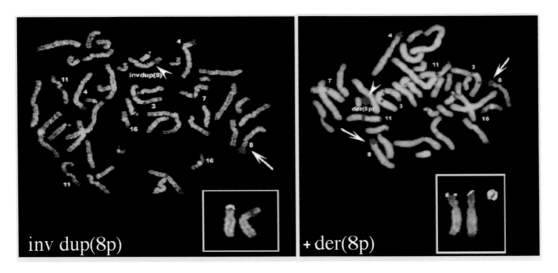

Fig. 4. The inv dup(8p) and the analphoid supernumerary chromosome +der(8p) are the two reciprocal products of the same abnormal recombination. Both fluorescent *in situ* hybridization images show the results obtained with the bacterial artificial chromosome (BAC) clone RP11-287P18 specific to the distal 8p olfactory receptor genes cluster. This clone gives signals on different chromosomes owing to high sequence identity of some of the olfactory receptor family members. Normal chromosome 8 and the inv dup(8p) are indicated by an arrow and an arrowhead, respectively. On the right image, the +der(8) appears completely covered by the signals. In the small squares, the green signals correspond to a single copy BAC clone (RP11-5E15) in distal 8p. The inv dup(8) lacks this signal, whereas the +der(8p) shows two opposite signals.

in the heterozygous state, renders misalignment and abnormal recombination more likely, just as it occurs in cytogenetically identifiable inversions *(7)*. In other words, the inversion predisposes the individual to a susceptibility to the formation of what were considered *de novo* chromosome rearrangements (inv dup[8p] and the + der[8p]) (Fig. 3).

CARRIERS OF THE 8P23 INVERSION: ARE THEY AT RISK FOR UNBALANCED OFFSPRING?

An unexpected finding is that both subjects with the inv dup(8p) or with +der(8) are single cases in their families, although the parent who has transmitted the anomalous chromosome is a carrier of the inversion and, therefore, one would have anticipated more than one unbalanced child. However, if we consider the analphoid chromosome, the occurrence of a neocentromere is a rare event *(25)*. Thus, most of the zygotes containing a +der(8p) will lose it very soon after acquiring a normal chromosome complement. As to the dicentric chromosome, we had assumed that it did undergo a breakage at the second meiotic division thus leading to a gamete having the inv dup(8p) and a gamete deleted for a portion of 8p. Floridia et al. *(22)* demonstrated that the size of the inv dup(8p) may differ according to the size of the 8p duplication which may involve even the centromere (from 8p22 to 8pcen) or may be much smaller (from 8p21.2 to 8p22) (Fig. 2). On the contrary, the inv dup(8p) size is remarkably constant as to the deletion region (8p23.2-pter) and the single copy region at 8p23.1 flanked by the two clusters of OR genes. These findings demonstrated that the dicentric breakage may occur in different positions between the two centromeres leading to a dicentric inv dup(8p) and a reciprocal acentric 8q, or to inv dup (8p)s with smaller duplications and reciprocal 8p- with different degrees of deletion (Fig. 2). It seems very likely that most of the deleted chromosomes 8 are not compatible with embryonic development resulting in premature termination of the pregnancy. Moreover, we demonstrated that in some cases the dicentric does not break at meiosis II but is inherited as such leading to an almost completely trisomic 8 zygote. Because of its instability, the dicentric may undergo breakage generating different cell lines in the embryo *(26)*. Should the inactivation of one centromere occur very early, thus stabilizing the dicentric 8, the resulting embryo will be trisomic for an almost entire chromosome 8. It has been clearly demonstrated that survival of trisomy 8 is possible when the aneuploid cell line arises relatively late in development *(27)*. Thus, embryos with trisomy 8 owing to the presence of a dicentric chromosome are expected to be prematurely aborted. Because no evidence of increased spontaneous abortions has been found in mothers of inv dup(8p) subjects (manuscript in preparation) we postulate that the trisomy 8 fetuses result in preclinical abortions. In conclusion, as Madan *(28)* and Sutherland et al. *(29)* already observed with paracentric inversion carriers, also subjects carrying the 8p23 cryptic inversion have a very low risk for unbalanced progeny.

OTHER CHROMOSOME REARRANGEMENTS MEDIATED
BY CRYPTIC PARACENTRIC INVERSION

Osborne et al. *(30)* observed a heterozygous inversion of the Williams-Beuren syndrome region in 4 of 12 parents transmitting the disease-related chromosome. Their data had been fully confirmed by Bayés et al. *(31)*, who found that one-third of the transmitting progenitors were heterozygous for an inversion between the centromeric and the telomeric segmental duplications at 7q11.23, which are in opposite orientation. The mechanism by which the inversion generates an interstitial deletion is probably owing to the fact that the normal and the inverted chromosome synapse for all their length and "balloon out" at the inversion region, thus allowing NAHR between the segmental duplications lying in opposite orientation (Fig. 5).

We also demonstrated that the t(4;8)(p16;p23) recurrent translocation, reported in several cases *(32)* either in the balanced or unbalanced form, is mediated by two pairs of homologous OR-gene clusters located at 4p16 and 8p23, respectively *(33)*. In five *de novo* cases of unbalanced and balanced translocations, all of maternal origin, we could demonstrate a double heterozygous inversion between the two pairs of OR-gene clusters at 4p16 and 8p23 in all the mothers. It seems likely that the two pairs of homologous chromosomes cannot synapse in their distal short arm regions involved in the inversion and this allows the occurrence of a crossingover between homologous regions located into nonhomologous chromosomes (Fig. 6). 4p16 and 8p23 heterozygous inversion was detected in 12.5% (4/40) and 26% (13/50) of control subjects, respectively, whereas 2.5% (1/40) were scored as double heterozygous.

Heterozygous cryptic inversions as the basis of unbalanced rearrangements have also been found in mothers having a 15q11-q13 deleted Angelman syndrome (AS) child *(34)*. The inversion was detected in the mothers of four out six AS cases with the breakpoint 2–3 (BP2/3) 15q11–q13 deletion, but not in seven mothers of AS because of paternal uniparental disomy 15. The BP2–BP3 chromosome 15q11–q13 inversion was detected in 4 of 44 subjects (9%) of the general population.

From these data it emerges that the heterozygous inversion between homologous segmental duplications is an important mechanism causing abnormal synapsis and NAHR and, thus, that

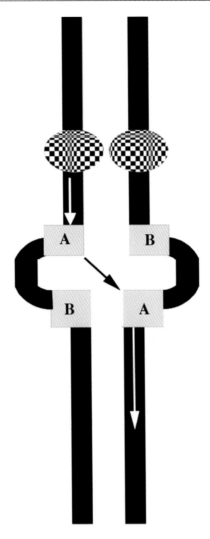

Fig. 5. Possible mechanism explaining how the paracentric inversion may lead to a deleted recombinant chromosome. The abnormal synapsis created by the inversion allows recombination between identical or nearly identical segmental duplications (gray blocks, A and B). Arrows indicate the occurrence of recombination. Chess-patterned circles indicate the centromeres.

these types of inversions constitute an important factor for susceptibility to the occurrence of unbalanced chromosome rearrangements. However, it is also clear that not all recurrent rearrangements can be explained by this mechanism: Saitta et al. *(35)* did not find evidence of inversion of 22q11.2 in the chromosome that becomes deleted in subjects with a DiGeorge/velocardiofacial syndrome phenotype. Similarly, several researchers could not find any inversion at 15q11-q13 in the fathers of deletion Prader-Willi syndrome subjects. Thus, it seems obvious that other mechanisms beyond to the inversion may cause synapsis displacement between homologous segmental duplications, in turn, leading to NAHR.

Recent studies *(36,37)* demonstrated the existence of large segments of the genome, ranging in size from 100 kb to 2 Mb, varying several folds in copy number in the human population and

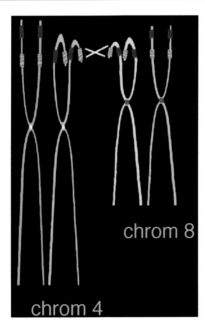

Fig. 6. The recurrent translocation t(4;8)(p16;p23) is mediated by two pairs of olfactory receptor gene clusters at 4p16 and 8p23 (yellow and orange blocks). Double heterozygous inversions between these two segmental duplications prevent a normal synapsis to occur along each pair of homologous chromosomes and allows nonallelic homologous recombination between nonhomologous chromosomes.

denominated large-scale copy number variations (LCVs). A higher than expected association between LCVs and known segmental duplications has been noted both by Iafrate et al. and Sebat et al. *(36,37)*. It has been demonstrated that the instability of some genomic regions is owing to the presence of segmental duplications *(38)*. This suggests that LCVs and genomic rearrangements might have a common mechanistic basis *(39)*.

CONCLUSIONS AND PROSPECTIVES

Inversions and more specifically cryptic inversions flanked by inversely oriented segmental duplications could be much more frequent than previously estimated. Segmental duplications represent approx 5% of our genome. A systematic study of the genomic regions flanked by segmental duplications *(40)* might reveal other inversion genomic polymorphisms. Ours and other studies revealed that cryptic inversions flanked by LCRs are an important but not the only susceptibility factor for the occurrence of unbalanced constitutional chromosome rearrangements. After years of darkness on the molecular causes of structural chromosome abnormalities and on the possible susceptibility factors behind them, it seems that the tangle begins to be unravelled. Segmental duplications are the cause of genomic instability and heterozygous carriers of cryptic inversions are at enhanced risk to form gametes with chromosome imbalances. Investigations on the presence of heterozygous variants with respect to LCVs in the parents transmitting structural chromosome abnormalities will likely determine whether these variants represent another risk factor.

REFERENCES

1. Yunis JJ, Sawyer JR, Dunham K. The striking resemblance of high-resolution G-banded chromosomes of man and chimpanzee. Science 1980;208:1145–1148.
2. Yunis JJ, Prakash O. The origin of man: a chromosomal pictorial legacy. Science 1982;215:1525–1530.
3. Nickerson E, Nelson DL. Molecular definition of pericentric inversion breakpoints occurring during the evolution of humans and chimpanzees. Genomics 1998;50:368–372.
4. Locke DP, Archidiacono N, Misceo D, et al. Refinement of a chimpanzee pericentric inversion breakpoint to a segmental duplication cluster. Genome Biol 2003;4:R50.
5. Youings S, Ellis K, Ennis S, Barber J, Jacobs P. A study of reciprocal translocations and inversions detected by light microscopy with special reference to origin, segregation, and recurrent abnormalities. Am J Med Genet 2004;126A:46–60.
6. Shaffer LG, Lupski JR. Molecular mechanisms for constitutional chromosomal rearrangements in humans. Annu Rev Genet 2000;34:297–329.
7. Gardner RJM, Sutherland GR. *Chromosome Abnormalities and Gentic Counselling*. Oxford, New York: Oxford University Press, 2004.
8. Jacobs PA, Frackiewicz A, Law P, Hilditch CJ, Morton NE. The effect of structural aberrations of the chromosomes on reproductive fitness in man II Results. Clin Genet 19758:169–178.
9. Jaarola M, Martin RH, Ashley T. Direct evidence for suppression of recombination within two pericentric inversions in humans: a new sperm-FISH technique. Am J Hum Genet 1998;63:218–224.
10. Zetka MC, Rose AM. The meiotic behavior of an inversion in Caenorhabditis elegans. Genetics 1992;131: 321–332.
11. Lakich D, Kazazian HH Jr, Antonarakis SE, Gitschier J. Inversions disrupting the factor VIII gene are a common cause of severe haemophilia A. Nat Genet 1993;5:236–241.
12. Bondeson ML, Dahl N, Malmgren H, et al. Inversion of the IDS gene resulting from recombination with IDS-related sequences is a common cause of the Hunter syndrome. Hum Mol Genet 1995;4:615–621.
13. Small K, Iber J, Warren ST. Emerin deletion reveals a common X-chromosome inversion mediated by inverted repeats. Nat Genet 1997;16:96–99.
14. Small K, Warren ST. Emerin deletions occurring on both Xq28 inversion backgrounds. Hum Mol Genet 1998;7:135–139.
15. Therman E, Sarto GE, Patau K. Apparently isodicentric but functionally monocentric X chromosome in man. Am J Hum Genet 1974;26:83–92.
16. Saunier S, Calado J, Benessy F, et al. Characterization of the NPHP1 locus: mutational mechanism involved in deletions in familial juvenile nephronophthisis. Am J Hum Genet 2000;66:778–789.
17. Skaletsky H, Kuroda-Kawaguchi T, Minx PJ, et al. The male-specific region of the human Y chromosome is a mosaic of discrete sequence classes. Nature 2003;423:825–837.
18. Jobling MA, Williams GA, Schiebel GA, et al. A selective difference between human Y-chromosomal DNA haplotypes. Curr Biol 1998;8:1391–1394.
19. Repping S, Skaletsky H, Brown L, et al. Polymorphism for a 16-Mb deletion of the human Y chromosome persists through balance between recurrent mutation and haploid selection. Nat Genet 2003;35:247–251.
20. Tyler-Smith C, McVean G. The comings and goings of a Y polymorphism. Nat Genet 2003;35:201–202.
21. Giglio S, Broman KW, Matsumoto N, et al. Olfactory receptor-gene clusters, genomic-inversion polymorphisms, and common chromosome rearrangements. Am J Hum Genet 2001;68:874–883.
22. Floridia G, Piantanida M, Minelli A, et al. The same molecular mechanism at the maternal meiosis I produces mono- and dicentric 8p duplications. Am J Hum Genet 1996;58:785–796.
23. Broman K, Matsumoto N, Giglio S, et al. Common long human inversion polymorphism on chromosome 8p. In: *Science and Statistics: A Festschrift for Terry Speed* (Goldstein DR, ed.). IMS Lecture Notes-Monograph Series, 2003; pp. 237–245.
24. Shimokawa O, Kurosawa K, Ida T, et al. Molecular characterization of inv dup del(8p): analysis of five cases. Am J Med Genet 2004;128A:133–137.
25. Amor DJ, Choo KH. Neocentromeres: role in human disease, evolution, and centromere study. Am J Hum Genet 2002;71:695–714.
26. Pramparo T, Giglio S, Gregato G, et al. Inverted duplications: how many of them are mosaic? Eur J Hum Genet 2004;12:713–717.

27. Robinson WP, Binkert F, Bernasconi F, Lorda-Sanchez I, Werder EA, Schinzel, AA. Molecular studies of chromosomal mosaicism: relative frequency of chromosome gain or loss and possible role of cell selection. Am J Hum Genet 1995;56:444–451.

28. Madan K. Paracentric inversions: a review. Hum Genet 1995;96:503–515.

29. Sutherland GR, Callen DF, Gardner RJ. Paracentric inversions do not normally generate monocentric recombinant chromosomes. Am J Med Genet 1995;59:390–392.

30. Osborne LR, Li M, Pober B, et al. A 15 million-basepair inversion polymorphism in families with Williams-Beuren syndrome. Nat Genet 2001;29:321–325.

31. Bayes M, Magano LF, Rivera N, Flores R, Perez Jurado LA. Mutational mechanisms of Williams-Beuren syndrome deletions. Am J Hum Genet 2003;73:131–151.

32. Wieczorek, D, Krause, M, Majewski, F, et al. Unexpected high frequency of de novo unbalanced translocations in patients with Wolf-Hirschhorn syndrome (WHS). J Med Genet 2000;37:798–804.

33. Giglio S, Calvari V, Gregato G, et al. Heterozygous submicroscopic inversions involving olfactory receptor-gene clusters mediate the recurrent t(4;8)(p16;p23) translocation. Am J Hum Genet 2002;71:276–285.

34. Gimelli G, Pujana MA, Patricelli MG, et al. Genomic inversions of human chromosome 15q11-q13 in mothers of Angelman syndrome patients with class II (BP2/3) deletions. Hum Mol Genet 2003;12:849–858.

35. Saitta SC, Harris SE, Gaeth AP, et al. Aberrant interchromosomal exchanges are the predominant cause of the 22q112 deletion. Hum Mol Genet 2004;13:417–428.

36. Iafrate AJ, Feuk L, Rivera MN, et al. Detection of large-scale variation in the human genome. Nat Genet 2004;36:949–951.

37. Sebat J, Lakshmi B, Troge J, et al. Large-scale copy number polymorphism in the human genome. Science 2004;305:525–528.

38. Lupski JR. Genomic disorders: structural features of the genome can lead to DNA rearrangements and human disease traits. Trends Genet 1998;14:417–422.

39. Carter NP. As normal as normal can be? Nat Genet 2004;36:931–932.

40. Bailey JA, Gu Z, Clark RA, et al. Recent segmental duplications in the human genome. Science 2002;297: 1003–1007.

21

Monosomy 1p36 As a Model for the Molecular Basis of Terminal Deletions

Blake C. Ballif, PhD and Lisa G. Shaffer, PhD

CONTENTS

BACKGROUND

Deletion of the most distal, telomeric band of human chromosomes can result in a variety of mental retardation and multiple congenital anomaly syndromes. These terminal deletions are some of the most commonly observed structural chromosome abnormalities detected by routine cytogenetic analysis. Terminal deletions of 1p36 occur in approx 1 in 5000 live births, making it the most frequently observed terminal deletion and one of the most commonly observed mental retardation syndromes in humans. Molecular characterization of subjects with monosomy 1p36 indicates that, like other terminal deletions, 1p36 deletions have breakpoints occurring in multiple locations over several megabases and are comprised of terminal truncations, interstitial deletions, complex rearrangements, and derivative chromosomes. In addition, cryptic interrupted inverted duplications have been observed at the end of terminally deleted chromosomes, suggesting premeiotic breakage–fusion–bridge (BFB) cycles can be intermediate steps in the process of generating and stabilizing terminal deletions of 1p36. Overall, these observations are identical to those made in yeast and other model systems in which a double-strand break (DSB) near a telomere can be repaired by a variety of mechanisms to stabilize the end of a broken chromosome. Furthermore, sequence analysis and fluorescent *in situ* hybridization (FISH) mapping of the terminal 10.5 Mb of 1p36 including a variety of terminal deletion breakpoint junctions indicate that segmental duplications, low-copy repeats (LCRs), and short repetitive DNA sequence elements may mediate the generation and stabilization of terminal deletions of 1p36. We hypothesize that nonallelic homologous recombination (NAHR) between palindromic or inverted LCRs in the subtelomeric region of

From: *Genomic Disorders: The Genomic Basis of Disease*
Edited by: J. R. Lupski and P. Stankiewicz © Humana Press, Totowa, NJ

1p36 could generate a dicentric chromosome that is broken at a random location during the subsequent anaphase as the centromeres move to opposite poles. This model suggests that the molecular basis of terminal deletions may be directly linked to genomic architectural features in the subtelomeric regions that generate the initial, variable-sized terminally deleted chromosome, and that stabilization of the broken chromosome occurs by one of a variety of competing DSB repair pathways.

INTRODUCTION

Telomere Structure and Function

The distal ends of all linear chromosomes are capped by a specialized protein–DNA complex known as the telomere. The term "telomere" was originally put forth by Muller in 1938 to describe the "terminal gene" required for "sealing the end" of a broken chromosome *(1)*. This work was subsequently expanded upon by McClintock *(2,3)*, who demonstrated that broken chromosomes that have lost a telomere form end-to-end fusions resulting in dicentric chromosomes that are inherently unstable. In addition to preventing chromosome fusions, telomeres have now been shown to play critical roles in a number of cellular processes, most notably in the replication of linear chromosome ends *(4)*. Furthermore, telomere associations during meiosis suggest that they may be involved in homolog pairing and recombination and that they are necessary for faithful segregation of the chromosomes *(5)*.

Telomeric DNA consists of tandem repeats of simple G-rich sequences that show remarkable conservation throughout eukaryotic evolution. All human chromosomes terminate with approx 2–20 kb of the simple tandem repeat $(TTAGGG)_n$ *(6)*. Proximal to this telomeric repeat tract is a structurally complex region of subtelomeric DNA that can extend several hundred kilobases from the end of most chromosomes and has been shown to be highly polymorphic *(7–10)*. These subtelomeric regions are enriched with segmental duplications interspersed with interstitial $(TTAGGG)_n$-like sequences and other subtelomeric repeat sequence blocks that can be shared by a number of different chromosome ends *(10)*.

In addition, early chromosome banding (G-banding) studies indicated that the telomeric regions of most human chromosomes stain G-negative and contain GC-rich isochores and are, therefore, thought to be regions that contain abundant genes *(11,12)*. Thus, telomeric deletions and/or rearrangements have been predicted to result in more significant and serious phenotypic abnormalities than similar-sized deletions and/or rearrangements at other chromosomal locations *(11,13,14)*. Analysis of the draft sequence of the Human Genome assembly has recently confirmed that telomeric regions are gene-rich, although not to the extent originally estimated *(10)*.

Telomeric Aberrations and Mental Retardation

Mental retardation affects approx 3% of the world's population *(15)*. Although chromosomal and genetic disorders are thought to account for 30–40% of all cases with an additional 10–30% accounted for by environmental factors, the cause of mental retardation in the vast majority of subjects is still unknown *(16–18)*. It has been estimated that approx 20% of mental retardation is caused by a cytogenetic abnormality, with aneuploidy, mainly trisomy 21, being the most common. Although estimating the second most common cytogenetic cause may have some biases, in recent years telomeric abnormalities have emerged as a major yet previously under-recognized cause of mental retardation in the population *(19)*.

In the past decade, numerous submicroscopic chromosomal abnormalities in subjects with apparently normal karyotypes and mental retardation or multiple congenital anomalies have been identified by molecular methods such as DNA polymorphism analysis *(20–22)*, FISH *(13,23,24)*, and microarray-based comparative genomic hybridization (array CGH) *(25,26)*. Although it is difficult to compare directly these various studies because of differences in patient selection criteria and variations in the subtelomeric screening methodologies, the combined data suggest that approx 5% of subjects with idiopathic mental retardation or dysmorphic features and apparently normal karyotypes may have submicroscopic deletions and/or cryptic rearrangements at the telomeres *(19,27)*.

Terminal Deletions and Monosomy 1p36

Telomeric regions of the genome are of particular interest in clinical cytogenetics because, owing to their light G-negative staining on G-banded chromosomes, rearrangements of these regions are difficult to identify by conventional cytogenetic methodology. Nonetheless, terminal deletions are one of the most commonly observed structural chromosomal abnormalities detected by routine chromosome analysis.

The first deletion identified in humans was the terminal deletion of 5p associated with Cri-du-chat syndrome (5p-) *(28)*. Shortly thereafter, terminal deletions of 4p were identified and the resulting syndrome, Wolf-Hirschhorn, was described *(29,30)*. With the advent of chromosome banding techniques and the more recent molecular cytogenetic technology, visible or subtle terminal deletions have been identified for every human chromosome *(14)*. This has allowed the delineation of a number of mental retardation syndromes associated with deletion of the telomeric bands of the chromosomes including Miller-Dieker (17p-) *(31)* and monosomy 1p36 (1p-) *(32)*. However, the molecular mechanism(s) that generates and stabilizes terminal deletions is only beginning to be elucidated.

Terminal deletions of 1p36 occur in approx 1 in 5000 live births, making it the most frequently observed terminal deletion and one of the most commonly occurring mental retardation syndromes in humans *(27,33)*. Monosomy 1p36 is characterized by distinct facial features including deep-set eyes, flat nasal bridge, asymmetric ears, and pointed chin. Other features include mild to severe mental retardation, seizures, hearing impairment, vision disorders, growth failure, hypothyroidism, oropharyngeal dysphagia, orofacial clefting, and cardiac defects *(34,35)*.

More than 100 subjects with deletions of 1p36 have now been systematically analyzed *(34* and unpublished data). Although the majority of cases of monosomy 1p36 have been identified through cytogenetic analysis, this deletion is difficult to visualize by routine chromosome analysis at the 400–550 band resolution. However, the majority (98%) of terminal deletions of 1p36 can be visualized retrospectively using good quality chromosomes at a resolution of 550 bands or greater, with careful attention to chromosome band 1p36 *(27)*. Nevertheless, nearly half of patients studied had at least one chromosome analysis, sometimes two, interpreted as normal *(27)*. Furthermore, the size and complexity of the deletion cannot be distinguished at the resolution of the light microscope. A variety of molecular cytogenetic techniques have revealed that deletion sizes in monosomy 1p36 vary widely with no single common breakpoint *(32,34,36)*. Additionally, terminal deletions, interstitial deletions, complex rearrangements, and derivative chromosomes have been identified among the study cell lines *(34,37,38)*. Given that 1p36 deletions are relatively common and, like other terminal deletions, comprise a heterogeneous group of submicroscopic rearrangements with breakpoints occurring in multiple locations over several megabases, monosomy 1p36 has proven to be a valuable model for investigating the molecular basis of terminal deletions.

MECHANISMS THAT GENERATE AND STABILIZE TERMINAL DELETIONS

Telomeres provide structural stability to the ends of all linear chromosomes. Loss of a telomere, by either a DNA DSB or by improper telomere maintenance can, if not properly repaired, lead to apoptosis, cell senescence, or severe genomic instability characterized by gene amplifications and deletions as a result of perpetual BFB cycles *(4,39)*. It is now clear that there are at least two general repair pathways that exist within the cell whereby a terminally deleted chromosome can acquire a new telomeric cap.

The first pathway is known as "telomere healing" and results in the stabilization of terminal deletions by the direct addition of telomeric repeats onto the end of a broken chromosome *(40)*. The results of telomere healing events are pure terminal truncations. Although true telomere healing events may occur by telomerase-mediated, *de novo* addition of telomeric repeats on the end of a chromosome *(37,40–43)*, pure terminal truncations can also result from telomerase-independent, recombination-based telomere capture mechanisms from a pre-existing telomere *(44,45)*.

The second general pathway has been termed "telomere capture" and refers to the process through which a terminally deleted chromosome acquires a new telomeric sequence from another chromosomal location *(46–48)*. Telomere capture events could potentially occur between sister chromatids, homologs, or nonhomologous chromosome ends and result in derivative chromosomes. Although a number of examples of what appear to be telomere healing and telomere capture events have now been described in a variety of model organisms *(37,42,49–54)*, relatively few cases have been reported for constitutional chromosome abnormalities in humans. Moreover, the precise mechanisms that mediate these pathways in humans are not understood. Furthermore, it is not clear why terminal deletions are so common and which mechanism of repair and stabilization is used most frequently.

Molecular studies on a large cohort of subjects with cytogenetically defined terminal deletions of 1p36 using microsatellite analysis, FISH, and array CGH indicate that deletion sizes range from approx 1 Mb to more than 10.5 Mb with the majority (40%) of breakpoints clustering between 3 and 5 Mb from the telomere *(26,34)*. Furthermore, telomere FISH studies have identified interstitial deletions (6%), derivative chromosomes (17%), complex rearrangements (5%), and apparently pure terminal deletions (72%) *(34,38)*.

Ten rearrangements of 1p36 have been examined at the DNA sequence level *(38,55,56)* and an additional two were examined by microarray analysis and FISH *(57)*. Based on the previous molecular analyses, seven were apparently pure terminal deletions, three were known derivative chromosomes 1 [der(1)t(1;1)(p36;q44)], and two were apparent duplications of 1p36. Analysis of the breakpoint junctions in these subjects uncovered evidence for BFB cycles, confirmed a telomere healing event, and clarified the mechanisms of telomere capture involved in terminal deletions of 1p36. In the next sections we discuss in detail the various mechanisms by which terminal deletions can be generated and stabilized, most of which have already been observed in terminal deletions of 1p36, and suggest that terminal deletions of 1p36 are a good model for understanding the breakage and stabilization of human chromosomes.

Breakage–Fusion–Bridge Cycles

Breakpoint junction sequences from two subjects with monosomy 1p36 identified terminal deletions associated with cryptic interrupted inverted duplications at the end of the chromosome *(37)*. These breakpoint sequences are identical in structure to those found in embryonic stem (ES) cell lines and tumor cell lines that have gone through BFB cycles as a result of uncapped sister chromatids being fused by nonhomologous end joining *(58,59)*. The analysis of two additional subjects with apparent duplications of 1p36 showed terminal deletions, duplications, and triplications *(57)*. The mechanisms postulated to result in these complex rearrangements involve BFB cycles *(57)*. These data represent the first evidence of a BFB cycle generating a constitutional chromosome rearrangement resulting in a human genetic disease. Furthermore, this suggests that the observed variability in size of terminal deletions of 1p36 (and other terminal deletions) may be the result of random breaks generated when a fused, dicentric chromosome is broken during anaphase separation of the centromeres. Perhaps most significant is that the identification of BFB cycles suggests that at least some terminal deletions of 1p36 are not generated and stabilized in a single step but pass through an intermediate phase as a broken chromosome that must then be stabilized by some other cellular mechanism.

Telomere Healing

Pure terminal truncations have been reported in at least 12 terminal deletion cases from a variety of human chromosome ends *(37 40,41,43,60–62)*. Recently, sequence analysis of the precise breakpoint junctions in subjects with monosomy 1p36 confirmed at least one case to be a pure terminal truncation stabilized by telomeric repeat sequences *(37)*. Telomere healing has also been identified in human tumor cell lines *(58)*, mouse ES cells *(42)*, and a number of other model organisms *(49,50,52,53)*. Although it is presumed that pure terminal truncations were stabilized by *de novo* telomere healing by telomerase, broken chromosomes stabilized by acquisition of telomeric sequences from another chromosome end could appear virtually identical to ones stabilized by *de novo* telomere synthesis. However, the reported findings of pure $(TTAGGG)_n$ telomeric repeats at the sites of healing, as opposed to the variant telomeric repeats that are commonly found in the proximal telomeric region of existing telomeres *(37,40,41,43,60,62–64)*, support *de novo* synthesis of telomere repeats by telomerase. Even though the lack of variant repeats is consistent with *de novo* addition, it is not definitive because greater than half of an existing telomere's 2–20 kb sequence consists of pure telomeric repeats *(63,64)*. In support of *de novo* synthesis, using an in vitro assay system, human telomerase was shown to preferentially recognize the sequence at the breakpoint of one 16p terminal truncation and to add $(TTAGGG)_n$ telomeric repeat sequences *(65)*.

Telomere Capture

In the past few years, a variety of cryptic telomeric aberrations have been identified, making it clear that many apparently pure terminal deletions, viewed at the resolution of the light microscope, are in fact terminal deletions/broken chromosomes stabilized by telomere capture events *(34,36,48,66,67)*. At least four models have been proposed for the molecular basis of telomere capture. First is the mechanism of NAHR between LCRs in nonhomologous telomeric regions *(68)*, which would predict the simultaneous generation and stabilization of a terminal deletion as a derivative chromosome. Analysis of der(1)t(1;1)(p36;q44) chromosomes from three subjects with monosomy 1p36 revealed variability in the breakpoint locations without any evidence for homologous sequences or LCRs between the 1p36 deletion and 1q translocation breakpoints *(56)*. This suggests that NAHR did not play a role in mediating these particular rearrangements. However, this does not preclude LCRs within the subtelomeric region of 1p36 from being involved in generating and/or stabilizing terminal deletions by other mechanisms such as subtelomeric pairing with proximal recombination.

The second major mechanism for telomere capture, which has been termed "subtelomeric pairing with proximal recombination" (SPPR), suggests that LCRs located within the complex subtelomeric regions can facilitate mispairing of nonhomologous chromosome ends *(69,70)*. A more proximal recombination event between the mispaired chromosomes at one of the more abundant and much shorter repetitive DNA sequence elements could generate a terminal deletion and stabilize it as a derivative chromosome in a single step. Although data from the three der(1)t(1;1)(p36;q44) chromosomes is consistent with a SPPR model in that no LCRs were identified at the breakpoints, microsatellite data from these subjects suggest that these telomere capture events were mediated by intrachromosomal rearrangements. Therefore, to remain consistent with a SPPR model, in these three der(1) cases 1qter sequences must have been translocated to 1pter from a sister chromatid *(56)*.

A third mechanism has recently been proposed for generating terminally deleted chromosomes that are stabilized by telomeric sequences originating from the opposite end of the chromosome, as seen in the three der(1)t(1;1)(p36;q44) chromosomes *(71)*. This model proposes that a premeiotic exchange between chromosome 1 homologs could result in the "transposition" of 1pter and 1qter sequences. If normal homolog pairing in meiosis occurred followed by a recombination event in 1p36 proximal to the site of interchromosomal "transposition," then the result could be both a deleted 1p, duplicated 1q chromosome and a duplicated 1p, deleted 1q chromosome *(56,71)*. Although technically possible, this mechanism does not account for the wide range of derivative chromosomes seen in monosomy 1p36 and in terminal rearrangements of other chromosomes.

The fourth, and most likely, model for telomere capture suggests that telomeric sequences from another chromosome end could be copied directly onto the end of a broken chromosome through a process known as break-induced replication (BIR) *(54)*. BIR has been studied in yeast systems and it has been recently shown to play a significant role in DSB repair and preventing gross chromosome instability by maintaining telomere integrity *(46,51,54,72,73)*. BIR is a very appealing mechanism in that a broken chromosome could theoretically be healed by copying telomeric DNA from any chromosome end. This could account for the wide range of derivative chromosomes seen in monosomy 1p36, as well as those in other terminal deletion syndromes, in addition to the lack of LCRs at or near the deletion/translocation breakpoints *(56)*.

Terminal Deletions of 1p36 As a Model for Mechanisms That Stabilize Broken Chromosomes

As a whole, the molecular analysis of terminal deletions of 1p36 is consistent with a number of recent reports that suggest a chromosome broken near the telomere can be stabilized by a variety of competing DSB repair pathways to provide the necessary telomeric cap *(54)*. In particular, telomere dysfunction because of improper telomere maintenance, chromosome breakage, or mutations in various DSB repair and/or S-phase checkpoint pathways results in severe genomic instability typical of cancer *(59,61,74–80)*. This genomic instability is characterized by chromosome fusions and BFB cycles that generate inverted duplications, terminal deletions, and nonreciprocal translocations that are stabilized by several telomere healing and telomere capture mechanisms *(54)*.

The recent studies by Kolodner et al. *(54)* of yeast are of particular interest because they suggest extensive and redundant DNA repair pathways function to keep genomic rearrangements at very low levels. Their data indicate that disruption of the S-phase checkpoints, compared to disruption of the G_1, G_2, or mitotic spindle checkpoints, significantly increases the rate of genome rearrangements *(54)*. These results indicate that replication errors play an important role in generating genomic instability. In addition, all of the genome rearrangements observed following inactivation of the S-phase checkpoint were terminal deletions stabilized by telomeric repeat sequences *(54)*. Kolodner et al. *(54)* have also shown that mutations in yeast that disrupt the BIR repair pathway, and not the classical DSB repair by homologous recombination, result in a significant increase in genome instability. Furthermore, telomerase-defective yeast show a dramatic increase in the number of BIR-induced nonreciprocal translocations and nonhomologous end-joining chromosome fusions *(54)*.

We propose that the diversity in rearrangements observed in terminal deletions of 1p36 illustrates a similar set of circumstances in human terminal deletions in that they reflect the various DSB repair pathways that were taken to stabilize a broken chromosome. Figure 1 shows a schematic representation of some of the known mechanistic pathways whereby a broken chromosome can be stabilized. Processing a broken chromosome through any one of these pathways can result in a terminal deletion coupled with a subtle telomeric rearrangement—all of which have been observed in monosomy 1p36 subjects *(34,37,55,56,81)*. Furthermore, these observations on terminal deletions of 1p36 suggest that the same variety of subtle telomeric rearrangements observed in other terminal deletion syndromes *(60,66,67,82)* are also likely to be the result of various DNA repair pathways stabilizing broken chromosomes.

GENOMIC ARCHITECTURE AND THE GENERATION OF TERMINAL DELETIONS OF 1P36

Repetitive DNA Sequence Elements

In recent years, numerous examples in the literature have documented repetitive DNA sequence elements as promoters of aberrant homologous recombination and DNA DSBs *(83,84)*. This is evidenced by the vast number of cases in which repetitive DNA sequence elements are found at the breakpoints in constitutional chromosomal aberrations that cause genetic disease and in sporadic chromosomal abnormalities that cause cancer *(83,84)*.

Presumably, aberrant homologous recombination between closely related repetitive DNA sequence elements (such as *Alu* and L1 sequences) can mediate these rearrangements without a prolonged period as a broken chromosome. In four subjects with apparently terminal deletions of 1p36, the breakpoints occurred in repetitive DNA sequence elements *(55)*. This suggests that aberrant homologous recombination may have been involved in generating and/or stabilizing these terminal deletions. Aberrant homologous recombination between *Alu* elements has also been attributed to the generation of two subtle interstitial deletions of 16p that were initially thought to be simple chromosomal truncations *(60,85)*. A similar situation has also been reported for a terminal deletion of 18q in which satellite III DNA sequences were located at the breakpoint *(86)*.

Some repetitive DNA sequence elements have also been shown to be susceptible to genomic rearrangements including deletions *(83,84)*. Microsatellite, minisatellite, and other short

Intact Normal Chromosome

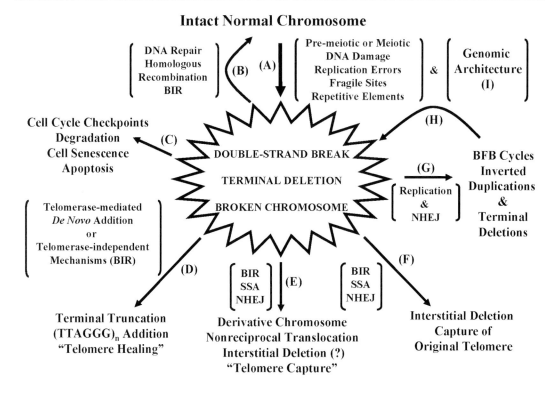

Fig. 1. Mechanisms for stabilizing a broken chromosome. (A) Premeiotic or meiotic DNA damage generates a double-strand break that converts an intact normal chromosome into a broken, terminally deleted chromosome. Although DNA repair pathways could function to restore an intact normal chromosome (B), cell-cycle checkpoints may recognize the damaged chromosome and target the cell for an apoptotic pathway (C). Thus, neither of these two possible pathways (B or C) would be observed in subjects with monosomy 1p36 because a restored normal chromosome (B) would not produce a phenotype and an apoptotic cell (C) would simply not survive. However, a variety of competing DNA repair pathways could function to stabilize a broken chromosome. Terminal truncations could be formed by telomerase-mediated *de novo* addition of telomeric repeats or through telomerase-independent mechanisms such as break-induced replication (BIR) (D). (E) Stabilization could also occur by telomere capture forming a derivative chromosome through BIR. If more than one broken chromosome is present in the cell, single-strand annealing or nonhomologous end-joining (NHEJ) could also generate a nonreciprocal translocation. If the original telomere were captured, a true interstitial deletion could also be formed (F). Alternatively, DNA replication and NHEJ could occur (G), resulting in breakage–fusion–bridge cycles that generate inverted duplications and terminal deletions that in turn require stabilization (H). All of these pathways have been proposed in terminal deletions of 1p36. In addition, genomic architectural features, such as palindromic low-copy repeats in the subtelomeric region of 1p36, could result in nonallelic homologous recombination, creating a dicentric chromosome that breaks at a random location during anaphase (I). These types of random breaks could be a source of variable-sized broken chromosomes that are then stabilized by one of several competing double-strand break repair pathways. A similar set of DNA repair pathways that safeguard against genomic instability has been described in yeast systems. (Adapted from ref. *54*.)

repetitive sequences are particularly susceptible to replication errors and can generate palindromic, hairpin structures that are prone to cleavage, resulting in DSBs and other chromosomal rearrangements *(87–90)*. Because the breakpoints of four subjects with terminal deletions of 1p36 were shown to be located within repetitive DNA sequence elements, it is reasonable to suggest that some terminal deletions of 1p36 may have been generated by DNA sequences that were susceptible to DNA DSBs *(55)*. These DSBs generate broken chromosomes that must then become stabilized by telomere healing or capture mechanisms to avoid potential BFB cycles. However, repetitive DNA sequence elements found at the end of a broken chromosome may also constitute a favorable site for stabilization by DNA repair mechanisms *(54)*.

Low-Copy Repeats and Segmental Duplications

What generates the initial broken chromosome and why terminal deletions of 1p36 are ascertained so frequently is still unknown. This could reflect higher instability in this particular region of the genome or increased survival of terminal deletions of 1p36 over other telomeric abnormalities. Interestingly, one method uses an inverted duplication of the short arm *(2)*. This was how McClintock originally formed a dicentric chromosome to generate broken chromosomes and initiate BFB cycles using a maize chromosome 9. A crossover between the normal homolog and the inverted portion of the duplicated chromosome, or between duplicated regions of sister chromatids, resulted in a dicentric chromosome that formed a bridge in anaphase with subsequent breakage *(2)*. Large-scale sequence analysis of the terminal 10.5 Mb of 1p36 indicates that segmental duplications along with palindromic and inverted LCRs may be present in the distal subtelomeric regions *(91)*. The region surrounding these LCRs forms a natural division between the interstitial deletion breakpoints of 1p36 and nearly all of the terminal deletion breakpoints (Ballif, Gajecka, and Shaffer, unpublished data). It is tempting to speculate that NAHR between palindromic or inverted LCRs in the subtelomeric region of 1p36 could be responsible for generating a dicentric chromosome that is broken at a random location during the subsequent anaphase as the centromeres move to opposite poles (Fig. 2).

Similar models have been proposed for generating inverted duplication/deficiency chromosomes, although those models were based on subtelomeric LCRs located in inverted orientations and positioned several megabases apart *(92–94)*. The palindromic repeats proposed in this model for terminal deletions of 1p36 would provide a single site for NAHR with subsequent breakage of the newly formed dicentric chromosome generating variable-sized terminally deleted and inverted duplication/deficiency chromosomes. Stabilization of the broken chromosomes could then occur by a variety of DSB repair pathways (Fig. 1). Although duplication/deletion chromosomes would also be expected to occur, it is likely that these reciprocal products have not been ascertained in studies of monosomy 1p36 because they would be predicted to have much smaller imbalances and may present with a mild phenotype that is not typical of the syndrome.

Because the genomic sequence of 1p36 is not in its finished form, the precise size and orientation of these putative LCRs is still under investigation *(91)*. However, regions of the genome that contain large duplications are notoriously difficult to map and sequence *(68,95,96)*. A closer examination of the subtelomeric regions of all chromosomes may be useful for understanding the molecular basis of other terminally deleted chromosomes.

SUMMARY

Combined, the data presented suggest that: (1) genomic architectural features may ultimately play a role in the generation of terminal deletions of 1p36 by generating the double-strand DNA breaks near the telomere, and (2) a variety of DNA repair pathways are responsible for stabilizing the broken chromosomes. Furthermore, based on the variety of rearrangements and the various mechanisms that generate and stabilize broken chromosomes ends, these

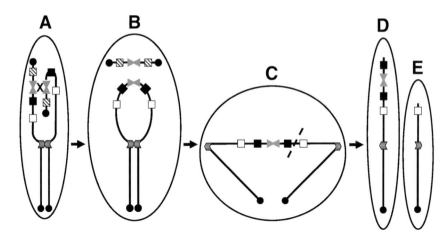

Fig. 2. Model for nonallelic homologous recombination (NAHR) between palindromic low-copy repeats (LCRs) in the subtelomeric region of 1p36. Palindromic LCRs are shown as arrowheads. Telomeric repeat sequences are shown as filled circles at the ends of the chromosomes. Unique sequences, shown as solid, hatched, and open boxes, are included for illustrative purposes. (A) Palindromic LCRs can promote misalignment of homologous chromosomes. (B) NAHR between misaligned palindromic LCRs results in the formation of a dicentric chromosome. (C) In anaphase, when the centromeres move to opposite poles, the resulting dicentric chromosome forms a bridge that will eventually break at a random location. (D) Random breakage results in one chromosome with an inverted duplication and a distal deletion and a second chromosome (E) with a terminal deletion. This random breakage could account for the variability in deletion size observed in terminal deletions of 1p36. However, these broken chromosomes must acquire a telomeric cap to be stabilized.

studies indicate that monosomy 1p36 provides a fundamental model for the molecular basis of constitutional terminal deletions in humans. In the future, the delineation of the structure of terminal deletions for other chromosome ends will determine whether the monosomy 1p36 model is representative of the molecular basis of all terminal deletions.

REFERENCES

1. Muller HJ. The remaking of chromosomes. Collecting Net 1938;13:181–195.
2. McClintock B. The behavior in successive nuclear divisions of a chromosome broken at meiosis. Proc Natl Acad Sci USA 1939;25:405–416.
3. McClintock B. The stability of broken ends of chromosomes in Zea mays. Genetics 1941;26:234–282.
4. Cervantes RB, Lundblad V. Mechanisms of chromosome-end protection. Curr Opin Cell Biol 2002;14: 351–356.
5. Cooper JP. Telomere transitions in yeast: the end of the chromosome as we know it. Curr Opin Genet Dev 2000;10:169–177.
6. Moyzis RK, Buckingham JM, Cram LS, et al. A highly conserved repetitive DNA sequence, (TTAGGG)n, present at the telomeres of human chromosomes. Proc Natl Acad Sci USA 1988;85:6622–6626.
7. Brown WR, MacKinnon PJ, Villasante A, Spurr N, Buckle VJ, Dobson MJ. Structure and polymorphism of human telomere-associated DNA. Cell 1990;63:119–132.
8. Cross SH, Allshire RC, McKay SJ, McGill NI, Cooke HJ. Cloning of human telomeres by complementation in yeast. Nature 1989;338:771–774.
9. Flint J, Bates GP, Clark K, et al. Sequence comparison of human and yeast telomeres identifies structurally distinct subtelomeric domains. Hum Mol Genet 1997;6:1305–1313.

10. Riethman H, Ambrosini A, Castaneda C, et al. Mapping and initial analysis of human subtelomeric sequence assemblies. Genome Res 2004;14:18–28.
11. Saccone S, De Sario A, Della Valle G, Bernardi G. The highest gene concentrations in the human genome are in telomeric bands of metaphase chromosomes. Proc Natl Acad Sci USA 1992;89:4913–4917.
12. Saccone S, De Sario A, Wiegant J, Raap AK, Della Valle G, Bernardi G. Correlations between isochores and chromosomal bands in the human genome. Proc Natl Acad Sci USA 1993;90:11,929–11,933.
13. National Institutes of Health and Institute of Molecular Medicine collaboration. A complete set of human telomeric probes and their clinical application. Nat Genet 1996;14:86–89.
14. Borgaonkar DS. Chromosomal Variation in Man. A Catalog of Chromosomal Variants and Anomalies. 4th ed. New York, NY: Alan R. Liss, Inc.,1984.
15. Roeleveld N, Zielhuis GA, Gabreels F. The prevalence of mental retardation: a critical review of recent literature. Dev Med Child Neurol 1997;39:125–132.
16. Elwood JH, Darragh PM. Severe mental handicap in Northern Ireland. J Ment Defic Res 1981;25:147–155.
17. Laxova R, Ridler MA, Bowen-Bravery M. An etiological survey of the severely retarded Hertfordshire children who were born between January 1, 1965 and December 31, 1967. Am J Med Genet 1977;1:75–86.
18. McDonald AD. Severely retarded children in Quebec: prevalence, causes, and care. Am J Ment Defic 1973;78:205–215.
19. Flint J, Knight S. The use of telomere probes to investigate submicroscopic rearrangements associated with mental retardation. Curr Opin Genet Dev 2003;13:310–316.
20. Flint J, Wilkie AO, Buckle VJ, Winter RM, Holland AJ, McDermid HE. The detection of subtelomeric chromosomal rearrangements in idiopathic mental retardation. Nat Genet 1995;9:132–140.
21. Slavotinek A, Rosenberg M, Knight S, et al. Screening for submicroscopic chromosome rearrangements in children with idiopathic mental retardation using microsatellite markers for the chromosome telomeres. J Med Genet 1999;36:405–411.
22. Wilkie AO. Detection of cryptic chromosomal abnormalities in unexplained mental retardation: a general strategy using hypervariable subtelomeric DNA polymorphisms. Am J Hum Genet 1993;53:688–701.
23. Knight SJ, Horsley SW, Regan R, et al. Development and clinical application of an innovative fluorescence in situ hybridization technique which detects submicroscopic rearrangements involving telomeres. Eur J Hum Genet 1997;5:1–8.
24. Knight SJ, Lese CM, Precht KS, et al. An optimized set of human telomere clones for studying telomere integrity and architecture. Am J Hum Genet 2000;67:320–332.
25. Veltman JA, Schoenmakers EF, Eussen BH, et al. High-throughput analysis of subtelomeric chromosome rearrangements by use of array-based comparative genomic hybridization. Am J Hum Genet 2002;70:1269–1276.
26. Yu W, Ballif BC, Kashork CD, et al. Development of a comparative genomic hybridization microarray and demonstration of its utility with 25 well-characterized 1p36 deletions. Hum Mol Genet 2003;12:2145–2152.
27. Heilstedt HA, Ballif BC, Howard LA, Kashork CD, Shaffer LG. Population data suggest that deletions of 1p36 are a relatively common chromosome abnormality. Clin Genet 2003;64:310–316.
28. Lejeune L, Lafourcade J, de Grouchy J, et al. Deletion partielle du bras court du chromosome 5. Individualisation d'un nouvel etat morbide. Sem Hop Paris 1963;18:1069–1079.
29. Hirschhorn K, Cooper HL, Firschein IL. Deletion of short arms of chromosomes 4-5 in a child with defects of midline fusion. Humangenetik 1965;1:479–482.
30. Wolf U, Reinwein H, Porsch R, Schroter R, Baitsch H. Defizienz an den kurzen armen eines chromosomes n 4. Humangenetik 1965;1:397–413.
31. Stratton RF, Dobyns WB, Airhart SD, Ledbetter DH. New chromosomal syndrome: Miller-Dieker syndrome and monosomy 17p13. Hum Genet 1984;67:193–200.
32. Shapira SK, McCaskill C, Northrup H, et al. Chromosome 1p36 deletions: the clinical phenotype and molecular characterization of a common newly delineated syndrome. Am J Hum Genet 1997;61:642–650.
33. Shaffer LG, Lupski JR. Molecular mechanisms for constitutional chromosomal rearrangements in humans. Annu Rev Genet 2000;34:297–329.
34. Heilstedt HA, Ballif BC, Howard LA, et al. Physical map of 1p36, placement of breakpoints in monosomy 1p36, and clinical characterization of the syndrome. Am J Hum Genet 2003;72:1200–1212.
35. Slavotinek A, Shaffer LG, Shapira SK. Monosomy 1p36. J Med Genet 1999;36:657–663.
36. Wu YQ, Heilstedt HA, Bedell JA, et al. Molecular refinement of the 1p36 deletion syndrome reveals size diversity and a preponderance of maternally derived deletions. Hum Mol Genet 1999;8:313–321.

37. Ballif BC, Kashork CD, Shaffer LG. The promise and pitfalls of telomere region-specific probes. Am J Hum Genet 2000;67:1356–1359.
38. Ballif BC, Yu W, Shaw CA, Kashork CD, Shaffer LG. Monosomy 1p36 breakpoint junctions suggest premeiotic breakage-fusion-bridge cycles are involved in generating terminal deletions. Hum Mol Genet 2003;12:2153–2165.
39. Gisselsson D. Chromosome instability in cancer: how, when, and why? Adv Cancer Res 2003;87:1–29.
40. Wilkie AO, Lamb J, Harris PC, Finney RD, Higgs DR. A truncated human chromosome 16 associated with alpha thalassaemia is stabilized by addition of telomeric repeat (TTAGGG)n. Nature 1990;346:868–871.
41. Flint J, Craddock CF, Villegas A, et al. Healing of broken human chromosomes by the addition of telomeric repeats. Am J Hum Genet 1994;55:505–512.
42. Sprung CN, Reynolds GE, Jasin M, Murnane JP. Chromosome healing in mouse embryonic stem cells. Proc Natl Acad Sci USA 1999;96:6781–6786.
43. Varley H, Di S, Scherer SW, Royle NJ. Characterization of terminal deletions at 7q32 and 22q13.3 healed by De novo telomere addition. Am J Hum Genet 2000;67:610–622.
44. Neumann AA, Reddel RR. Telomere maintenance and cancer; look, no telomerase. Nat Rev Cancer 2002;2:879–884.
45. Varley H, Pickett HA, Foxon JL, Reddel RR, Royle NJ. Molecular characterization of inter-telomere and intra-telomere mutations in human ALT cells. Nat Genet 2002;30:301–305.
46. Bosco G, Haber JE. Chromosome break-induced DNA replication leads to nonreciprocal translocations and telomere capture. Genetics 1998;150:1037–1047.
47. Meltzer PS, Guan XY, Trent JM. Telomere capture stabilizes chromosome breakage. Nat Genet 1993;4:252–255.
48. Ning Y, Liang JC, Nagarajan L, Schrock E, Ried T. Characterization of 5q deletions by subtelomeric probes and spectral karyotyping. Cancer Genet Cytogenet 1998;103:170–172.
49. Bottius E, Bakhsis N, Scherf A. Plasmodium falciparum telomerase: de novo telomere addition to telomeric and nontelomeric sequences and role in chromosome healing. Mol Cell Biol 1998;18:919–925.
50. Friebe B, Kynast RG, Zhang P, Qi L, Dhar M, Gill BS. Chromosome healing by addition of telomeric repeats in wheat occurs during the first mitotic divisions of the sporophyte and is a gradual process. Chromosome Res 2001;9:137–146.
51. Hackett JA, Feldser DM, Greider CW. Telomere dysfunction increases mutation rate and genomic instability. Cell 2001;106:275–286.
52. Kramer KM, Haber JE. New telomeres in yeast are initiated with a highly selected subset of TG1-3 repeats. Genes Dev 1993;7:2345–2356.
53. Muller F, Wicky C, Spicher A, Tobler H. New telomere formation after developmentally regulated chromosomal breakage during the process of chromatin diminution in Ascaris lumbricoides. Cell 1991;67:815–822.
54. Kolodner RD, Putnam CD, Myung K. Maintenance of genome stability in Saccharomyces cerevisiae. Science 2002;297:552–557.
55. Ballif BC, Gajecka M, Shaffer LG. Monosomy 1p36 breakpoints indicate repetitive DNA sequence elements may be involved in generating and/or stabilizing some terminal deletions. Chromosome Res 2004;12:133–141.
56. Ballif BC, Wakui K, Gajecka M, Shaffer LG. Translocation breakpoint mapping and sequence analysis in three monosomy 1p36 subjects with der(1)t(1;1)(p36;q44) suggest mechanisms for telomere capture in stabilizing de novo terminal rearrangements. Hum Genet 2004;114:198–206.
57. Gajecka M, Yu W, Ballif BC, et al. Delineation of mechanisms and regions of dosage imbalance in complex rearrangements of 1p36 leads to a putative gene for regulation of cranial suture closure. Eur J Hum Genet 2005;13:139–149.
58. Fouladi B, Sabatier L, Miller D, Pottier G, Murnane JP. The relationship between spontaneous telomere loss and chromosome instability in a human tumor cell line. Neoplasia 2000;2:540–554.
59. Lo AW, Sabatier L, Fouladi B, Pottier G, Ricoul M, Murnane JP. DNA amplification by breakage/fusion/bridge cycles initiated by spontaneous telomere loss in a human cancer cell line. Neoplasia 2002;4:531–538.
60. Horsley SW, Daniels RJ, Anguita E, et al. Monosomy for the most telomeric, gene-rich region of the short arm of human chromosome 16 causes minimal phenotypic effects. Eur J Hum Genet 2001;9:217–225.
61. Lamb J, Harris PC, Wilkie AO, Wood WG, Dauwerse JG, Higgs DR. De novo truncation of chromosome 16p and healing with (TTAGGG)n in the alpha-thalassemia/mental retardation syndrome (ATR-16). Am J Hum Genet 1993;52:668–676.

62. Wong AC, Ning Y, Flint J, et al. Molecular characterization of a 130-kb terminal microdeletion at 22q in a child with mild mental retardation. Am J Hum Genet 1997;60:113–120.

63. Allshire RC, Dempster M, Hastie ND. Human telomeres contain at least three types of G-rich repeat distributed non-randomly. Nucleic Acids Res 1989;17:4611–4627.

64. Baird DM, Jeffreys AJ, Royle NJ. Mechanisms underlying telomere repeat turnover, revealed by hypervariable variant repeat distribution patterns in the human Xp/Yp telomere. Embo J 1995;14:5433–5443.

65. Morin GB. Recognition of a chromosome truncation site associated with alpha-thalassaemia by human telomerase. Nature 1991;353:454–456.

66. Brkanac Z, Cody JD, Leach RJ, DuPont BR. Identification of cryptic rearrangements in patients with 18q-deletion syndrome. Am J Hum Genet 1998;62:1500–1506.

67. Marinescu RC, Johnson EI, Grady D, Chen XN, Overhauser J. FISH analysis of terminal deletions in patients diagnosed with cri-du-chat syndrome. Clin Genet 1999;56:282–288.

68. Stankiewicz P, Lupski JR. Genome architecture, rearrangements and genomic disorders. Trends Genet 2002;18:74–82.

69. Ledbetter DH. Minireview: cryptic translocations and telomere integrity. Am J Hum Genet 1992;51:451–456.

70. Mefford HC, Trask BJ. The complex structure and dynamic evolution of human subtelomeres. Nat Rev Genet 2002;3:91–102.

71. Daniel A, Baker E, Chia N, et al. Recombinants of intrachromosomal transposition of subtelomeres in chromosomes 1 and 2: a cause of minute terminal chromosomal imbalances. Am J Med Genet A 2003;117:57–64.

72. Malkova A, Ivanov EL, Haber JE. Double-strand break repair in the absence of RAD51 in yeast: a possible role for break-induced DNA replication. Proc Natl Acad Sci USA 1996;93:7131–7136.

73. Morrow DM, Connelly C, Hieter P. "Break copy" duplication: a model for chromosome fragment formation in Saccharomyces cerevisiae. Genetics 1997;147:371–382.

74. Artandi SE, Chang S, Lee SL, et al. Telomere dysfunction promotes non-reciprocal translocations and epithelial cancers in mice. Nature 2000;406:641–645.

75. Difilippantonio MJ, Petersen S, Chen HT, et al. Evidence for replicative repair of DNA double-strand breaks leading to oncogenic translocation and gene amplification. J Exp Med 2002;196:469–480.

76. Myung K, Chen C, Kolodner RD. Multiple pathways cooperate in the suppression of genome instability in Saccharomyces cerevisiae. Nature 2001;411:1073–1076.

77. Myung K, Datta A, Kolodner RD. Suppression of spontaneous chromosomal rearrangements by S phase checkpoint functions in Saccharomyces cerevisiae. Cell 2001;104:397–408.

78. Myung K, Kolodner RD. Suppression of genome instability by redundant S-phase checkpoint pathways in Saccharomyces cerevisiae. Proc Natl Acad Sci USA 2002;99:4500–4507.

79. Pipiras E, Coquelle A, Bieth A, Debatisse M. Interstitial deletions and intrachromosomal amplification initiated from a double-strand break targeted to a mammalian chromosome. Embo J 1998;17:325–333.

80. Smogorzewska A, Karlseder J, Holtgreve-Grez H, Jauch A, de Lange T. DNA ligase IV-dependent NHEJ of deprotected mammalian telomeres in G1 and G2. Curr Biol 2002;12:1635–1644.

81. Ballif BC, Kashork CD, Shaffer LG. FISHing for mechanisms of cytogenetically defined terminal deletions using chromosome-specific subtelomeric probes. Eur J Hum Genet 2000;8:764–770.

82. Christ LA, Crowe CA, Micale MA, Conroy JM, Schwartz S. Chromosome breakage hotspots and delineation of the critical region for the 9p-deletion syndrome. Am J Hum Genet 1999;65:1387–1395.

83. Deininger PL, Batzer MA. Alu repeats and human disease. Mol Genet Metab 1999;67:183–193.

84. Kolomietz E, Meyn MS, Pandita A, Squire JA. The role of Alu repeat clusters as mediators of recurrent chromosomal aberrations in tumors. Genes Chromosomes Cancer 2002;35:97–112.

85. Flint J, Rochette J, Craddock CF, et al. Chromosomal stabilisation by a subtelomeric rearrangement involving two closely related Alu elements. Hum Mol Genet 1996;5:1163–1169.

86. Katz SG, Schneider SS, Bartuski A, et al. An 18q- syndrome breakpoint resides between the duplicated serpins SCCA1 and SCCA2 and arises via a cryptic rearrangement with satellite III DNA. Hum Mol Genet 1999;8:87–92.

87. Bois P, Jeffreys AJ. Minisatellite instability and germline mutation. Cell Mol Life Sci 1999;55:1636–1648.

88. Bzymek M, Lovett ST. Instability of repetitive DNA sequences: the role of replication in multiple mechanisms. Proc Natl Acad Sci USA 2001;98:8319–8325.

89. Edelmann L, Spiteri E, Koren K, et al. AT-rich palindromes mediate the constitutional t(11;22) translocation. Am J Hum Genet 2001;68:1–13.

90. Kurahashi H, Shaikh T, Takata M, Toda T, Emanuel BS. The constitutional t(17;22): another translocation mediated by palindromic AT-rich repeats. Am J Hum Genet 2003;72:733–738.

91. Gajecka M, Ballif BC, Glotzbach CD, Bailey KA, Shaffer LG. Low-copy repeats and monosomy 1p36. The American Society of Human Genetics Annual Meeting. Toronto, ON, Canada, 2004.

92. Bonaglia MC, Giorda R, Poggi G, et al. Inverted duplications are recurrent rearrangements always associated with a distal deletion: description of a new case involving 2q. Eur J Hum Genet 2000;8:597–603.

93. Giglio S, Broman KW, Matsumoto N, et al. Olfactory receptor-gene clusters, genomic-inversion polymorphisms, and common chromosome rearrangements. Am J Hum Genet 2001;68:874–883.

94. Jenderny J, Poetsch M, Hoeltzenbein M, Friedrich U, Jauch A. Detection of a concomitant distal deletion in an inverted duplication of chromosome 3. Is there an overall mechanism for the origin of such duplications/deficiencies? Eur J Hum Genet 1998;6:439–444.

95. Bailey JA, Yavor AM, Massa HF, Trask BJ, Eichler EE. Segmental duplications: organization and impact within the current human genome project assembly. Genome Res 2001;11:1005–1017.

96. Eichler EE. Segmental duplications: what's missing, misassigned, and misassembled—and should we care? Genome Res 2001;11:653–656.

22 inv dup(15) and inv dup(22)

Heather E. McDermid, PhD and Rachel Wevrick, PhD

INTRODUCTION

The presence of a small supernumerary marker chromosome (SMC) in a karyotype creates a diagnostic dilemma, because the resulting duplications/triplications may cause abnormal development, depending on the location and size of the extra material. The most common SMC is the inv dup(15), the effect of which varies with size of triplication as well as the parent of origin. inv dup(22) is associated with the highly variable cat eye syndrome. Both are thought to be caused by U-type recombination between neighboring low-copy repeats (LCRs), resulting in both symmetric and asymmetric bisatellited dicentric supernumerary chromosomes. Studies are underway to associate the abnormal features of each syndrome with specific genes in the duplicated regions.

SMALL MARKER CHROMOSOMES

SMCs, detected prenatally or postnatally, have presented a diagnostic dilemma since the birth of cytogenetics nearly 50 years ago. SMCs, also referred to as extra structurally abnormal chromosomes, are present in addition to the normal chromosome complement, usually not identifiable by standard staining techniques, and typically smaller than the smallest autosome (1–4).

In a landmark study of almost 400,000 amniocenteses, 0.04% had an SMC of cytogenetically unidentifiable origin (reviewed in ref. 1). The incidence of SMCs at live birth has been variously reported as 0.05% (2) and 0.07% (3). SMCs can also exist as rings and occasionally may be present in multiple copies per cell. Mosaicism has been seen in 59% of all SMC cases, but is higher (69%) for SMCs derived from nonacrocentric chromosomes (4). In any case, the presence of an SMC may lead to an imbalance for whatever genes are duplicated in the SMC.

From: *Genomic Disorders: The Genomic Basis of Disease*
Edited by: J. R. Lupski and P. Stankiewicz © Humana Press, Totowa, NJ

When studied using fluorescence *in situ* hybridization (FISH), the chromosomal origin of most SMCs can be identified by the presence of chromosome-specific α-satellite DNA (although commercial satellite probes to differentiate chromosomes 13 from 21 and 14 from 22 are not available). More recent variants of the FISH technique, such as spectral karyotyping, centromere-specific multicolor FISH, and subcentromeric multicolor-FISH have allowed finer identification, the latter technique determining the presence of specific subcentromeric euchromatin *(5–7)*. SMCs derived from chromosome 15 can also be identified by specific staining with DAPI, a DNA-binding dye.

In a study of 112 autosomal SMCs ascertained both prenatally and postnatally, 68% were derived from acrocentric autosomes, and of those, 51% were derived from chromosome 15 (35% of all SMCs) *(4)*. The risk of an abnormal phenotype associated with the 32% of SMCs that are nonacrocentric-derived has been calculated as approx 28%, whereas SMCs derived from acrocentric autosomes, excluding chromosome 15, carry a lower risk (approx 7%) of abnormal phenotype *(8)*. Correlations between the SMC origin and phenotype have been attempted *(7,8)*. SMCs derived from chromosome 15 are associated with defined risk and distinct phenotype, depending on their genetic composition. As described below, imprinting of the proximal region of the chromosome 15 long arm also alters gene dosage effects. Specific SMCs derived from chromosome 22 cause a distinct phenotype, the cat eye syndrome (OMIM 115470).

INV DUP SMALL MARKER CHROMOSOMES

SMCs containing two copies of a centromere, arranged in an apparent mirror image symmetry around a central axis, have been referred to as isodicentric (idic), pseudoisodicentric (psu dic) or, more correctly, inverted duplication (inv dup) (Fig. 1). The best studied, recurrent inv dup SMCs are derived from chromosomes 15 or 22. These chromosomes are bisatellited because of an acrocentric p-arm on each end. They also contain two centromeres, usually separated by at least several megabases of euchromatin. Such chromosomes are often stable, presumably because one centromere is inactivated (hence the term pseudoisodicentric). An inv dup SMC associated with an otherwise normal karyotype results in a total of four copies of the excess region, and is therefore a triplication or partial tetrasomy.

inv dup SMCs have been referred to as isodicentric, but this term is appropriate only if the duplications on each side are symmetrical (Fig. 1). inv dup chromosomes have been found often to be asymmetrical, with one side of the chromosome considerably larger than the other. This results in a total of four copies of some regions and only three copies of others *(9)*.

inv dup SMCs can also originate from the other acrocentric chromosomes, but with less frequency and are associated with a less well-defined phenotype than that for chromosomes 15 and 22. Nonacrocentric chromosomes are also a source for inv dup SMCs. These may contain no α-satellite DNA and yet are stable, providing an opportunity to address the question of centromeric function in the absence of the DNA normally present at centromeres *(10)*. These unusual inv dup SMCs are C-band negative, yet have a G-banded primary constriction, which acts as an active kinetochore and reacts with CENP-C antibodies *(11)*. It is presumed that these SMCs activate noncentromeric sequences that function as neocentromeres.

It has long been suggested that inv dup chromosomes are derived from a "U-type" rather than the normal "X-type" exchange between nonsister or sister chromatids at meiosis I *(12,13)*. Mediated by LCRs on chromosomes 15 or 22, a U-type exchange between repeats in opposite

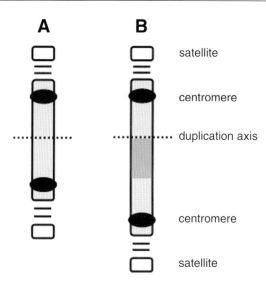

Fig. 1. Structure of bisatellited and dicentric inv dup chromosomes. These chromosomes can have a symmetrical duplication (A) or be asymmetrical, where one side of the duplication is larger than the other (B). In an asymmetric inv dup, the region nearest the centromere is present in two extra copies (light gray), whereas the more distal region is present in only one extra copy (dark gray).

orientation would lead to a dicentric SMC as well as an acentric fragment composed of two copies of the rest of each chromatid. The acentric fragment would be lost, whereas the SMC would be retained through nondisjunction and inactivation of one centromere. Each LCR in chromosome 22q11 is composed of complex blocks of repeats *(14)*. LCR2 and LCR4, in which most rearrangements occur, contain shared repeat blocks in both the same and opposite orientations, which facilitate U-type exchanges. If a U-type exchange occurs between elements of the same LCR (allelic), the resulting inv dup chromosome would essentially be symmetrical. A U-type exchange between similar elements of different LCRs (nonallelic) would produce an asymmetric SMC. Asymmetric inv dup SMCs could also result from a paracentric inversion of a region between LCRs, followed by recombination within the inversion loop *(15)*. This would similarly result in a dicentric SMC and an acentric fragment that is lost.

INV DUP(15)

inv dup chromosomes derived from chromosome 15 account for approx 35% of SMCs *(4)*, and, after trisomy 21, are the most common autosomal chromosomal aberration *(16)*. Although the phenotype associated with the inv dup(15) itself can be variable, uniparental disomy or deletion of the normal chromosome 15 can accompany the inv dup chromosome with additional clinical consequences *(17,18)*. The presence of abnormalities on the "normal" chromosomes 15, the size of the inv dup(15), and the parental origin of the chromosomal abnormalities all affect the severity of the outcome. This information is critical in the context of genetic counseling, particularly in the setting of prenatal ascertainment of a *de novo* inv dup(15).

Because of their relatively common frequency, chromosome 15 rearrangements have provided a rich source of information for the study of chromosomal abnormalities. The presence of a set of LCRs on the proximal long arm of chromosome 15 predisposes this region to a

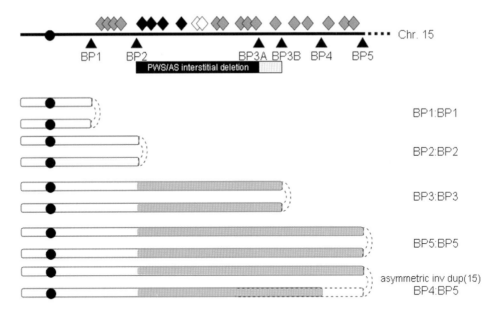

Fig. 2. Examples of various types of inv dup(15)s. Chromosome 15q11-q14 contains a set of genes that are expressed only from the paternally inherited allele (black diamonds, Prader-Willi syndrome [PWS] candidate genes), from the maternal allele in a tissue-specific fashion (white diamonds, including the Angelman syndrome [AS] gene *UBE3A*) or from both alleles (not imprinted, gray diamonds). Rearrangements of chromosome 15q11-q14 generally involve a set of low-copy repeats labeled BP1 through BP5; the PWS/AS interstitial deletions typically occur between BP2 and BP3A/3B. inv dup(15) chromosomes can involve any of the breakpoint regions, and can be symmetrical or asymmetrical, as in the bottom example. inv dup(15)s that contain material telomeric to BP2 (shaded gray) are associated with an adverse outcome. The centromere is represented by the black circle toward the left.

heterogeneous group of inter- and intrachromosomal rearrangements *(19,20)*. The nonallelic copies of these LCRs can misalign during meiosis, and the resulting nonallelic homologous recombination or unequal crossover event gives rise to structurally abnormal chromosomes. The LCRs are present in the breakpoint regions involved in the rearrangements, and are named in ascending order from the most centromeric, as break point (BP)1 to BP5 (Fig. 2).

The chromosomal disorders Prader-Willi syndrome (PWS; OMIM 176270) and Angelman syndrome (AS; OMIM 105830) most commonly involve a deletion of the genetic material between BP2 and BP3A/3B, with PWS deletions occurring on the paternally derived chromosome, and AS deletions occurring on the maternally derived chromosome *(19,20)* (Fig. 2). Although both syndromes include developmental delay, PWS individuals typically have a neonatal failure to thrive and hyperphagic obesity, among other neurodevelopmental findings *(21)*, whereas AS individuals typically have seizures and absent speech *(22)*. The difference between the phenotypes is owing to the presence of imprinted genes in the deletion region, which are expressed on only one chromosome in a manner dependent on parent of origin. The paternally expressed genes responsible for PWS are clustered toward the centromeric end of the BP2-BP3A/3B deletion region. Four of the PWS candidate genes, *MKRN3*, *NDN* (necdin), *MAGEL2*, and *SNURF/SNRPN*, are protein-coding and expressed in the nervous system during development *(23–26)*. Another PWS candidate gene encodes a functional RNA, the imprinting center transcript *(27)*. This transcript also contains a set of small nucleolar RNAs as well as acting as an antisense RNA for a more telomeric gene, *UBE3A*. In tissues in which the imprinting center transcript is active, this antisense regulation imparts paternal allele-specific gene silencing of *UBE3A*. Chromosomal deletions or other types of mutations that inactivate the maternal allele of *UBE3A* causes AS.

In addition to deletions, unequal recombination events can give rise to rare interstitial duplications and triplications, and to the more common inv dup(15). Maternally derived interstitial duplications of 15q11-q14 give rise to a phenotype, characterized by various types of intellectual impairment, which is distinct from the deletion syndromes, whereas paternally derived interstitial duplications are significantly less likely to be associated with abnormal phenotype *(28)*. There is at least one case where a paternally derived interstitial duplication was not associated with an adverse outcome, whereas the same duplication causes severe abnormalities upon maternal transmission *(29)*. *De novo* inv dup(15)(q11-q14) chromosomes also show a parent of origin bias, being almost exclusively maternal in origin *(30)*, and are associated with late maternal age *(4,31)*. This emphasizes the fact that the parental origin and size of the duplication region are important in predicting clinical outcome.

The smallest inv dup(15)s contain no duplicated material from the PWS/AS deletion region between BP2 and BP3 and carry a low risk of adverse outcome, despite the presence of at least four protein coding genes in the region centromeric to BP2 *(32,33)* (Fig. 2). The largest interstitial and supernumerary duplications contain extra copies of the chromosomal material extending distally to the PWS/AS BP3 region, and are associated with dysmorphic features, severe developmental delay, autism, seizures, strabismus, and abnormal dermatoglyphics *(28)*. inv dup(15)s, because of their derivation from an imprinted region, can present an unusual situation in terms of gene activity. A PWS or AS phenotype has been found in individuals who, in addition to the inv dup(15), carry either a deletion or uniparental disomy for chromosome 15, leading to the parent of origin phenotypes associated with loss of one parental copy of imprinted genes *(17,18)*.

The inv dup(15)s carrying duplicated PWS/AS region material are categorized according to the breakpoints involved, with examples given in Fig. 2. Several groups have identified the repeat regions involved in inv dup(15)s and interstitial duplications, using FISH, somatic cell hybrids and array comparative genomic hybridization to detect the dosage and position of single genomic sequences *(16,19,20,34,35)*. At high resolution, some inv dup(15)s that were thought to be symmetrical are in fact asymmetrical, and involve recombination between two different BP repeat clusters *(35)*. The most common of the larger inv dup(15)s involves BP4 and BP5, whereas most of the remainder are the result of a symmetrical BP3 to BP3 rearrangement. Individuals with this latter class of inv dup(15) carry one paternally derived and three maternally derived copies of the PWS/AS region, whereas individuals carrying the BP4:BP5 inv dup(15)s carry this genetic material plus additional copies of maternally inherited genes distal to the PWS/AS region *(35)*. Clear phenotypic differences among these latter classes, if they exist, have yet to emerge. A dosage effect associated with inv dup(15)s is evident, however, with reports of individuals with hexasomy for 15q11-q14 at the severe end of the phenotypic spectrum *(36)*.

The high frequency of chromosomal rearrangements is undoubtedly related to the presence of the "BP" LCRs (Fig. 2), but rearrangements appear to arise from a variety of recombinational mechanisms. Reciprocal recombination events of the PWS/AS deletion region likely cause interstitial duplications involving the same LCRs. Studies using probes located near the chromosome 15 centromere suggest that aberrant U-type exchange resulting in inv dup(15) can occur between sister chromatids, or between homologous chromosomes either during or after recombination *(34)*. The development of informative markers closer to the centromere of chromosome 15 and sequencing of the breakpoints will facilitate further analyses of the structure and mechanism of origin of these structurally abnormal chromosomes.

INV DUP(22)

The consequence of inv dup(22) for clinical phenotype is in one way simpler than that for the inv dup(15) since chromosome 22 does not appear to be influenced by genomic imprinting. No convincing sex bias has been seen in chromosome 22 rearrangements *(37)*, and three cases of maternal uniparental disomy 22 have shown normal phenotype *(38–40)*. However, the remarkable phenotypic variation of the associated syndrome results in diagnostic problems of its own.

inv dup(22)(q11) is associated with cat eye syndrome (CES), which is characterized by abnormalities of the eye, heart, anus, kidneys, skeleton, gastrointestinal tract, and face *(41–43)*. Patients may show mild mental retardation, but many are within the normal intelligence quotient (IQ) range. The syndrome derives its name from ocular coloboma, although only about half of CES patients show this feature. Preauricular skin tags or pits are the most constant feature. The CES phenotype is surprisingly variable, ranging from apparently normal to multiple severe and life-threatening malformations. The incidence of CES has been estimated to be 1/50–150,000 (OMIM 115470). Because some patients are mildly affected, there are numerous cases of inheritance of the CES chromosome, sometimes through multiple generations *(44)*.

Although the CES chromosome is often stable, it is not uncommon to detect mosaicism *(42)*. There are also cases where the inv dup(22) has shown instability within a family, resulting in secondary rearrangements *(45)*. The parental origin of few inv dup(22)s has been determined. By comparing Q-banded polymorphisms, two cases were shown to originate from both maternal homologs *(46)*. A similar analysis identified a third case of maternal origin, but from the same chromosome 22 homolog *(47)*. Thus, both intra- and interchromosomal recombination can be involved in the production of inv dup(22).

The 22q11 region has a variety of chromosomal rearrangements that are mediated by LCRs (reviewed in ref. *48*). Most prominent is the common deletion associated with DiGeorge syndrome/velocardiofacial syndrome (DGS/VCFS). The majority of DGS/VCFS deletions localize between LCR22-2 and LCR22-4, spanning approx 3 Mb (Fig. 3). A small percentage of deletions occur between LCR22-2 and LCR22-3a, spanning approx 1.5 Mb. CES chromosomes also appear to break at these LCRs *(9,49)*.

An inv dup(22) is formed from breakpoints in two chromatids. In a type I CES chromosome, both breakpoints are at LCR22-2, only the CES region (proximal to LCR22-2) is included and the inv dup(22) is symmetrical *(9)*. In type II CES chromosomes, the DGS/VCFS region is also included in the duplication. Type II chromosomes can be symmetrical, with both breakpoints in LCR22-4 and two additional copies of the DGS/VCFS region (type IIb), or asymmetrical, with breakpoints at LCR22-2 and LCR22-4 and with only one extra copy of the DGS/VCFS region (type IIa). A case has also been found with at least one breakpoint at LCR22-3a *(50)*.

The CES phenotype results from overexpression of dosage sensitive genes in the CES critical region. The critical region for CES was determined by the analysis of an unusual patient with a relatively stable, supernumerary double r(22) *(51)*. This child had all major physical

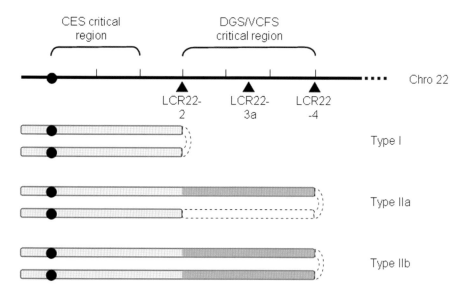

Fig. 3. Composition of various inv dup(22)s associated with cat-eye syndrome (CES). The inv dup(22) breakpoints coincide with the location of the of low copy repeats associated with DGS/VCFS deletions. Type I and IIb chromosomes are symmetrical duplications, with the latter containing the DGS/VCFS critical region as well as the CES region. Type IIa chromosomes are asymmetrical, with only one extra copy of the DiGeorge syndrome/velocardiofacial syndrome region, but two extra copies of the CES region. There is also one reported case of a CES chromosome with a LCR22-3a breakpoint, although in this case the location of the second breakpoint is not clear (50, case 2).

features of CES, although development could not be assessed as the child died at 17 days. The ring contained approx 2 Mb of proximal 22q11 from the centromere to a region distal to the *ATP6E* gene. A typical inv dup(22) contain at least an additional 1 Mb. The first 1–1.5-Mb from the 22 centromere contain pericentromeric repeats that are unlikely to contain active and unique genes *(52)*. Thus, the majority, if not all, of the genes in the CES critical region lie within an approx 700-kb interval that contains at least 14 predicted or known genes *(52)*. The gene or genes causative for CES features has yet to be determined. Candidates identified include a secreted growth factor predicted to have adenosine deaminase activity (*CECR1*) *(53,54)*, and a transcription factor involved in chromatin remodeling *(55)*.

A proportion of CES chromosomes have one or two copies of the DGS/VCFS region in additional to four copies of the CES region. Duplications of the DGS/VCFS region have been associated recently with variable symptoms including learning disabilities, cognitive and behavioral abnormalities, palate defects, hearing loss, heart defects, growth deficiency, developmental and motor delays, and urogenital anomalies *(56)*. This likely represents only a spectrum of the microduplication 22q11.2 syndrome, because the patients were ascertained during testing specific for the DGS/VCFS deletion. In any case, one would assume that the addition of extra copies of the DGS/VCFS region would worsen the phenotype of CES, but this has not been observed. However, because only 10 CES patients have been characterized in this way *(9)*, this lack of correlation is likely to be because of the extreme variability of the overall syndrome masking more subtle changes brought on by additional copies of the DGS/VCFS

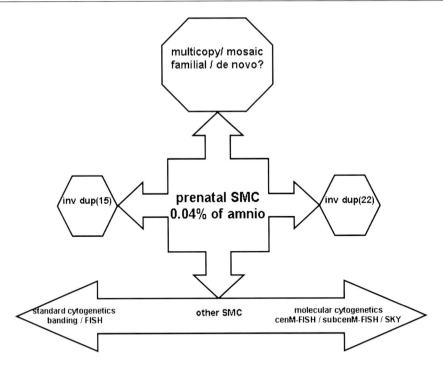

Fig. 4. Prenatal identification of small marker chromosomes—a diagnostic predicament. Prenatally identified small marker chromosomes (SMCs) involving chromosomes 15 and 22 have partially predictable outcomes. The phenotypic outcome for a fetus with an SMC can depend on its molecular composition, whether the SMC is familial or *de novo*, and whether it is present in multiple copies or only in some cells. Overall, molecular and cytogenetic tests have been or are being developed that should unequivocally identify the extra material present in the SMC.

region. Only the analysis of a much larger cohort of CES patients will determine whether a correlation exists between phenotype and the size of the CES chromosome.

CES is usually associated with the inv dup(22), however interstitial duplications have also been reported *(57–59)*. Again, because of phenotypic variability and problems of ascertaining mild cases, it is not yet clear whether three copies of the CES region produce less susceptibility to malformations than four copies. Interestingly, the father and grandfather of the child with the supernumerary double r(22) both had a single supernumerary r(22) and appeared normal, stressing the variability of this syndrome even within families *(51)*.

There is also a class of inv dup(22) associated with a normal phenotype *(3,60,61)*. These chromosomes are often familial, and presumably contain no dosage-sensitive genes. The size in comparison to CES chromosomes has not been determined yet, and no commercial probe exists to differentiate the two. The cytogenetic appearance of these small inv dup(22)s is not always helpful in distinguishing them from CES chromosomes. This makes the prenatal discovery of an inv dup(22) a serious genetic counseling dilemma.

SUMMARY

inv dup chromosomes 15 and 22, along with recurrent deletions and duplications, appear to be the inevitable consequence of the presence of LCRs relatively close to the centromere of acrocentric chromosomes 15 and 22. Formation of an inv dup chromosome results in a combination of duplication and triplication of variable regions, depending on the LCRs involved and whether the chromosome is symmetrical or asymmetrical. The phenotypic consequences of such rearrangements also vary with the LCR used.

The finding of an acrocentric-derived inv dup chromosome or other SMC at prenatal diagnosis presents a diagnostic dilemma (Fig. 4). Identification of the chromosomal origin of the SMC can be achieved using centromere-specific FISH probes, although the commercially available probe for chromosomes 13/21 and 14/22 does not distinguish the two. Chromosome painting, or more complex molecular cytogenetic methods can now identify the extraneous material, and additional analysis is then required to determine the size of the SMC. Prediction of clinical outcome remains problematic, especially for inv dup(22). Overall, further investigation of the frequency and clinical outcomes of the more commonly occurring SMCs should enable the development of algorithms for genetic counseling after cytogenetic identification of an SMC.

REFERENCES

1. Warburton D. De novo balanced chromosome rearrangements and extra marker chromosomes identified at prenatal diagnosis: clinical significance and distribution of breakpoints. Am J Hum Genet 1991;49:995–1013.
2. Buckton KE, Spowart G, Newton MS, Evans HJ. Forty four probands with an additional "marker" chromosome. Hum Genet 1985;69:353–370.
3. Gravholt CH, Friedrich U. Molecular cytogenetic study of supernumerary marker chromosomes in an unselected group of children. Am J Med Genet 1995;56:106–111.
4. Crolla JA, Youings SA, Ennis S, Jacobs PA. Supernumerary marker chromosomes in man: parental origin, mosaicism and maternal age revisited. Eur J Hum Genet 2005;13:154–160.
5. Haddad BR, Schrock E, Meck J, et al. Identification of de novo chromosomal markers and derivatives by spectral karyotyping. Hum Genet 1998;103:619–625.
6. Nietzel A, Rocchi M, Starke H, et al. A new multicolor-FISH approach for the characterization of marker chromosomes: centromere-specific multicolor-FISH (cenM-FISH). Hum Genet 2001;108:199–204.
7. Starke H, Nietzel A, Weise A, et al. Small supernumerary marker chromosomes (SMCs): genotype-phenotype correlation and classification. Hum Genet 2003;114:51–67.
8. Crolla JA. FISH and molecular studies of autosomal supernumerary marker chromosomes excluding those derived from chromosome 15: II. Review of the literature. Am J Med Genet 1998;75:367–381.
9. McTaggart KE, Budarf ML, Driscoll DA, Emanuel BS, Ferreira P, McDermid HE. Cat eye syndrome chromosome breakpoint clustering: identification of two intervals also associated with 22q11 deletion syndrome breakpoints. Cytogenet Cell Genet 1998;81:222–228.
10. Depinet TW, Zackowski JL, Earnshaw WC, et al. Characterization of neo-centromeres in marker chromosomes lacking detectable alpha-satellite DNA. Hum Mol Genet 1997;6:1195–1204.
11. Amor DJ, Choo KH. Neocentromeres: role in human disease, evolution, and centromere study. Am J Hum Genet 2002;71:695–714.
12. Van Dyke DL, Weiss L, Logan M, Pai GS. The origin and behavior of two isodicentric bisatellited chromosomes. Am J Hum Genet 1997;29:294–300.
13. Schreck RR, Breg WR, Erlanger BF, Miller OJ. Preferential derivation of abnormal human G-group-like chromosomes from chromosome 15. Hum Genet 1997;36:1–12.
14. Babcock M, Pavlicek A, Spiteri E, et al. Shuffling of genes within low-copy repeats on 22q11 (LCR22) by Alu-mediated recombination events during evolution. Genome Res 2003;13:2519–2532.
15. Emanuel BS, Shaikh TH. Segmental duplications: an 'expanding' role in genomic instability and disease. Nat Rev Genet 2001;2:791–800.
16. Wandstrat AE, Schwartz S. Isolation and molecular analysis of inv dup(15) and construction of a physical map of a common breakpoint in order to elucidate their mechanism of formation. Chromosoma 2000;109:498–505.
17. Spinner NB, Zackai E, Cheng SD, Knoll JH. Supernumerary inv dup(15) in a patient with Angelman syndrome and a deletion of 15q11-q13. Am J Med Genet 1995;57:61–65.

18. Robinson WP, Wagstaff J, Bernasconi F, et al. Uniparental disomy explains the occurrence of the Angelman or Prader-Willi syndrome in patients with an additional small inv dup(15) chromosome. J Med Genet 1993;30:756–760.

19. Christian SL, Fantes JA, Mewborn SK, Huang B, Ledbetter DH. Large genomic duplicons map to sites of instability in the Prader- Willi/Angelman syndrome chromosome region (15q11-q13). Hum Mol Genet 1999;8:1025–1037.

20. Amos-Landgraf JM, Ji Y, Gottlieb W, et al. Chromosome breakage in the Prader-Willi and Angelman syndromes involves recombination between large, transcribed repeats at proximal and distal breakpoints. Am J Hum Genet 1999;65:370–386.

21. Gunay-Aygun M, Schwartz S, Heeger S, O'Riordan MA, Cassidy SB. The changing purpose of Prader-Willi syndrome clinical diagnostic criteria and proposed revised criteria. Pediatrics 2001;108:E92.

22. Clayton-Smith J, Laan L. Angelman syndrome: a review of the clinical and genetic aspects. J Med Genet 2003;40:87–95.

23. Lee S, Walker CL, Wevrick R. Prader-Willi syndrome transcripts are expressed in phenotypically significant regions of the developing mouse brain. Gene Expr Patterns 2003;3:599–609.

24. Jong MT, Gray TA, Ji Y,et al. A novel imprinted gene, encoding a RING zinc-finger protein, and overlapping antisense transcript in the Prader-Willi syndrome critical region. Hum Mol Genet 1999;8:783–793.

25. MacDonald HR, Wevrick R. The necdin gene is deleted in Prader-Willi syndrome and is imprinted in human and mouse. Hum Mol Genet 1997;6:1873–1878.

26. Gray TA, Saitoh S, Nicholls RD. An imprinted, mammalian bicistronic transcript encodes two independent proteins. Proc Natl Acad Sci USA 1999;96:5616–5621.

27. Runte M, Huttenhofer A, Gross S, Kiefmann M, Horsthemke B, Buiting K. The IC-SNURF-SNRPN transcript serves as a host for multiple small nucleolar RNA species and as an antisense RNA for UBE3A. Hum Mol Genet 2001;10:2687–2700.

28. Bolton PF, Dennis NR, Browne CE, et al. The phenotypic manifestations of interstitial duplications of proximal 15q with special reference to the autistic spectrum disorders. Am J Med Genet 2001;105:675–685.

29. Cook EH Jr, Lindgren V, Leventhal BL, et al. Autism or atypical autism in maternally but not paternally derived proximal 15q duplication. Am J Hum Genet 1997;60:928–934.

30. Mignon C, Malzac P, Moncla A, et al. Clinical heterogeneity in 16 patients with inv dup 15 chromosome: cytogenetic and molecular studies, search for an imprinting effect. Eur J Hum Genet 1996;4:88–100.

31. Maraschio P, Zuffardi O, Bernardi F, et al. Preferential maternal derivation in inv dup(15): analysis of eight new cases. Hum Genet 1981;57:345–350.

32. Chai JH, Locke DP, Greally JM, et al. Identification of four highly conserved genes between breakpoint hotspots BP1 and BP2 of the Prader-Willi/Angelman syndromes deletion region that have undergone evolutionary transposition mediated by flanking duplicons. Am J Hum Genet 2003;73:898–925.

33. Huang B, Crolla JA, Christian SL, et al. Refined molecular characterization of the breakpoints in small inv dup(15) chromosomes. Hum Genet 1997;99:11–17.

34. Wandstrat AE, Leana-Cox J, Jenkins L, Schwartz S. Molecular cytogenetic evidence for a common breakpoint in the largest inverted duplications of chromosome 15. Am J Hum Genet 1998;62:925–936.

35. Wang NJ, Liu D, Parokonny AS, Schanen NC. High-resolution molecular characterization of 15q11-q13 rearrangements by array comparative genomic hybridization (array CGH) with detection of gene dosage. Am J Hum Genet 2004;75:267–281.

36. Mann SM, Wang NJ, Liu DH, et al. Supernumerary tricentric derivative chromosome 15 in two boys with intractable epilepsy: another mechanism for partial hexasomy. Hum Genet 2004;115:104–111.

37. Morrow B, Goldberg R, Carlson C, et al. Molecular definition of the 22q11 deletions in velo-cardio-facial syndrome. Am J Hum Genet 1995;56:1391–1403.

38. Kirkels VG, Hustinx TW, Scheres JM. Habitual abortion and translocation (22q;22q): unexpected transmission from a mother to her phenotypically normal daughter. Clin Genet 1980;18:456–461.

39. Palmer CG, Schwartz S, Hodes ME. Transmission of a balanced homologous t(22q;22q) translocation from mother to normal daughter. Clin Genet 1980;17:418–422.

40. Schinzel AA, Basaran S, Bernasconi F, Karaman B, Yuksel-Apak M, Robinson WP. Maternal uniparental disomy 22 has no impact on the phenotype. Am J Hum Genet 1994;54:21–24.

41. Schinzel A, Schmid W, Fraccaro M, et al. The "cat eye syndrome": dicentric small marker chromosome probably derived from a no.22 (tetrasomy 22pter to q11) associated with a characteristic phenotype. Report of 11 patients and delineation of the clinical picture. Hum Genet 1981;57:148–158.

42. Berends MJ, Tan-Sindhunata G, Leegte B, van Essen AJ. Phenotypic variability of Cat-Eye syndrome. Genet Couns 2001;12:23–34.
43. Rosias PR, Sijstermans JM, Theunissen PM, et al. Phenotypic variability of the cat eye syndrome. Case report and review of the literature. Genet Couns 2001;12:273–282.
44. Luleci G, Bagci G, Kivran M, Luleci E, Bektas S, Basaran S. A hereditary bisatellite-dicentric supernumerary chromosome in a case of cat-eye syndrome. Hereditas 1989;111:7–10.
45. Urioste M, Visedo G, Sanchis A, et al. Dynamic mosaicism involving an unstable supernumerary der(22) chromosome in cat eye syndrome. Am J Med Genet 1994;49:77–82.
46. Magenis RE, Sheehy RR, Brown MG, et al. Parental origin of the extra chromosome in the cat eye syndrome: evidence from heteromorphism and in situ hybridization analysis. Am J Med Genet 1988;29:9–19.
47. Tupler R, Hoeller A, Pezzolo A, Maraschio P. Maternal derivation of inv dup (22) and clinical variation in cat-eye syndrome. Ann Genet 1994;37:153–155.
48. McDermid HE, Morrow BE. Genomic disorders on 22q11. Am J Hum Genet 2002;70:1077–1088.
49. Edelmann L, Pandita RK, Spiteri E, et al. A common molecular basis for rearrangement disorders on chromosome 22q11. Hum Mol Genet 1999;8:1157–1167.
50. Crolla JA, Howard P, Mitchell C, Long FL, Dennis NR. A molecular and FISH approach to determining karyotype and phenotype correlations in six patients with supernumerary marker(22) chromosomes. Am J Med Genet 1997;72:440–447.
51. Mears AJ, el-Shanti H, Murray JC, McDermid HE, Patil SR. Minute supernumerary ring chromosome 22 associated with cat eye syndrome: further delineation of the critical region. Am J Hum Genet 1995;57:667–673.
52. Footz T.K, Brinkman-Mills P, Banting GS, et al. Analysis of the cat eye syndrome critical region in humans and the region of conserved synteny in mice : a search for candidate genes at or near the human chromosome 22 pericentromere. Genome Res 2001;11:1053–1070.
53. Riazi MA, Brinkman-Mills P, Nguyen T, et al. The human homolog of insect-derived growth factor, CECR1, is a candidate gene for features of cat eye syndrome. Genomics 2000;64:277–285.
54. Maier SA, Podemski L, Graham SW, McDermid HE, Locke J. Characterization of the adenosine deaminase-related growth factor (ADGF) gene family in Drosophila. Gene 2001;280:27–36.
55. Banting GS, Barak O, Ames TM, et al. CECR2, a protein involved in neurulation, forms a novel chromatin remodeling complex with SNF2L. Hum Mol Genet 2005;14:513–524.
56. Ensenauer RE, Adeyinka A, Flynn HC, et al. Microduplication 22q11.2, an emerging syndrome: clinical, cytogenetic, and molecular analysis of thirteen patients. Am J Hum Genet 2003;73:1027–1040.
57. Reiss JA, Weleber RG, Brown MG, Bangs CD, Lovrien EW, Magenis RE. Tandem duplication of proximal 22q: a cause of cat-eye syndrome. Am J Med Genet 1985;20:165–171.
58. Knoll JH, Asamoah A, Pletcher BA, Wagstaff J. Interstitial duplication of proximal 22q: phenotypic overlap with cat eye syndrome. Am J Med Genet 1995;55:221–224.
59. Lindsay EA, Shaffer LG, Carrozzo R, Greenberg F, Baldini A. De novo tandem duplication of chromosome segment 22q11-q12: clinical, cytogenetic, and molecular characterization. Am J Med Genet 1995;56:296–299.
60. Brondum-Nielsen K, Mikkelsen M. A 10-year survey, 1980-1990, of prenatally diagnosed small supernumerary marker chromosomes, identified by FISH analysis. Outcome and follow-up of 14 cases diagnosed in a series of 12,699 prenatal samples. Prenat Diagn 1995;15:615–619.
61. Engelen JJ, Tuerlings JH, Albrechts JC, Schrander-Stumpel CT, Hamers AJ, De Die-Smulders CE. Prenatally detected marker chromosome identified as an i(22)(p10) using (micro)FISH. Genet Couns 2000;11:13–17.

23 Mechanisms Underlying Neoplasia-Associated Genomic Rearrangements

Thoas Fioretos, MD, PhD

CONTENTS

BACKGROUND
INTRODUCTION
GENOMIC ABNORMALITIES IN TUMORS
LCR-MEDIATED i(17Q) FORMATION
ARE LCRs COMMON MEDIATORS OF GENOMIC ALTERATIONS IN CANCER?
SUMMARY
REFERENCES

BACKGROUND

Neoplastic disorders are characterized by recurrent somatically acquired chromosomal aberrations that alter the structure and/or expression of a large number of genes. Most "cancer genes" discovered to date in human neoplasms have been identified through isolation of genes at the breakpoints of balanced chromosomal translocations. Although functional studies of such cancer-causing genes have demonstrated their causal role in tumorigenesis, the mechanisms underlying the formation of recurrent chromosomal changes in cancer remain enigmatic. Low-copy repeats (LCRs) are important mediators of erroneous meiotic recombination, resulting in constitutional chromosomal rearrangements. Recently, LCRs have been implicated in the formation of the frequent and characteristic neoplasia-associated chromosomal aberrations t(9;22)(q34;q11) and i(17q), suggesting that similar genome architecture features may play an important role in generating also other somatic chromosomal rearrangements.

INTRODUCTION

Neoplasia originates in a single cell through acquired somatic genetic changes. To date, approx 300 "cancer genes" (i.e., genes causally implicated in oncogenesis), have been identified *(1)*. These cancer-causing genes encode proteins that normally regulate cellular proliferation, differentiation, and/or cell death. A probably too simplistic, but generally accepted, way of classifying cancer genes is based on the way they act at the cellular level. So-called oncogenes act dominantly (i.e., a single-mutated allele is sufficient to contribute to oncogenesis), whereas so-called tumor suppressor genes (TSGs) are recessive (i.e., both genes need to

From: *Genomic Disorders: The Genomic Basis of Disease*
Edited by: J. R. Lupski and P. Stankiewicz © Humana Press, Totowa, NJ

be mutated). It has also become clear over the last few years that, haploinsufficiency, which is loss of only one allele, also may be an important factor in tumor development and progression *(2)*.

Several types of mutations in cancer genes have been identified *(1)*, including point mutations within coding and non-coding regions, small insertions/deletions altering the open reading frame, as well as gene copy-number changes and rearrangements resulting from chromosomal abnormalities. The latter group of aberrations has been studied extensively, with more than 300 recurrent balanced chromosomal abnormalities reported *(3)*. Most cancer genes discovered to date have been identified at the breakpoints of balanced chromosomal translocations that result in either chimeric fusion genes or deregulation of genes at the breakpoints by juxtaposition of regulatory elements to another gene *(4,5)*. Most likely, however, there is a heavy bias towards fusion genes in the current estimation of the total number of cancer genes not only because of methodological limitations in the past to detect subtle changes at the DNA level on a genome-wide basis (e.g., point mutations or small deletions), but also because of difficulties in identifying single cancer genes in neoplasias characterized by complex and/or unbalanced chromosomal aberrations affecting multiple genes.

Although functional studies of individual cancer genes using various transformation assays or transgenic animal models have demonstrated their causal role in tumorigenesis *(6)*, the mechanisms underlying the formation of recurrent chromosomal changes in neoplasia remain elusive. Most of our knowledge is based on cloning individual fusion genes and looking for repeat elements or putative recombinogenic sequence motifs at the vicinity of the breakpoints. In many instances, however, it has been difficult to determine whether the presence of a certain motif at a chromosomal breakpoint represents a chance occurrence or a bona fide association. This lack of knowledge seems to contrast with the rapid progress made recently in the field of constitutional genomic abnormalities, exemplified by the increasing number of microdeletion syndromes being identified and the involvement of LCRs in generating such disorders *(7)*. However, LCRs have been implicated recently in the formation of the most common isochromosome, i(17q), in human neoplastic disorders *(8)* and also in the balanced translocation, t(9;22)(q34;q11), the cytogenetic hallmark of chronic myeloid leukemia (CML) *(9)*. This chapter focuses on mechanisms involved in the generation of somatically acquired structural chromosomal aberrations with an emphasis on recent advances made in elucidating how i(17q) is formed. Whenever applicable, conceptual and mechanistic differences between somatically and constitutionally acquired genetic changes are also discussed.

GENOMIC ABNORMALITIES IN TUMORS

At the chromosomal level, genomic changes in tumor cells are visible either as balanced abnormalities (reciprocal translocations, inversions, and insertions) or unbalanced changes, including nonreciprocal translocations, deletions, duplications, numerical aberrations, and amplifications (visible as double minutes, or homogenously staining regions) *(10)*. Individual cancer genes become altered through several different mechanisms; oncogenes are typically activated by point mutations, structural rearrangements, and amplifications, whereas TSGs become inactivated by mutations, deletions, or silencing through methylation.

The overwhelming majority of oncogenes in human malignancies have been identified by isolating genes located at the breakpoints of balanced chromosomal translocations that result in tumor-specific fusion genes. To date, 271 fusion genes have been described and because many genes recombine with shared partner genes (e.g., *ETV6*, *MLL*, *EWSR1*), the number of rearranged genes (275 unique genes) is smaller than expected from the number of fusion genes *(4)*. Fusion genes are particularly common in hematologic malignancies and in mesenchymal tumors and are considered key mediators of malignant transformation in these tumor entities *(5,11)*. In contrast, tumors of epithelial origin, the most common tumor type in man, are generally believed to originate through loss of TSGs or activation of oncogenes by genomic amplification *(12)*. This dichotomy, suggesting a fundamental tissue-specific difference in the genetic mechanisms by which neoplasia is initiated, has been challenged recently, however, and it has been suggested that fusion genes in epithelial tumors may be more frequent than previously anticipated *(4)*.

What are the mechanisms underlying the formation of balanced chromosomal translocations resulting in fusion genes? In hematologic malignances, two qualitatively different types of rearrangements have been identified, each probably arising through different mechanisms *(13,14)*. In a subset of malignancies of B- or T-cell origin, illegitimate recombinations result in the juxtaposition of a variety of structurally intact oncogenes to enhancer elements of the immunoglobulin (*Ig*)- or the T-cell receptor (*TCR*) loci. A paradigmatic example of this category is the Burkitt lymphoma-associated t(8;14) translocation, which brings the *MYC* oncogene into the vicinity of regulatory elements of the *IgH* locus, resulting in deregulated expression of *MYC (15,16)*. In this subset of malignancies the mechanism behind the chromosomal breakpoint in one of the partner genes seems apparent as double strand breaks arise normally in the *Ig* and *TCR* loci during V(D)J recombination. However, little is known about the underlying mechanisms of chromosomal breaks in *MYC*. The breakpoints occur at sites with no homology to V(D)J or switch recombinase recognition sequences, suggesting that they are unlikely to be dependent upon these activities *(17)*. Interesting progress has been made recently in elucidating the mechanism behind the t(14;18), which is characteristic of follicular lymphoma. Through this translocation, the *BCL2* gene is relocated into the *IgH* locus. The breakpoints in *BCL2* occur within a confined 150 basepair region (Mbr) and it has been shown that the RAG complex, which is the normal enzyme for DNA cleavage at V(D)J segments, is capable of introducing nicks in the Mbr *(18)*. Importantly, the *BCL2* Mbr is not a V(D)J recombination signal. Instead, the RAG complex nicks the Mbr because it adopts a nonB DNA structure, providing a basis for the fragility of the *BCL2* locus *(18)*. Whether similar structural features may explain the juxtaposition of other oncogenes to the *Ig* or *TCR* loci remains to be investigated.

The second and by far the most common outcome of balanced translocations in neoplasia is the creation of fusion genes, resulting in the expression of chimeric fusion proteins *(4,13)*. In such fusion genes, double-strand breaks typically (but not exclusively) occur in introns within so called "breakpoint clusters regions" that can vary in size from a few basepairs to hundreds of kilobases. So far, no consistent consensus sequences or specific repetitive elements have been identified within the many breakpoint clusters identified. Many recombinogeneic motifs and repetitive elements have been reported to coincide with translocation breakpoints in neoplasia *(13,19–21)*, e.g., *Alu* sequences, topoisomerase II cleavage sites, and chi-like elements, but given their frequent genome-wide occurrence it is difficult, with a few exceptions, to currently ascribe them a direct role in generating reciprocal translocations. Only a few systematic studies on the importance of the nucleotide composition and the occurrence of recombination-associated motifs in neoplasia-associated translocation breakpoints are currently available. A recent survey examined up to 125 bp on either side of translocation and gross deletion breakpoints in neoplasia and constitutional disorders *(20)*. The majority of the breakpoints were derived from translocations in hematologic malignancies and polypyrimidine tracts and specific recombination-associated motifs (e.g., DNA polymerase pause sites/frame-shift hotspots, *IgH* class s with sites, heptamer/nonamer V[D]J recombination signal sequences, translin binding sites, and chi elements) were found to be over-represented in the translocation breakpoints *(20)*.

Specific DNA breakage has been implicated in the genesis of some translocations, mainly those involving the *MLL* gene, known to fuse to a wide variety of partner genes in acute myeloid and lymphocytic leukemias *(22)*. Rearrangement of *MLL* is also frequent in therapy-related leukemias, occurring in patients previously treated with topoisomerase II inhibitors *(23)*. The genomic breakpoints in *MLL* in therapy-related cases often coincide with topoisomerase II cleavage sites, DNase I-hypersensitive sites, and scaffold attachment regions, indicating that these chromatin structural elements may influence the location of these translocation breakpoints *(24–26)*. Data are also at hand suggesting that sublethal apoptotic signals, through the activation of endonucleases, may result in site-specific cleavage of *MLL* and other genes forming fusion genes *(21,27)*.

The great majority of all translocations that have been studied to date, mainly in leukemias and mesenchymal tumors, show no extensive regions of homology at the breakpoints, and are, hence, believed to arise through (error-prone) nonhomologous end joining *(13,21,28)*. A prerequisite for end joining to take place is, of course, a spatial proximity of the broken chromosome ends. Available data on several genes involved in frequent and specific translocations, e.g., *IgH/MYC* and *BCR/ABL1*, show that, indeed, such genes are preferentially positioned in close proximity relative to each other in the nucleus, suggesting that the formation of translocations also is determined in part by higher order of spatial organization of the genome *(29–31)*.

When trying to understand the features underlying the observed confinement of chromosomal breakpoints into clusters, it is important to consider that they represent the result of selection on the protein level. In fact, transcription factors and tyrosine kinase-encoding proteins are overrepresented among proteins involved in fusion genes *(4)*, and critical functional domains of these have to remain intact to provide a selective advantage. Hence, numerous chromosomal breaks, with scattered distribution, may occur in somatic cells, either because of endogenous or exogenous genotoxic factors, but are never brought to our attention because of their failure to provide a selective edge.

It is likely that other genome structural features of importance for generating neoplasia-associated genomic rearrangements will be identified in the near future. An entirely novel mechanism that may prove important will be discussed in detail in the following sections.

LCR-MEDIATED i(17q) FORMATION

Isochromosome 17q [i(17q)] constitutes the most common isochromosome in human neoplasia and has been described both as a primary and as a secondary abnormality, suggesting an important pathogenetic role in tumor development as well as in progression *(32)*. The i(17q) is frequent in hematologic malignancies, in particular as a secondary abnormality in addition to the characteristic t(9;22)(q34;q11) in CML, but is also the most common chromosomal aberration in primitive neuroectodermal tumors and medulloblastomas *(33)*.

Fioretos et al. *(33)* characterized the i(17q) in more detail, using fluorescence *in situ* hybridization (FISH) with several yeast artificial chomosome (YAC) clones on a series of leukemias, and showed that the i(17q), in most cases, was a dicentric isochromosome (isodicentric), and

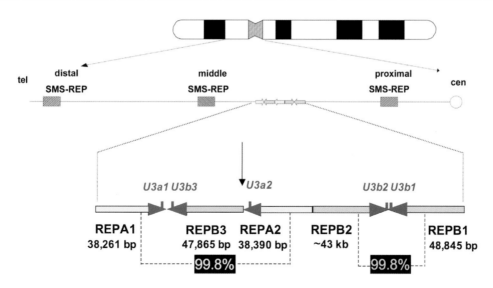

Fig. 1. Schematic representation of the Isochromosome 17q [i(17q)] breakpoint region. At the top, an ideogram of chromosome 17 is depicted. In the middle, the localization of the breakpoint region with respect to the Smith-Magenis syndrome-REPs is shown. Below, the complex genome architecture of the breakpoint is shown with yellow and gray arrows referring to the REPA and REPB copies, respectively. The REPA and REPB copies are arranged according to their suggested orientation and structure. REPB2 is truncated when compared to REPB1 and REPB3 copies. Both REPA copies contain exons 1–3 of the *GRAP* gene, the remaining exons map telomeric to the REPA1 (not shown). This indicates that REPA2 originated from REPA1, the position of the putative evolutionary breakpoint is depicted with a vertical black arrow. Three *U3b* and two *U3a* genes map to the arrowhead portion of REPB and REPA, respectively. The blue arrowheads of REPAs and REPBs represent a nearly identical approx 4-kb sequence shared among both REPAs and REPBs. (Reproduced from ref. *8* with permission.)

not monocentric as suggested by conventional G-banding *(34)*. Consistent with this observation, the breakpoints were shown to cluster within 17p11 implying that the i(17q) formally should be designated idic(17)(p11). Because of its less cumbersome and more descriptive designation, and also for historical reasons, "i(17q)" prevails in the literature. Interestingly, the majority of the 17p11 breakpoints were shown to occur within a 900 kb YAC clone (828b9) located in the Smith-Magenis syndrome (SMS) common deletion region *(34,35)*, suggesting that this germ line genetically unstable region also could be of importance in generating the i(17q) somatic event.

Given the genetically unstable nature of the SMS common deletion region, further efforts were undertaken to delineate the i(17q) breakpoint region in 17p11. FISH mapping using a large set of bacterial artificial chromosome (BAC), P1 artificial chromosome, and fosmid clones covering the breakpoint, together with extensive sequence comparison and the analysis of restriction maps of individual clones, enabled the establishment of a physical map of an approx 240-kb genomic interval including the i(17q) breakpoint cluster region (Fig. 1). This region, localized between the middle and proximal SMS-REPs (Fig. 1), was shown to contain several interesting features. First, two types of distinct LCRs, designated REPA and REPB, present in two and three copies, respectively, were identified within this region. Secondly, their location and orientation with respect to each other strongly suggested that they play an important role in the formation of the i(17q) rearrangement. As outlined in Fig. 1, the two copies of REPA (REPA1 and REPA2) are both approx 38 kb in size, display 99.8% sequence identity, are arrayed inversely with respect to each other, and are separated by another LCR, the approx 48 kb REPB3. The organization of the three REPB copies (REPB1, -2, and -3) is more complex. REPB1 (approx 49 kb) and the truncated REPB2 (approx 43 kb) share 99.8% sequence identity and are inverted with respect to one another (inverted repeats [IRs]). They are separated by an approx 400-bp spacer region and, hence, represent a palindrome or cruciform structure. REPB3 (approx 48 kb) is oriented inversely with respect to REPB2 (99.8% identity). Another interesting feature is the presence of two *U3b* genes (*U3b2* and *U3b1*) that are located in an inverted orientation in the center of this palindromic structure. A similar DNA structure of 8731 bp is present in the junction region between REPA1 and REPB3. The *U3a* or *U3b* genes are located at the head-portion of each REPA and REPB. They display more than 98.5% identity and belong to the *U3* (*RNU3*) evolutionary conserved gene family of small nuclear RNAs required for the processing of pre-18S rRNA *(36,37)*. The very high degree of similarities among the three REPBs and independently among two REPAs indicates that the segmental duplication events that generated these LCRs are of recent origin, as suggested by evolutionary studies of other highly homologous LCRs *(38)*, or alternatively, undergo frequent gene conversion. A final remarkable feature of this region is the high content (approx 30%) of *Alu* repeats. Greater than 80% of the 4 kb flanking the center of the cruciform are repetitive sequences, with 50% consisting of *Alu* sequences. Furthermore, each of the five REPs is flanked by *Alu* sequences. Thus, as recently suggested *(39)*, the high *Alu* repeat content could be important in the genesis of the large segmental duplications present in this region.

The large approx 86-kb long cruciform generated by REPB1 and REPB2 is a genomic architectural feature that potentially could trigger a recombination event resulting in the i(17q)-formation. Indeed, IRs or cruciforms are known to generate hairpins, facilitated by intrastrand pairing of complementary single-strand DNA sequences assembled in the lagging strand during DNA replication *(40,41)*. A double-strand break (DSB) introduced in such a hairpin can result in deletions, or either inter- or intrachromosomal recombination events, mediated by the homologous recombination machinery *(42)*. Critical factors implicated in the rate of such rearrangements are the extent of sequence identity between the inverted repeats, their size, and the length of the spacer (sequences present between the cruciform sequences). The rate of genomic rearrangements rises as the length of the repeat increases and the spacer sequence length decreases *(43)*. The cruciform identified in the i(17q) breakpoint cluster region is characterized by two inverted repeats, approx 48 kb and approx 43 kb in length, separated by a 400-bp spacer. If broken, DNA ends generated in the hairpin/cruciform structures of the i(17q) breakpoint can trigger the DSB-repair (DSBR) machinery. A subsequent nonallelic homologous recombination (NAHR) event between the repeats with opposite orientations located in the two sister chromatids (i.e., sister chromatid exchange) can result in the formation of an isodicentric chromosome 17 and of an acentric fragment (Fig. 2) *(8)*.

Similar to i(17q), breakpoint analyses of constitutional isochromosomes of the long arm of the X chromosome, "i(Xq)," and of the most common constitutional isodicentric chromosomes, i.e., "inv dup(15)" and "inv dup(22)," suggest that these isodicentric abnormalities also may result from NAHR between inverted LCRs *(7)*. As to the role of IRs or cruciform in constitutional genomic rearrangements, such genome architecture features, albeit of smaller size, have been identified at the breakpoints of the most common non-Robertsonian translocation, t(11;22)(q23;q11) *(44,45)* and of the translocation t(17;22)(q11;q11) described in two

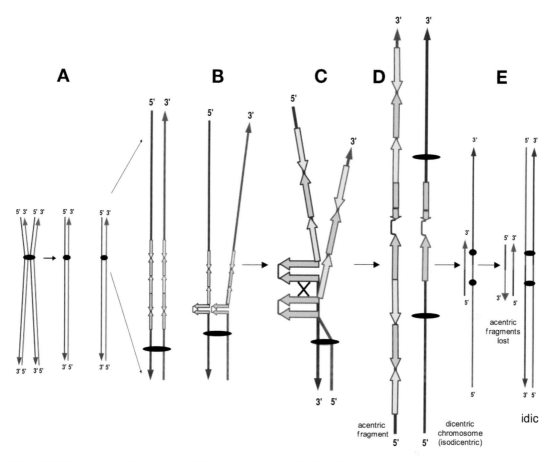

Fig. 2. Molecular mechanism for i(17q)-formation. (A) The division of a metaphase chromosome is shown. The double strand DNA of each chromatid is depicted in red and blue and the orientation with 3' and 5'. (B) The formation of a REPB1 and REPB2 palindrome with (C) subsequent breakage and (D) reunion between palindromes on sister chromatids results in the origin of both dicentric and acentric structures. (E) The dicentric and acentric structures after replication. The acentric material is lost in dividing cells because of the lack of a centromere. The (iso-) dicentric structure (isochromosome) is retained and will not become disrupted during anaphase because one of the two centromeres are inactivated as a result of their close proximity. Yellow and gray arrows refer to REPA and REPB copies, respectively, whereas the X depicts interchromatid mispairing of direct repeats. According to this model, i(17q) should formally be designated idic(17)(p11.2). (Reproduced from ref. 8 with permission.)

patients with neurofibromatosis type 1 (46,47). Moreover, genomic characterization of the AZFc region on chromosome Y, which is deleted in close to 20% of patients with oligo- or azoospermia, revealed a 3-Mb sequence that is deleted via homologous recombination events mediated by two direct repeats, present at the edges of this structure (48).

The breakpoint region of i(17q) resides within the SMS commonly deleted region and is flanked by the middle and proximal SMS-REPs. Furthermore, several other repeat elements have been reported telomeric and centromeric to the i(17q) breakpoint region (49–51). It is unclear why the breakpoints in i(17q) are clustered in the delineated 240-kb region and not in the other closely located repeats, but it could well be that only the complex nature of the breakpoint region allows this chromosomal abnormality to be formed, or, alternatively, that only such rearrangements provide a selective advantage to the neoplastic cells. The i(17q) breakpoint region could, of course, also facilitate erroneous meiotic recombination, but the resulting gross genomic imbalances (i.e., whole arm deletion of 17p and duplications of 17q), are unlikely to be compatible with normal embryonic development.

ARE LCRS COMMON MEDIATORS OF GENOMIC ALTERATIONS IN CANCER?

LCRs have, thus, been shown to be important mediators of rearrangements in constitutional genomic disorders. An important question in this context is whether they also play an equally important role in generating neoplasia-associated genomic changes. Unfortunately, only limited knowledge on this aspect is currently available. It is likely, however, that an increasing awareness of such genome architectural features will yield important insights in the near future.

Indeed, apart from a role in i(17q)-formation, LCRs have been implicated recently also in the generation of one of the most common neoplasia-associated reciprocal chromosomal translocation, the t(9;22)(q34;q11) in CML (9). Not only the vicinity of the breakpoints of this chromosomal abnormality, but also the entire *BCR* and *ABL1* genes have been extensively searched in the past for the presence of repetitive elements or recombinogeneic motifs, that could provide a mechanism for the translocation, but no convincing support for their role in generating this aberration has been forthcoming. In light of this, the finding reported by Saglio et al. (9) is particularly interesting. Studying the *BCR/ABL1* fusion at the mRNA level, they identified a rare case with an insertion of 126 nucleotides at the junction between the two genes (9). This junction fragment was shown to derive from a region 1.4 Mb 5' of *ABL1*. Using a BAC clone covering this region as a probe in FISH experiments, a weak signal was identified distal to the *BCR* gene at 22q11 in addition to the expected signal at 9q34. This finding suggested the existence of significantly homologous sequences in the proximity of both genes involved in the translocation. Sequence comparison finally revealed the presence of a 76-kb duplicated genomic region present on 9q34 and on 22q11, 150 kb 3' of *BCR*. Thus, in contrast to i(17q), where the presence of LCRs coincides with the actual breakpoint, the duplicated genomic region is located outside the *BCR* and *ABL1* breakpoints. This suggests another potential role of LCRs in facilitating mitotic chromosomal exchange: by bringing two genes into proximity of each other, the likelihood for recombination between them would be dramatically increased. Subsequent random breakage and end-joining of the two genes, possibly guided by repetitive elements or sequence motifs in the vicinity of the breakpoints, followed by selection for cells producing in-frame *BCR/ABL1* fusion products, would result in a clonal expansion and clinically manifest leukemia. To date, no systematic study investigating the presence of LCRs in the proximity of genes reported to form fusion genes has been reported, but in light of the t(9;22) example, such analyses may well prove fruitful.

Could LCRs also play a role in mediating other chromosomal abnormalities characterizing human neoplasia? Although far from proven, it has been suggested that the amplification of candidate oncogenes in high-grade ostesarcoma could be LCR-mediated, because the amplification profiles in these tumors coincide with the genomic localization of LCRs in the Charcot-Marie-Tooth disease type 1A and SMS regions (52).

Another question that arises is whether genomic regions known to be deleted, or less frequently duplicated, in constitutional genomic disorders could be rearranged also in neoplastic disorders. Genomic regions known to be meiotically unstable and resulting in the well-known constitutional microdeletion syndromes may be unstable also in cancer cells, not least because of the dysfunctional DNA repair and decreased apoptotic activity characterizing such cells in general. It is important to stress, however, that fundamentally different selection mechanisms are likely to be active in neoplastic cells and congenital microdeletion syndromes. Whereas neoplastic cells will become selected because of growth advantage at the cellular level allowing gross genomic alterations, imbalances in congenital disorders have to be compatible with embryonic development. It cannot be excluded, however, that genes contained within regions lost in microdeletion syndromes, in the haploinsufficient state may confer selective advantage to tumor cells.

Finally, an interesting, but entirely speculative, aspect to address in the future will be if certain LCRs, yet to be detected or already implicated in neoplasia, display copy number and/or structural polymorphisms that could render certain individuals more prone to acquire structural somatic chromosomal changes of importance for tumor development or progression. Most likely, such polymorphisms or "risk alleles" would be of low penetrance, but could nevertheless provide important additional information in a clinical setting.

SUMMARY

It seems clear that LCRs, like in constitutional disorders, may play an important, previously unrecognized, role in mediating chromosomal rearrangements also in neoplasia. However, it is still too early to postulate a more general role for their involvement in cancers. Such conclusions will have to await more systematic studies comparing their genomic localization and organization with that of chromosomal breakpoints in neoplasia. In principle, this should be possible already at this stage for balanced chromosomal translocations, which, to date, have been shown to involve more than 250 genes. High-resolution array-based comparative genomic hybridization methods and improvement of other technologies, allowing genome-wide detection of subtle genomic imbalances in the cancer genome, are likely to yield further insights into commonly lost or gained chromosomal regions. With improved annotations of the human genome, this will facilitate the identification of genome structural features that may be critical mediators of tumor type-specific genomic rearrangements or of genetic changes occurring in several tumor entities. Having identified such features, their isolation and introduction into various experimental systems will be important further steps to undertake in order to validate their suggested involvement in generating neoplasia-associated genetic alterations.

ACKNOWLEDGMENTS

The author would like to thank Bertil Johansson and Felix Mitelman for providing valuable comments to this work, and Aikaterina Barbouti and Pawel Stankiewicz for their critical role in experimentally elucidating the i(17q) breakpoint region. The original work described in this article was supported by grants from the Swedish Cancer Society and the Swedish Children's Cancer Foundation.

REFERENCES

1. Futreal PA, Coin L, Marshall M, et al. A census of human cancer genes. Nat Rev Cancer 2004;4:177–183.
2. Santarosa M, Ashworth A. Haploinsufficiency for tumour suppressor genes: when you don't need to go all the way. Biochim Biophys Acta 2004;1654:105–122.

3. Mitelman F, Johansson B, Mertens F. Mitelman Database of Chromosome Aberrations in Cancer: http://cgap.nci.nih.gov/Chromosomes/Mitelman; 2005.

4. Mitelman F, Johansson B, Mertens F. Fusion genes and rearranged genes as a linear function of chromosome aberrations in cancer. Nat Genet 2004;36:331–334.

5. Rabbitts TH. Chromosomal translocations in human cancer. Nature 1994;372:143–149.

6. Hahn WC, Weinberg RA. Modelling the molecular circuitry of cancer. Nat Rev Cancer 2002;2:331–341.

7. Stankiewicz P, Lupski JR. Genome architecture, rearrangements and genomic disorders. Trends Genet 2002;18:74–82.

8. Barbouti A, Stankiewicz P, Nusbaum C, et al. The breakpoint region of the most common isochromosome, i(17q), in human neoplasia is characterized by a complex genomic architecture with large, palindromic, low-copy repeats. Am J Hum Genet 2004;74:1–10.

9. Saglio G, Storlazzi CT, Giugliano E, et al. A 76-kb duplicon maps close to the BCR gene on chromosome 22 and the ABL gene on chromosome 9: possible involvement in the genesis of the Philadelphia chromosome translocation. Proc Natl Acad Sci USA 2002;99:9882–9887.

10. Heim S, Mitelman F. *Cancer Cytogenetics.* Second ed. New York NY: Wiley-Liss, 1995.

11. Helman LJ, Meltzer P. Mechanisms of sarcoma development. Nat Rev Cancer 2003;3:685–694.

12. Albertson DG, Collins C, McCormick F, Gray JW. Chromosome aberrations in solid tumors. Nat Genet 2003;34:369–376.

13. Rowley JD. Chromosome translocations: dangerous liaisons revisited. Nat Rev Cancer 2001;1:245–250.

14. Look AT. Oncogenic transcription factors in the human acute leukemias. Science 1997;278:1059–1064.

15. ar-Rushdi A, Nishikura K, Erikson J, Watt R, Rovera G, Croce CM. Differential expression of the translocated and the untranslocated c-myc oncogene in Burkitt lymphoma. Science 1983;222:390–393.

16. Taub R, Kirsch I, Morton C, et al. Translocation of the c-myc gene into the immunoglobulin heavy chain locus in human Burkitt lymphoma and murine plasmacytoma cells. Proc Natl Acad Sci USA 1982;79:7837–7841.

17. Hecht JL, Aster JC. Molecular biology of Burkitt's lymphoma. J Clin Oncol 2000;18:3707–3721.

18. Raghavan SC, Swanson PC, Wu X, Hsieh CL, Lieber MR. A non-B-DNA structure at the Bcl-2 major breakpoint region is cleaved by the RAG complex. Nature 2004;428:88–93.

19. Kolomietz E, Meyn MS, Pandita A, Squire JA. The role of Alu repeat clusters as mediators of recurrent chromosomal aberrations in tumors. Genes Chromosomes Cancer 2002;35:97–112.

20. Abeysinghe SS, Chuzhanova N, Krawczak M, Ball EV, Cooper DN. Translocation and gross deletion breakpoints in human inherited disease and cancer I: nucleotide composition and recombination-associated motifs. Hum Mutat 2003;22:229–244.

21. Greaves MF, Wiemels J. Origins of chromosome translocations in childhood leukaemia. Nat Rev Cancer 2003;3:639–649.

22. Daser A, Rabbitts TH. Extending the repertoire of the mixed-lineage leukemia gene MLL in leukemogenesis. Genes Dev 2004;18:965–974.

23. Felix CA. Leukemias related to treatment with DNA topoisomerase II inhibitors. Med Pediatr Oncol 2001;36:525–535.

24. Aplan PD, Chervinsky DS, Stanulla M, Burhans WC. Site-specific DNA cleavage within the MLL breakpoint cluster region induced by topoisomerase II inhibitors. Blood 1996;87:2649–2658.

25. Felix CA, Hosler MR, Winick NJ, Masterson M, Wilson AE, Lange BJ. ALL-1 gene rearrangements in DNA topoisomerase II inhibitor-related leukemia in children. Blood 1995;85:3250–3256.

26. Strissel PL, Strick R, Tomek RJ, Roe BA, Rowley JD, Zeleznik-Le NJ. DNA structural properties of AF9 are similar to MLL and could act as recombination hot spots resulting in MLL/AF9 translocations and leukemogenesis. Hum Mol Genet 2000;9:1671–1679.

27. Betti CJ, Villalobos MJ, Diaz MO, Vaughan AT. Apoptotic triggers initiate translocations within the MLL gene involving the nonhomologous end joining repair system. Cancer Res 2001;61:4550–4555.

28. Zucman-Rossi J, Legoix P, Victor JM, Lopez B, Thomas G. Chromosome translocation based on illegitimate recombination in human tumors. Proc Natl Acad Sci USA 1998;95:11,786–11,791.

29. Neves H, Ramos C, da Silva MG, Parreira A, Parreira L. The nuclear topography of ABL, BCR, PML, and RARalpha genes: evidence for gene proximity in specific phases of the cell cycle and stages of hematopoietic differentiation. Blood 1999;93:1197–1207.

30. Kozubek S, Lukasova E, Mareckova A, et al. The topological organization of chromosomes 9 and 22 in cell nuclei has a determinative role in the induction of t(9,22) translocations and in the pathogenesis of t(9,22) leukemias. Chromosoma 1999;108:426–435.

31. Roix JJ, McQueen PG, Munson PJ, Parada LA, Misteli T. Spatial proximity of translocation-prone gene loci in human lymphomas. Nat Genet 2003;34:287–291.
32. Mertens F, Johansson B, Mitelman F. Isochromosomes in neoplasia. Genes Chromosomes Cancer 1994;10: 221–230.
33. Biegel JA, Rorke LB, Janss AJ, Sutton LN, Parmiter AH. Isochromosome 17q demonstrated by interphase fluorescence in situ hybridization in primitive neuroectodermal tumors of the central nervous system. Genes Chromosomes Cancer 1995;14:85–96.
34. Fioretos T, Strömbeck B, Sandberg T, et al. Isochromosome 17q in blast crisis of chronic myeloid leukemia and in other hematologic malignancies is the result of clustered breakpoints in 17p11 and is not associated with coding TP53 mutations. Blood 1999;94:225–232.
35. Chen KS, Manian P, Koeuth T, et al. Homologous recombination of a flanking repeat gene cluster is a mechanism for a common contiguous gene deletion syndrome. Nat Genet 1997;17:154–163.
36. Gao L, Frey MR, Matera AG. Human genes encoding U3 snRNA associate with coiled bodies in interphase cells and are clustered on chromosome 17p11.2 in a complex inverted repeat structure. Nucleic Acids Res 1997;25:4740–4747.
37. Dragon F, Gallagher JE, Compagnone-Post PA, et al. A large nucleolar U3 ribonucleoprotein required for 18S ribosomal RNA biogenesis. Nature 2002;417:967–970.
38. Bailey JA, Gu Z, Clark RA, et al. Recent segmental duplications in the human genome. Science 2002;297: 1003–1007.
39. Bailey JA, Liu G, Eichler EE. An Alu transposition model for the origin and expansion of human segmental duplications. Am J Hum Genet 2003;73:823–834.
40. Mizuuchi K, Mizuuchi M, Gellert M. Cruciform structures in palindromic DNA are favored by DNA supercoiling. J Mol Biol 1982;156:229–243.
41. Nasar F, Jankowski C, Nag DK. Long palindromic sequences induce double-strand breaks during meiosis in yeast. Mol Cell Biol 2000;20:3449–3458.
42. Akgun E, Zahn J, Baumes S, et al. Palindrome resolution and recombination in the mammalian germ line. Mol Cell Biol 1997;17:5559–5570.
43. Lobachev KS, Shor BM, Tran HT, et al. Factors affecting inverted repeat stimulation of recombination and deletion in Saccharomyces cerevisiae. Genetics 1998;148:1507–1524.
44. Edelmann L, Spiteri E, Koren K, et al. AT-rich palindromes mediate the constitutional t(11;22) translocation. Am J Hum Genet 2001;68:1–13.
45. Kurahashi H, Emanuel BS. Long AT-rich palindromes and the constitutional t(11;22) breakpoint. Hum Mol Genet 2001;10:2605–2617.
46. Kehrer-Sawatzki H, Haussler J, Krone W, et al. The second case of a t(17;22) in a family with neurofibromatosis type 1: sequence analysis of the breakpoint regions. Hum Genet 1997;99:237–247.
47. Kurahashi H, Shaikh T, Takata M, Toda T, Emanuel BS. The constitutional t(17;22): another translocation mediated by palindromic AT-rich repeats. Am J Hum Genet 2003;72:733–738.
48. Kuroda-Kawaguchi T, Skaletsky H, Brown LG, et al. The AZFc region of the Y chromosome features massive palindromes and uniform recurrent deletions in infertile men. Nat Genet 2001;29:279–286.
49. Park SS, Stankiewicz P, Bi W, et al. Structure and evolution of the Smith-Magenis syndrome repeat gene clusters, SMS-REPs. Genome Res 2002;12:729–738.
50. Stankiewicz P, Shaw CJ, Dapper JD, et al. Genome architecture catalyzes nonrecurrent chromosomal rearrangements. Am J Hum Genet 2003;72:1101–1116.
51. Stankiewicz P, Shaw CJ, Withers M, Inoue K, Lupski JR. Serial segmental duplications during primate evolution result in complex human genome architecture. Genome Res 2004;14:2209–2220.
52. van Dartel M, Hulsebos TJ. Amplification and overexpression of genes in 17p11.2 ~ p12 in osteosarcoma. Cancer Genet Cytogenet 2004;153:77–80.

V FUNCTIONAL ASPECTS OF GENOME STRUCTURE

24

Recombination Hotspots in Nonallelic Homologous Recombination

Matthew E. Hurles, PhD
and James R. Lupski, MD, PhD

INTRODUCTION

Rearrangement breakpoints resulting from nonallelic homologous recombination (NAHR) are typically clustered within small, well-defined portions of the segmental duplications that promote the rearrangement. These NAHR "hotspots" have been identified in every NAHR-promoted rearrangement in which breakpoint junctions have been sequenced in sufficient numbers. Enhancement of recombinatorial activity in NAHR hotspots varies from 3 to 237 times more than in the surrounding "cold" duplicated sequence. NAHR hotspots share many features in common with allelic homologous recombination (AHR) hotspots. Both AHR and NAHR hotspots appear to be relatively small (<2 kb) and are initiated by double-strand breaks. Gene conversion events as well as crossovers are enhanced at NAHR hotspots. Recent work has improved our understanding of the origins of NAHR and AHR hotspots, with both appearing to be relatively short-lived phenomena. Our present understanding of NAHR hotspots comes from a limited number of locus-specific studies. In the future, we can expect genome-wide analyses to provide many further insights.

During meiosis, AHR occurs between homologous chromosomes, generating haplotypic diversity in the succeeding generation. The distribution of these recombination events throughout the genome has been known to be nonrandom for decades, but in the past 5 years ever-finer spatial resolutions have revealed dramatic heterogeneity in AHR rates at the DNA sequence level. These studies have demonstrated the existence of recombination hotspots, where AHR

From: *Genomic Disorders: The Genomic Basis of Disease*
Edited by: J. R. Lupski and P. Stankiewicz © Humana Press, Totowa, NJ

rates can be several orders of magnitude more than in surrounding "cold" regions. In parallel to these developments, sufficient numbers of breakpoints of selected NAHR rearrangements have been characterized at the DNA sequence level to resolve the distribution of crossovers in these cases. This has similarly led to the identification of NAHR hotspots within paralogous sequences. This chapter profiles AHR and NAHR hotspots and discusses their similarities with a view to understanding the molecular mechanisms underpinning pathogenic NAHR.

It is necessary to be clear when defining what constitutes a recombination hotspot. In the most general sense, a hotspot is a region of elevated activity relative to its surroundings. However, activity in the "surroundings" can be quantified in a number of ways. We consider a recombination hotspot to be an interval of DNA, defined at the sequence level, which manifests elevated recombinatorial activity relative to its immediate flanking sequences. In principle, a recombination hotspot could alternatively be defined as exhibiting elevated recombinatorial activity relative to the genome average. It is worth noting that the DNA1 hotspot identified experimentally in the major histocompatibility complex (MHC) region (1) using the former criterion actually exhibits lower recombinatorial activity than the genome average. Likewise, crossover in the NAHR hotspot in the Charcot-Marie-Tooth disease type 1A (CMT1A)-REP (2) does not appear to be significantly more frequent than the average genome-wide recombination rate and has been referred to as a positional specificity for strand exchange (3). Nonetheless, studies of both regions revealed that not all homologous sequences are equal and a "punctate" pattern of crossovers is revealed for both AHR and NAHR.

In addition, homologous recombination is a process that can result in one of two outcomes: a crossover event or a gene conversion. Consequently, we consider that a recombination hotspot may become apparent because of elevated levels of either outcome.

The Importance of Recombination Hotspots

There are a handful of pathogenic mutation processes that operate in the human genome (e.g., base substitution, replication slippage, NAHR). For some of these mutational mechanisms we have a good understanding of the rates and locations at which these mutations arise (e.g., base substitution and replication slippage), whereas for NAHR we do not. Examining the distribution of recombination events at the sequence level is perhaps one of the most important clues we can have for understanding the basis of pathogenic NAHR. In a more general sense, the fine-mapping of all homologous recombination (HR) processes can only help our admittedly basic comprehension of what is a fundamental cellular process.

In recent years there has been a growing desire to be able to use patterns of linkage disequilibrium (LD) throughout the genome to design more efficient association studies for the detection of genes predisposing to complex diseases (4). These patterns of LD have been investigated at high resolution at several sites within the genome and a common finding is that the physical distance over which LD persists in the genome is highly variable (5). This variability leads to a "block-like" haplotypic structure in which regions of high LD are separated by shorter sequences across which LD is minimal (6). One of the main causal mechanisms by which this block-like structure might arise is the existence of extreme AHR rate heterogeneity. The idea being that recombination rates are low or absent within haplotype blocks but that hotspots of recombinatorial activity map between blocks. Other possible causal mechanisms of these haplotypic structures exist, however these alternative processes are dependent on population-specific demographic factors. Given the immense effort it is taking to map haplotypic structures in four human populations in the HapMap project (7), it is important to know to what degree it is possible to predict haplotypic structures in other populations from the data on these four. If the distribution of LD is determined mainly by population demography then haplotype structures are likely to differ markedly between populations. If, however, recombination hotspots, a molecular rather then population-based process, accounts for patterns of LD and these hotspots are shared between populations, then haplotype structures are much more likely to be shared between populations.

In addition, accurate estimates of recombination rates are required when drawing evolutionary inferences from autosomal variation, for example, the estimation of the very recent age of the HIV-resistant CCR5-Δ32 mutation *(8)*. The apparent recent origin of this variant has lead to further work examining the possible role of the CCR5-Δ32 mutation in conferring resistance to recent plagues within the past 1000 years *(9,10)*. This dating estimation is almost entirely predicated on an assumption of recombination rate homogeneity across a 46-Mb portion of chromosome 3.

IDENTIFICATION OF RECOMBINATION HOTSPOTS

The most obvious means to examine recombination rate heterogeneity is to identify a sufficient number of individual recombination events within a set of defined physical intervals, such that the frequency of recombination in one interval can be compared with that in another. This can be achieved at a variety of different spatial resolutions. Despite this conceptual similarity, the methods used to identify AHR and NAHR hotspots have traditionally been very different.

Finding NAHR Hotspots

NAHR events are generally ascertained as a result of their deleterious phenotypic outcomes; usually conveyed by gene dosage effects secondary to DNA rearrangements (e.g., deletion or duplication). In this sense they are similar to phenotype-based screens in model organisms. *De novo* NAHR events are subsequently identified by comparing the genomes of patients and their parents. A collection of *de novo* NAHR events can then be fine-mapped to identify and ultimately sequence the rearrangement breakpoints. Not all recurrent rearrangements result from NAHR *(11)* and so the preliminary identification of similar sized rearrangements must be followed by the mapping of breakpoints to blocks of duplicated sequence.

Most NAHR breakpoints have been mapped to a pair of duplicated sequences (also referred to as low-copy repeats, segmental duplications, or duplicons), but not to a specific interval within these duplicated sequences. There are two major complicating factors that hinder the fine-mapping of NAHR breakpoints within duplicated sequences: the presence of the duplicated sequences in multiple copies, and the complex sequence variation within duplicated sequences.

Somatic cell hybrids that retain only the rearranged copy of a chromosome and not its unrearranged homolog have been found to be extremely useful in disentangling the signals from the multiple copies of the duplicated sequences that have driven the NAHR events. Reducing the copy number of the sequences flanking the breakpoint interval enables the isolation of a junction-specific breakpoint that can be subsequently sequenced.

The complex pattern of sequence variation within duplicated sequences means that variants apparent within the reference sequence that distinguish between proximal and distal copies of a duplicated sequence (known as *cis*-morphisms or paralogous sequence variants [PSVs]) may exhibit multi-site variation *(12)*. In other words, rather than being diagnostic of the proximal copy of a duplicated sequence a variant may be absent from either copy, present in both copies or even present only in the distal copy. Sequencing parental chromosomes to characterize sequence variation in the duplicated sequences prior to NAHR can be critical to defining the precise interval between two PSVs between which the breakpoint must map.

Finding AHR Hotspots

In contrast to NAHR, AHR events are generally ascertained through their generation of recombinant haplotypes rather than any phenotypic effects. Initially, recombinant haplotypes were identified though the pedigree analysis of haplotypes of sparsely distributed markers. Unfortunately, the relatively low frequency of recombination events across the genome as a whole (approx 50 crossovers per male meiosis) means that to obtain accurate estimates over even relatively large physical distances requires large numbers of meioses. It is not feasible to type the number of meioses required to get accurate estimates of recombination frequency for the shorter distances (tens of kilobases) over which the patterns of LD described above are observed *(13)*.

In recent years, researchers have taken advantage of the fact that the 50 million sperm in every milliliter of semen each represent an independent product of meiosis to characterize male AHR at much finer resolution. By amplifying recombinant-specific haplotypes by PCR from pools of accurately quantified numbers of sperm it has become possible to estimate recombination frequencies over intervals of hundreds of bases (*see* Fig. 1) *(14)*. However, the painstaking optimization required to achieve the levels of sensitivity necessary to detect single recombinant haplotypes (spanning <10 kb) against a background of thousands of nonrecombinant haplotypes renders it difficult to expand the initial locus-specific studies of recombination rate heterogeneity across the whole genome.

More recently, a new class of statistical methods have been devised that can infer recombination rate heterogeneity from the patterns of sequence variation within a population *(15,16)*. Rather than collect individual recombination events this approach relies on being able to detect the cumulative impact of recombination on haplotypic structures. Having been verified against known, experimentally determined hotspots, these methods provide the prospect of being able to scan across the entire genome using datasets of haplotype diversity that are already being generated in the HapMap project.

FEATURES OF AHR AND NAHR HOTSPOTS

Known NAHR Hotspots

Only for a minority of genomic disorders have the breakpoints of the disease-causing rearrangements been mapped to specific intervals within duplicated sequences. However, for every case in which sufficient numbers of breakpoints have been precisely mapped, substantial NAHR rate heterogeneity within the duplicated sequence is observed. Table 1 documents the known NAHR hotspots. It can be seen that the list of rearrangements is only a small subset of the comprehensive list of genomic disorders given elsewhere in this book.

Known AHR Hotspots

The number of experimentally determined AHR hotspots is similarly limited and are highly nonrandomly distributed throughout the genome. Some were initially identified at low resolution in pedigree analysis of a few well-characterized loci (e.g., β-globin, the MHC and the pseudo-

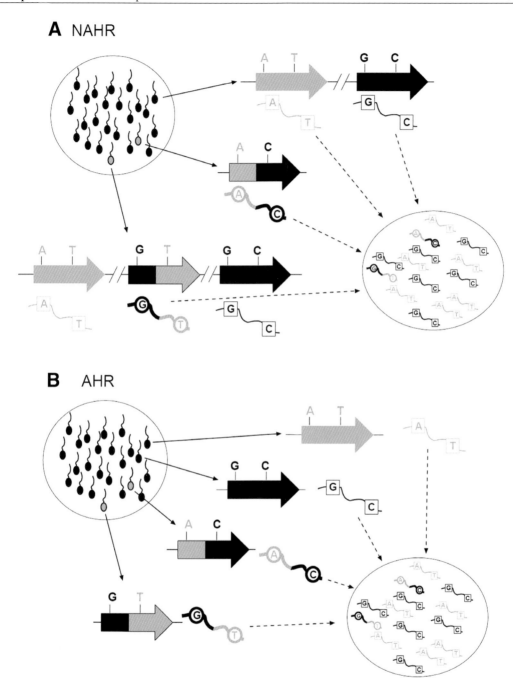

Fig. 1. Rare recombination events in spermatogenesis generate a low frequency of recombinant haplotypes. Rare sperm in which selected allelic homologous recombination (AHR) or nonallelic homologous recombination (NAHR) events have occurred are shown in gray. Gray/black arrows indicate homologous sequences. Variants that differ between the homologous sequences are shown above the arrow. Novel haplotypes diagnostic of different reciprocal recombination events are show for (A) NAHR: deletion and duplication and (B) AHR. The problem of identifying recombination (AHR or NAHR) events in sperm can, therefore, be reduced to one of identifying recombinant haplotypes in sperm DNA against a high background of nonrecombinant haplotypes.

Table 1
Known NAHR Hotspots

Disease	Chr.	Repeats	Hotspot	Maximum size of hotspot	Size of contiguous homology block	Factor of enhancement[a]	Refs.
Azoospermia (AZFa)	Y	HERV15	ID1	1.3 kb	10 kb	5X	47–50
Azoospermia (AZFa)	Y	HERV15	ID2	1.7 kb	10 kb	3X	47–50
Azoospermia	Y	Distal P1/P5	—	933 bp	92 kb	66X	51
NF1	17	NF1-REPs	—	2 kb	85 kb	20X	52
HNPP	17	CMT1A-REPs	—	557 bp	24 kb	31X	53
CMT1A	17	CMT1A-REPs	—	741 bp	24 kb	18X	20
SMS	17	SMS-REPs	Block A hotspot	1.1 kb	170 kb	29X	54
SMS	17	SMS-REPs	Block C hotspot	1.6 kb	170 kb	26X	54
SMS	17	LCR17pA and LCR17pD	—	524 bp	124 kb	237X	55
Williams-Beuren syndrome (WBS)	7	WBS-LCRs Bc/Bm	Block B hotspot on normal (not inverted) background	3.4 kb	143 kb	9–18X	56

a The factor of enhancement (F) is calculated according to the equation below, which takes into account the size of the hotspot (H), the size of the contiguous duplicated block of appreciable homology (R), and the proportion of breakpoints found within the hotspot (q); $F = Rq/H$.

HERV, human endogenous retrovirus; NF1, neurofibromatosis 1; HNPP, hereditary neuropathy with liability to pressure palsies; CMT1A, Charcot-Marie-Tooth disease type 1A; SMS, Smith-Magenis syndrome; LCR, low-copy repeat; Chr., chromosome.

autosomal region) or from patterns of LD (e.g., the MHC) and were subsequently fine-mapped in males using sperm typing methods. Other AHR hotspots were identified in sequences flanking minisatellites during studies of minisatellite mutation dynamics in sperm (reviewed by ref. *17*).

Properties of AHR and NAHR Hotspots

Despite the relative paucity of well-characterized AHR and NAHR hotspots, a number of shared features of both types of hotspots have been observed *(18)*. Three characteristics shared by both NAHR and AHR hotspots are: (1) they occupy clearly delimited short intervals less than 2 kb in size; (2) there are no obvious sequence similarities either within each class of hotspot or between them; and (3) they appear to be coincident with gene conversion events.

In addition to the absence of sequence conservation between hotspots of both HR classes, there is no apparent shared sequence context (e.g., GC content, CpG dinucleotide frequency, poly[A]/poly[T] fraction, dispersed repeats or the presence of [AC]$_n$ repeats) that is consistently associated with the presence of hotspots. It may be that recombination hotspots have more similar properties in higher levels of chromatin organization (e.g., chromatin conformation, epigenetic marks, histone modification, intranuclear organization) than they do in pri-

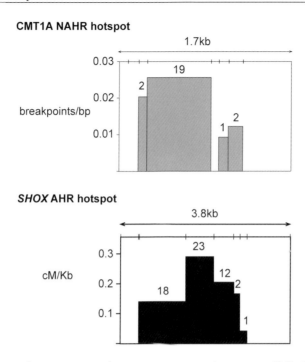

Fig. 2. Crossover frequencies across two sites, one encompassing an nonallelic homologous recombination (NAHR) and the other an allelic homologous recombination (AHR) hotspot. The number of crossover events observed in neighbouring intervals of homologous sequences separated by single nucleotide polymorphisms (AHR) or paralogous sequence variants (NAHR) demonstrate the existence of tightly confined hotspots for both AHR and NAHR. The CMT1A-REP data come from ref. *20* and the *SHOX* data come from ref. *46*. The number above each column indicates the number of individual events detected.

mary sequence. Alternatively, a non-B DNA conformation may initiate breaks that stimulate recombinatorial activity. Most of the NAHR hotspots listed in Table 1 are associated with longer stretches of identity between the paralogous sequences in which they reside. This is not surprising given the known dependence of HR rate on levels of sequence similarity and the presence of much greater variation in sequence identity between paralogous sequences than between allelic sequences in the human genome. This has lead to the idea that gene conversion between paralogous sequences could potentiate subsequent rearrangements as a result of generating greater similarity between the paralogs (homogenization). Such gene conversion events could be considered "premutations" for genomic disorders, analogous to those apparent for triplet repeat disorders.

The morphology of AHR hotspots is better characterized than for NAHR hotspots and it appears that for AHR hotspots a central peak in activity is surrounded by symmetrical tails (*see* Fig. 2). This commonality among AHR hotspots has lead to suggestions that they reflect underlying similarities between hotspots in the initiation and processing of recombination events *(19)*.

The intensity of recombination hotspots can be measured in a variety of different ways. Intensity can be considered to be relative, for example the enhancement in activity in hotspots over flanking cold regions, or absolute intensities, for example recombination rate per meiosis. It has been estimated that the *SHOX* AHR hotspot in the pseudo-autosomal region has a recombination rate of 3/1000 meioses, which is considerably lower than the intensity of some of the most intense hotspots in yeast (10–100/1000 meioses) *(19)*. We can use the incidence of autosomal dominant genomic disorders that result from NAHR to estimate an absolute intensity of their associated NAHR hotspots. Mutations in the 741-bp CMT1A-REP hotspot are found in 56% of all CMT1A duplications, which occur at a *de novo* rate of approx 1/2500 meioses, indicating an absolute intensity of 0.22/1000 meioses *(20)*.

Limited evidence on sex-specific AHR and NAHR rates suggest that there are sex-dependent differences in NAHR hotspot intensities that mirror the well-studied sex-specific differences in the chromosome-wide distribution and frequency of AHR. For example, *de novo* CMT1A duplications occur preferentially in the paternal germline *(21)*, whereas the *TAP2* AHR hotspot appears to be much more active in the female germline *(22)*.

Further complexities in the variability of NAHR hotspot activity are suggested by the finding that the preferential location of breakpoints of neurofibromatosis 1 deletions are different in meiotic and mitotic events *(23)*, and that the intensity of the CMT1A-REP hotspot varies among individuals *(3)*. Disentangling the various factors that underlie quantitative differences in NAHR and AHR hotspot intensity between individuals, between hotspots, and between haplotypes should lead to improved understanding of the mechanistic basis underlying recombination rate heterogeneity.

MECHANISTIC BASIS OF RECOMBINATION HOTSPOTS

Our understanding of the mechanistic basis of homologous recombination in mammals has been driven primarily by the correlation of theoretical models with the roles played by homologs of the well-characterized proteins involved in recombination processes in yeast and bacteria. However, HR is involved in a multiplicity of tightly regulated processes in both soma and germline. In addition, it appears likely that HR can proceed via a number of related, but distinct, pathways. Therefore, it is reasonable to suspect that different subsets of HR proteins are recruited during these different processes. Despite these caveats, we can characterize HR as a process initiated by a double-strand break (DSB), which is subsequently processed to facilitate a homology search, which results in the formation of an intermediate comprising at least one Holliday junction that is then resolved to generate either a crossover or a gene conversion event *(24)*. In principle, a recombination hotspot could result from biases at any one of these stages (i.e., initiation, processing, and resolution) that favor a resulting crossover.

The Machinery of HR

Meiotic recombination hotspots in yeast result primarily from a biased distribution of DSBs introduced by the protein Spo11 *(25)*. Targeting Spo11 in a sequence-specific manner by fusing it with a DNA-binding domain is sufficient to generate a recombination hotspot in a previously cold region *(26)*. Furthermore, it has been shown that a pre-existing hotspot can be repressed by changes in chromatin structure *(27)*. In yeast, as in other eukaryotes, homologs of the bacterial RecA protein catalyze the invasion of the processed DSB into homologous sequences. Components of the mismatch repair machinery are involved in the assessment of the degree of homology. The ratio of gene conversion to crossover at a hotspot has been found to differ both between mitosis and meiosis, and between different hotspots in the same genome. Moreover, it has been argued that there may be different classes of hotspot in yeast *(28)*.

What relevance do these findings have for mammalian HR? There is recent evidence that DSBs form preferentially in hotspot regions in mice *(29)*, but otherwise it remains to be proven that mammalian HR hotspots also result from preferential initiation by DSBs. Evidence from sperm-typing *(30)* and population genetic studies suggest that the majority of recombination intermediates at meiotic AHR hotspots are resolved as gene conversions rather than as crossovers, but there is also evidence of variation in the gene conversion/crossover ratio between hotspots *(30)*. This suggests that hotspot activity is not solely determined by initiation, but also by subsequent events in HR.

The sequential recruitment of different proteins to sites of HR during mammalian meiotic recombination has been mapped cytogenetically *(31)*. This mapping has shown that the number of initial sites of DNA–DNA interactions as revealed by foci of RecA homologs seems to be 10-fold larger than the number of eventual crossover events. Only the minority of sites that recruit the mismatch repair protein MLH1 are thought to undergo crossovers. The majority of sites that do not appear to be associated with crossovers recruit a different mismatch repair protein, MSH4. Perhaps this excess of MSH4-recruiting sites reflects the ratio of gene conversion to crossover events observed in the sperm-typing study.

Evidence From Additional Observations

Additional observations from diverse sources provide further insights into the nature of HR hotspots. In mice it has been demonstrated that AHR hotspot activity declines as sequence similarity lessens *(32)*. This mirrors the enrichment of NAHR hotspots in the more similar portions of paralogous sequences. Clearly, some kind of sequence similarity threshold is necessary, but not sufficient for hotspot activity, although this threshold is poorly understood at present. The situation in NAHR may be complicated by the competition between nonallelic and allelic homologs to a DSB arising within a sequence that is duplicated elsewhere in the genome. Competition between these alternate substrates may determine the ratio of AHR to NAHR and could reflect such factors as the sequence similarity, orientation, and spatial separation between potential substrates in the meiotic nucleus.

Could it be that an NAHR hotspot merely reflects an AHR hotspot within a paralogous sequence, which its paralog is of similar sequence identity to the allelic homolog? In this regard the NAHR hotspots residing in the male-specific portion of the Y (MSY) chromosome are particularly interesting given that this region of the genome is constitutively haploid. Paralogous sequences in the MSY that contain these hotspots lack an allelic pairing partner during meiosis. Consequently, these sequences do not undergo AHR, although some of them are known to undergo frequent paralogous gene conversion *(33)*.

EVOLUTIONARY ORIGINS OF HOTSPOTS

The evolution of recombination hotspots both within humans and between humans and higher primates has been studied only minimally. The evolutionary origins of recombination hotspots is closely related both to the underlying mechanisms of HR, and also to the factors that modulate HR rates. We argue that if we were to have a better understanding of the origins of hotspots, we would also more fully understand their underlying mechanism.

In humans, there is conflicting evidence on the issue of whether recombination hotspots are shared between populations. The CMT1A NAHR hotspot appears to be conserved between populations *(34,35)*, as do the AHR hotspots in the class II region of the MHC *(36)*, whereas a study identifying AHR hotspots from large-scale population genetic data finds support for the existence of population-specific hotspots *(15)*. Looking deeper into evolutionary history, it appears that the *TAP2* AHR hotspot at least, is not conserved in chimpanzees *(37)*.

DSB models for HR suggests that hotspots should be ephemeral phenomena *(38)*. A sequence variant that acts as preferential site for the initiation of HR through the generation of a DSB is likely to be preferentially removed during HR as the initiating strand is gene converted to the state of the less active variant on the homologous sequence. This bias would reduce the frequency of the recombinogenic variant in the population in a process known as "meiotic drive" (a biased inheritance of alleles). This prediction of meiotic drive has been verified experimentally in both human and mouse AHR hotspots *(32,39)*.

This leads to the obvious question, if recombinogenic variants are doomed to extinction, how do recombination hotspots arise in the first place? One suggestion is that the number of potential recombination hotspots is more than the number of active hotspots, and that the focusing of activity on a single location allows the other "cryptic" hotspots to evolve neutrally. Once an active hotspot wanes, a nearby cryptic hotspot could become active. This suggests a dynamic relationship between frequency and activity of recombinogenic variants and recombination hotspot location. An intriguing situation that may have a bearing on this relationship is the finding that alternate hotspots exist in the mouse MHC depending on the haplotypes that are recombining *(32)*. Additional insights into the transient nature of recombination hotspots comes from the observations of large inter-individual variation in the intensity of specific AHR hotspots *(39,40)* that is associated with single base changes in and around the hotspots. It has yet to be demonstrated that inter-individual variation in NAHR hotspot activity can be ascribed to single base changes in the locality of the hotspot.

Comparative Studies: Evolutionary Origins of NAHR Hotspots

The likely dependence of NAHR rates on levels of sequence similarity between paralogs suggests that monitoring the evolution of this similarity may inform our understanding of the time-depth of NAHR hotspots. One recent study of NAHR between paralogous human endogenous retrovirus (HERV) proviral sequences, flanking the Y-chromosome *Azoospermia Factor a (AZFa)* locus that when deleted causes male infertility, provided evidence for several hominid-specific gene conversion events that may have rendered the associated hotspots better substrates for chromosomal rearrangements in humans than in either chimpanzees or gorillas *(41)*. Gene conversion generates signatures of concerted evolution in alignments of comparative sequences (*see* Fig. 3) and in the *AZFa*-HERVs these signatures are coincident with the location of the NAHR hotspots. If we continue the "premutation" analogy, homogenizing permutations have occurred on the hominid lineage and become fixed in an ancestral species to modern humans. However, because gene conversion and chromosomal rearrangement reflect the alternative products of a common intermediate, it may be that a recombinogenic sequence motif/structure underpins the association and the increased sequence identity resulting from gene conversion plays only a minor role in determining the frequency of chromosomal rearrangement. Nevertheless, the coincidence of signatures of concerted evolution and recurrent breakpoints of chromosomal rearrangements (mapped at the DNA sequence level) may enable the identification of putative rearrangement hotspots from analysis of comparative sequences from great apes.

Why Do Recombination Hotspots Exist?

Our lack of understanding of recombination rate heterogeneity in the human genome is emphasised by our ignorance as to why recombination hotspots exist in the first place. Recombination rate heterogeneity seems to be a general feature of sexually reproducing eukaryotic

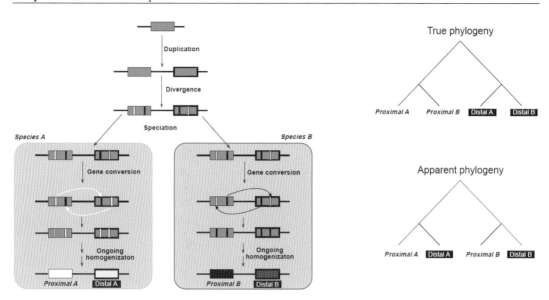

Fig. 3. The effect of concerted evolution on phylogeny. Independent gene conversion events between paralogous sequences in two sequences lead to the sequences being homogenized within a species. As a consequence, phylogenies constructed from these sequences exhibit a different topology from that expected given the sequence of duplication and speciation events. This phylogenetic pattern can be used to detect regions of the genome undergoing "concerted evolution." The "true phylogeny" shows the actual evolutionary relationships among the four sequence as a result of duplication preceding speciation. The "apparent phylogeny" is the phylogeny that would be reconstructed from an alignment of the four sequences after undergoing concerted evolution.

species. Are AHR hotspots themselves of benefit to such organisms or are they a by-product of the need to regulate recombination events to ensure correct segregation of chromosomes? There are a number of plausible evolutionary scenarios that explain why hotspots themselves might be beneficial. For example: AHR hotspots might ensure that advantageous linkage groups are maintained together, or they might facilitate the operation of selection by ensuring that selective pressures operate independently at two loci under selection on either side of a hotspot *(42)*. It is less easy to find reasons to explain why NAHR hotspots might exist, other than the fact that they are related mechanistically to AHR hotspots.

One intriguing prospect is that if NAHR and AHR hotspots are linked by a common mechanism, then the two processes are likely to co-evolve. Given the often pathogenic nature of NAHR, it could be that the machinery of AHR evolved to minimize NAHR. This certainly seems possible. Although individual pathogenic NAHR-promoted rearrangements are so rare that locus-specific selective pressures are likely to be too weak to affect evolutionary change, cumulatively these rearrangements may well assert an appreciable selective pressure. Is there any evidence that AHR has evolved to minimize NAHR? In a hypothetical 3-Gb genome comprised of only single copy sequences, the minimal length of sequence identity between recombining partners required to ensure that HR occurs between allelic sequences needs only be approx 20-bp long (frequency of random reoccurrence of a 20mer is 4^{20}, which is much more than 3 Gb). This length is at least an order of magnitude shorter than the apparent minimal length in mammals, which seems likely to be more than 200 bp *(43)*. This could well reflect the presence of so many dispersed repeats (and, hence, potential for NAHR) in the human genome. It is also possible that the lower rate of AHR in males reflects enhancement of NAHR on the sex chromosomes in the heterogametic germline, where a lack of meiotic pairing partner outside of the pseudo-autosomal regions may facilitate pathogenic intrachromosomal rearrangements *(44)*. An additional possibility to take into account when extrapolating from studies dissecting HR processes in model organisms is that the apparently recent proliferation of segmental duplications in primate genomes *(45)* may have imposed further modification on AHR processes, such that significant differences exist between AHR in primates and in other, less-duplicated, mammalian genomes.

CONCLUSIONS AND FUTURE WORK

Currently, only a small number of NAHR and AHR hotspots have been characterized in detail at the molecular level. However, whenever NAHR hotspots have been sought, they have been found. Despite this paucity of well-characterized HR hotspots, we have seen that NAHR and AHR hotspots share several important features in common, which may suggest that they share similar molecular mechanisms. However, there are no obvious shared sequence motifs between AHR or NAHR hotspots that might allow us to predict the position of hotspots on the basis of the single reference sequence at our disposal. Although it is difficult to draw firm conclusions from so few data, it seems that NAHR hotspots are likely to be less intense (in terms of locus-specific events per generation) than AHR hotspots. This is not altogether surprising given: (1) competition between allelic and paralogous sequences and (2) a requirement for chromosomal gymnastics for NAHR to proceed. In contrast to many other fundamental processes in the human genome, there are good mechanistic reasons, and limited evidence, that individual NAHR and AHR hotspots are not likely to be highly conserved over large evolutionary distances.

Undoubtedly, what is required for a quantum leap in our understanding of HR hotspots are methods that allow these hotspots to be identified in a high-throughput manner. At present, all NAHR hotspots have been identified on the basis of phenotypes associated with the rearrangements they promote. This requirement to collect sufficient numbers of rare rearrangements from the population represents the major barrier to such high-throughput methods. A haplotype-driven (as opposed to a phenotype-driven) assay for NAHR in sperm could be the answer. Sperm-typing methods have been successful in recent years in characterising novel AHR hotspots *(13)*. Candidate locations to test for NAHR hotspot activity could be identified by scanning comparative sequences of segmental duplications in great ape species for signals of concerted evolution.

Sperm-typing methods of assaying genome "rearrangeability" would also help to address many of the outstanding fundamental questions concerning NAHR hotspots, which include:

- To what degree do rates of NAHR vary between loci, individuals, and populations, and what factors underscore this variation?
- What is the relationship between gene conversion hotspots and rearrangement hotspots?
- Are NAHR hotspots simply AHR hotspots within paralogous sequences?
- Are there different classes of NAHR and AHR hotspots?
- Are NAHR and AHR hotspots necessarily short-lived?

Although our focus on a specific class of mutational mechanisms underlying relatively rare genetic diseases may appear to be of esoteric interest, we would argue that the role played by NAHR in other more common diseases with a genetic component is likely to have been under-ascertained. We think that it is reasonable to assume that every mutational mechanism in the human genome contributes to Mendelian *and* complex diseases, albeit to varying extents. Currently, NAHR has only been convincingly linked to the former. It has been well recognized that our ability to dissect the genetic basis of complex disease susceptibility will depend greatly on the underlying allelic architecture. This allelic architecture is itself dependent on assumptions about the dynamics of the underlying mutation process. Consequently, our ability to detect the contribution of NAHR to complex disease will depend in large degree on the presently unknown rates and locations of NAHR in the human genome. For example, the widespread existence of NAHR hotspots suggests that chromosomal rearrangements that are indistinguishable at the DNA sequence level may arise recurrently on diverse haplotypic backgrounds. Such haplotypic heterogeneity within a population could hinder the detection of any such etiologically important variants. Greater comprehension of the mutation dynamics of NAHR (and other mutational processes) should be used to improve the experimental design of searches for variants conferring susceptibility to complex diseases.

SUMMARY

NAHR hotspots within duplicated sequences that promote rearrangements have been found whenever they have been sought with sufficient resolution. AHR and NAHR hotspots share a number of important features in common, implying that they share the same underlying mechanism. Many questions remain regarding the numbers and locations of NAHR hotspots and new methodologies will be needed to gain a genome-wide understanding of this fundamental mutational process.

REFERENCES

1. Jeffreys AJ, Kauppi L, Neumann R. Intensely punctate meiotic recombination in the class II region of the major histocompatibility complex. Nat Genet 2001;29:217–222.
2. Reiter LT, Murakami T, Koeuth T, et al. A recombination hotspot responsible for two inherited peripheral neuropathies is located near a mariner transposon-like element. Nat Genet 1996;12:288–297.
3. Han LL, Keller MP, Navidi W, Chance PF, Arnheim N. Unequal exchange at the Charcot-Marie-Tooth disease type 1A recombination hot-spot is not elevated above the genome average rate. Hum Mol Genet 2000;9: 1881–1889.
4. Pritchard JK, Przeworski M. Linkage disequilibrium in humans: models and data. Am J Hum Genet 2001;69: 1–14.
5. Dawson E, Abecasis GR, Bumpstead S, et al. A first-generation linkage disequilibrium map of human chromosome 22. Nature 2002;418:544–548.
6. Gabriel SB, Salomon R, Pelet A, et al. The structure of haplotype blocks in the human genome. Science 2002;296:2225–2229.
7. The International HapMap Consortium. The International HapMap Project. Nature 2003;426:789–796.
8. Stephens JC, Reich DE, Goldstein DB, et al. Dating the origin of the CCR5-Delta32 AIDS-resistance allele by the coalescence of haplotypes. Am J Hum Genet 1998;62:1507–1515.
9. Mecsas J, Franklin G, Kuziel WA, Brubaker RR, Falkow S, Mosier DE. Evolutionary genetics: CCR5 mutation and plague protection. Nature 2004;427:606.
10. Galvani AP, Slatkin M. Evaluating plague and smallpox as historical selective pressures for the CCR5-Delta 32 HIV-resistance allele. Proc Natl Acad Sci USA 2003;100:15,276–15,279.
11. Kurahashi H, Emanuel BS. Long AT-rich palindromes and the constitutional t(11;22) breakpoint. Hum Mol Genet 2001;10:2605–2617.
12. Fredman D, White SJ, Potter S, Eichler EE, Den Dunnen JT, Brookes AJ. (2004) Complex SNP-related sequence variation in segmental genome duplications. Nat Genet 2004;36:861–866.
13. Arnheim N, Calabrese P, Nordborg M. Hot and cold spots of recombination in the human genome: the reason we should find them and how this can be achieved. Am J Hum Genet 2003;73:5–16.

14. Jeffreys AJ, Murray J, Neumann R. High-resolution mapping of crossovers in human sperm defines a minisatellite-associated recombination hotspot. Molecular Cell 1998;2:267–273.

15. Crawford DC, Bhangale T, Li N, et al. Evidence for substantial fine-scale variation in recombination rates across the human genome. Nat Genet 2004;36:700–706.

16. McVean GA, Myers SR, Hunt S, Deloukas P, Bentley DR, Donnelly P. The fine-scale structure of recombination rate variation in the human genome. Science 2004;304:581–584.

17. de Massy B. Distribution of meiotic recombination sites. Trends Genet 2003;19:514–522.

18. Lupski JR. Hotspots of homologous recombination in the human genome: not all homologous sequences are equal. Genome Biology 2004;5:242.

19. Kauppi L, Jeffreys AJ, Keeney S. Where the crossovers are: recombination distributions in mammals. Nat Rev Genet 2004;5:413–424.

20. Lopes J, Ravise N, Vandenberghe A, et al. Fine mapping of de novo CMT1A and HNPP rearrangements within CMT1A-REPs evidences two distinct sex-dependent mechanisms and candidate sequences involved in recombination. Hum Mol Genet 1998;7:141–148.

21. Palau F, Lofgren A, De Jonghe P, et al. Origin of the de novo duplication in Charcot-Marie-Tooth disease type 1A: unequal nonsister chromatid exchange during spermatogenesis. Hum Mol Genet 1993;2:2031–2035.

22. Jeffreys AJ, Ritchie A, Neumann R. High resolution analysis of haplotype diversity and meiotic crossover in the human TAP2 recombination hotspot. Hum Mol Genet 2000;9:725–733.

23. Kehrer-Sawatzki H, Kluwc L, Sandig C, et al. High frequency of mosaicism among patients with neurofibromatosis type 1 (NF1) with microdeletions caused by somatic recombination of the JJAZ1 gene. Am J Hum Genet 2004;75:410–423.

24. Szostak JW, Orr-Weaver TL, Rothstein RJ, Stahl FW. The double-strand-break repair model for recombination. Cell 1983;33:25–35.

25. Baudat F, Nicolas A. Clustering of meiotic double-strand breaks on yeast chromosome III. Proc Natl Acad Sci USA 1997;94:5213–5218.

26. Pecina A, Smith KN, Mezard C, Murakami H, Ohta K, Nicolas A. Targeted stimulation of meiotic recombination. Cell 2002;111:173–184.

27. Ben-Aroya S, Mieczkowski PA, Petes TD, Kupiec M. The compact chromatin structure of a Ty repeated sequence suppresses recombination hotspot activity in Saccharomyces cerevisiae. Mol Cell 2004;15:221–231.

28. Petes TD. Meiotic recombination hot spots and cold spots. Nat Rev Genet 2001;2:360–369.

29. Qin J, Richardson LL, Jasin M, Handel MA, Arnheim N. Mouse strains with an active H2-Ea meiotic recombination hot spot exhibit increased levels of H2-Ea-specific DNA breaks in testicular germ cells. Mol Cell Biol 2004;24:1655–1666.

30. Jeffreys AJ, May CA. Intense and highly localized gene conversion activity in human meiotic crossover hot spots. Nat Genet 2004;36:151–156.

31. Moens PB, Kolas NK, Tarsounas M, Marcon E, Cohen PE, Spyropoulos B. The time course and chromosomal localization of recombination-related proteins at meiosis in the mouse are compatible with models that can resolve the early DNA-DNA interactions without reciprocal recombination. J Cell Sci 2002;115:1611–1622.

32. Yauk CL, Bois PR, Jeffreys AJ. High-resolution sperm typing of meiotic recombination in the mouse MHC Ebeta gene. Embo J 2003;22:1389–1397.

33. Rozen S, Skaletsky H, Marszalek JD, et al. Abundant gene conversion between arms of palindromes in human and ape Y chromosomes. Nature 2003;423:873–876.

34. Timmerman V, Rautenstrauss B, Reiter LT, et al. Detection of the CMT1A/HNPP recombination hotspot in unrelated patients of European descent. J Med Genet 1997;34:43–49.

35. Warner LE, Reiter LT, Murakami T, Lupski JR. Molecular mechanisms for Charcot-Marie-Tooth disease and related demyelinating peripheral neuropathies. Cold Spring Harb Symp Quant Biol 1996;61:659–671.

36. Kauppi L, Sajantila A, Jeffreys AJ. Recombination hotspots rather than population history dominate linkage disequilibrium in the MHC class II region. Hum Mol Genet 2003;12:33–40.

37. Ptak SE, Roeder AD, Stephens M, Gilad Y, Paabo S, Przeworski M. Absence of the TAP2 human recombination hotspot in chimpanzees. PLoS Biol 2004;2:849–855.

38. Boulton A, Myers RS, Redfield RJ. The hotspot conversion paradox and the evolution of meiotic recombination. Proc Natl Acad Sci USA 1997;94:8058–8063.

39. Jeffreys AJ, Neumann R. Reciprocal crossover asymmetry and meiotic drive in a human recombination hot spot. Nat Genet 2002;31:267–271.

40. Monckton DG, Neumann R, Guram T, et al. Minisatellite mutation-rate variation associated with a flanking DNA sequence polymorphism. Nat Genet 1994;8:162–170.
41. Hurles ME, Willey D, Matthews L, Hussain SS. Origins of chromosomal rearrangement hotspots in the human genome: evidence from the AZFa deletion hotspots. Genome Biol 2004;5:R55.
42. Hey J. What's so hot about recombination hotspots? PLoS Biol 2004;2:730–733.
43. Waldman AS, Liskay RM. Dependence of intrachromosomal recombination in mammalian cells on uninterrupted homology. Mol Cell Biol 1988;8:5350–5357.
44. Hurles ME, Jobling MA. A singular chromosome. Nat Genet 2003;34:246–247.
45. Bailey JA, Gu Z, Clark RA, et al. Recent segmental duplications in the human genome. Science 2002;297:1003–1007.
46. May CA, Shone AC, Kalaydjieva L, Sajantila A, Jeffreys AJ. Crossover clustering and rapid decay of linkage disequilibrium in the Xp/Yp pseudoautosomal gene SHOX. Nat Genet 2002;31:272–275.
47. Kamp C, Hirschmann P, Voss H, Huellen K, Vogt PH. Two long homologous retroviral sequence blocks in proximal Yq11 cause AZFa microdeletions as a result of intrachromosomal recombination events. Hum Mol Genet 2000;9:2563–2572.
48. Blanco P, Shlumukova M, Sargent CA, Jobling MA, Affara N, Hurles ME. Divergent outcomes of intrachromosomal recombination on the human Y chromosome: male infertility and recurrent polymorphism. J Med Genet 2000;37:752–758.
49. Bosch E, Jobling MA. Duplications of the AZFa region of the human Y chromosome are mediated by homologous recombination between HERVs and are compatible with male fertility. Hum Mol Genet 2003;12:341–347.
50. Sun C, Skaletsky H, Rozen S, et al. Deletion of azoospermia factor a (AZFa) region of human Y chromosome caused by recombination between HERV15 proviruses. Hum Mol Genet 2000;9:2291–2296.
51. Repping S, Skaletsky H, Lange J, et al. Recombination between palindromes P5 and P1 on the human Y chromosome causes massive deletions and spermatogenic failure. Am J Hum Genet 2002;71:906–922.
52. Lopez-Correa C, Dorschner M, Brems H, et al. Recombination hotspot in NF1 microdeletion patients. Hum Mol Genet 2001;10:1387–1392.
53. Reiter LT, Hastings PJ, Nelis E, De Jonghe P, Van Broeckhoven C, Lupski JR. Human meiotic recombination products revealed by sequencing a hotspot for homologous strand exchange in multiple HNPP deletion patients. Am J Hum Genet 1998;62:1023–1033.
54. Bi W, Park SS, Shaw CJ, Withers MA, Patel PI, Lupski JR. Reciprocal crossovers and a positional preference for strand exchange in recombination events resulting in deletion or duplication of chromosome 17p11.2. Am J Hum Genet 2003;73:1302–1315.
55. Shaw CJ, Withers MA, Lupski JR. Uncommon deletions of the Smith-Magenis syndrome region can be recurrent when alternate low-copy repeats act as homologous recombination substrates. Am J Hum Genet 2004;75:75–81.
56. Bayes M, Magano LF, Rivera N, Flores R, Perez Jurado LA. Mutational mechanisms of Williams-Beuren syndrome deletions. Am J Hum Genet 2003;73:131–151.

25 Position Effects

Paweł Stankiewicz, MD, PhD

CONTENTS

BACKGROUND

Position effects describe the observed alteration in protein-coding gene expression that may accompany a change in genomic position of a given gene. A position effect may result from chromosomal translocation or other genomic rearrangements. Recent advances in chromatin studies in several different species including yeast, *Drosophila*, and mouse have contributed significantly to better understanding of human diseases resulting from abnormal epigenetic effects. Molecular models attempting to explain position effects in humans have been proposed; however, none of them adequately addresses a variety of mechanisms. According to the noncontact models, the *cis-* or *trans*-regulatory elements, or locus control regions, are physically separated from the target gene and act either at the RNA level, by protein interactions, or by mediation of boundary elements, termed insulators. On the contrary, the contact models invoke spatial-temporal modifications of chromatin structure (e.g., active chromatin hub). In both models, the conserved nongenic sequences (CNGs) may play an important role in genomic regulation of gene expression. The recent introduction of new techniques including tagging and recovery of associated proteins (RNA-TRAP) and capturing chromatin conformation (CCC or 3C), has provided powerful tools to investigate position effects in humans.

INTRODUCTION

Chemical modifications to DNA or histones that alter the structure of chromatin without changing the DNA coding sequence are described as epigenetic. Change in histone code, DNA

From: *Genomic Disorders: The Genomic Basis of Disease*
Edited by: J. R. Lupski and P. Stankiewicz © Humana Press, Totowa, NJ

methylation, or genes packaging in the nucleus can result in altered regulation of gene expression that has been referred to as a position effect.

Early studies of heterochromatin in *Drosophila* have led to the discovery of the phenomenon of position effect variegation (PEV), a juxtaposition of a euchromatic gene in a novel *cis*-acting heterochromatin environment wherein the gene becomes epigenetically silenced *(1)*. Subsequently, PEV has been described also in yeast *(2)* and mammals *(3–5)*. The molecular mechanisms for PEV have remained elusive, but recent progress in chromatin studies has begun to illuminate molecular aspects of this phenomenon. It has been speculated that the spreading of heterochromatic packaging protects the cell against the invading retrotransposons and transposable elements *(6)*. In addition to well known features of heterochromatin, e.g., histone deacetylation, histone methylation (histone H3 on lysine 9, H3-mK9), and heterochromatin-associated protein HP1, small RNAs, RNAi, and siRNAs have been shown in yeast to play important roles in heterochromatin assembly through the RNA-induced initiation of a transcriptional gene silencing complex *(7–9)*.

The infrequently described *trans*-regulation is probably best represented in *Drosophila* by the transvection phenomenon, a pairing-dependent interallelic complementation, or the ability of one locus to affect the expression of the allele, on the homologous chromosome *(10)*. In recent years, transvection has been reported in *Drosophila* at a rapidly growing number of loci, and transvection-like phenomena have been described in a number of different organisms, including plants, fungi, and mammals *(11)*.

Despite the near completion of the human genome sequence, little is known about genomic aspects of gene regulation in humans. Kleinjan and van Heyningen *(12)* reviewed position effects of chromosomal rearrangements in humans and proposed a few potential mechanisms: (1) separation of the gene from its enhancer or promoter region (locus control region); (2) juxtaposition with an enhancer element from another gene; (3) removal of the long-range insulator or boundary elements; (4) competition with another enhancer; and (5) PEV. A useful model for studying such regulation is provided by genomic rearrangements resulting in diseases, in which chromosome breakpoints do not disrupt the causative gene but instead map outside the intact gene.

CONTACT VS NONCONTACT MODELS OF POSITION EFFECT

Many of the balanced chromosome aberration breakpoints associated with abnormal phenotype in humans have been mapped up to 400 kb both upstream and downstream from the causative gene *(13)*. Remarkably, a few cases with putative *cis*-acting regulatory elements have been described as distant as 1 Mb upstream from the target gene (Table 1). Interestingly, no chromosome breakpoints have been found in the genomic regions approx 400–800 kb from the disease-causative gene. This statistically significant bimodal distribution of breakpoints suggests the role of a chromatin structure, rather than the noncontact mechanisms.

Preaxial Polydactyly and Sonic Hedgehog SHH

Preaxial polydactyly (PPD) (MIM 190605) is one of the most common limb malformation in humans. Belloni et al. *(14)* and Roessler et al. *(15)* reported a position effect approx 250 kb upstream of the *SHH* gene, responsible for PPD. By analyzing a chromosome breakpoint of an apparently balanced reciprocal translocation t(5;7)(q11;q36) in a patient with PPD and a transgenic insertion site in a polydactylous mouse mutant sasquatch (*Ssq*) (supernumerary

Table 1
Long-Range Position Effects in Humans

Gene affected	Maximal distance of breakpoint from gene		Rearrangement type	References
	Upstream	Downstream		
SOX9	~900 kb	1.3 Mb	Translocation	28,36,37
POU3F4	~900 kb			111
FKHL7	~1.2 Mb			112
MAF	~1 Mb			113
SHH	~1 Mb			18
DACH	~1Mb			114
OTX2				115
PLP1				116,117
NSD1				118

preaxial digits of the hind fcct) *(16)*, Lettice et al. *(17)* identified an evolutionary conserved non-coding regulatory element termed ZRS. The ZRS regulatory site is located approx 1-Mb 5' from the sonic hedgehog gene *SHH*, in intron 5 of the *LMBR1* gene. Using a *cis-trans* genetic test in mice, Lettice et al. *(18)* and Sagai et al. *(19)* demonstrated *cis-* and not *trans*-interactions between the *Ssq* locus and the *Shh* gene. These findings further suggested the presence of a long-range *cis*-regulating enhancer of *SHH*, capable of causing congenital abnormalities. Supporting these findings, Lettice et al. *(17)* identified four different point mutations in the ZRS in unrelated Dutch, Belgian, and Cuban families with PPG that did not have coding mutations in *SHH*. Further genomic comparison using the computer program VISTA among human, mouse, and teleost fish medaka revealed the mammals-fishes-conserved-sequences MFCS1 (corresponding to ZRS), MFCS2, and MFCS3 in and around *LMBR1 (20)*. Interestingly, these elements are located only approx 100 kb from *Shh* in medaka fish. When deleted in mouse, MCFS1 resulted in a complete loss of *Shh* expression and truncation of the mouse limb *(20)*.

Blepharophimosis and FOXL2 *and Aniridia and* PAX6

Evolutionarily conserved long-range *cis*-regulatory elements have been found also in introns of other genes. Three chromosome translocation breakpoints were mapped within introns 6, 11, and 12 of *MRPS22* in patients with blepharophimosis/ptosis/epicanthus inversus syndrome (BPES). These breakpoints are located approx 170 kb upstream to the BPES-causitive *FOXL2 (21)*. In addition, four microdeletions with a 126-kb overlap were identified more distal to these breakpoints, 230 kb upstream to *FOXL2*. Interestingly, the shortest region of deletion overlap contains several CNGs with putative transcription-factor binding sites that represent potential candidate *cis*-regulatory elements *(21a)*. Moreover, translocation breakpoints have been identified within the last intron of *PAXNEB*, more than 150 kb downstream of *PAX6*, the gene responsible for aniridia *(22)*.

Campomelic Dysplasia and SOX9

Haploinsufficiency of *SOX9* on 17q24.3 causes campomelic dysplasia (CD), (MIM 114290), a clinically distinct syndrome characterized by semilethal skeletal malformation syndrome with or without XY sex reversal *(23–26)*. The two mechanisms responsible for *SOX9* haploinsufficiency are intragenic mutations *(27)* and chromosome rearrangements including translocations, inversions, and deletions *(28)*. The analysis of 12 patients with CD and apparently balanced chromosome rearrangements showed the breakpoints scattered up to approx 900 kb upstream of *SOX9*, whereas the gene itself was intact *(29–30)*. Recently, Pop et al. *(31)* reported an approx 1.5-Mb microdeletion located approx 380 kb upstream of *SOX9*.

Huang et al. *(32)* described a chromosome duplication dup(17)(q24.1q24.3) associated with XX female-to-male sex reversal and Bishop et al. *(33)* reported XX female-to-male sex reversal in a transgenic *Odd Sex* mouse with a 134-kb insertional deletion, resulting from a recombinant construct insertion 0.98 Mb upstream of *SOX9*. The authors proposed that a Dct promoter of the inserted construct interacted with gonad-specific enhancer elements, yielding sex reversal *(34)*. Thus, both the chondrogenic and gonadal functions of *SOX9* appear to be precisely regulated by elements located as far as 1 Mb away from the gene itself.

Detailed DNA analysis of the genomic region extending up to 1 Mb proximal to *SOX9* failed to uncover any protein-coding genes, suggesting that the chromosomal rearrangements remove one or more *cis*-regulatory elements from an extended *SOX9* region *(28,31,34,35)*. Recently, four independent 17q chromosome breakpoints were mapped 786–809, 899, 900, and 932 kb upstream of *SOX9* *(36–38)*. In addition, in a prenatal identification of acampomelic CD with male-to-female sex reversal in a fetus with a *de novo* balanced complex karyotype, the 17q breakpoint mapped approx 1.3 Mb downstream of *SOX9*. This is perhaps the longest-range position effect described in the field of human genetics, and the first report of CD with the chromosome breakpoint mapping 3' to *SOX9* *(37)*.

Using a regulatory potential computer program in conjunction with the analysis of the rearrangement breakpoints, highly conserved genomic sequences that potentially represent *cis*-regulatory elements, were identified both upstream (1.1 kb *SOX9* evolutionarily conserved regulatory element 1 [SOX9cre1]) and downstream of *SOX9*. These were shown to co-localize with *SOX9* in the interphase nucleus despite being located 1.1 Mb upstream and 1.3 Mb downstream to it, respectively *(37)*. This suggests that the murine SOX9cre1 element has been modified by the inserted Dct promoter in *Odd Sex* mice *(34)* and that in humans SOX9cre1 is responsible for the isolated Robin sequence phenotype cosegregating with a balanced t(2;17)(q24.1;24.3) translocation reported recently by Jamshidi et al. *(39)*. The 17q breakpoint in this family maps very close and proximal to SOX9cre1 *(36)*. It is also likely that some patients with isolated Robin sequence have mutations involving SOX9cre1 or other regulatory elements of *SOX9*. Thus, the mild campomelic dysplasia phenotype found in patients with translocation breakpoints near *SOX9* *(36,37,40,41)* may be the result of slightly modified expression of chondrocyte-specific genes, secondary to altered *SOX9* regulation as a result of spatial dissociation from the distal SOX9cre1.

GENOMIC INSULATORS

Insulators, or boundary elements, are DNA elements that have the potential to block the function of enhancers on gene promoters as well as spreading of chromatin silencing *(42)*. Almost all reported insulators have been shown to require the regulatory chromatin insulator protein CTCF.

CTCF also binds to several sites in the unmethylated imprinted-control regions that are essential for blocking the enhancers. Recently, Yu et al. *(43)* demonstrated that a post-translational modification, poly(ADP-ribosyl)ation of CTCF, regulates its activity as a transcriptional insulator.

Insulators are considered a very promising and useful tool in gene therapy applications for ensuring high-level and stable expression of transgenes *(42,44)*. The structure and function of insulators have been studied best on the chicken β-*globin* locus and in the *Igf2* and *H19* region on human chromosome 11p15.5.

Chicken β-Globin Locus

Pioneering work by Felsenfeld and colleagues on the chicken β-*globin* locus has led to the identification of an HS4 insulator element and demonstrated the important role of CTCF protein in boundary elements *(45)*. They were also able to show the blocking activity of insulators in an in vitro construct *(46)*. Yusufzai et al. *(47)* showed that, together with CTCF, the nucleolar protein nucleophosmin tethers the insulator to the nucleolus and, thus, may generate chromatin loop structures separating promoters from their enhancer. Recent chromatin studies revealed that, similar to observations made in yeast *(6)*, histone modifications (acetylation and H3K4 methylation) in human appear to be pivotal for the insulator function *(48–50)*.

Beckwith-Wiedemann Syndrome

Beckwith-Wiedemann syndrome (BWS) is caused by deregulation of expression of imprinted genes in chromosome 11p15.5. BWS is characterized by prenatal overgrowth, midline abdominal wall defects, macroglossia, and embryonal tumors. *H19* and *Igf2* genes implicated in the BWS are expressed from the maternal or the paternal chromosome, respectively. Webber et al. *(51)* described the unmethylated imprinted-control region (ICR) that acts as a chromatin boundary between differently imprinted *Igf2* and *H19*. Two independent groups showed that the binding of the enhancer-blocking protein CTCF to the ICR depends on its methylation status *(52,53)*. The binding of CTCF to ICR on maternal chromosome averts interaction between the *Igf2* promoter and its enhancer, leading to *Igf2* silencing. On the paternal allele, spreading of methylation of the ICR inhibits *H19* and eliminates the CTFC-ICR assembly, resulting in normal *Igf2* expression *(54)*. Thus, DNA methylation- and CTCF-dependent enhancer blocking mediate genomic imprinting of *H19* and *Igf2* loci. Supporting this notion, Prawitt et al. *(54a)* described a 2.2-kb familial microdeletion involving three CTCF-target sites in the *H19/IGF2*-imprinting center and proposed that it is causitive for BWS and Wilms tumor.

Myotonic Dystrophy

CTG trinucleotide repeat expansion in the DM1 locus on chromosome 19q13.32 affects the expression of two adjacent genes *DMPK* and *SIX5* and leads to myotonic dystrophy, an autosomal dominant disorder characterized by myotonia, muscular dystrophy, cataracts, hypogonadism, frontal balding, and electrocardiogram changes. Filippova et al. *(55)* demonstrated that CTCF binding sites flank the CTG repeat and act as insulator element between *DMPK* and *SIX5*. Similar to the *H19* and *Igf2* genes, methylation of these sites eliminates binding of CTCF. Thus, methylation of the DM1 locus in myotonic dystrophy disrupts the insulator function. The role of CTCF in the insulator function has been proposed also in establishing a regulatable epigenetic switch for X chromosome inactivation *(56,57)* and in cancer *(58)*.

NONGENIC INTERSPECIES SEQUENCE CONSERVATION

Comparative genomics studies of several different species enabled identification of conserved non-coding DNA sequences that appear to have important biological functions. Several computer programs have been developed to perform such comparative analyses *(59,60)*. In addition to the anticipated protein-coding genes and non-coding RNA genes, the multispecies comparison of human chromosome 21 sequence revealed the presence of a large number of highly conserved DNA sequence blocks of unknown function *(61,62)*. Intriguingly, these potentially functional CNGs, or multispecies conserved sequences, are significantly more conserved than protein-coding genes *(62)*. In addition, it has been estimated that in the human genome there are approx 60,000 CNGs, approximately twice as many as the number of coding genes and that CNGs may constitute 0.3–1% of the human genome. It is tempting to speculate that these elements may play a role in long-distance functional or structural gene regulation (e.g., in chromatin folding/loop formation by matrix scaffold attachment regions) *(63,64)*.

Non-Coding RNAs

Recently, by studying the α-*globin* gene, Tufarelli et al. *(65)* described a novel mechanism of position effect-related gene regulation, "antisense-mediated *cis*-acting methylation utilizing non-coding RNA (ncRNA)," that is similar to the *XIST/TSIX*–mediated X chromosome inactivation *(66)*. It has been estimated that at least 20% of human genes have antisense transcripts *(67,68)*. Several non-coding transcripts have been found associated with human diseases including B-cell lymphoma, lung cancer, prostate cancer, cartilage-hair hypoplasia, spinocerebellar ataxia type 8, DiGeorge syndrome, autism, and schizophrenia *(69)*. ncRNAs-based gene regulation may be an important mechanism of cell function particularly in more complex organisms; however, the molecular mechanisms still await elucidation.

CHROMATIN STRUCTURE AND FUNCTION

Active Chromatin Hub

Distal enhancers have been hypothesized to interact with gene promoters through a set of proteins that act by bending DNA to bring the enhancers within physical proximity of their respective target gene, thus, regulating its function (chromatin loop contact model) *(70–72)*. After analyzing the β-*globin* locus using the 3C technique *(73)*, Tolhuis et al. *(74)* proposed an "active chromatin hub (ACH)" model, wherein active genes and DNAse I hypersensitive sites are in close spatial proximity forming a three-dimensional (3D) hub of hyperaccessible chromatin and the remaining fragments loop out. Interestingly, this structure was found only in gene-expressing erythroid tissues and was linearized in nonexpressing brain tissue *(74)*. Moreover, during erythroid differentiation, *cis*-regulatory elements of the β-*globin* locus form a nuclear compartmentalization with RNA polymerase II representing ACH *(75)*. Subsequently, the same group proved that multiple interactions between *cis*-regulatory elements and the target gene are required to maintain the ACH structure *(76)*. Supporting this notion, Horike et al. *(77)* demonstrated that formation of a silent-chromatin loop is a novel mechanism underlying *MECP2* gene regulation in the Rett syndrome.

Matrix-Scaffold Attachment Regions (M/SARs)

By attaching chromatin to the nuclear matrix, matrix-scaffold attachment regions (M/SARs) are thought to participate in chromatin loop formation *(77,78)* and represent initiation sites for chromosome condensation *(79)*. Recently, Ioudinkova et al. *(80)* hybridized a DNAse I digested nuclear matrix containing the M/SAR elements to a 60mer oligonucleotide arrays covering the chicken α-*globin* locus and identified a co-localization of 40-kb α-*globin* chromatin loop attachment region with the nuclear M/SAR and the previously described CTCF-dependent enhancer blocker elements *(81)*.

Transcription Sites and Nuclear Territories: Functional Organization of Interphase Nuclei

Transcriptionally active chromatin is believed to be markedly compartmentalized in chromosome territories *(82)*. Active loci are located predominantly at or near the surface of compact chromatin domains, depositing newly synthesized RNA directly into the interchromatin space *(83,84)*. Tanabe et al. *(85)* showed evolutionary conservation of chromosome territory arrangements in cell nuclei from higher primates.

Using chromatin precipitation, sucrose gradient sedimentation, and array comparative genomic hybridization (aCGH) techniques, Gilbert et al. *(86)* showed that gene-rich domains are enriched in open chromatin fibers and suggested that domains of open chromatin may create an environment that facilitates transcriptional activation and could provide an evolutionary constraint to maintain clusters of genes together along chromosomes.

A growing number of human diseases have been shown to result from abnormal chromatin structure *(87)*. Dysfunctions in proper chromatin remodeling can affect epigenetic interactions and in turn lead to gene expression multi-system disorders and neoplasias *(88)*. The importance of chromatin-nuclear envelope interactions has been emphasized further in laminopathies, a new group of genetic diseases, wherein mutations in *lamin A/C*, a constituent of the nuclear envelope, can presumably deregulate chromatin-nuclear envelope interactions that manifest with a broad spectrum of disorders. These include Emery–Dreifuss and limb-girdle muscular dystrophies (skeletal muscles), Charcot–Marie–Tooth neuropathy (peripheral nerves), dilated cardiomyopathy (heart), Dunnigan familial partial lipodystrophy (adipose tissue), and mandibuloacral dysplasia (skeletal system) *(89,90)*. The best known example of disease resulting from abnormal chromatin structure or function is probably facioscapulohumeral muscular dystrophy (FSHD). FSHD has been included also in a novel group of genetic diseases associated with transcriptional derepression *(91,92)*.

Facioscapulohumeral Muscular Dystrophy

FSHD is the third most common muscular dystrophy and usually manifests in the second decade of life with progressive wasting of facial, upper arm, and shoulder muscles. FSHD is caused by interstitial deletion involving polymorphic heterochromatic 3.3 kb *D4Z4* repeats in 4q35. The number of repeats varies between 11 and 100 copies in normal individuals. In patients affected with FSHD, the number of *D4Z4* repeats is lower than 11 (<35 kb) and is associated with derepression and altered methylation of *ANT1*, *FRG1*, and *FRG2* and hypomethylation of *D4Z4* *(93)*. An element within *D4Z4* has been proposed to bind a multi-protein complex and mediate transcriptional repression of the 4q35 genes, *ANT1*, *FRG1*, and *FRG2 (94)*. Consequently, an epigenetic PEV-like mechanism with *D4Z4* acting as a silencer element has been proposed *(92,95,96)*.

Recently, four models attempting to explain the pathomechanism of FSHD have been postulated *(97)*. In a *cis*-spreading scenario, interstitial deletion of *D4Z4* leads to local chromatin relaxation with spreading of upregulation *(94,98,99)*. The insulator mechanism predicts inefficiency of the contracted *D4Z4* boundary element to the distally located heterochromatin *(100)* and in the chromatin *cis*-loop model, the number of *D4Z4* repeats determines the 3D chromatin structure and, thus, direct interactions between *D4Z4* and the upstream genes *(95)*. The fourth model supplements the third one and implies the perturbation of 4qter with nuclear lamina and subsequent misbalance of chromatin and transcription factors *(101–102)*.

NOVEL METHODS

Recently, a number of molecular techniques that enable insight into chromatin structure and function have been developed.

Capturing Chromosome Confirmation

Dekker et al. *(73)* described a methodology that can estimate the spatial organization and frequency of interactions between two genomic regions in organisms from bacteria to human. After formaldehyde-induced crosslinking, *Eco*RI digestion, intramolecular ligation, and reverse crosslinking, the frequency of different loci being connected is assessed by quantitative polymerase chain reaction (PCR) with primers specific to gene promoter and other investigated loci.

RNA-TRAP

To identify the locus control regions that directly interacts with the investigated gene (contact model), Carter et al. *(103)* developed a RNA fluorescence *in situ* hybridization method called RNA-TRAP. The tissue to be analyzed is attached to poly-L-lysine coated glass slides and fixed with formaldehyde. Intron-specific oligonucleotide probe labeled with digoxigenin is hybridized to the expressed pre-mRNA, followed by addition of anti-digoxigenin antibody labeled with horse radish and subsequently biotin-tyramide that on contact with horse radish, covalently attaches to neighbor proteins (tyrosines). Such prepared cells are removed from slides, fragmented by sonication, and purified by affinity chromatography on a streptavidin-agarose column. Finally, similar to the 3C technique, the gene-interacting DNA fragment can be identified by PCR.

Both 3C and RNA-TRAP techniques have proven to be sensitive and specific and have been used successfully for assessment of the distances between long-range gene enhancers and promoters *(104)*, the influence of 3D organization of a gene locus for its regulation *(105)*, and dynamic organization of genes into shared nuclear compartments *(106)*.

ChIP-on-Chip Analysis

The combination of aCGH with chromatin precipitation (ChIP) techniques enabled the development of a novel useful methodology, termed ChIP-on-chip or ChIP-chip. Like in the two above techniques, in the first step, the DNA and proteins are crosslinked using formaldehyde. Subsequently, the specimen is sonicated and immunoprecipitated with an antibody against the investigated protein. The separated DNA-protein complex is cohybridized with the reference DNA using aCGH with target DNA of interest to determine the localization of the associated DNA *(107)*.

Microscopy

Bussiek et al. *(108)* applied scanning force microscopy to analyze DNA loop formation on nucleosomes. Another tool that proved to be useful in decoding the human chromatin structure on the genomic level is electron immunomicroscopy *(109)*.

Real-Time PCR

McArthur et al. *(110)* showed that real-time PCR enabled quantification of the sensitivity of chromatin to digestion by DNase I from small amounts of tissue samples. Such an approach provides the potential to achieve accurate and detailed mapping of chromatin structure.

SUMMARY

Studies of position effects contributed significantly to a better understanding of gene regulation; however, we are only beginning to understand the epigenetic effects of chromatin. 3D chromatin dynamics, evolutionarily conserved nongenic sequences, and boundary elements (insulators) appear to be the major factors responsible for position effect in humans.

ACKNOWLEDGMENTS

I appreciate the critical review by Dr. Cornelius Boerkoel.

REFERENCES

1. Muller HJ. Types of visible variations induced by X-rays in Drosophila. J Genet 1930;22:299–334.
2. Allshire RC, Javerzat JP, Redhead NJ, Cranston G. Position effect variegation at fission yeast centromeres. Cell 1994;76L157–169.
3. Cattanach BM. Position effect variegation in the mouse. Genet Res Camb 1974;23:291–306.
4. Festenstein R, Tolaini M, Corbella P, et al. Locus control region function and heterochromatin-induced position effect variegation. Science 1996;271:1123–1125.
5. Milot E, Fraser P, Grosveld F. Position effects and genetic disease. Trends Genet 1996;12:123–126.
6. Elgin SC, Grewal SI. Heterochromatin: silence is golden. Curr Biol 2003;13:R895–R898.
7. Hall IM, Noma K, Grewal SI. RNA interference machinery regulates chromosome dynamics during mitosis and meiosis in fission yeast. Proc Natl Acad Sci USA 2003;100:193–198.
8. Grewal SI, Rice JC. Regulation of heterochromatin by histone methylation and small RNAs. Curr Opin Cell Biol 2004;16:230–238.
9. Pal-Bhadra M, Leibovitch BA, Gandhi SG, et al. Heterochromatic silencing and HP1 localization in Drosophila are dependent on the RNAi machinery. Science 2004;303:669–672.
10. Lewis EB. The theory and application of a new method of detecting chromosomal rearrangements in Drosophila melanogaster. Am Nat 1954;88:225–239.
11. Duncan IW. Transvection effects in Drosophila. Annu Rev Genet 2002;36:521–556.
12. Kleinjan D-J, van Heyningen V. Position effect in human genetic disease. Hum Mol Genet 1998;7: 1611–1618.
13. Kleinjan DA, van Heyningen V. Long-range control of gene expression: emerging mechanisms and disruption in disease. Am J Hum Genet 2005;76:8–32.
14. Belloni E, Muenke M, Roessler E, et al. Identification of Sonic hedgehog as a candidate gene responsible for holoprosencephaly. Nat Genet 1996;14:353–356.
15. Roessler E, Ward DE, Gaudenz K, et al. Cytogenetic rearrangements involving the loss of the Sonic Hedgehog gene at 7q36 cause holoprosencephaly. Hum Genet 1997;100:172–181.
16. Sharpe J, Lettice L, Hecksher-Sorensen J, Fox M, Hill R, Krumlauf R. Identification of sonic hedgehog as a candidate gene responsible for the polydactylous mouse mutant Sasquatch. Curr Biol 1999;9:97–100.

17. Lettice LA, Heaney SJ, Purdie LA, et al. A long-range Shh enhancer regulates expression in the developing limb and fin and is associated with preaxial polydactyly. Hum Mol Genet 2003;12:1725–1735.

18. Lettice LA, Horikoshi T, Heaney SJH, et al. Disruption of a long-range cis-acting regulator for Shh causes preaxial polydactyly. Proc Natl Acad Sci USA 2002;99:7548–7553.

19. Sagai T, Masuya H, Tamura M, et al. Phylogenetic conservation of a limb-specific, cis-acting regulator of Sonic hedgehog (Shh). Mamm Genome 2004;15:23–34.

20. Sagai T, Hosoya M, Mizushina Y, Tamura M, Shiroishi T. Elimination of a long-range cis-regulatory module causes complete loss of limb-specific Shh expression and truncation of the mouse limb. Development 2005;132:797–803.

21. Crisponi L, Uda M, Deiana M, et al. FOXL2 inactivation by a translocation 171 kb away: analysis of 500 kb of chromosome 3 for candidate long-range regulatory sequences. Genomics 2004;83:757–764.

21a. Betsen D, Raes J, Leroy BP, et al. Deletions involving long-range conserved nongenic sequences upstream and downstream of *FOXL2* as a novel disease-causing mechanism blepharophimosis syndrome. Am J Hum Genet 2005;77:205–218.

22. Kleinjan DA, Seawright A, Schedl A, Quinlan RA, Danes S, van Heyningen V. Aniridia-associated translocations, DNase hypersensitivity, sequence comparison and transgenic analysis redefine the functional domain of PAX6. Hum Mol Genet 2001;10:2049–2059.

23. Houston CS, Opitz JM, Spranger JW, et al. The campomelic syndrome: review, report of 17 cases, and follow-up on the currently 17-year-old boy first reported by Maroteaux et al in 1971. Am J Med Genet 1983;15:3–28.

24. Foster JW, Dominguez-Steglich MA, Guioli S, et al. Campomelic dysplasia and autosomal sex reversal caused by mutations in an SRY-related gene. Nature 1994;372:525–530.

25. Wagner T, Wirth J, Meyer J, et al. Autosomal sex reversal and campomelic dysplasia are caused by mutations in and around the SRY-related gene SOX9. Cell 1994;79:1111–1120.

26. Mansour S, Hall CM, Pembrey ME, Young ID. A clinical and genetic study of campomelic dysplasia. J Med Genet 1995;32:415–420.

27. Meyer J, Südbeck P, Held M, et al. Mutational analysis of the SOX9 gene in campomelic dysplasia and autosomal sex reversal: lack of genotype/phenotype correlations. Hum Mol Genet 1997;6:91–98.

28. Pfeifer D, Kist R, Dewar K, et al. Campomelic dysplasia translocation breakpoints are scattered over 1 Mb proximal to SOX9: evidence for an extended control region. Am J Hum Genet 1999;65:111–124.

29. Wunderle VM, Critcher R, Hastie N, Goodfellow PN, Schedl A. Deletion of long-range regulatory elements upstream of SOX9 causes campomelic dysplasia. Proc Natl Acad Sci USA 1998;95:10,649–10,654.

30. Erdel M, Lane A.H., Fresser F, Probst P, Utermann G, Scherer G. A new campomelic dysplasia translocation breakpoint maps 400 kb from SOX9. [abstract P0249]. European Society of Human Genetics Munich. Eur J Hum Genet Suppl 2004;12:136.

31. Pop R, Conz C, Lindenberg KS, et al. Screening of the 1 Mb SOX9 5' control region by array CGH identifies a large deletion in a case of campomelic dysplasia with XY sex reversal. J Med Genet 2004;41:e47.

32. Huang B, Wang S, Ning Y, Lamb AN, Bartley J. Autosomal XX sex reversal caused by duplication of SOX9. Am J Med Genet 1999;87:349–353.

33. Bishop CE, Whitworth DJ, Qin Y, et al. A transgenic insertion upstream of Sox9 is associated with dominant XX sex reversal in the mouse. Nat Genet 2000;26:490–494.

34. Qin Y, Kong Lk, Poirier C, Truong C, Overbeek PA, Bishop CE. Long-range activation of Sox9 in Odd Sex (Ods) mice. Hum Mol Genet 2004;13:1213–1218.

35. Bagheri-Fam S, Ferraz C, Demaille J, Scherer G, Pfeifer D. Comparative genomics of the SOX9 region in human and Fugu rubripes: conservation of short regulatory sequence elements within large intergenic regions. Genomics 2001;78:73–82.

37. Hill-Harfe KL, Kaplan L, Stalker H, et al. Acampomelic campomelic dysplasia and a mild skeletal dysplasia associated with chromosome 17 translocations 900-932 kb upstream of SOX9: Implications for campomelic dysplasia diagnosis and SOX9 regulation. Am J Hum Genet 2004;76:663–671.

37. Velagaleti GVN, Bien-Willner GA, Northup JK, et al. Position effects due to chromosome breakpoints mapping ~ 900 Kb upstream and ~ 1.3 Mb downstream of SOX9 in two cases with campomelic dysplasia. Am J Hum Genet 2005;76:652–662.

38. Stankiewicz P, Hill-Harfe KL, Velagaleti GVN, et al. Position effects due to four chromosome breakpoints mapping ~786-809, 899, 900, and 932 kb upstream and one ~1.3 Mb downstream of SOX9 in patients with campomelic dysplasia. 5th European Cytogenetics Conference. Madrid, Spain. June 4–7, 2005.

39. Jamshidi N, Macciocca I, Dargaville PA, et al. Isolated Robin sequence associated with a balanced t(2;17) chromosomal translocation. J Med Genet 2004;41:e1.

40. Stalker HJ, Zori RT. Variable expression of rib, pectus, and scapular anomalies with Robin-type cleft palate in a 5-generation family: a new syndrome? Am J Med Genet 1997;73:247–250.

41. Stalker HJ, Gray BA, Zori RT. Dominant transmission of a previously unidentified 13/17 translocation in a five-generation family with Robin cleft and other skeletal defects. Am J Med Genet 2001;103:339–341.

42. Kuhn EJ, Geyer PK. Genomic insulators: connecting properties to mechanism. Curr Opin Cell Biol 2003;15:259–265.

43. Yu W, Ginjala V, Pant V, et al. Poly(ADP-ribosyl)ation regulates CTCF-dependent chromatin insulation. Nat Genet 2004;36:1105–1110.

44. Recillas-Targa F, Valadez-Graham V, Farrell CM. Prospects and implications of using chromatin insulators in gene therapy and transgenesis. Bioessays 2004;26:796–807.

45. West AG, Gaszner M, Felsenfeld G. Insulators: many functions, many mechanisms. Genes Dev 2002;16:271–288.

46. Burgess-Beusse B, Farrell C, Gaszner M, et al. The insulation of genes from external enhancers and silencing chromatin. Proc Natl Acad Sci USA 2002;99:16,433–16,437.

47. Yusufzai TM, Tagami H, Nakatani Y, Felsenfeld G. CTCF tethers an insulator to subnuclear sites, suggesting shared insulator mechanisms across species. Mol Cell 2004;13:291–298.

48. Litt MD, Simpson M, Gaszner M, Allis CD, Felsenfeld G. Science 2001;293:2453–2455.

49. West AG, Huang S, Gaszner M, Litt MD, Felsenfeld G. Recruitment of histone modifications by USF proteins at a vertebrate barrier element. Mol Cell 2004;16:453–463.

50. Zhou J, Berger SL. Good fences make good neighbors: barrier elements and genomic regulation. Mol Cell 2004;16:500–502.

51. Webber A, Ingram RI, Levorse J, Tilghman SM. Location of enhancers is essential for imprinting of H19 and Igf2. Nature 1998;391:711–715.

52. Bell AC, Felsenfeld G. Methylation of a CTCF-dependent boundary controls imprinted expression of the Igf2 gene. Nature 2000;405:482–485.

53. Hark AT, Schoenherr CJ, Katz DJ, Ingram RS, Levorse JM, Tilghman SM. CTCF mediates methylation-sensitive enhancer-blocking activity at the H19/Igf2 locus. Nature 2000;405:486–489.

54. Reik W, Murrell A. Genomic imprinting. Silence across the border. Nature 2000;405:408–409.

54a. Prawitt D, Enklaar T, Gärtner-Rupprecht B, et al. Microdeletion of target sites for insulator protein CTCF in a chromosome 11p15 imprinting center in Beckwith-Wiedemann syndrome and Wilms' tumor. Proc Natl Acad Sci USA 2005;102:4085–4090.

55. Filippova GN, Thienes CP, Penn BH, et al. CTCF-binding sites flank CTG/CAG repeats and form a methylation-sensitive insulator at the DM1 locus. Nat Genet 2001;28:335–343.

56. Chao W, Huynh KD, Spencer RJ, Davidow LS, Lee JT. CTCF, a candidate trans-acting factor for X-inactivation choice. Science 2002;295:345–347.

57. Pugacheva EM, Tiwari VK, Abdullaev Z, et al. Familial cases of point mutations in the XIST promoter reveal a correlation between CTCF binding and pre-emptive choices of X chromosome inactivation. Hum Mol Genet 2005;14:953–965.

58. Ohlsson R, Renkawitz R, Lobanenkov V. CTCF is a uniquely versatile transcription regulator linked to epigenetics and disease. Trends Genet 2002;1:520–527.

59. Nobrega MA, Pennacchio LA. Comparative genomic analysis as a tool for biological discovery. J Physiol 2004;55:31–39.

60. Miller W, Makova KD, Nekrutenko A, Hardison RC. Comparative genomics. Annu Rev Genomics Hum Genet 2004;5:15–56.

61. Dermitzakis ET, Reymond A, Lyle R, et al. Numerous potentially functional but non-genic conserved sequences on human chromosome 21. Nature 2002;420:578–582.

62. Dermitzakis ET, Reymond A, Scamuffa N, et al. Evolutionary discrimination of mammalian conserved non-genic sequences (CNGs). Science 2003;302:1033–1035.

62. Thomas JW, Touchman JW, Blakesley RW, et al. Comparative analyses of multi-species sequences from targeted genomic regions. Nature 2003;424:788–793.

63. Gaffney DJ, Keightley PD. Unexpected conserved non-coding DNA blocks in mammals. Trends Genet 2004;20:332–337.

63. Glazko GV, Koonin EV, Rogozin IB, Shabalina SA. A significant fraction of conserved noncoding DNA in human and mouse consists of predicted matrix attachment regions. Trends Genet 2003;19:119–124.

65. Tufarelli C, Stanley JA, Garrick D, et al. Transcription of antisense RNA leading to gene silencing and methylation as a novel cause of human genetic disease. Nat Genet 2003;34:157–165.

66. Kleinjan DJ, van Heyningen V. Turned off by RNA. Nat Genet 2003;34:125–126.

67. Kiyosawa H, Yamanaka I, Osato N, Kondo S, Hayashizaki Y. Antisense transcripts with FANTOM2 clone set and their implications for gene regulation. Genome Res 2003;13:1324–1334.

68. Yelin R, Dahary D, Sorek R, et al. Widespread occurrence of antisense transcription in the human genome. Nature Biotechnol 2003;21:379–386.

69. Mattick JS. RNA regulation: a new genetics? Nat Rev Genet 2004;5:316–323.

70. Ptashne M. Gene regulation by proteins acting nearby and at a distance. Nature 1986;322:697–701.

71. Mueller HP, Schaffner W. Transcriptional enhancers can act in trans. Trends Genet 1990;6:300–304.

72. Hanscombe O, Whyatt D, Fraser P, et al. Importance of globin gene order for correct developmental expression. Genes Dev 1991;5:1387–1394.

73. Dekker J, Rippe K, Dekker M, Kleckner N. Capturing chromosome conformation. Science 2002;295:1306–1311.

74. Tolhuis B, Palstra RJ, Splinter E, Grosveld F, de Laat W. Looping and interaction between hypersensitive sites in the active beta-globin locus. Mol Cell 2002;10:1453–1465.

75. Palstra R-J, Tolhuis B, Splinter E, Nijmeijer R, Grosveld F, de Laat W. The β-globin nuclear compartment in development and erythroid differentiation. Nat Genet 2003;35:190–194.

76. Patrinos GP, de Krom M, de Boer E, et al. Multiple interactions between regulatory regions are required to stabilize an active chromatin hub. Genes Dev 2004;18:1495–1509.

77. Horike S, Cai S, Miyano M, Cheng J-F, Kohwi-Shigematsu T. Loss of silent-chromatin looping and impaired imprinting of DLX5 in Rett syndrome. Nat Genet 2005;37:31–40.

77. Saitoh Y, Laemmli UK. Metaphase chromosome structure: bands arise from a differential folding path of the highly AT-rich scaffold. Cell 1994;76:609–622.

78. Heng HH, Goetze S, Ye CJ, et al. Chromatin loops are selectively anchored using scaffold/matrix-attachment regions. J Cell Sci 2004;117:999–1008.

79. Strick R, Laemmli UK. SARs are cis DNA elements of chromosome dynamics: synthesis of a SAR repressor protein. Cell 1995;83:1137–1148.

80. Ioudinkova E, Petrov A, Razin SV, Vassetzky YS. Mapping long-range chromatin organization within the chicken alpha-globin gene domain using oligonucleotide DNA arrays. Genomics 2005;85:143–151.

81. Valadez-Graham V, Razin SV, Recillas-Targa F. CTCF-dependent enhancer blockers at the upstream region of the chicken alpha-globin gene domain. Nucleic Acids Res 2004;32:1354–1362.

82. Cremer T, Kupper K, Dietzel S, Fakan S. Higher order chromatin architecture in the cell nucleus: on the way from structure to function. Biol Cell 2004;96:555–567.

83. Verschure PJ, van Der Kraan I, Manders EM, van Driel R. Spatial relationship between transcription sites and chromosome territories. J Cell Biol 1999;147:13–24.

84. Spector DL. The dynamics of chromosome organization and gene regulation. Annu Rev Biochem 2003;72:573–608.

85. Tanabe H, Müller S, Neusser M, et al. Evolutionary conservation of chromosome territory arrangements in cell nuclei from higher primates. Proc Natl Acad Sci USA 2002;99:4424–4429.

86. Gilbert N, Boyle S, Fiegler H, Woodfine K, Carter NP, Bickmore WA. Chromatin architecture of the human genome: gene-rich domains are enriched in open chromatin fibers. Cell 2004;118:555–666.

87. Bickmore WA, van der Maarel SM. Perturbations of chromatin structure in human genetic disease: recent advances. Hum Mol Genet 2003;12:R207–R213.

88. Cho KS, Elizondo LI, Boerkoel CF. Advances in chromatin remodeling and human disease. Curr Opin Genet Dev 2004;14:308–315.

89. Mounkes L, Kozlov S, Burke B, Stewart CL. The laminopathies: nuclear structure meets disease. Curr Opin Genet Dev 2003;13:223–230.

90. Maraldi NM, Squarzoni S, Sabatelli P, et al. Laminopathies: involvement of structural nuclear proteins in the pathogenesis of an increasing number of human diseases. J Cell Physiol 2004;203:319–327.

91. Gabellini D, Tupler R, Green MR. Transcriptional derepression as a cause of genetic diseases. Curr Opin Genet Dev 2003;13:239–245.

92. Gabellini D, Green MR, Tupler R. When enough is enough: genetic diseases associated with transcriptional derepression. Curr Opin Genet Dev 2004;14:301–307.

93. van Overveld PG, Lemmers RJ, Sandkuijl LA, et al. Hypomethylation of D4Z4 in 4q-linked and non-4q-linked facioscapulohumeral muscular dystrophy. Nat Genet 2003;35:315–317.

94. Gabellini D, Green MR, Tupler R. Inappropriate gene activation in FSHD: a repressor complex binds a chromosomal repeat deleted in dystrophic muscle. Cell 2002;110:339–348.

95. Jiang G, Yang F, Van Overveld PG, Vedanarayanan V, van der MS, Ehrlich M. Testing the position-effect variegation hypothesis for facioscapulohumeral muscular dystrophy by analysis of histone modification and gene expression in subtelomeric 4q. Hum Mol Genet 2003;12:2909–2921.

96. Tupler R, Gabellini D. Molecular basis of facioscapulohumeral muscular dystrophy. Cell Mol Life Sci 2004;61:557–566.

97. van der Maarel SM, Frants RR. The D4Z4 repeat-mediated pathogenesis of facioscapulohumeral muscular dystrophy. Am J Hum Genet 2005;76:375–386.

98. Hewitt JE, Lyle R, Clark LN, et al. Analysis of the tandem repeat locus D4Z4 associated with facioscapulohumeral muscular dystrophy. Hum Mol Genet 1994;3:1287–1295.

99. Winokur ST, Bengtsson U, Feddersen J, et al. The DNA rearrangement associated with facioscapulohumeral muscular dystrophy involves a heterochromatin-associated repetitive element: implications for a role of chromatin structure in the pathogenesis of the disease. Chromosome Res 1994;2:225–234.

100. van Deutekom JCT. Towards the molecular mechanism of facioscapulohumeral muscular dystrophy. PhD thesis, Leiden University, Leiden, 1996.

101. Masny PS, Bengtsson U, Chung SA, et al. Localization of 4q35.2 to the nuclear periphery: is FSHD a nuclear envelope disease? Hum Mol Genet 2004;13:1857–1871.

102. Tam R, Smith KP, Lawrence JB. The 4q subtelomere harboring the FSHD locus is specifically anchored with peripheral heterochromatin unlike most human telomeres. J Cell Biol 2004;167:269–279.

103. Carter D, Chakalova L, Osborne CS, Dai YF, Fraser P. Long-range chromatin regulatory interactions in vivo. Nat Genet 2002;32:623–626.

104. Vakoc CR, Letting DL, Gheldof N, et al. Proximity among distant regulatory elements at the beta-globin locus requires GATA-1 and FOG-1. Mol Cell 2005;17:453–462.

105. Drissen R, Palstra RJ, Gillemans N, et al. The active spatial organization of the beta-globin locus requires the transcription factor EKLF. Genes Dev 2004;18:2485–2490.

106. Osborne CS, Chakalova L, Brown KE, et al. Active genes dynamically colocalize to shared sites of ongoing transcription. Nat Genet 2004;36:1065–1071.

107. Carter NP, Vetrie D. Applications of genomic microarrays to explore human chromosome structure and function. Hum Mol Genet 2004;13:R297–R302.

108. Bussiek M, Toth K, Brun N, Langowski J. DNA-loop formation on nucleosomes shown by in situ scanning force microscopy of supercoiled DNA. Mol Biol 2005;345:695–706.

109. Cmarko D, Verschure PJ, Otte AP, van Driel R, Fakan S. Polycomb group gene silencing proteins are concentrated in the perichromatin compartment of the mammalian nucleus. J Cell Sci 2003;116:335–343.

110. McArthur M, Gerum S, Stamatoyannopoulos G. Quantification of DNaseI-sensitivity by real-time PCR: quantitative analysis of DNaseI-hypersensitivity of the mouse beta-globin LCR. J Mol Biol 2001;313:27–34.

111. de Kok YJM, Vossenaar ER, Cremers CWRJ, et al. Identification of a hot spot for microdeletions in patients with X-linked deafness type 3 (DFN3) 900 kb proximal to the DFN3 gene POU3F4. Hum Mol Genet 1996;5:1229–1235.

112. Davies AF, Mirza G, Flinter F, Ragoussis J. An interstitial deletion of 6p24-p25 proximal to the FKHL7 locus and including AP-2alpha that affects anterior eye chamber development. J Med Genet 1999;36:708–710.

113. Jamieson RV, Perveen R, Kerr B, et al. Domain disruption and mutation of the bZIP transcription factor, MAF, associated with cataract, ocular anterior segment dysgenesis and coloboma. Hum Mol Genet 2002;11:33–42.

114. Kimura-Yoshida C, Kitajima K, Oda-Ishii I, et al. Characterization of the pufferfish Otx2 cis-regulators reveals evolutionarily conserved genetic mechanisms for vertebrate head specification. Development 2004;131:57–71.

115. Nobrega MA, Ovcharenko I, Afzal V, Rubin EM. Scanning human gene deserts for long-range enhancers. Science 2003;302:413.

116. Lee JA, Madrid RE, Sperle K, Ritterson C, Hobson GM, Garbern J, Lupski JR, Inoue K. Spastic paraplegia type 2 associated with axonal neuropathy and apparent PLP1 position effect. Ann Neurol 2005;in press.

117. Muncke N, Wogatzky BS, Breuning M, et al. Position effect on PLP1 may cause a subset of Pelizaeus-Merzbacher disease symptoms. J Med Genet 2004;41:e121.

118. Shen JJ, Kurotaki N, Patel A, Lupski JR, Brown CW. Low factor XII level in an individual with Sotos syndrome. Pediatr Blood Cancer 2005;44:187–189.

VI Genomic Disorders: Modeling and Assays

26 Chromosome-Engineered Mouse Models

Pentao Liu, PhD

CONTENTS

INTRODUCTION

Chromosome rearrangements cause genomic disorders and cancer in human. Region-specific low-copy repeats (LCRs) can mediate nonallelic homologous recombination (NAHR) that results in chromosome rearrangements. Using the Cre-*lox*P site-specific recombination system, chromosome rearrangements that cause genomic disorders and cancer can be recapitulated in the mouse. Technology advancements in mouse genetics, such as recombineering, will undoubtedly facilitate modeling genetic changes associated with genomic disorders in the mouse.

GENOMIC DISORDERS

In the last decade, a novel class of human disorders caused by chromosome rearrangements owing to regional structural characteristics of the genome has been recognized. These conditions are referred to as genomic disorders *(1)*. A common biological consequence of the chromosome rearrangements in genomic disorders is copy number change of dosage-sensitive gene(s) within the rearranged region.

The unique genomic architectures associated with genomic disorders include complex region-specific LCRs that are usually 10–500 kb in size and greater than 95% in sequence identity *(2,3)*. LCRs can stimulate and mediate NAHR, which in turn leads to unstable genomic regions that are prone to chromosome rearrangements *(4)*. It is estimated that as much as 5–10% of the human genome might be duplicated, reflecting the recent evolution of LCRs in the primate lineage *(5)*. In contrast to the human genome, preliminary analysis of the mouse genome suggests that only 1.7–2.0% is part of recent large segmental duplications (less than

From: *Genomic Disorders: The Genomic Basis of Disease*
Edited by: J. R. Lupski and P. Stankiewicz © Humana Press, Totowa, NJ

half of what is observed for the human genome) *(6)*. In general chromosome rearrangements caused by NAHR are usually relatively small in size (i.e., <2–3 Mb) and often difficult to detect cytogenetically. However, these rearrangements are large from a molecular viewpoint. Therefore, molecular approaches, such as pulsed-field gel electrophoresis, fluorescent *in situ* hybridization, and more recently array-based comparative genomic hybridization (aCGH), are used for their detection and analysis.

TRANSGENESIS AND GENE TARGETING IN THE MOUSE

The mouse is the most widely used experimental organism to model human disease and to study mammalian development. One important reason is that humans and mice share remarkable genetic similarity. These two species diverged from a common ancestor approx 75 million years ago *(7,8)* but share a similar genome size (3×10^{-9} bp), have a similar number of genes (25,000–30,000), and display a high homology between individual genes. Furthermore, the two genomes share extensive syntenic regions with orthologous genes present in the same order on the chromosomes *(9)*. For example, the whole human chromosome 17 is syntenic to the distal part of the mouse chromosome 11. Similarities between the mouse and human extend to anatomical, embryological, physiological, and other biological traits. Additional advantages of mice include small size, short life span, and rapid reproductive cycle. Perhaps the biggest advantage of using mice to model human disease is the availability of tremendous genetic resources. For example, there are many inbred mouse strains available that have strain-specific characteristics and show striking differences in many biological traits. William Castle and Clarence Cook Little developed the concept of inbred strains of mice where mice are generated by a minimum of 20 consecutive generations of brother–sister mating *(10)*. As a result, all the loci in the genome of an inbred mouse strain are homozygous. The pure genetic background in inbred mice is essential for performing genetic analyses.

Genetically modified mice became available when transgenic technologies were developed *(11–15)*. To generate a transgenic mouse line, a tissue-specific promoter linked to a DNA fragment (usually the cDNA of a gene) is microinjected into the pronuclei of fertilized mouse egg to produce founder lines. In general, transgenic mouse technology is primarily used to determine the phenotypic consequence associated with overexpression or ectopic expression of a studied gene *(16)*. A wealth of knowledge of gene function has been obtained from studying transgenic mice, however, the conventional transgenic mouse technology has its limitations. For instance, in addition to being unable to generate loss of function mutations, conventional transgenesis does not allow one to control either transgene copy number or integration site. Furthermore, the expression of a transgene is often affected by position effects from surrounding chromatin.

The ability to precisely engineer the mouse genome is the breakthrough that has brought mice to the forefront of biological research. This breakthrough combined two technology fronts: first, embryonic stem (ES) cells derived from the inner cell mass of normal mouse embryos were isolated in cell culture *(17,18)* and were later found to retain their pluripotency including the ability to colonize the mouse germline *(19)*. Second, it became possible to perform homologous recombination in mammalian cells *(20,21)*, and later in mouse ES cells *(22)*, thus, enabling genetic manipulation at a specific locus- targeting. Since the first true knockout mice were born *(23)*, gene targeting technology has revolutionized mouse genetics and disease-modeling. It is estimated that more than 3000 mouse genes have been targeted in

ES cells and knockout mice derived. These mutant mice have provided fundamental insights into gene function in mammals.

CHROMOSOME ENGINEERING IN THE MOUSE

The conventional gene knockout technology can generate identifiable genomic deletions up to 19 kb *(24)*. However, this is not sufficient to model large chromosome rearrangements found in human genomic disorders. Chromosome rearrangements can be induced by either X-ray or chemicals in the mouse *(25–27)*. However, the randomness of the endpoints in the irradiation-induced chromosome rearrangements has hampered broader applications for such genetic approaches to produce research resources. Chromosome engineering technology was developed to enable the construction of rearrangements of defined sizes in specific genomic locations. It combines gene targeting that defines chromosome rearrangement endpoints, and a site-specific recombination system from bacteriaphage P1, Cre-*lox*P, that can mediate recombination between two *lox*P sites. Cre is a 38-kDa recombinase that alone can catalyse recombination between two 34-bp *lox*P sites in mammalian cells *(28)*. Prior to its application in chromosome engineering, Cre-*lox*P system had been used to make small genomic deletions in conditional knockout mice *(29,30)*.

In 1993, while a graduate student in the laboratory of Professor Allan Bradley, together with Ramiro Ramirez-Solis, a postdoctoral fellow in the lab, I tested the Cre-*lox*P system for its ability to induce large chromosomal rearrangements. It was known that the Cre-*lox*P system is capable of efficiently inducing smaller deletions of a few thousands basepairs in mammalian cells. We anticipated that the intrachromosomal recombination efficiencies between two *lox*P sites that are millions of basepairs away, or that are on two different chromosomes, could be very low and a positive selection might, therefore, be required to detect and to recover the large recombination products. In an ideal positive selection system, a selection marker would be activated on Cre-*lox*P recombination and the recombinants could, thus, be selected out in appropriate medium. We chose the human hypoxanthine phosphoribosyl transferase (HPRT) minigene as the positive selection marker for two reasons. First, an *Hprt* deficient ES cell line, AB2.2, was available in the lab and it had been shown to be capable of highly efficient germline transmission. The second reason is the unique structure of the *HPRT* minigene which contains intron 2 of the human *HPRT* gene that is required for efficient expression in mouse ES cells. A *lox*P site can therefore be conveniently inserted into the middle of this intron (*Xba*I site) without affecting the *HPRT* minigene activity. We subsequently divided the *HPRT* minigene into two non-functional parts, the 5' and the 3' cassettes with the intronic *lox*P site embedded in both cassettes (Fig. 1). On recombination mediated by *lox*P sites and catalyzed by Cre, a full-length *HPRT* minigene is reconstituted and the recombinant can be selected out using hypoxanthine amniopterin thymidine (HAT) medium (Fig. 1).

To generate a defined chromosome rearrangement, the recombination cassettes need to be targeted, on a sequential manner, to two endpoints. We tested the ability of the *HPRT* selection system to generate chromosome rearrangements between the *Hsd17β* and the *Gastrin* loci separated by approx 1 Mb on the mouse chromosome 11 *(31)*. As illustrated in Fig. 1, the 5' *HPRT* cassette was targeted to the *Hsd17β* locus in ES cells. The 3' *HPRT* cassette was then targeted to the *Gastrin* locus in ES cells with the 5' *HPRT* cassette already targeted into the *Hsd17β* locus. To induce the recombination, double-targeted ES cells were transfected with a plasmid that transiently expressed Cre. We recovered all of the expected recombinants in

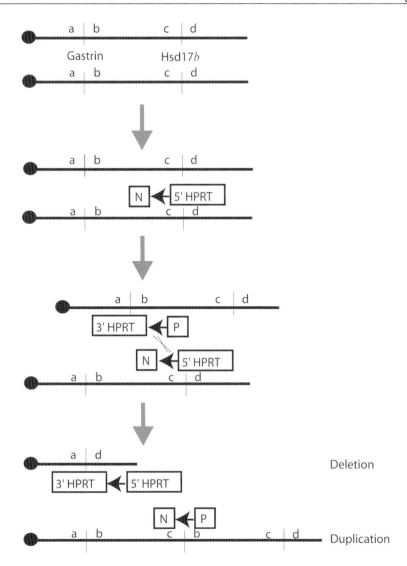

Fig. 1. Chromosome engineering between *Hsd17β* and *Gastrin* loci on the mouse chromosome 11. (A) Loci on the chromosome 11 are represented by *a*, *b*, *c*, and *d*. (B) The two recombination cassettes (5' and 3') are targeted consecutively to the two desired rearrangement endpoints (*Hsd17β* and *Gastrin*) in embryonic stem (ES) cells. (C) Recombination between the two *lox*P sites catalyzed by Cre recombinase regenerates a full-length *HPRT* minigene that enables the deletion to be selected for in HAT medium. (D) When the two cassettes are targeted to the two chromosome 11 homologous, both the deletion and the duplication can be recovered in a single ES cell. Filled arrow, *lox*P site; *P*, puromycin resistance cassette; *N*, neomycin resistant cassette.

HAT medium and confirmed the anticipated rearranged genomic structures by Southern hybridization *(31)*.

In order to generate a desired chromosome rearrangement, it is critical to know the orientation of two endpoints relative to each other on the chromosome and to the centromere because of the nature of the selection. As we described in the initial chromosome engineering experiments *(31)*, to obtain a deletion without prior knowledge of the endpoint orientation, four types of double-targeted ES cells had to be generated and tested. For example, generation of a deletion requires the two recombination cassettes in the correct orientation so that after recombination the *HPRT* minigene is reconstituted on the deletion chromosome in order to survive HAT selection. The finished mouse genome sequence *(9)* now enables one to obtain the information regarding the position and orientation of the two endpoints for a specific rearrangement. As a result, the recombination substrates can be targeted to the endpoints and the desired rearrangement can be obtained reliably and diagnosed readily.

Cre-*lox*P-mediated recombination can occur either *in cis* (two *lox*P sites are on the same chromosome) or *in trans* (two *lox*P sites are on different chromosomes). Figure 1 shows that when two recombination cassettes are targeted to two homologous chromosomes, both the deletion and the duplication can potentially be generated and recovered in a single ES cell. When these genetically balanced ES cells contribute to the mouse germline, from one chimaera, offspring with either the deletion or the duplication chromosomes can be recovered *(32)*.

Following the initial success with 1-Mb chromosomal rearrangements, we found that even larger chromosomal rearrangements could be successfully induced and recovered with the *HPRT* minigene selection system, with sizes ranging from 3 to 22 cM *(32)*. Most importantly, after multiple rounds of manipulation, ES cells harboring the engineered chromosomal rearrangements still retained the competence for germline transmission. This finding is often overlooked but represents a key step in chromosome engineering because, after multiple rounds of manipulation, ES cells were originally thought to lose germline competence. Further extension of the *HPRT* minigene selection system has facilitated the development of induced mitotic recombination in mouse ES cells *(33)*.

The ability to generate designed chromosomal rearrangements opens a new research field and offers new genetic resources. For example, in addition to modeling human disease, chromosome deletions can be used to uncover recessive mutations in genetic screens in vitro and in vivo *(34)*. Chromosome inversions can be engineered to function as balancers to facilitate *N*-ethyl-*N*-nitrosourea mutagenesis screens and to maintain mutant mouse lines *(35)*.

In addition to Cre-*lox*P-mediated chromosome engineering, other approaches have been developed to generate chromosome rearrangements. One of these approaches is to irradiate F1 hybrid mouse ES cells *(36)*. The irradiated ES cells have a negative selection marker, Herpes simplex virus thymidine kinase *(HSV-TK)*, targeted by homologous recombination to a defined locus. If deletions caused by irradiation encompass the *TK*-tagged locus, the cells will survive in 2'-fluoro-2'-deoxy-5-iodo-1-β-D-arabinofuranosyluracil medium. The advantage of this approach is that from a single experiment, multiple deletions of various sizes centered on the tagged locus can potentially be recovered. These deletions are useful for estimating haploinsufficiency tolerance of various chromosome regions in ES cells and may be used directly for in vitro genetic screens *(37)*. Importantly, ES cells carrying these irradiation-induced deletions still retain their ability to contribute to germline development in chimaeras. Thus, large genomic deletions from these experiments are useful for estimating haploinsufficiency in the mouse prior to making precise chromosomal rearrangements in this genomic region using Cre-*lox*P and for modeling certain genomic disorders. For instance, several deletions on the mouse chromosome 5 syntenic to human 4p16.3 were produced in one experiment *(38)*. The mice heterozygous for these deletions have phenotype similar to Wolf-Hirschhorn syndrome caused by monosomy 4p16.3. Thus, these deletion mice can directly serve as the mouse models for human disease syndromes *(38)*.

Compared to the *TK*-anchored deletion strategy, chromosome engineering using Cre-*lox*P has advantages. First, defined chromosome rearrangements can only be obtained with the precisely engineered endpoints (preselected loci). Second, other types of rearrangements, such as duplications, inversions, and translocations, can also be generated with chromosome engineering. Third, when a large chromosome rearrangement needs to be induced only in somatic cells, site-specific recombination is much more efficient.

MICER and Insertion Vectors

One important practical limitation for chromosome engineering is construction of targeting vectors to introduce the recombination cassettes to the rearrangement endpoints. Previously, genomic DNA libraries in λ-phage were screened with specific probes in order to isolate genomic DNA fragments to serve as the homology regions in gene targeting. Targeting vectors are then constructed by ligating two homology arms to one of the recombination substrates (5' or 3' *HPRT-lox*P cassettes). However, it could take one person a couple of months to build a targeting vector with this approach. To improve the efficiency of this step, the Bradley laboratory at Baylor College of Medicine constructed two mouse genomic phage libraries in which 10-kb genomic DNA fragments are cloned into two complementary backbones (Fig. 2) *(39)*. The cloning backbone for the first library has the 5' *HPRT-lox*P cassette, a *PGKNeobpA* positive selection cassette, and the *Tyrosinase* coat color gene for easy identification of the mice (Fig. 2A). On the other hand, the 3' *HPRT-lox*P cassette, the *PGKpurobpA* selection cassette, and the *Agouti* coat color gene are cloned into the backbone of the 3' *HPRT* library (Fig. 2B) *(39)*. As a result, clones from these two libraries can be used directly as premade gene targeting vectors for chromosome engineering. Recently, The Wellcome Trust Sanger Institute has sequenced the two *HPRT-lox*P genomic libraries (Mutagenic Insertion and Chromosome Engineering Resource [MICER]) (http://www.sanger.ac.uk/PostGenomics/mousegenomics/) *(40)*. Individual MICER clones can now be viewed directly on the Ensembl website and ordered through the Sanger Institute (http://www.sanger.ac.uk/cgi-bin/teams/team38/CloneRequest/CloneRequest).

To make a defined chromosome rearrangement, MICER clones corresponding to the two endpoints are linearized within the genomic inserts to generate a DNA double strand-break that stimulates efficient homologous recombination (Fig. 2). Gene targeting in ES cells with these vectors has been shown to be very efficient *(40)*. Targeting events in ES cells using MICER clones can be identified using a DNA fragment that is removed from the genomic DNA insert in the linearization process, or using an external probe, in Southern hybridization *(39,41)*.

Although MICER clones provide a convenient way to make targeting vectors for chromosome engineering, they are all insertion targeting vectors that can introduce challenges compared to replacement vectors *(42)*. Because there is no negative selection marker present on insertion vectors, on homologous recombination, these vectors can potentially form concatemers that may greatly complicate analysis of targeted events. Concatemerization of the recombination substrates may also complicate the ensuing Cre-*lox*P recombination because multiple *lox*P sites in a concatemer might have different orientations.

To obtain clean targeting events, replacement vectors are usually used. Genomic DNA fragments serving as the two homology-arms are isolated so that the recombination cassettes can be placed between them. This can be difficult in many cases because appropriate restriction enzyme sites have to be found or engineered in order to ligate all the DNA fragments together.

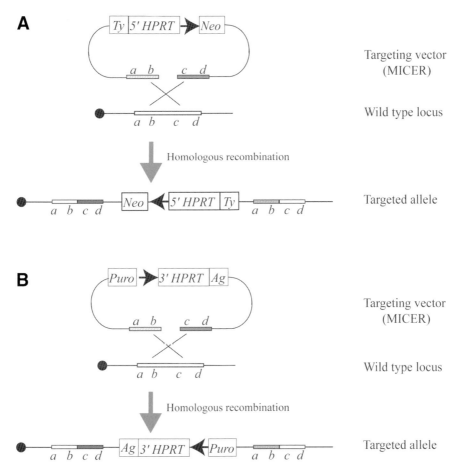

Fig. 2. Mutagenic Insertion and Chromosome Engineering Resource (MICER) clones for chromosome engineering. (A) Clones from the first MICER library carry the *5' HPRT* cassette, *Neo* and a *Tyrosinase* minigene (*Ty*). (B) Clones from the second MICER library have the *3' HPRT* cassette, Puromycin resistance cassette (*Puro*) and a *K14-agouti* (*Ag*) cassette. Vectors are linearized in the middle of the genomic fragments (*a, b, c, d*) to create a DNA double strand break for homologous recombination. Filled arrow, *lox*P site.

Recombineering

In the last few years, a highly efficient approach to manipulate DNA in *Escherichia coli*, termed recombineering *(43,44)*, has become available. This technology utilizes the bacteria phage λ-homologous recombination system, called Red. Recombineering allows DNA with homology as short as 50 bp to be recombined efficiently in *E. coli* and as a result has facilitated many kinds of genomic manipulations and experiments that previously were difficult to implement.

Three phage proteins are required for the λ-Red functions: Exo, Beta, and Gam *(45)*. Exo is a 5'>3' exonuclease that acts on linear double-strand DNA (dsDNA) to generate 3' single-strand DNA (ssDNA) overhangs for recombination. β protein binds to the ssDNA overhangs created by Exo and stimulates complementary strand annealing. The recombination is further enhanced by Gam, which inhibits the RecBCD activity of the host cell. RecBCD is a major nuclease that degrades exogenous double strand DNA in *E. coli*. In 1998, Francis Stewart's laboratory first discovered that homologous recombination function encoded by a prophage (Rac, encodes RecE and RecT) can be used to engineer cloned DNA *(43)*. Soon after this seminal work, an alternative system was developed in a collaboration between Court et al. and Copeland et al. *(46,47)*. In this new system, a defective λ-phage with a temperature sensitive repressor, *cI857*, is inserted into the *E. coli* genome. As a result, the λ-Red functions can be induced by shifting culture temperature from 32 to 42°C for 10–15 minutes. Experience from many laboratories showed that this system appears more efficient than the original RecET system *(48)*.

To construct targeting vectors for chromosome engineering using recombineering, the original *HPRT* minigene cassettes are modified with selection markers that are functional in both ES cells and in *E. coli* (Chan et al. unpublished). For example, the 5' *HPRT* cassette is linked to an engineered *Neo* gene that is selectable in ES cells and in *E. coli (49)*. Similarly, the 3' *HPRT* cassette is linked with a *Bsd* cassette that is selectable with Blasticidin in both ES cells and in *E. coli*. The next step is to transform a bacterial artificial chromosome (BAC) containing one rearrangement endpoint into recombineering-competent *E. coli* cells such as DY380 (Fig. 3) *(47)*. Alternatively, a mini-λ construct can be transformed to the original BAC containing host *E. coli* cells *(50)*. Once the BAC is established in DY380 cells, the recombination cassette (for example the *5' HPRT-Neo*) flanked by short homology sequences can be targeted to a precise position on the BAC by recombineering (Fig. 3). The final targeting vector can subsequently be constructed by retrieving the genomic DNA fragment containing the corresponding recombination substrate to a plasmid backbone. This process has proven to be very efficient and reliable *(49)*. The major advantage of using recombineering over premade targeting vector libraries is that more flexible designs can be easily introduced to a precise genomic location. The prerequisite for using recombineering is that the genomic sequence of a given locus is known. The availability of the mouse genome sequences greatly facilitates the broader use of recombineering in mouse genetics. Nevertheless, the current mouse genome sequence in the public database is from the C57BL6 strain, whereas most mouse ES cell lines are derived from various 129 strains. It is therefore essential that genomic resources based on the 129 strains of mice should be established and made available to the research community. For instance, at least one BAC library from a 129 strain should be end-sequenced and placed into public databases. These BACs would best serve the research community if they are already in recombineering-competent host cells.

Stewart's lab has shown recently that a BAC carrying multiple selection cassettes engineered using recombineering can be used to target multiple linked loci simultaneously *(51)*. This approach can be potentially modified to target the 5' and 3' recombination cassettes to the two rearrangement endpoints simultaneously in one cell transfection experiment. The success of this strategy can further reduce the laborious serial targeting required for chromosome engineering and increase the likelihood that the manipulated cells are still competent for germline transmission.

MOUSE MODELS GENERATED BY CHROMOSOME ENGINEERING

During the last decade, technology advances have already made generating large chromosome rearrangements possible in the mouse. Continuous development of new technologies will undoubtedly further facilitate our ability to engineer many kinds of chromosome changes associated with human disorders. Some of the recent successes that utilized chromosome engineering to model genomic disorders and to genetically dissect human disease are briefly described.

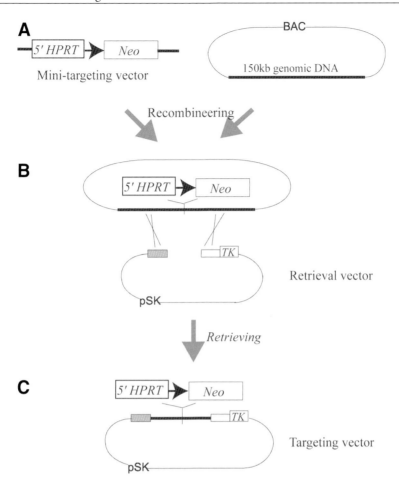

Fig. 3. Construction of targeting vectors by recombineering. (A) A bacterial artificial chromosome (BAC) with an approx 150-kb genomic DNA insert is transformed to recombineering competent *Escherichia coli* cells (DY380). The recombination substrate, 5'*HPRT* cassette, together with a *Neo/Kan* cassette, can be recombined using short homology arms (200–500 bp) to a precise position in the BAC with recombineering. (B) In the next step, a retrieval vector, which has two short homology arms (200–500 bp) corresponding to the ends of the interested genomic region, is linearized and electroporated to the BAC containing DY380 cells. (C) Homologous recombination (gap repair) between the two homology arms on the retrieval vector and the sequences on the BAC results in cloning of the genomic DNA and the targeted 5' *HPRT-Neo* cassette from the BAC to the retrieval vector. Different genetic elements such as a *TK* cassette (Herpes simplex virus thymidine kinase gene) for negative selection in embryonic stem cells can be engineered to the retrieval vector. A detailed description of this approach can be found in ref. *49*. pSK, plasmid pBluescript SK.

del22q11.2 *Syndrome*

del22q11.2 syndrome (also known as DiGeorge syndrome [DGS], velocardiofacial syndrome [VCFS], and conotruncal anomaly face syndrome) with an incidence of 1 in every 4000–5000 births, is the most frequent chromosomal microdeletion syndrome known *(52)*. The common deletion is caused by LCR-mediated recombination *(53–55)*. Typical patient phenotype includes cardiovascular defects, thymic, parathyroid, craniofacial anomalies, and learning disabilities. Many of the features (e.g., heart outflow tract, craniofacial, velopharyngeal, ear, thymic, and parathyroid abnormalities) are attributable to developmental defects of the embryonic pharyngeal apparatus.

Although at least 30 genes have been mapped to the common deletion region of *del22q11.2*, until recently, none of these genes had been shown to carry genetic mutations in the patients who do not have the common deletion. The mouse syntenic region of the *del22q11.2* genomic region is located on the mouse chromosome 16. Using chromosome engineering, a 1.2-Mb deletion (*Es2-Ufd1l*) was generated and the deletion was subsequently established in the mouse germline *(56)*. Some of the embryos and adult mice carrying the deletion in heterozygous status manifested cardiovascular defects on a mixed genetic background. However, these deletion mice did not have other phenotypes associated with the 22q11.2 deletion in the human patients. Nevertheless, the mutant mice did recapitulate one important phenotype of the *del22q11.2* syndrome, confirming that the disease-causing gene(s) is within this deletion interval.

To narrow the critical genomic region, Lindsay et al. *(57)* generated several smaller deletions and found that one deletion containing the transcription factor gene, *Tbx1*, is responsible for the cardiovascular defects in the mouse. Two additional evidences supported *Tbx1* is the causal gene. First, a P1 artificial chromosome containing *Tbx1* rescued the cardiovascular defects in the deltion mice. Second, a *Tbx1* hypomorphic allele confirmed that *Tbx1* is a dosage sensitive gene in the mouse and is required for normal development of the pharyngeal arch arteries *(57)*. In an independent study, a chromosomal deletion encompassing the *Tbx1* locus was generated by crossing two *lox*P sites, that were in the *del22q11.2* critical region but located on the two homologous chromosome 16, to *cis* configuration *(58)*. The deletion generated by Cre-*lox*P spanned approx 1 Mb and the heterozygous deletion mice had similar cardiovascular defects as found in the mice engineered by Lindsay et al. *(57)*.

To further confirm the role of *TBX1* in *del22q11.2*, a null allele of *Tbx1* was generated by gene targeting. Interestingly, although mice heterozygous for this null allele of *Tbx1* only had cardiac outflow tract anomalies (identical to the phenotype in the deletion heterozygotes), the *Tbx1* –/– mice displayed a wide range of developmental anomalies encompassing almost all of the common DGS/VCFS features, including hypoplasia of the thymus and parathyroid glands, cardiac outflow tract abnormalities, abnormal facial structures, abnormal vertebrae, and cleft palate *(59)*. Taken these data together, analysis of the genetically engineered mice strongly supported that haploinsufficiency of *TBX1* is responsible for most clinical findings in *del22q11.2* patients. This hypothesis has been confirmed by recent studies that identified *TBX1* mutations in patients with a typical *del22q11.2* phenotype but with no apparent genomic deletions *(60)*.

The *Tbx1* analyses represent an excellent demonstration of the power of using genetically modified mice to dissect the molecular basis of a human disease. It is interesting to note that the *Tbx1* gene appears to be more sensitive to dosage reduction in human than in the mouse. This may reflect species difference, an important aspect that should be taken into account when interpreting data obtained from genetically modified mouse models. It has been postulated that humans are more sensitive than the mouse to lower levels of the dosage-sensitive gene products and, thus, display increased phenotype penetrance *(59)*. In support of this view, in several other cases, including *MSX2* and *PAX9*, heterozygous effects are evident in humans but not in the mouse, but the homozygous effects in mouse are similar in nature to the human heterozygous effects *(61–64)*. Another important lesson learned from genetic dissection of *del22q11.2* in the mouse is that genetic heterogeneity may be common for human disease. Analyses of hundreds of patients with apparent *del22q11.2* phenotype but without the deletion failed to identify any *TBX1* mutations in several previous studies *(57,58)*. Identifying the *TBX1* mutations became possible only when the studies were implemented in the potential mutation-carrying patients with extremely careful clinical examination *(60)*.

Smith-Magenis Syndrome Deletion and the Reciprocal Dup(17)(p11.2p11.2)

Smith-Magenis syndrome (SMS) is a genomic disorder associated with a deletion within sub-band p11.2 of chromosome 17 *(65)*. The common deletion is caused by NAHR mediated by LCRs named SMS-REPs *(66)*. The clinical phenotypes of SMS includes craniofacial abnormalities, brachydactyly, self-injurious behavior, sleep abnormalities, and mental retardation *(65)*. Patients with the predicted reciprocal duplication recombination product have less severe clinical phenotype: mild to borderline mental retardation and behavioral difficulties *(67)*.

Using the Cre-*lox*P chromosome engineering technology, Walz et al. *(68)* generated mice that carry a deletion on the mouse chromosome 11, which is partially syntenic to the genomic interval frequently deleted in SMS patients. Heterozygous mice carrying this deletion have craniofacial abnormalities, seizures, marked obesity, and male-specific reduced fertility.

On the other hand, mice heterozygous for a duplication of the same genomic region are underweight, do not have seizures, craniofacial abnormalities or fertility defects, but are hyperactive, and have impaired contextual fear conditioning *(68,69)*. Importantly, mice that have the deletion and the duplication (compound heterozygous) do not have any of the major phenotypes consistent with the hypothesis that the traits expression is caused by gene dosage effects and most probably not by position effects from altered chromosomal structures in both rearrangements.

Retinoic acid-induced gene 1 (*RAI1*) has been found recently mutated in rare patients with many features of SMS but without a recognizable deletion. Therefore, *RAI1* has been proposed to be the major player in the SMS phenotype *(70)*. Analysis of *RAI1* knockout mice and mice with increased dosage of *RAI1* should identify the in vivo biological function of this gene and confirm its role in SMS. In the meantime, it is also necessary to generate nested deletions and duplications within the SMS genomic region to identify genes that might cause minor phenotypes or are genetic modifiers of the phenotypes caused by *RAI1* mutations.

Modeling Chromosomal Rearrangements of Cancer

Genomic rearrangements also play critical role in cancer. Recurrent genomic aberrations have been found in both human lymphomas and solid tumors *(71,72)*. For technical reasons, one type of genomic aberrations, recurrent balanced chromosomal translocations, are better characterized in human leukaemia and lymphomas *(73)*. Among the most common chromosomal translocation breakpoint regions in human leukaemia is chromosome 11q23. These translocations involve the mixed-lineage leukaemia gene, *MLL*, and greater than 30 different *MLL* fusion partners *(74)*, whereas the identity of these partners determines the etiology of the subsequent leukaemia in humans. Based on the Cre-*lox*P technology, a chromosomal translocation between *MLL* and eleven nineteen leukaemia (*Enl*) was induced specifically in haematopoietic cells in mice. These translocation mice developed a rapid onset and high penetrance of leukemogenesis that models many key aspects of the human disease *(75)*.

Other chromosomal aberrations found in human cancer include interstitial deletions and amplifications. In general, a deletion indicates the presence of a tumor suppressor gene, whereas an amplified region contains one or more oncogenes. The chromosomal deletions can be modeled relatively easily using chromosome engineering. Because most of the homozygous genomic deletions found in human tumors are large, establishing similar size deletions in the mouse would be difficult owing to possible embryonic lethality. To overcome this technical difficulty, large chromosome rearrangements can be induced by expressing Cre temporally and/or spatially in somatic cells. It is estimated that Cre can induce up to 10 cM rearrangements in the mouse without significantly reducing the recombination efficiency *(76)*. Using chromosome engineering, mice with four copies of a chromosome region can be generated. This copy number change is small compared to amplification of a chromosome region in cancer. However, it has been shown that moderate increase of copy number (three to eight absolute copies) of *PI3CA* is associated with activation of PI3 kinase activities and ovarian cancer *(77)*. It is also known that people with trisomy of certain chromosomes have greater cancer risk and poor clinical outcomes in leukaemia *(78)*. Therefore the genomic regions that are found to have moderate copy number increase from array-CGH can potentially be assessed for their relevance to cancer in the mouse with chromosome engineering.

Cancer is a complex genetic disease and multiple genetic events are usually required for cancer development. Mice harboring the engineered chromosomal rearrangements should be either put on a sensitized genetic background, or be challenged with mutagens to facilitate tumor development in order to assess the relevance of these genetic mutations to cancer development.

CONCLUSION

During the last decade, the ability to precisely engineer the mouse genome in ES cells and to establish the mutations in the mouse germline has revolutionized mouse genetics and human disease modeling. In particular, chromosome engineering has allowed us to model gross chromosomal changes found in human genomic disorders and in cancer.

Microarray-based CGH has become a powerful method for the genome-wide detection of genomic DNA copy number changes quantitatively and for mapping them directly onto the sequence of the human genome *(79–82)*. It is very likely that, with these genomic technologies being more widely applied in clinical diagnosis and analysis, many other submicroscopic genomic rearrangements as well as population-specific polymorphisms mediated by LCRs/NAHR will be detected. Similarly, more recurrent chromosomal changes will be found to be involved in cancer initiation and progression. Furthermore, with systematic analysis of finished human genome sequence, more genomic regions will be predicted to be prone to genomic rearrangements. Modeling these genomic changes in the mouse is exciting and will undoubtedly provide us important clues to the biological consequences of these genomic mutations.

ACKNOWLEDGMENTS

The author thanks Kathryn Chapman for critical comments on the manuscript.

REFERENCES

1. Lupski JR. Genomic disorders: structural features of the genome can lead to DNA rearrangements and human disease traits. Trends Genet 1998;14:417–422.
2. Inoue K, Lupski JR. Molecular mechanisms for genomic disorders. Annu Rev Genomics Hum Genet 2002;3: 199–242.
3. Stankiewicz P, Lupski JR. Genome architecture, rearrangements and genomic disorders. Trends Genet 2002;18:74–82.

4. Shaw CJ, Lupski JR. Implications of human genome architecture for rearrangement-based disorders: the genomic basis of disease. Hum Mol Genet 2004;13:R57–R64.

5. Samonte RV, Eichler EE. Segmental duplications and the evolution of the primate genome. Nat Rev Genet 2002;3:65–72.

6. Bailey JA, Church DM, Ventura M, Rocchi M, Eichler EE. Analysis of segmental duplications and genome assembly in the mouse. Genome Res 2004;14:789–801.

7. Madsen O, Scally M, Douady CJ, et al. Parallel adaptive radiations in two major clades of placental mammals. Nature 2001;409:610–614.

8. Murphy WJ, Eizirik E, Johnson WE, Zhang YP, Ryder OA, O'Brien SJ. Molecular phylogenetics and the origins of placental mammals. Nature 2001;409:614–618.

9. Waterston RH, Lindblad-Toh K, Birney E, et al. Initial sequencing and comparative analysis of the mouse genome. Nature 2002;420:520–562.

10. Morse H. *Origins of Inbred Mice*. New York, NY: Academic Press, 1978.

11. Gordon JW, Scangos GA, Plotkin DJ, Barbosa JA, Ruddle FH. Genetic transformation of mouse embryos by microinjection of purified DNA. Proc Natl Acad Sci USA 1980;77:7380–7384.

12. Brinster RL, Chen HY, Trumbauer M, Senear AW, Warren R, Palmiter RD. Somatic expression of herpes thymidine kinase in mice following injection of a fusion gene into eggs. Cell 1981;27:223–231.

13. Costantini F, Lacy E. Introduction of a rabbit beta-globin gene into the mouse germ line. Nature 1981;294: 92–94.

14. Wagner EF, Stewart TA, Mintz B. The human beta-globin gene and a functional viral thymidine kinase gene in developing mice. Proc Natl Acad Sci USA 1981;78:5016–5020.

15. Wagner TE, Hoppe PC, Jollick JD, Scholl DR, Hodinka RL, Gault JB. Microinjection of a rabbit beta-globin gene into zygotes and its subsequent expression in adult mice and their offspring. Proc Natl Acad Sci USA 1981;78:6376–6380.

16. Hanahan D. Transgenic mice as probes into complex systems. Science 1989;246:1265–1275.

17. Evans MJ, Kaufman MH. Establishment in culture of pluripotential cells from mouse embryos. Nature 1981;292:154–156.

18. Martin GR. Isolation of a pluripotent cell line from early mouse embryos cultured in medium conditioned by teratocarcinoma stem cells. Proc Natl Acad Sci USA 1981;78:7634–7638.

19. Bradley A, Evans M, Kaufman MH, Robertson E. Formation of germ-line chimaeras from embryo-derived teratocarcinoma cell lines. Nature 1984;309:255–256.

20. Smithies O, Gregg RG, Boggs SS, Koralewski MA, Kucherlapati RS. Insertion of DNA sequences into the human chromosomal beta-globin locus by homologous recombination. Nature 1985;317:230–234.

21. Thomas KR, Capecchi MR. Introduction of homologous DNA sequences into mammalian cells induces mutations in the cognate gene. Nature 1986;324:34–38.

22. Thomas KR, Capecchi MR. Site-directed mutagenesis by gene targeting in mouse embryo-derived stem cells. Cell 1987;51:503–512.

23. Thompson S, Clarke AR, Pow AM, Hooper ML, Melton DW. Germ line transmission and expression of a corrected HPRT gene produced by gene targeting in embryonic stem cells. Cell 1989;56:313–321.

24. Zhang H, Hasty P, Bradley A. Targeting frequency for deletion vectors in embryonic stem cells. Mol Cell Biol 1994;14:2404–2410.

25. Russell WL. X-ray-induced mutations in mice. Cold Spring Harb Symp Quant Biol 1951;16:327–336.

26. Russell LB, Hunsicker PR, Cacheiro NL, Bangham JW, Russell WL, Shelby MD. Chlorambucil effectively induces deletion mutations in mouse germ cells. Proc Natl Acad Sci USA 1989;86:3704–3708.

27. Stubbs L, Carver EA, Cacheiro NL, Shelby M, Generoso W. Generation and characterization of heritable reciprocal translocations in mice. Methods 1997;13:397–408.

28. Sauer B, Henderson N. Site-specific DNA recombination in mammalian cells by the Cre recombinase of bacteriophage P1. Proc Natl Acad Sci USA 1988;85:5166–5170.

29. Gu H, Zou YR, Rajewsky K. Independent control of immunoglobulin switch recombination at individual switch regions evidenced through Cre-loxP-mediated gene targeting. Cell 1993;73:1155–1164.

30. Gu H, Marth JD, Orban PC, Mossmann H, Rajewsky K. Deletion of a DNA polymerase beta gene segment in T cells using cell type-specific gene targeting. Science 1994;265:103–106.

31. Ramirez-Solis R, Liu P, Bradley A. Chromosome engineering in mice. Nature 1995;378:720–724.

32. Liu P, Zhang H, McLellan A, Vogel H, Bradley A. Embryonic lethality and tumorigenesis caused by segmental aneuploidy on mouse chromosome 11. Genetics 1998;150:1155–1168.

33. Liu P, Jenkins NA, Copeland NG. Efficient Cre-loxP-induced mitotic recombination in mouse embryonic stem cells. Nat Genet 2002;30:66–72.

34. Kile BT, Hentges KE, Clark AT, et al. Functional genetic analysis of mouse chromosome 11. Nature 2003;425:81–86.

35. Zheng B, Sage M, Cai WW, et al. Engineering a mouse balancer chromosome. Nat Genet 1999;22:375–378.

36. You Y, Bergstrom R, Klemm M, et al. Chromosomal deletion complexes in mice by radiation of embryonic stem cells. Nat Genet 1997;15:285–288.

37. Chen Y, Yee D, Dains K, et al. Genotype-based screen for ENU-induced mutations in mouse embryonic stem cells. Nat Genet 2000;24:314–317.

38. Naf D, Wilson LA, Dergstrom RA, et al. Mouse models for the Wolf-Hirschhorn deletion syndrome. Hum Mol Genet 2001;10:91–98.

39. Zheng B, Mills AA, Bradley A. A system for rapid generation of coat color-tagged knockouts and defined chromosomal rearrangements in mice. Nucleic Acids Res 1999;27:2354–2360.

40. Adams DJ, Biggs PJ, Cox T, et al. Mutagenic nsertion and chromosome engineering resource (MICER). Nat Genet 2004;36:867–871.

41. Mills AA, Bradley A. From mouse to man: generating megabase chromosome rearrangements. Trends Genet 2001;17:331–339.

42. Hasty P, Rivera-Perez J, Chang C, Bradley A. Target frequency and integration pattern for insertion and replacement vectors in embryonic stem cells. Mol Cell Biol 1991;11:4509–4517.

43. Zhang Y, Buchholz F, Muyrers JP, Stewart AF. A new logic for DNA engineering using recombination in Escherichia coli. Nat Genet 1998;20:123–128.

44. Copeland NG, Jenkins NA, Court DL. Recombineering: a powerful new tool for mouse functional genomics. Nat Rev Genet 2001;2:769–779.

45. Court DL, Sawitzke JA, Thomason LC. Genetic engineering using homologous recombination. Annu Rev Genet 2002;36:361–388.

46. Yu D, Ellis HM, Lee EC, Jenkins NA, Copeland NG, Court DL. An efficient recombination system for chromosome engineering in Escherichia coli. Proc Natl Acad Sci USA 2000;97:5978–5983.

47. Lee EC, Yu D, Martinez de Velasco J, et al. A highly efficient Escherichia coli-based chromosome engineering system adapted for recombinogenic targeting and subcloning of BAC DNA. Genomics 2001;73:56–65.

48. Muyrers JP, Zhang Y, Buchholz F, Stewart AF. RecE/RecT and Redalpha/Redbeta initiate double-stranded break repair by specifically interacting with their respective partners. Genes Dev 2000;14:1971–1982.

49. Liu P, Jenkins NA, Copeland NG. A highly efficient recombineering-based method for generating conditional knockout mutations. Genome Res 2003;13:476–484.

50. Court DL, Swaminathan S, Yu D, et al. Mini-lambda: a tractable system for chromosome and BAC engineering. Gene 2003;315:63–69.

51. Testa G, Zhang Y, Vintersten K, et al. Engineering the mouse genome with bacterial artificial chromosomes to create multipurpose alleles. Nat Biotechnol 2003;21:443–447.

52. Scambler PJ. The 22q11 deletion syndromes. Hum Mol Genet 2000;9:2421–2426.

53. Edelmann L, Pandita RK, Morrow BE. Low-copy repeats mediate the common 3-Mb deletion in patients with velo-cardio-facial syndrome. Am J Hum Genet 1999;64:1076–1086.

54. Edelmann L, Pandita RK, Spiteri E, et al. A common molecular basis for rearrangement disorders on chromosome 22q11. Hum Mol Genet 1999;8:1157–1167.

55. Shaikh TH, Kurahashi H, Emanuel BS. Evolutionarily conserved low copy repeats (LCRs) in 22q11 mediate deletions, duplications, translocations, and genomic instability: an update and literature review. Genet Med 2001;3:6–13.

56. Lindsay EA, Botta A, Jurecic V, et al. Congenital heart disease in mice deficient for the DiGeorge syndrome region. Nature 1999;401:379–383.

57. Lindsay EA, Vitelli F, Su H, et al. Tbx1 haploinsufficieny in the DiGeorge syndrome region causes aortic arch defects in mice. Nature 2001;410:97–101.

58. Merscher S, Funke B, Epstein JA, et al. TBX1 is responsible for cardiovascular defects in velo-cardio-facial/ DiGeorge syndrome. Cell 2001;104:619–629.

59. Jerome LA, Papaioannou VE. DiGeorge syndrome phenotype in mice mutant for the T-box gene, Tbx1. Nat Genet 2001;27:286–291.

60. Yagi H, Furutani Y, Hamada H, et al. Role of TBX1 in human del22q11.2 syndrome. Lancet 2003;362: 1366–1373.

61. Stockton DW, Das P, Goldenberg M, D'Souza RN, Patel PI. Mutation of PAX9 is associated with oligodontia. Nat Genet 2000;24:18–19.

62. Peters H, Neubuser A, Kratochwil K, Balling R. Pax9-deficient mice lack pharyngeal pouch derivatives and teeth and exhibit craniofacial and limb abnormalities. Genes Dev 1998;12:2735–2747.

63. Satokata I, Ma L, Ohshima H, et al. Msx2 deficiency in mice causes pleiotropic defects in bone growth and ectodermal organ formation. Nat Genet 2000;24:391–395.

64. Wilkie AO, Tang Z, Elanko N, et al. Functional haploinsufficiency of the human homeobox gene MSX2 causes defects in skull ossification. Nat Genet 2000;24:387–390.

65. Greenberg F, Guzzetta V, Montes de Oca-Luna R, et al. Molecular analysis of the Smith-Magenis syndrome: a possible contiguous-gene syndrome associated with del(17)(p11.2). Am J Hum Genet 1991;49:1207–1218.

66. Chen KS, Manian P, Koeuth T, et al. Homologous recombination of a flanking repeat gene cluster is a mechanism for a common contiguous gene deletion syndrome. Nat Genet 1997;17:154–163.

67. Potocki L, Chen KS, Park SS, et al. Molecular mechanism for duplication 17p11.2- the homologous recombination reciprocal of the Smith-Magenis microdeletion. Nat Genet 2000;24:84–87.

68. Walz K, Caratini-Rivera S, Bi W, et al. Modeling del(17)(p11.2p11.2) and dup(17)(p11.2p11.2) contiguous gene syndromes by chromosome engineering in mice: phenotypic consequences of gene dosage imbalance. Mol Cell Biol 2003;23:3646–3655.

69. Walz K, Spencer C, Kaasik K, Lee CC, Lupski JR, Paylor R. Behavioral characterization of mouse models for Smith-Magenis syndrome and dup(17)(p11.2p11.2). Hum Mol Genet 2004;13:367–378.

70. Slager RE, Newton TL, Vlangos CN, Finucane B, Elsea SH. Mutations in RAI1 associated with Smith-Magenis syndrome. Nat Genet 2003;33:466–468.

71. Albertson DG, Collins C, McCormick F, Gray JW. Chromosome aberrations in solid tumors. Nat Genet 2003;34:369–376.

72. Rabbitts TH. Chromosomal translocations in human cancer. Nature 1994;372:143–149.

73. Rowley JD. The critical role of chromosome translocations in human leukemias. Annu Rev Genet 1998;32: 495–519.

74. Daser A, Rabbitts TH. Extending the repertoire of the mixed-lineage leukemia gene MLL in leukemogenesis. Genes Dev 2004;18:965–974.

75. Forster A, Pannell R, Drynan LF, et al. Engineering de novo reciprocal chromosomal translocations associated with Mll to replicate primary events of human cancer. Cancer Cell 2003;3:449–458.

76. Zheng B, Sage M, Sheppeard EA, Jurecic V, Bradley A. Engineering mouse chromosomes with Cre-loxP: range, efficiency, and somatic applications. Mol Cell Biol 2003;20:648–655.

77. Shayesteh L, Lu Y, Kuo WL, et al. PIK3CA is implicated as an oncogene in ovarian cancer. Nat Genet 1999;21:99–102.

78. Farag SS, Archer KJ, Mrozek K, et al. Isolated trisomy of chromosomes 8, 11, 13 and 21 is an adverse prognostic factor in adults with de novo acute myeloid leukemia: results from Cancer and Leukemia Group B 8461. Int J Oncol 2002;21:1041–1051.

79. Solinas-Toldo S, Lampel S, Stilgenbauer S, et al. Matrix-based comparative genomic hybridization: biochips to screen for genomic imbalances. Genes Chromosomes Cancer 1997;20:399–407.

80. Pinkel D, Segraves R, Sudar D, et al. High resolution analysis of DNA copy number variation using comparative genomic hybridization to microarrays. Nat Genet 1998;20:207–211.

81. Pollack JR, Perou CM, Alizadeh AA, et al. Genome-wide analysis of DNA copy-number changes using cDNA microarrays. Nat Genet 1999;23:41–46.

82. Cai WW, Mao JH, Chow CW, Damani S, Balmain A, Bradley A. Genome-wide detection of chromosomal imbalances in tumors using BAC microarrays. Nat Biotechnol 2002;20:393–396.

27

Array-CGH for the Analysis
of Constitutional Genomic Rearrangements

Nigel P. Carter, DPhil, Heike Fiegler, PhD,
Susan Gribble, PhD, and Richard Redon, PhD

CONTENTS

BACKGROUND
INTRODUCTION
ARRAY-CGH
ANALYSIS OF COPY NUMBER CHANGES
ARRAY PAINTING
HIGHER RESOLUTION ANALYSIS OF REARRANGEMENTS
OLIGONUCLEOTIDE ARRAYS
CONCLUSIONS
SUMMARY
REFERENCES

BACKGROUND

Rapid, high-resolution analysis of genomic rearrangements has become possible using array-comparative genomic hybridization (aCGH), a combination of CGH with DNA microarray technology. Using aCGH, genome copy number changes and rearrangement breakpoints can now be mapped and analyzed at resolutions down to a few kilobases or even less in a single hybridization. This technology is enabling us to identify previously hidden rearrangements in patients with suspected genomic disorders for which no karyotype aberrations could be identified using conventional cytogenetic analysis. Furthermore, the development of array painting has revealed a surprising level of rearrangement complexity in patients with apparently balanced translocations.

INTRODUCTION

The introduction of CGH *(1)* for the genome wide analysis of copy number changes opened up new opportunities for the study of genome rearrangement. In CGH, DNA from a test genome is fluorescently labeled in one color (e.g., red) and cohybridized with a reference, normal genome labeled in a second color (e.g., green) onto normal metaphase spreads. The

From: *Genomic Disorders: The Genomic Basis of Disease*
Edited by: J. R. Lupski and P. Stankiewicz © Humana Press, Totowa, NJ

labeled probes are prehybridized with Cot1 DNA to suppress repetitive elements to allow the hybridization to represent largely unique sequences in the genome. Where there is equal copy number between the two genomes, equal amounts of test and reference DNA hybridize and the region appears as a mixture of red and green. Where a region of the test genome is deleted, the corresponding region on the normal metaphase spreads hybridizes more reference DNA than test DNA so that the region appears green. Where a region of the test genome is gained or amplified, the corresponding region on the normal metaphase spreads hybridizes more test DNA than reference DNA and so appears red. By measuring the ratio of the fluorescences, orthogonal to and along each metaphase chromosome, ratio profiles are generated where a high ratio indicates copy number gain and a low ratio copy number loss.

The main application of this technology has been in the study of solid tumors, where it is difficult or impossible to access metaphase chromosomes for direct analysis of rearrangements *(2,3)*. CGH has also found application in the analysis of constitutional abnormalities particularly in nonrecurrent rearrangements where the genome scanning ability of CGH is particularly suited to identifying *de novo* abnormalities *(4)*. However, the resolution with which gains and losses can be identified is restricted by the use of normal metaphase chromosomes as the substrate for the comparative hybridization. In routine use this resolution is limited such that a single-copy loss needs to be in the order of 3–5 Mb in size to be detected *(5)*. With the availability of well-mapped clone resources as a product of the public domain effort to sequence the human genome, it became possible to replace and represent the metaphase chromosome with an arrayed series of large insert clones spotted onto glass slides. This methodology was described in 1997 as matrix-CGH *(6)* and shortly afterwards as aCGH *(7)*, a name which has fallen into common usage.

ARRAY-CGH

aCGH is performed essentially in the same way as metaphase CGH. Test and reference DNA are differentially labeled, preannealed with Cot1 DNA and then hybridized to the microarray. After washing, the slide is scanned and the intensity of each fluorescent DNA for each clone on the array measured. The fluorescence ratio is then plotted along the length of each chromosome using the mapped position of the clones (*see* Fig. 1). Again, gains are represented by increased ratios and losses by decreased ratios. With aCGH, analysis resolution is determined by the insert size and the density along the genome of the clones spotted onto the slide.

Clone DNA was originally extracted from large scale cultures for direct spotting onto slides *(6,7)*. Carrying out such large scale cultures quickly becomes a costly and time consuming process when expanded to the number of clones required to construct an array with a resolution of one clone every 1 Mb of the human genome (approx 3000 clones). To overcome this problem, several approaches have been applied to amplify the clone DNA enzymatically for spotting, thus removing the requirement for large-scale DNA preparations. These have included methods such as linker adapter polymerase chain reaction (PCR) *(8)*, rolling circle PCR using bacteriophage Phi29 *(9)*, or degenerate oligonucleotide primed PCR (DOP-PCR) *(10)* using an amine modified version of the standard DOP-PCR primer 6MW *(11,12)*. *Escherichia coli* genomic DNA however is a common contaminant of DNA preparations of large insert clones. The degree of contamination has been estimated by real-time PCR to be between 6 and 26% dependent on the method used for purification *(13)*. This contaminating *E. coli* DNA will reduce the capacity of each probe spotted on the array to hybridize with the DNA of interest and may contribute to increased nonspecific background signal. In order to overcome this

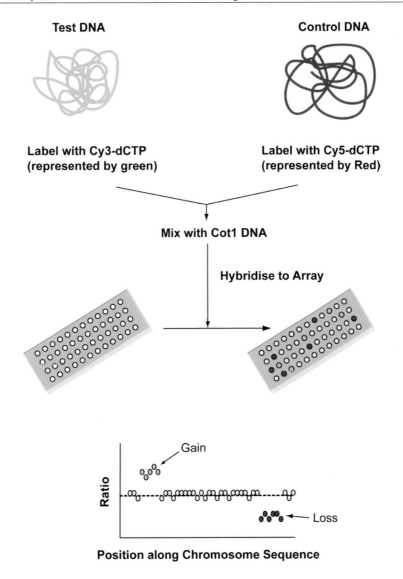

Fig. 1. Principle of array-comparative genomic hybridization.

problem, we designed three new DOP-PCR primers (DOP1, -2, and -3) that were chosen to be efficient in amplifying human genomic DNA but inefficient in amplifying the contaminating *E. coli* DNA *(14)*. The use of these three new DOP-PCR primers, particularly in combination, revealed a significant increase in sensitivity and reproducibility in genomic hybridizations compared to arrays constructed with the standard DOP-PCR primer 6MW *(14)*.

ANALYSIS OF COPY NUMBER CHANGES

aCGH, typically using arrays with a resolution of one clone per megabase, has been widely applied to the analysis of copy number alterations in solid tumors *(3)*. Figure 2 shows a typical result for a renal cell carcinoma cell line where the terminal part of chromosome 1p shows

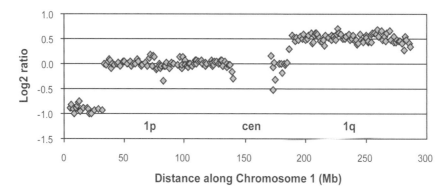

Fig. 2. Array-comparative genomic hybridization analysis of a renal cell carcinoma cell line. A single copy number loss of the distal part of the short arm of chromosome 1 and a single-copy gain of the distal part of the long arm.

single copy loss, whereas the terminal part of 1q shows single copy number gain. More recently, the improved resolution of aCGH has been applied to the identification of submicroscopic gains (microduplications) and losses (microdeletions) in patients with learning disability and/or dysmorphology. In a study of 50 patients with cytogenetically normal karyotypes but with learning disability and dysmorphology, we identified 12 small copy number changes in 12 patients *(15)* ranging in size from a single clone to as large as 14 Mb. Seven of these copy number changes were deletions (six *de novo* and one inherited from a phenotypically normal parent) and the remaining five copy number changes were duplications (one *de novo* but four inherited from phenotypically normal parents). Although it is reasonable to suggest that the *de novo* copy number changes are likely to be associated with the phenotype, the role of the inherited copy number changes is unclear. The inheritance of copy number changes that do not segregate with the phenotype may simply be the consequence of normal human variation, as suggested by recent reports of widespread large scale copy number variations in the normal population *(16,17)*, but we cannot rule out that such changes in the context of the other allele might be associated with the phenotype.

Of particular interest is that none of the copy number changes we observed in these patients were recurrent or overlapped with each other. Indeed, microduplications and microdeletions in similar patients reported by others *(18,19)* are similarly unique. From this it is clear that the study of many more patients will be required before we will be able to define new microdeletion and microduplication syndromes, provide clinicians with information on probable outcome and dissect out genotype-phenotype associations. To aid collection of such data and collaboration on an international scale, we have developed a Web-based interactive database, DECIPHER (http://decipher.sanger.ac.uk). DECIPHER not only holds microdeletion or microduplication data with detailed patient phenotype information but also displays the genomic position of all copy number changes in the database (including known microdeletion/microduplication syndromes and normal copy number polymorphisms) within the genome browser Ensembl, with all of its tools relating to the annotation of the human genome available for analysis.

ARRAY PAINTING

Although aCGH can identify copy number changes associated with chromosome rearrangement, aberrations that involve no loss or gain of DNA (inversions, balanced translo-

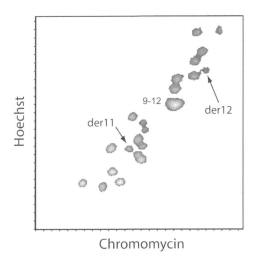

Fig. 3. Flow karyotype of a t(11;12) lymphoblastoid cell line. The derivative chromosomes are easily distinguished from the unaffected homologs by a change in DNA content and basepair ratio. (Adapted from ref. *20.*)

cations) remain undetected. We have developed a modification of aCGH, which allows balanced translocations and their breakpoints to be analyzed on the microarrays. The method, which we have called array painting, involves the separation of the derivative chromosomes from the rest of the genome using flow sorting *(20)*. On the flow cytometer, chromosomes in suspension and stained with two DNA-binding dyes can be identified using a combination of DNA content and basepair ratio. Most balanced translocations involve an unequal exchange of DNA between the two derivatives such that the derivative chromosomes are different in size and/or basepair ratio from the normal homologs (*see* Fig. 3). In this way, the derivative chromosomes can be sorted as purified fractions away from each other and their normal homologs, differentially labeled and hybridized to an array (*see* Fig. 4). On the array, fluorescence will only be detected on clones corresponding to the sequences present in the sorted chromosomes. The fluorescence ratio for these clones will either be high or low depending on which derivative chromosome the sequence of the clone corresponds (*see* Fig. 3). Should a clone on the array span a breakpoint, sequences from both the derivatives will hybridize generating intermediate ratio values.

We have used array painting together with aCGH to study patients with apparently balanced translocations expecting to map rapidly the translocation breakpoints and discover genes which might be disrupted by the rearrangement. However, we have discovered an unexpected level of complexity in these patients with as many as 60% of cases showing deletion at or near the translocation breakpoint, the involvement of additional chromosomes in the rearrangement or microdeletion/microduplication on chromosomes not involved in the translocation *(21)*. The power of this methodology is its ability to screen the whole genome (aCGH) and the entire length of the derivative chromosomes (array painting) for rearrangement. This contrasts with the use of fluorescence *in situ* hybridization (FISH) for analysis of translocation breakpoints, which owing to the time and effort involved in performing FISH studies have focused primarily on the breakpoints, thus, potentially missing rearrangements elsewhere in the genome.

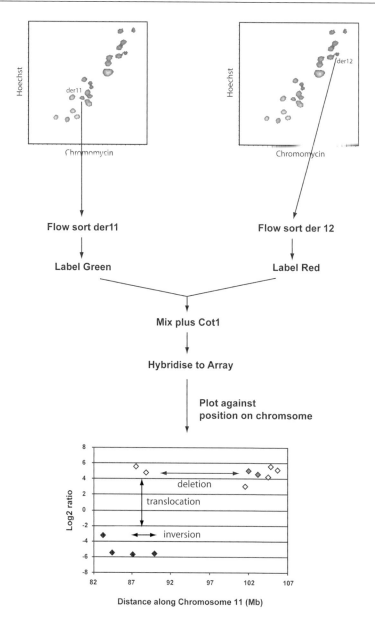

Fig. 4. Principle of Array painting. The graph shows a detail of the ratio plot for chromosome 11 close to the rearrangement breakpoint. Low ratios indicate sequences present on the derivative 11 and high ratios on the derivative 12. The analysis showed that the rearrangement involved an inversion/deletion event followed by translocation (for details, *see* ref. *20*). (Adapted from ref. *20*.)

HIGHER RESOLUTION ANALYSIS OF REARRANGEMENTS

To date, most published analyses of genomic rearrangements using microarrays have utilized arrays which sample the genome with one clone of 100- to 200-kb in length every 1 Mb *(14,22,23)*. Although these arrays greatly improve on the resolution of analyses possible with metaphase chromosomes as targets for hybridization, higher resolution arrays would allow more detailed analysis of rearrangements. In particular, we are interested in the molecular mechanisms involved in the generation of the rearrangements we identify and for this we require DNA sequence across the breakpoint regions. The sequence from junction regions is most efficiently and cost-effectively generated from PCR or long range PCR products for which primers need to be designed to within a few kilobases of the breakpoints, thus, requiring high resolution analysis of breakpoint position.

One way of improving resolution is to increase the density of clones on the array. Several groups have generated arrays of overlapping clones to targeted regions or whole chromosomes *(9,24–28)*. We have used an array of overlapping clones for the whole of chromosome 1 to analyze patients with constitutional 1p36 deletion syndrome *(29)*. We found two patients where the first had a deletion restricted to the most terminal 2.5 Mb of 1p36.33, whereas the second had a deletion of 6.9 Mb in length, starting 3 Mb from the terminal region. As these two patients showed overlapping phenotypes but nonoverlapping 1p36 deletions, we believe that 1p36 deletion syndrome may be caused by positional effects as well as more conventional contiguous gene deletion. Recently, the first whole genome, bacterial artificial chromosome (BAC) tiling path array, comprising approx 32,000 fingerprint-mapped RPCI-11 BAC clones, has been described *(30)*. Although this array is initially being applied to solid tumors *(31)*, it is clear that such arrays would similarly improve the resolution of the analysis of constitutional rearrangements. In particular, the largely overlapping nature of the clone inserts ensures that breakpoints will be identified to within a clone. Our own genome tiling path array of more than 30,000 clones largely selected from the clones used to generate the reference human sequence (the Golden Path) is in validation and we intend to implement this array as our initial tool for the analysis of constitutional rearrangements.

A second way of improving array resolution is to reduce the length of the genomic sequences spotted onto the arrays. For a first increase in resolution, we routinely utilize fosmid libraries whose clones have been mapped onto the reference sequence. These clones show a high degree of overlap (*see* Fig. 5) and this redundancy can be used to improve the resolution of the array even beyond the size of the clones as was originally described by Albertson *(32)*. Figure 6 shows a microdeletion on chromosome 9 analyzed using a 1-Mb array and with a custom high density fosmid array targeted to the deletion breakpoints. With such fosmid arrays breakpoints can be positioned to within 20–40 kb.

Clones with inserts of even smaller size are also useful for breakpoint mapping. We have utilized small insert libraries from flow-sorted chromosomes, which have been sequenced in an effort to identify single nucleotide polymorphisms in the human genome. Although these libraries only have a two- to threefold coverage of each chromosome, their small insert size compensates for occasional gaps in tile paths. Figure 7 shows aCGH profiles delineating the proximal breakpoint of the previously shown chromosome 9 microdeletion, using the 1-Mb array, the custom high density fosmid array and finally a high density small insert clones array (1 to 4 kb in length). Custom arrays of this type enable breakpoints to be mapped to well within the distance required for long-range PCR products to be generated from junction regions and sequencing of breakpoints.

OLIGONUCLEOTIDE ARRAYS

Although the discussion in this chapter has concerned genomic clone arrays, some groups have used oligonucleotide arrays for analysis of copy number changes in tumors *(33,34)* and large-scale copy number variation in normal individuals *(16)*. The signal to noise ratio for

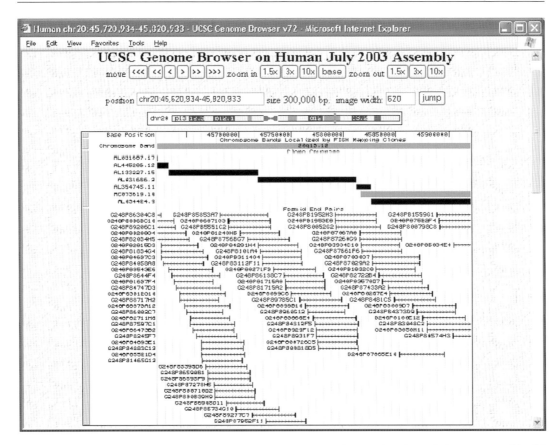

Fig. 5. High-density fosmid clones. Example of the coverage of a small region of chromosome 20 with fosmid clones as shown in the UCSC genome browser.

genomic hybridizations to these arrays is generally low producing a large level of measurement variation such that direct hybridization of complete genomic DNA requires considerable data smoothing (e.g., running averages of eight data points) and statistical calling of copy number trends *(34)*. However, reducing the complexity of the hybridization, typically by using restriction digestion with catch linker PCR, which favors only the smaller fragments, copy number information can be generated. Affymetrix arrays designed for SNP analysis *(33)* as well as custom long-oligonucleotide arrays (ROMA technology *[35]*) have been used in this way. Data generated from such arrays is still inherently noisy as differences in the restriction pattern of the test and reference DNAs produce artifactual differences, which might be interpreted as copy number changes. To overcome this, averaging or more sophisticated statistical analysis is used to identify copy number trends. In practice, three or more oligonucleotides within a genomic region are required to report a copy number change in order for this to be accepted as valid *(16,33)*. Thus, although an array comprising 100,000 oligonucleotides would appear to have an average resolution of 30 kb, in practice the resolution is three times this, i.e., 90 kb. The advantage of oligonucleotide arrays is that each sequence can be designed to be unique and repeat free. Inevitably for tiling path arrays using large insert clones, many clones will include segmental duplications or high levels of repeat sequence which compromise the level and specificity of response of such clones to copy number changes.

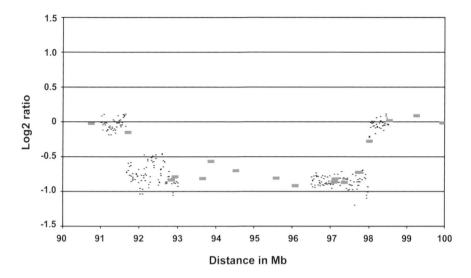

Fig. 6. Array-comparative genomic hybridization (aCGH) analysis using different resolution arrays. aCGH profile of a microdeletion on chromosome 9 analyzed using a 1 Mb array (large gray bars) and with a custom high density fosmid array (small black bars) targeted to the deletion breakpoints.

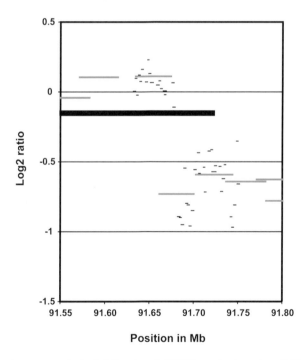

Fig. 7. Array-comparative genomic hybridization (aCGH) analysis using different resolution arrays. aCGH profiles of the proximal breakpoint of the chromosome 9 microdeletion shown in Fig. 6, using the 1 Mb array (large black bar), the custom high density fosmid array (medium gray bars) and a high density small insert clones array (short black bars).

CONCLUSIONS

As DNA microarrays become more widely available and, hopefully, less expensive we will see an increasing application of this technology for the study of chromosome rearrangements. The methodology is amenable to automation, both for hybridization and analysis, so is particularly suited for clinical applications. At the moment this technology largely remains a research tool. However, as aCGH becomes more established and in particular, as we understand the consequences of copy number changes in both normal individuals and patients, we would predict that this technology will become a very efficient method for prenatal as well as postnatal diagnosis. In clinical practice, microarray technology will have limitations. For example, inversions, translocations, and ploidy changes would not be detected by aCGH. However, the vast majority of prenatal samples are reported as normal by current methods and there is a considerable need for a rapid method to screen out these cases leaving more resources available for the analysis of patients with chromosome rearrangements. Only time will tell if DNA microarray technology will be adopted as a routine method in the cytogenetics laboratory.

SUMMARY

In this chapter, we have illustrated how the combination of CGH and DNA microarray technology (aCGH) enables rapid, high-resolution analysis of genome rearrangements. aCGH allows the whole genome to be scanned for submicroscopic copy number changes and to define precisely rearrangement breakpoints. We demonstrate how, by choice of clone size and separation across the genome, rearrangements can be analyzed genome-wide with resolutions of 200 kb and, for targeted regions, to within a few kilobases.

REFERENCES

1. Kallioniemi A, Kallioniemi OP, Sudar D, et al. Comparative genomic hybridization for molecular cytogenetic analysis of solid tumors. Science 1992;258:818–821.
2. Forozan F, Karhu R, Kononen J, Kallioniemi A, Kallioniemi OP. Genome screening by comparative genomic hybridization. Trends Genet 1997;13:405–409.
3. Lichter P, Fischer K, Joos S, et al. Efficacy of current molecular cytogenetic protocols for the diagnosis of chromosome aberrations in tumor specimens. Cytokines Mol Ther 1996;2:163–169.
4. Ness GO, Lybaek H, Houge G. Usefulness of high-resolution comparative genomic hybridization (CGH) for detecting and characterizing constitutional chromosome abnormalities. Am J Med Genet 2002;113:125–136.
5. Kirchhoff M, Rose H, Lundsteen C. High resolution comparative genomic hybridisation in clinical cytogenetics. J Med Genet 2001;38:740–744.
6. Solinas-Toldo S, Lampel S, Stilgenbauer S, et al. Matrix-based comparative genomic hybridization: biochips to screen for genomic imbalances. Genes Chromosomes Cancer 1997;20:399–407.
7. Pinkel D, Segraves R, Sudar D, et al. High resolution analysis of DNA copy number variation using comparative genomic hybridization to microarrays. Nat Genet 1998;20:207–211.
8. Snijders AM, Nowak N, Segraves R, et al. Assembly of microarrays for genome-wide measurement of DNA copy number. Nat Genet 2001;29:263–264.
9. Buckley PG, Mantripragada KK, Benetkiewicz M, et al. A full-coverage, high-resolution human chromosome 22 genomic microarray for clinical and research applications. Hum Mol Genet 2002;11:3221–3229.
10. Hodgson G, Hager JH, Volik S, et al. Genome scanning with array CGH delineates regional alterations in mouse islet carcinomas. Nat Genet 2001;29:459–464.
11. Telenius H, Carter NP, Bebb CE, Nordenskjold M, Ponder BA, Tunnacliffe A. Degenerate oligonucleotide-primed PCR: general amplification of target DNA by a single degenerate primer. Genomics 1992;13:718–725.

12. Telenius H, Pelmear AH, Tunnacliffe A, et al. Cytogenetic analysis by chromosome painting using DOP-PCR amplified flow-sorted chromosomes. Genes Chromosomes Cancer 1992;4:257–263.
13. Foreman PK, Davis RW. Real-time PCR-based method for assaying the purity of bacterial artificial chromosome preparations. Biotechniques 2000;29:410–412.
14. Fiegler H, Carr P, Douglas EJ, et al. DNA microarrays for comparative genomic hybridization based on DOP-PCR amplification of BAC and PAC clones. Genes Chromosomes Cancer 2003;36:361–374.
15. Shaw-Smith C, Redon R, Rickman L, et al. Microarray based comparative genomic hybridisation (array-CGH) detects submicroscopic chromosomal deletions and duplications in patients with learning disability/mental retardation and dysmorphic features. J Med Genet 2004;41:241–248.
16. Sebat J, Lakshmi B, Troge J, et al. Large-scale copy number polymorphism in the human genome. Science 2004;305:525–528.
17. Iafrate AJ, Feuk L, Rivera MN, et al. Detection of large-scale variation in the human genome. Nat Genet 2004;36:949–951.
18. Vissers LE, de Vries BB, Osoegawa K, et al. Array-based comparative genomic hybridization for the genomewide detection of submicroscopic chromosomal abnormalities. Am J Hum Genet 2003;73:1261–1270.
19. Tyson C, McGillivray B, Chijiwa C, Rajcan-Separovic E. Elucidation of a cryptic interstitial 7q31.3 deletion in a patient with a language disorder and mild mental retardation by array-CGH. Am J Med Genet 2004;129A:254–260.
20. Fiegler H, Gribble SM, Burford DC, et al. Array painting: a method for the rapid analysis of aberrant chromosomes using DNA microarrays. J Med Genet 2003;40:664–670.
21. Gribble SM, Prigmore E, Burford DC, et al. The complex nature of constitutional de novo apparently balanced translocations in patients presenting with abnormal phenotypes. J Med Genet 2005;42:8–16.
22. Snijders AM, Nowee ME, Fridlyand J, et al. Genome-wide-array-based comparative genomic hybridization reveals genetic homogeneity and frequent copy number increases encompassing CCNE1 in fallopian tube carcinoma. Oncogene 2003;22:4281–4286.
23. Greshock J, Naylor TL, Margolin A, et al. 1-Mb resolution array-based comparative genomic hybridization using a BAC clone set optimized for cancer gene analysis. Genome Res 2004;14:179–187.
24. Woodfine K, Fiegler H, Beare DM, et al. Replication timing of the human genome. Hum Mol Genet 2004;13:575.
25. Wang NJ, Liu D, Parokonny AS, Schanen NC. High-resolution molecular characterization of 15q11-q13 rearrangements by array comparative genomic hybridization (array CGH) with detection of gene dosage. Am J Hum Genet 2004;75:267–281.
26. Zafarana G, Grygalewicz B, Gillis AJ, et al. 12p-amplicon structure analysis in testicular germ cell tumors of adolescents and adults by array CGH. Oncogene 2003;22:7695–7701.
27. Yu W, Ballif BC, Kashork CD, et al. Development of a comparative genomic hybridization microarray and demonstration of its utility with 25 well-characterized 1p36 deletions. Hum Mol Genet 2003;12:2145–2152.
28. Shaw CJ, Shaw CA, Yu W, et al. Comparative genomic hybridisation using a proximal 17p BAC/PAC array detects rearrangements responsible for four genomic disorders. J Med Genet 2004l;41:113–119.
29. Redon R, Rio M, Gregory SG, et al. Tiling path resolution mapping of constitutional 1p36 deletions by array-CGH: contiguous gene deletion or 'deletion with positional effect' syndrome? J Med Genet 2005;42:166–171.
30. Ishkanian AS, Malloff CA, Watson SK, et al. A tiling resolution DNA microarray with complete coverage of the human genome. Nat Genet 2004;36:299–303.
31. de Leeuw RJ, Davies JJ, Rosenwald A, et al. Comprehensive whole genome array CGH profiling of mantle cell lymphoma model genomes. Hum Mol Genet 2004;13:1827–1837.
32. Albertson DG, Ylstra B, Segraves R, et al. Quantitative mapping of amplicon structure by array CGH identifies CYP24 as a candidate oncogene. Nat Genet 2000;25:144–146.
33. Bignell GR, Huang J, Greshock J, et al. High-resolution analysis of DNA copy number using oligonucleotide microarrays. Genome Res 2004;14:287–295.
34. Carvalho B, Ouwerkerk E, Meijer GA, Ylstra B. High resolution microarray comparative genomic hybridisation analysis using spotted oligonucleotides. J Clin Pathol 2004;57:644–646.
35. Lucito R, Healy J, Alexander J, et al. Representational oligonucleotide microarray analysis: a high-resolution method to detect genome copy number variation. Genome Res 2003;13:2291–2305.

VII APPENDICES

A

Well-Characterized Rearrangement-Based Diseases and Genome Structural Features at the Locus

Paweł Stankiewicz, MD, PhD
and James R. Lupski, MD, PhD

The following table provides details of well-characterized genomic disorders. It lists the position of the disease locus in the genome, potential dosage-sensitive genes, type and size of the rearrangement, and genome architectural features at the locus involved.

From: *Genomic Disorders: The Genomic Basis of Disease*
Edited by: J. R. Lupski and P. Stankiewicz © Humana Press, Totowa, NJ

Disorders	OMIM	Inheritance pattern	Chromosome	Gene(s)	Rearrangement		Recombination substrates				
					Type	Size (kb)	Repeat size (kb)	Identity (%)	Recombination hotspot	Orientation	Type
Bartter syndrome type III	601678	AD	1p36.13	*CLCNKA/B*	del	11	14			D	G/y
Gaucher disease	230800	AR	1q22	*GBA*	del	16				D	G/y
Familial juvenile nephronophthisis	256100	AR	2q13	*NPHP1*	del	290	45	>97		D	G
3q29 microdeletion syndrome	609425		3q29	*PAK2, DLG1?*	del	1500	>30	>97.5		D	
Fascioscapulohumeral muscular dystrophy/polymorphic copy number	158900	AD	4q35.2	*FRG1?*	del	25–222	3.3			D	
Spinal muscular atrophy	253300	AR	5q13.2	*SMN1*	inv, dup	900	500			I	
Sotos syndrome	117550	AD	5q35	*NSD1*	del	2000	400	99	2.5 kb	D	GC
Congenital adrenal hyperplasia III/21 hydroxylase deficiency	201910	AR	6p21.32	*CYP21*	del	30		96–98		D	G/y
Williams-Beuren syndrome	194050	AD	7q11.23	*ELN, LIMK1*	del, inv	1600	>320	98	3.4 kb	C	GC
inv dup(8p); der(8)(pterp23.1::p23.2pter); del(8)(p23.1p23.2)			8p23		inv/dup/del	400		95–97		I	OR-GC
Glucocorticoid-remediable aldosteronism	103900	AD	8q24.3	*CYP11B1/2*	dup	45	10	95		D	G
δβ-thalassemia (Hb variants Lepore and Miyada)	141900	AR	11p15.4	δ- and β-globin	del	7				D	G
Prader-Willi syndrome	176270	AD	15q11.2q13	*SNRPN, NDN, necdin, SnoRNAs?*	del	3500	400			C	GC
Angelman syndrome	105830	AD	15q11.2q13	*UBE3A*	del	3500	400			C	GC
dup(15)(q11.2q13) syndrome			15q11.2q13	?	dup	3500	400			C	GC
triplication 15q11.2q13			15q11.2q13	?	trip	3500	400			C	GC
inv dup(15)(q11q13)			15q11.2q13	?	inv dup	3500	400			D	GC
α-thalassemia	141800		16p13.3	α-globin	del	3.7	4			D	S
Polycystic kidney disease 1	601313	AD	16p13.3	*PKD1*			50	95			

Charcot-Marie-Tooth type 1A disease	118220	AD	17p12	PMP22	dup	1400	24	98.7	741 bp	D	S
Hereditary neuropathy with liability to pressure palsies	162500	AD	17p12	PMP22	del	1400	24	98.7	557 bp	D	S
Smith-Magenis syndrome	182290	AD	17p11.2	RAI1	del	4000	200	98	524 bp/1.1 kb	D	GC
dup(17)(p11.2p11.2) syndrome		AD	17p11.2	RAI1?	dup	4000	200	98		D	GC
Neurofibromatosis type 1	162200	AD	17q11.2	NF1	del	1400	85		2 Kb	D	G
Breast cancer	114480	AD	17q21.3	BRCA1	del	37	14	92	624 bp	D	G
Pituitary dwarfism	262400	AR	17q23.3	GH1	del	6.7	2.24	99		D	S
Frontotemporal demetia	600274	AD	17q21.3	MAPT?	inv	570	120–500	90–99		C	S
DiGeorge syndrome/velocardio-facial syndrome	188400/192430	AD	22q11.2	TBX1	del	3000/1500	225–400	97–98		C	GC
dup(22)(q11.2q11.2) syndrome			22q11.2	?	dup	3.000	225–400	97–98		C	GC
triplication 22q11.2q11.2			22q11.2	?	trip	≥3000	225–400	97–98		C	GC
Cat-eye syndrome, inv dup(22)(q11.2)			22q11.2	?	inverted dup	225–400	225–400	97–98		C	GC
CYP2D6 pharmacogenetic trait	124030	AR	22q13.2	CYP2D6	del/dup	9,3	2.8			D	S
Ichthyosis	308100	XL	Xp22.31	STS	del	1900	11	95		D	S
idic(X)(p11.2)					isodicentric					?	
Hunter syndrome (mucopolysaccharidosis type II)	309900	XL	Xq28	IDS	inv del	20	3	>88			G/ψ
Rett syndrome/duplication of MECP2	312750	XL	Xq28	MECP2	del/dup						
Red–green color blindness, polymorphic copy number	303800	XL	Xq28	RCP and GCP	del	0	39	98		D	G
Emery-Dreifuss muscular dystrophy/polymorphic inversion of 38 kb	310300	XL	Xq28	Emerin and FLN1	del/dup/inv	48	11.3	99.2			
Incontinentia pigmenti	308300	XL	Xq28	NEMO	del	10	0.870			D	
Hemophilia A	306700	XL	Xq28	Factor VIII	inv	300–500	9.5	99.9		I	
Male infertility, AZFa microdeletion	415000	YL	Yq11.21	USP9Y, DBY ?	del	800	10	94	1.3 kb		R
Male infertility, AZFc microdeletion	415000	YL	Yq11.23	RBMY, DAZ ?	del	3.500	229	99.97	933 bp		P1/P3

D, autosomal dominant; AR, autosomal recessive; XL, X chromosome-linked; YL, Y chromosome-linked; del, deletion; dup, duplication; trip, triplication; inv, inversion; I, inverted; D, direct; G, gene; ψ, pseudogene; S, segment of genome, C, complex; P, palindromes; R, retrovirus; OMIM, Online Mendelian Inheritance in Man database (http://www3.ncbi.nlm.nih.gov/Omim/). (Adapted and expanded from ref. 1.)

REFERENCES

1. Stankiewicz P, Lupski JR. Genome architecture, rearrangements, and genomic disorders. Trends Genet 2002;18:74–82.

B | Diagnostic Potential for Chromosome Microarray Analysis

Paweł Stankiewicz, MD, PhD, Sau Wai Cheung, PhD, and Arthur L. Beaudet, MD

To overcome the approx 3–10 Mb resolution limitation of conventional, chromosome-based cytogenetic banding and comparative genomic hybridization (CGH) diagnostic methods, arrays of large insert bacterial artificial chromosome (BAC) and P1-derived artificial chromosome (PAC) clones for selected rearrangement-prone genomic regions were immobilized on glass slides. This approach enables detection of copy number changes throughout the genome at virtually whatever resolution desired. CGH arrays have been designed initially for the analysis of constitutional abnormalities involving specific targeted chromosome regions and subtelomeric regions of all chromosomes. Arrays have also been constructed for complete coverage of the human genome with overlapping BAC clones. The latter approach, however, has been tempered by high cost associated with array production, challenges in clinical interpretation of newly discovered rare variants, and current limitations of the knowledge and clinical relevance of large segmental copy number variants. To circumvent these challenges, a limited number (360–850) of BAC clones have been selected specifically for clinically relevant regions of the genome known to be responsible for genomic disorders and the locations for each of these clones has been verified by fluorescence *in situ* hybridization. This novel high-resolution custom chromosome microarray analysis (CMA) allows screening of 41 subtelomeric regions, and more than 40 microdeletion/microduplication syndromes and other well-established gene dosage-sensitive genomic disorders in a single test *(1,2)*. The detection rate for abnormalities has been estimated as 8.4% in the current version 5. Furthermore, the approach enables the detection of several genomic changes not visualized by conventional clinical chromosome G-banding techniques. Targeted arrays have also been clinically applied in prenatal diagnosis *(3)*.

This appendix delineates the clinical phenotypes wherein CMA may be useful. Each of these conditions can be owing to a DNA rearrangement of the human genome. In some diseases, a rearrangement represents the major mutational mechanism, whereas in others genomic changes account for a smaller proportion of the cases. It is anticipated that this list may expand substantially as high-resolution analysis of the human genome is systematically applied to individuals with diverse phenotypes in both clinical research and medical practice.

The information in the following table is intended to help clinicians in the use of interpretation of array CGH in genetic diagnosis. The material covered is very complex and this table is necessarily a simplification to some extent. Users should consult the primary literature and other sources for more detailed information. An updated electronic version of the table with links can be found at http://www.bcm.edu/geneticlabs/tests/cyto/cmaregionsv5/html.

From: *Genomic Disorders: The Genomic Basis of Disease*
Edited by: J. R. Lupski and P. Stankiewicz © Humana Press, Totowa, NJ

OMINI	Phenotype	Genes	Cytogenetics	Detection (%)	Selected refs. PMID	GeneTests/ GeneReviews
General properties						
Various	Various	Various	Deletions and duplications of subtelomeric regions	High	11951177 14628292 15904506 15834244 15723295 16024975	−
Various	Various	Various	Deletions and duplications of pericentromeric regions	High	13680362 15508017	+
Various	Various	Various	Aneuploidy for any chromosome	High		−
Disorders with high detection rates (>50%)						
607872	1p36 deletion syndrome	Multiple	1p36 deletion	>95–99%	10507720 12915473	−
256100	*NPHP1* Familial juvenile nephronophthisis	*NPHP1*, nephrocystin	2q13 homozygous deletion	60–70% homozygous	9361039 9326933	+
609425	3q29 microdeletion syndrome	*PAK2, DLG1?*	3q29 deletion	>95%	15918153	−
194190	*WHS* Wolf-Hirschhorn syndrome	Multiple	4p16.3 deletion	>95–99%	11480768 15734578	+
123450	Cri-du-chat syndrome	Multiple	5p15.2-p13.3 deletion	>95–99%	11238681 15635506	+
194050	*WBS* Williams–Beuren syndrome	*ELN* elastin, *LIMK1* LIM kinase 1	7q11.23 deletion	>95–99%	11701637 12796854	+
	inv dup(8p): der(8)(pterp23.1::p23.2pter); del(8)(p23.1p23.2)	Unknown	Deletion, inverted duplication 8p23	>95%	8533823 11231899	−
150230	*LGS* Langer-Giedion syndrome	*TRPS1* zinc finger transcription *TRPS1* and *EXT1* exostosin 1	8q23.3-q24.11 deletion	>95%	7711731 8530105	+
	9q34.3 deletion syndrome	Multiple	9q34.4 deletion	>95%	15805169 15805155	−

601362	*DGS2* DiGeorge syndrome 2	Unknown	10p14 deletion	>95%	9781025 15253763	+
601224	*PSS* Potocki-Shaffer syndrome	*ALX4* Aristaless-like-4 and/or *EXT2* exostosin 2	11p11.2 deletion	>95%	8644736 15852040	+
147791	*JBS* Jacobsen (11q25 deletion) syndrome		11q24-q25	~65%	14597985 15266616	−
176270	*PWS* Prader-Willi syndrome	*SNRPN*, *NDN* necdin, snoRNAs	15q11.2-q13 deletion	~70%	8651269 11694676	+
105830	*AS* Angelman syndrome	*UBE3A* ubiquitin ligase 3A	15qa11.2-q13 deletion	~70%	7625452 8651269	+
	dup(15)(q11.2q13) syndrome		15q11.2-q13	~99%	9106540 15318025	−
	15q21 deletion syndrome		15q21 deletion	~99%	12684692	−
247200	*MDLS* Miller-Dieker lissencephally syndrome	*LIS1* and/or *YWHAE*	17p13.3 deletion	>90% for full syndrome	11115846 12621583	+
118220	*CMT1A* Charcot-Marie-Tooth type 1A disease	*PMP22* peripheral myelin protein 22	17p12 duplication	>98%	11835373 16106622	+
162500	*HNPP* Heredity neuropathy with liability to pressure palsies	*PMP22* perioheral myelin protein 22	17p12 deletion	~85%	8422677 10586225	+
182290	*SMS* Smith-Magenis syndrome	*RAI1* reinoic acid-induced gene 1	17p11.2 deletion	~99%	15148657 14614393	+
	dup(17)(p11.2p11.2) syndrome		17p11.2 duplication	~99%	10615134	−
115470	*CES* cat-eye syndrome		inv dup(22)(q11.2)	>90%	15756300 11381032	+
188400/ 192430	*DGS1* DiGeorge, *VCFS* velocardiofacial syndrome	*TBX1* T-box 1 22q11.2 deletion	>95%		1349199 9350810	+
608363	dup(22)(q11.2q11.2) syndrome	Possibly *TBX1* T-box 1	22q11.2 duplication	~99%	14526392 15800846	−
127300	*LWD* Leri-Weill dyschondrosteosis	*SHOX/SHOXY* shory stature homeobox	Xp22.23/Yp11.32	60–80% in LWD, less in short stature	11739418 16103983	+
308100	*STS* steroid sulfatase deficiency	*ARSC2* aryl sulfatase C	Xp22.31 deletion	>95%	2644167 3480263	+

(continued)

OMNI no.	Phenotype	Genes	Cytogenetics	Detection (%)	Selected refs. PMID	GeneTests/ Gene Reviews
	STS dup Xp22.31 Unclear if benign or disease related		Xp22.31 duplication	>95%	15060094 16175506	–
300200	AHC Congenital adrenal hypoplasia	NROB1 nuclear receptor family 0 B1	Xp21.2 deletion	High in contiguous, low isolated gene	11032329 15684452	+
300018	DSS Dosage-sensitive sex reversal	NROB1 nuclear receptor family 0 B1	Xp21.2 duplication	>95%	7951319 15216557	–
312080	PMD Pelizaeus-Merzbacher disease	PLP1 proteolipid protein 1	Xp22 duplication or deletion	60–70%/<2%	12297985 15627202	+

Disorders with intermediate or uncertain detection rates

OMNI no.	Phenotype	Genes	Cytogenetics	Detection (%)	Selected refs. PMID	GeneTests/ Gene Reviews
	2q22.3 deletion	2q22.3 deletion				
220200	DWS Dandy-Walker syndrom	ZIC1, Zic4 zinc finger protein of the cerebellum 1, 4	3q24 deletion	Uncertain	15591274 15338008	–
180500	RIEG1 Rieger syndrome, type 1	PITX2	4q25 deletion	Uncertain	8944018 12647202	+
101400	SCS Saethre-Chotzen syndrome	TWIST homolog of Drosophila TWIST	7p21.1 deletion	10–30%	1746608 8988166	+
190350	TRPS1 trichorhinophalangeal syndrome 1	TRSP1 zinc finger transcription TRPS1	8q23.3 deletion	<30%	9150732 11112658	+
1462555	HDR Hypoparathyroidism, sensorineural deafness, and renal disease	GATA3 GATA-binding protein 3	10p14 duplication	Uncertain	10633131 10935639	–
608071	SHFM3 split-hand/foot malformation 3		10p14 duplication		12913067	+
106210	AN2 aniridia II	PAX6 paired box gene 6	11p13 deletion	20–35% overall; higher in WAGR	9482572 11479730	+
607102	Wilms tumor	WT1 Wilms tumor 1 gene	11p13 deletion	20–35% overall; higher in WAGR	9090524 15150775	+
194072	WAGR syndrome	PAX6 and WT1	11p13 deletion	20–35% overall; higher in WAGR	9132491 12386836	+

OMIM	Disorder	Gene	Location	Detection rate	References	
	Luekodystrophy		11q14.2-q14.3	Uncertain	14722582	–
180200	RB1 retinoblastoma	RB1 retinoblastoma 1	13q14.2 deletion	Low except contiguous gene cases	10450867 15642837	+
180849	RSTS Rubinstein-Taybi syndrome	CREBBP CREB-binding protein	16p13.3 deletion	~10%	12070251 14974086	+
309801	MLS Micophthalmia with linear skin defects		Xp22.2 deletion	Uncertain	16059943	–
191092	TSC2 tuberous sclerosis 2	TSC2 tuberin	16p13.3 deletion	17%	8269512 10205261	+
300474	GK Glycerol kinase deficiency	GK glycerol kinase	Xp22 deletion	High in contiguous, low isolated gene	11032329 11479736	+
480000	Sex reversal X/Y translocations	SRY sex-determining region Y	Yp11.31 deletion	Moderate in XX males and XY females	11480910 11479736	–
415000	AZFa Azoospermia factora		Yq11 deletion	Uncertain	15474244 15890785	–
415000	AZFb Azoospermia factora		Yq11 deletion	Uncertain	15474244 15890785	–
415000	AZFc Azoopermia factora		Yq11.23 deletion	5–10%	15474244 15890785	+

Disorders with low or very low detection rates

OMIM	Disorder	Gene	Location	Detection rate	References	
164280	Feingold syndrome	MYCN	2p24.3 deletion	Very low	8989454	–
157170	HPE2 holoprosencephaly 2	SIX3 sine oculis homolog 3	2p21 deletion	Low	8824878 10369266	+
122470	CDLS Cornelia de Lange syndrome	NIPBL nipped-B-like	5p13.2 deletion	Very very low	15146185 16075459	+
117550	Sotos syndrome	NSD1 nuclear receptor binding Su-var	5q35 deletion	Low except in Japanese	15942875 15805156	+
119600	CCD cleidocranial dysplasia	RUNX2 runt-related transcription factor 2	6p21.1 deletion	Very low	8533817 9182765	+
1757000	GCPS Greig cephalopoly-syndactyly syndrome	GLI3 GLI-Kruppel family 3	7p14.1 deletion	5–10%	14608643 1650914	+

(continued)

OMINI no.	Phenotype	Genes	Cytogenetics	Detection (%)	Selected refs. PMID	GeneTests/ Gene Reviews
142945	HPE3 holoprosencephaly 3	SHH sonic hedgehog	7q36.3 deletion	Low ~5%	8896571 9254845	+
214800	CHARGE syndrome	CHD7 Chromo-domain helicase DNA-binding 7	8q12.2 deletion	Very low	15300250 15666308	+
See basal cell nevus	HPE7 holoprosencephaly 7	Missense mutations		0%	11941477	−
109400	BCNS basal cell nevus syndrome	PTCH patched Drosophila homolog	9q22.32 deletion	<5%	8681379 8755929	+
161200	NPS Nail-patella syndrome	LMS1B LIM-homeo box factor 1β	9q33.3 deletion	Very low	9590287 10094193	+
130650	BWS Beckwith-Wiedmann syndrome	IGF2 insulin-like growth factor II, CDKN1C cyclin-dependent kinase inhibitor 1C	11p15.5 deletion/duplication	1–2%	9350814 9781904	+
163950	NS1 Noonan syndrome	PTPN11	12q24.13 deletion	Very low	9412792 10636744	+
603073	HPE5 holoprosencephaly 5	ZIC2 zinc finger protein cerebellum 2	13q32.3 deletion	<5%	7573047 8418661	+
209850	Autism	Uncertain	15q11.2-q13 maternal duplication	1–3%	11803514 15197683	+
142340	HCD hernia, congenital diaphragmatic		15q26.1-q26.2 deletion	Low	15057983 15750894	+
191100	TSC1 tuberous sclerosis 1	TSC1 hamartin	9q34.2	2%	9328481	+
600273	PKDTS polycystic kidney disease 1/tuberous sclerosis 2	PKD1 polycystin 1, TSC2 tuberin	16p13.3 deletion	1–2% high for two gene deletion	9306341 14695542	+
162200	NF1 neurofibromatosis type 1	NF1 neurofibromin 1	17q11.2 deletion	2–5%	15236313 15944227	+
114290	CMPD Campomelic dysplasia	SOX9 SRY-box 9	17q24.3 deletion	Low	9724758 15060123	−
142946	HPE4 holoprosencephaly 4	TGIF transforming growth factor-β induced factor	18p11.31 deletion	<5%	10835638 12522553	+
118450	AGS Alagille syndrome	JAG1 jagged 1	20p12.2 deletion	5–7%	11180599	−

190685	Down syndrome critical region	Multiple	21q22 duplication	Rare compared to trisomy 21	11745040 2143053 11280955	+
236100	HPE1 holosencephaly 1	TMEM1? transmembrane protein 1	21q22.3 deletion	<5%	7633421	+
101000	NF2 neurofibromatosis II	NF2 neurofibromin 2	22q12.2 deletion	<10%	15645494 15681480	+
300495	AUTSX2 autism, X-linked susceptibility to, 2	Possibly NLGN4	Xp22.32 deletion	Very low, uncertain	10071191	+
308700	KAL1 Kallmann syndrome 1	KAL1 Kallmann syndrome 1	Xp22.31 deletion	Low exccept contiguous gene	2602357 9727739	+
300300	Bruton agammaglobulinemia	BTK Bruton agammaglobulinemia tyrosine kinase	Xq22.1 deletion	Very low except contiguous gene	11338284	+
306955	X-linked heterotaxy	ZIC3 zinc finger protein cerebellum 3	Xq26.3 deletion	Very low	9311745	–
300123	MRGH mental retardation X-linked with growth hormone deficiency	SOX3 SRY-box 3	Xq27.1 deletion or duplication	Very low of all MR	15800844	–
312750	RTT Rett syndrome	MECP2 methyul-CpG-binding protein-2	Xq28 deletion/duplication	5%?	15841480 16080119	+

aThe azoospermia regions are not evaluated in prenatal samples.

REFERENCES

1. Bejjani BA, Saleki R, Ballif BD, et al. Use of targeted array-based CGH for the clinical diagnosis of chromosomal imbalance: is less more? Am J Med Genet 2005;134:259–267.
2. Cheung SW, Shaw CA, Yu W, et al. Development and validation of a CGH microarray for clinical cytogenetic diagnosis. Genet Med 2005;7:422–432.
3. Rickman L, Fiegler H, Shaw-Smith C, et al. Prenatal detection of unbalanced chromosomal rearrangements by array-CGH. J Med Genet 2005; in press.

Index

415

About the Editors

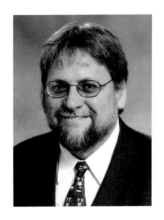

Jim Lupski received his initial scientific training at the Cold Spring Harbor Laboratory as an Undergraduate Research Participant (URP) and at New York University, completing the MD/PhD program in 1985 in bacterial genetics. In 1986, he moved to Houston, TX for clinical training in pediatrics (1986–1989) and medical genetics (1989–1992), later establishing his own laboratory at Baylor College of Medicine where he remains as the Cullen Professor of Molecular and Human Genetics since 1995. His laboratory determines molecular mechanisms for disease using molecular biological, genomic, and human genetic approaches to investigate clinical phenotypes. Through studies of Charcot-Marie-Tooth peripheral neuropathy, a common autosomal dominant trait owing to a submicroscopic 1.4-Mb duplication, and Smith-Magenis syndrome, a microdeletion syndrome, his laboratory has delineated the concept of "genomic disorders" and established the critical role of gene dosage in conveying human disease phenotypes. An increasing number of human diseases are recognized as the result of recurrent DNA rearrangements involving unstable genomic regions and have thus been classified as genomic disorders. Dr. Lupski's laboratory has also developed mouse models for genomic disorders. He recently completed a sabbatical at the Wellcome Trust Sanger Institute (2004–2005) in Cambridge, England where he studied mouse genetics and genomics.

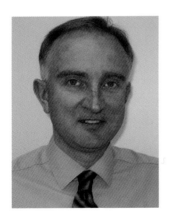

Paweł Stankiewicz graduated Medical University of Warsaw in 1991. He received his scientific training in clinical cytogenetics in the Department of Medical Genetics, National Research Institute of Mother and Child in Warsaw, Poland (1994–2000), in the Institute of Human Genetics, University of Göttingen, Göttingen, and in the Institute of Human Genetics and Medical Biology, University Halle-Wittenberg, in Halle/Saale, Germany (1996–1997, German Academic Exchange Service, DAAD). He obtained his PhD in molecular cytogenetics in 1999. In 2000, he moved to Houston, TX where he worked as a postdoctoral fellow in Dr. Lupski's laboratory in the Department of Molecular & Human Genetics at Baylor College of Medicine. His research focused on elucidation of molecular mechanisms of genomic rearrangements in proximal chromosome 17p. While characterizing the breakpoints of chromosome aberrations in patients with Smith-Magenis syndrome using fluorescence *in situ* hybridization, pulsed-field gel electrophoresis, and computational analyses, he identified the role of complex genomic architecture involving low-copy repeats in formation of constitutional, evolutionarily, and somatic rearrangements. Since 2003, he has been working as an Assistant Professor in the Department of Molecular & Human Genetics, Baylor College of Medicine, Houston, TX.